Mult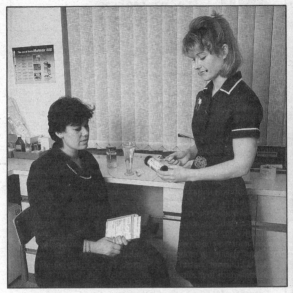SG

Reagent Strips

KT-599-390

for comprehensive urinalysis

 Ames Division, Miles Limited, P.O. Box 37,
Stoke Court, Stoke Poges,
SLOUGH SL2 4LY. Tel: (0753) 645151

* Trademark of Miles Inc. USA

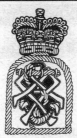

QARNNS

The Royal Navy's Nurses

They are a dedicated team of professionals who care for Royal Naval personnel, their families and also civilians.

It is possible to join QARNNS as a Medical Assistant, Student Nurse, Staff Nurse, Enrolled Nurse (G) or Nursing Officer.

If you would like further information please write to The Director, Naval Careers Service, Old Admiralty Building, Spring Gdns., London SW1A 2BE.

Orthopaedic Nursing 2/e

Anne Footner

Fully revised and expanded, this authoritative text provides a complete guide to orthopaedic nursing care. Covering all major innovations and recent developments, each chapter now also features helpful learning objectives and comprehensive suggestions for further reading. The full spectrum of nursing problems from caring for the patient before and after an operation, to caring for those requiring special considerations are discussed. A major new chapter focuses on nursing models in depth.

0 7020 1602 0   256pp   140 ills   Pb
June 1992   Baillière Tindall   £10.95

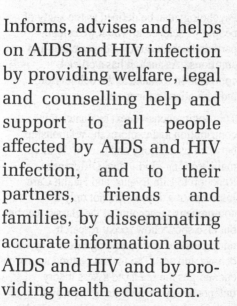

Robert W. Oliver
Psychology and Health Care

Psychology can be defined as the study of people - a science in which we can all participate with our own experiences and emotions. As such, it has a crucial contribution to make to the delivery of individualised patient care.

This comprehensive text evaluates this contribution and explores the relationship between psychology and health. In three main sections - Individual Differences, Reaction to Life Events, and Health Care Interventions, it provides not only a comprehensive account of the classic theories, but also shows how recent research underpins our understanding of the way we behave and act. The patient centred approach encourages the reader to assess theory independently in the light of their own individual practice, and provides a valuable insight into the delivery and experience of care.

0 7020 1601 2   ca 320pp   ca 146 Ills   Pb Jan 1993   Baillière Tindall   ca £12.95

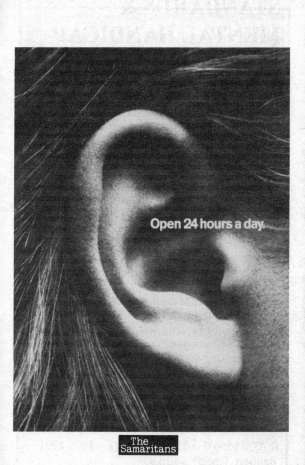

Open 24 hours a day.

The Samaritans

STANDARDS & MENTAL HANDICAP

KEYS TO COMPETENCE

Tony Thompson & Peter Mathias (Eds)

The authors of this new text are innovators in policy, practice and education in the field of mental handicap and learning difficulties. Here they lucidly explore the implications which the recent policy changes in the educational, health and social services will have for standards and for professionals in nursing and social work. This multidisciplinary text asserts that the raising of standards must be a collective enterprise, and guides the reader through four main issues -

- changes in policy
- competences required to help those with learning difficulties and to acquire skills
- requirements of professionals working in a multicultural society
- continuing professional development

Encompassing the competences required for the Diploma in Social Work and Project 2000, this text will appeal particularly to students of mental handicap nursing, social work and integrated courses.

0 7020 1566 0   512pp   30 ills   Pb   1991
Baillière Tindall   £13.95

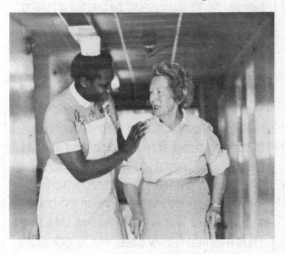

Susan Hinchliff & Susan Montague (Eds)
Physiology for Nursing Practice

"The entire approach in this excellent book confirms the importance of a 'bionursing' view of the relation between the life sciences and the practice of nursing"
Nursing Times

This exciting and imaginative text enables the reader to understand the principles and mechanisms of normal body function and how these mechanisms alter in illness. The reader is provided with a rational basis for assessing patients' health problems and the planning, delivery and evaluation of care. The book is divided into sections which logically illustrate the functions of the body as a complex homeostatic system. Multi-choice format review questions, suggestions for practical work and references of particular relevance enable readers to test and develop their knowledge.

0 7020 1194 0   695pp   384 ills   Pb   1988   Baillière Tindall   £15.95

PERSONAL INFORMATION

Name _____

Address _____

_____

_____

Tel No _____

Training School/College of Nursing _____

_____

_____

Date of Entry _____

Date of Completion _____

Personal Identification No. _____

Examination pass date _____

Additional qualifications and dates

Baillière's
Nurses'
Dictionary

Baillière's Nurses' Dictionary

Revised by

BARBARA F. WELLER
RGN RSCN RNT

Paediatric Nurse Tutor, Norfolk College of Nursing and Midwifery, Norwich, Norfolk; formerly Nursing Officer, Department of Health, Elephant and Castle, London

RICHARD J. WELLS
BA SRN RMN ONC FETC FRSH FRCN

Head of Rehabilitation Services, Royal Marsden Hospital, London SW3 6JJ; formerly Advisor in Oncology Nursing, the Royal College of Nursing, London

Baillière Tindall Limited
London   Philadelphia   Toronto
Sydney   Tokyo

This book is printed on acid free paper.

Baillière Tindall   24–28 Oval Road
W. B. Saunders   London NW1 7DX

The Curtis Center
Philadelphia, PA 19106-3399

55 Horner Avenue
Toronto, Ontario M8Z 4X6, Canada

Harcourt Brace Jovanovich (Australia) Pty Ltd,
30–52 Smidmore Street
Marrickville, NSW 2204, Australia

Harcourt Brace Jovanovich Japan Inc.
Ichibancho Central Building, 22–1 Ichibancho
Chiyoda-ku, Tokyo 102, Japan

Twenty-first edition 1990
   Third printing 1992

English Language Book Society edition of 20th edition 1984
Spanish edition of 18th edition (Elicien, Barcelona) 1977
Italian edition of 18th edition (Editorial Ermes, Milan) 1977
French edition of 18th edition (Libraire Maloine, Paris) 1978
English Language Book Society edition of 21st edition 1990

Typeset by Photo-graphics, Honiton, Devon
Printed and bound in Great Britain by
HarperCollins Manufacturing, Glasgow

British Library Cataloguing in Publication Data is available
ISBN (paperback) 0-7020-1456-7
ISBN (cased) 0-7020-1505-9
ISBN (ELBS) 0-7020-1460-5

CONTENTS

PREFACE

A twenty-first birthday is a time for celebration: time to think about the past and to consider the future.

As the editors of this 21st edition we have been very conscious of the proud history of *Baillière's Nurses' Dictionary*, especially as it was the first comprehensive pocket dictionary to recognize the special needs of nurses in 1912. This innovative approach to nursing lexicography by the Publishers has continued to lead the way, with revisions of the text every four or five years. Language and the use of words is like a living organism that reacts to change and to style. This applies to every day colloquial usage and also to the language of the professional with the need to incorporate the terminology of the latest developments.

Browsing through past editions of the dictionary serves as an illustration of our own nursing history. Entries in the past were primarily anatomical, or related to obscure instruments (who has now heard of a Jube's two-way syringe for blood transfusion?) and dated materia medica – very relevant and useful to the practising nurse of that time but not for today.

With a twenty-first celebration comes emancipation. Nursing, perhaps more than any other health care profession, is an integrative discipline that borrows, blends, modifies and adapts knowledge from many subjects. It is also essentially an applied discipline continually concerned with improving patient care, and *improvement* implies *change*. Nursing knowledge and care practices thus require their own distinct definitions which in turn acknowledge that such change is at the frontier of our professional development. One frontier, however, we have not crossed is the use of gender. We have followed well-established practice of assuming the patient to be male and the nurse to be female. The sexism is unintentional and unavoidable in certain instances.

The Appendices have continued to be included by popular demand and have been substantially revised in the light of changes in our profession and society. Both authors consider that such issues as acquired immune deficiency syndrome (AIDS) and transcultural nursing merited new appendices to take the user into the 1990s, and to date this is the only dictionary to cover such subjects in this way. Many new illustrations have also been included.

Acknowledgements
Revising a dictionary is rather like painting the Forth Bridge in that it is 'on-going' and requires a team to keep the objectives in sight. We should like to acknowledge the support of colleagues and friends who contributed new definitions and other material, especially Jenny Barclay,

Lizzie Janes and Tim Root who assisted with some Appendices. Nigel Turton provided many new pronunciations for this edition, and we are extremely grateful to him for his involvement in the project. The contribution of David Proudfoot in the typing of the Appendices is greatly appreciated. We should also like to acknowledge the support of partners who kept 'the home fires burning' whilst definitions and entries were considered. Finally, we should like to acknowledge with considerable gratitude Sarah Smith, Senior Editor at Baillière Tindall, who made things possible for us in a tight time-table and prevented us from straying too far!

BARBARA F. WELLER
RICHARD J. WELLS

PUBLISHER'S ACKNOWLEDGEMENTS

The publishers would like to thank the following for their kind permission to reproduce material in this dictionary: W. B. Saunders Company for figures in Æsculapius, airway, cell, fluid, haemodialysis, intussusception, leukocytes, and Trousseau's sign; American College of Surgeons, figure in Lund and Browder chart; Laerdal Medical, figure in intubation; McGraw-Hill, figure in injection.

We are also grateful to the following Baillière Tindall authors for their kind permission to use material from their texts: Margaret Adams, for figures in graafian follicle and ectopic gestation (from Adams M: *Baillière's Midwives' Dictionary*, Seventh Edition, 1983); Doug Blood and Virginia Studdert, for *Brunus edwardii* entry (from Blood DO and Studdert VP: *Baillière's Comprehensive Veterinary Dictionary*, 1988); Ann Faulkner, for figures in alimentary canal and Maslow's hierarchy of needs (from Faulkner A: *Nursing: A Creative Approach*, 1985); Sheila Jackson and Penelope Bennett, for figures in bone (compact), ear, endometrium, hair and heart (from Jackson S and Bennet P: *Physiology with Anatomy for Nurses*, 1988); Betty Kershaw, Stephen G. Wright, and Pauline Hammonds for figure in Australian lift (from Kershaw B et al: *Helping to Care: A Handbook for Carers at Home and in Hospital*, 1989); Jack Lyttle, for figure in social class (from *Mental Disorder: Its Care and Treatment*, 1986); and Jeannette Watson and Joan Royle for figure in haemodialysis (from Watson JE and Royle JR: *Watson's Medical-Surgical Nursing and Related Physiology*, Third Edition, 1987).

Every effort has been made to contact copyright holders of material reproduced in this dictionary. In the few instances where this has not been possible, the publishers invite such copyright holders to contact them.

PRONUNCIATION GUIDE

Introduction:

The pronunciations are transcribed using ordinary English-spelling letters. So that the guide is consistent and unambiguous, these characters have been combined together in precise ways (see below). The avoidance of the use of phonetic symbols (with the exception of the upside-down 'e' or 'schwa' (ə) ensures that the guide is more-or-less immediately, and to some extent intuitively, understandable.

Style of transcription

All pronunciations are found in parentheses immediately following the bold main entry word (or variant, if one exists). The pronunciations reflect what could be called 'unaccented' or 'neutral' British English. Furthermore, transcriptions given reflect *current, spoken usage* of the terms rather than how the term 'should' be pronounced, i.e. the guide does not attempt to be didactic or prescriptive.

Variant pronunciations and spellings. Where alternative pronunciations for a word are given, or where alternative spellings or synonyms are given, these are separated by commas. For example:

> **medicine** ('medisin, 'medsin)
> **neurone** (**neuron**) ('nyooə·rohn, 'nyooə·ron)

Alternative pronunciations are often given in a truncated form with the use of hyphens. For example:

> **encephalic** (ˌenkə'falik,- ˌensə-)

Entries with repeated words. Note that once a transcription for a particular word has been given, subsequent entries that use the same word do not have a repeated transcription of that word again.

Characters and combinations used to represent sound. In the pronunciation guide, single letters represent single sounds and where two or more characters are combined, as in the accompanying tables, these also represent precise sounds.

Pronunciation style guide

	Vowel sounds	Nearest International Phonetic Alphabet Character
a	as in **bad** (bad)	æ
ah	as in **father** ('fahdhə)	a:
air	as in **hair** (hair)	εə or eə

	Vowel sounds	*Nearest International Phonetic Alphabet Character*
aw	as in **water** ('wawtə)	ɔː (cf. **or**)
ay	as in **fatal** ('fayt'l)	eɪ
e	as in **bed** (bed)	ɛ or e
ee	as in **fetus** ('feetəs)	iː
i	as in **film** (film)	ɪ
ie	as in **bite** (biet)	aɪ
i·ə	as in **chloropsia** klor'ropsi·ə)	ɪə
iə	as in **fear** (fiə)	ɪə
ieə	as in **diet** ('dieət)	aɪə
o	as in **body** (,bodee)	ɒ
oh	as in **choke** (chohk)	əʊ
oo	as in **boot** (boot)	uː
ooə	as in **cure** (kyooə)	ʊə
or	as in **claw** (klor)	ɔː (cf. **aw**)
ow	as in **now** (now)	aʊ
owə	as in **hour** (owə)	aʊə
oy	as in **goitre** ('goytə)	ɔɪ
oyə	as in **soya** ('soyə)	ɔɪə
u	as in **tongue** (tung)	ʌ
uh	as in **put** (puht)	ʊ
ə	as in **mother** ('mudhə)	ə
ər	as in **bird** (bərd)	ɜː
y	as in **yet** ('yet)	j (semi vowel)

Consonant sounds

b	as in **baby** ('baybee)	b
ch	as in **chat** (chaht)	tʃ
d	as in **digit** ('dijit)	d
dh	as in **they** (dhay)	ð
f	as in **fever** ('feevə)	f
g	as in **gag** (gag)	g
h	as in **heal** (heel)	h
j	as in **jump** (jump)	dʒ
k	as in **king** (king)	k
kh	as in **loch** (lokh)	χ or x
l	as in **light** (liet)	l
m	as in **man** (man)	m
n	as in **need** (need)	n
ng	as in **sung** (sung)	ŋ
nh	as in **restaurant** ('restəronh)	õŋ or ɓ
ny	as in **nutrition** (nyoo'trishən)	nj

	Vowel sounds	*Nearest International Phonetic Alphabet Character*
p	as in **pelvis** ('pelvis)	p
r	as in **rod** (rod)	r
s	as in **sack** (sak)	s
sh	as in **fish** (fish)	ʃ
t	as in **test** (test)	t
th	as in **thirst** (thərst)	θ
v	as in **vein** (vayn)	v
w	as in **weight** (wayt)	w
z	as in **zero** ('ziə·roh)	z
zh	as in **pleasure** ('plezhə)	ʒ

Stress marks. These are used where the word or term has more than one syllable, with the stress mark placed *before* the syllable to be stressed. The primary stressed syllable is indicated by superior stress mark (') and secondary stress by a subscript stress mark (ˌ). For example:

> **respiration** (ˌrespi'rayshən)
> **respirator** ('respiˌraytə)
> **respiratory** ('respirətree)

Syllabic apostrophe. Where a consonant is preceded by an apostrophe, this indicates that the consonant should be pronounced. For example:

> **hospital** ('hospit'l)

The used of the centred dot. Where two letters occur together that may be mistaken for a different sound from that intended, a centred full point is added to separate the characters. For example:

> **myopia** (mie'ohpi·ə)

Sub-entries

The term being sought may be a main entry or a sub-entry under the main entry. Sub-entries are listed alphabetically under the main entry, with the initial letter(s) of the main entry repeated. For example:

> **abdomen** . . .
>   *Acute a.* . . . .
>   *Pendulous a.* . . . .
>   *Scaphoid (navicular) a.* . . . .

Cross-referencing

Throughout the dictionary, cross-references are given within the text as SMALL CAPITALS. For example:

fibrin ('fiebrin) an insoluble protein that is essential to CLOTTING of blood, formed from fibrinogen by action of thrombin.

There are also situations where it is simply more convenient to define the word in a different location, to which the reader is then referred.

Translations. Where a translation of a foreign term occurs, it is indicated in *italic type* immediately following the abbreviation for the language (which is in square brackets). For example:

acus ('akəs) [L.] *a needle*

Abbreviations used in this dictionary

b. born
L. Latin
Fr. French

Drug names. Where possible, only generic names are used. However, some proprietary drug names and names for preparations are included with information (and sometimes cross-references) concerning the generic drug(s) involved. Inclusion of a drug in the dictionary does not imply endorsement.

A

A accommodation; adenine; anode (anodal); anterior axial; symbol for ampere and mass number.

abacterial (,aybak'tiə·ri·əl) indicating a condition not caused by bacteria.

abarticulation (,abah,tikyuh'layshən) dislocation of a joint.

abatement (ə'baytmənt) a decrease in the severity of a pain or a symptom.

abdomen ('abdəmən,'ab'doh-) the belly. The cavity between the diaphragm and the pelvis, lined by a serous membrane, the peritoneum, and containing the stomach, intestines, liver, gallbladder, spleen, pancreas, kidneys, suprarenal glands, ureters and bladder. For descriptive purposes, its area can be divided into nine regions (see Figure). *Acute a.* any abdominal condition urgently requiring treatment, usually surgical. *Pendulous a.* a condition in which the anterior part of the abdominal wall hangs down over the pubis. *Scaphoid (navicular) a.* a hollowing of the anterior wall commonly seen in grossly emaciated people.

abdominal (ab'domin'l) pertaining to the abdomen. *A. aneurysm* a dilatation of the abdominal aorta. *A. aorta* that part of the aorta below the diaphragm. *A. breathing* deep breathing; hyper-

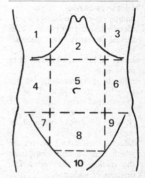

1. *Right hypochondriac;* 2. *epigastric;* 3. *left hypochondriac;* 4. *right lumbar;* 5. *umbilical;* 6. *left lumbar;* 7. *right iliac;* 8. *hypogastric;* 9. *left iliac;* 10. *pubic.*

ABDOMEN

pnoea. *A. reflex* reflex contraction of abdominal wall muscles observed when skin is lightly stroked. *A. section* incision through the abdominal wall.

abdominopelvic (ab,dominoh'pelvik) concerning the abdomen and the pelvic cavity.

abdominoperineal (ab,dominoh-,peri'neeəl) pertaining to the abdomen and the perineum. *A. excision* an operation performed through the abdomen and the perineum for the excision of the rectum or bladder. Often done as a synchronized operation by two surgeons, one working at each approach.

abdominoposterior (ab,dominohpo'stiə·ri·ə) indicating a position of the fetus with its abdomen turned towards the maternal back.

abduce (ab'dyoos) to abduct or to draw away.

abducent (ab'dyoosənt) leading away from the midline. *A. muscle* the external rectus muscle of the eye, which rotates it outward. *A. nerve* the cranial nerve which supplies this muscle.

abductor (ab'duktə) a muscle which draws a limb away from the midline of the body. The opposite of adductor.

Aberdeen formula ('abədeen) a method developed in Aberdeen in 1974 of estimating the number of nurses needed on a ward, based on the number and dependency of the patients. The formula is W = N (B + T) + A + D + E where:

W = average weekly nursing workload in hours.

N = average number of patients in ward.

B = time in hours per week required to maintain the standard of basic nursing care for a totally helpless bedfast patient.

T = time required for technical nursing of the ward speciality expressed as a percentage of the time spent on basic nursing.

A = time per patient per week for administrative duties.

D = time per patient per week for domestic work.

E = patient dependency factor for ward speciality.

aberrant (a'berənt) taking an unusual course. Used of blood vessels and nerves.

aberration (,abə'rayshən) deviation from the normal. In optics, failure to focus rays of light. *Mental a.* mental disorder of an unspecified kind.

ability (ə'bilitee) the power to perform an act, either mental or physical, with or without training. *Innate a.* the ability with which a person is born.

ablation (ab'layshən) removal or destruction by surgical or radiological means of neoplasms or other body tissue.

ablepharia (,ayble'fair·riə,ablə-) congenital reduction or absence of eyelids.

ablutomania (ə'blootoh'mayni·ə) compulsion to wash oneself frequently.

abnormal (,ab'nawm'l) varying from what is regular or usual.

abort (ə'bawt) 1. to terminate a process or disease before it has run its normal course. 2. to give birth to a fetus earlier than the 28th week of pregnancy.

abortifacient (ə,bawti'fayshənt) an agent or drug which may induce abortion.

abortion (ə'bawshən) 1. premature cessation of a normal process. 2. emptying of the pregnant uterus before the end of the 28th week. 3. the product of such an abortion. *Complete a.* one in which the contents of the uterus are expelled intact. *Criminal a.* the termination of pregnancy for reasons other than those permitted by law (i.e. danger to mental or physical health of mother or child or family), and without medical approval. *Incomplete a.* that in which some part of the fetus or placenta is retained in the uterus. *Induced a.* the intentional emptying of the uterus. *Inevitable a.* abortion where bleeding is profuse and accompanied by pains, the cervix is dilated and the contents of the uterus can be felt. *Missed a.* one where all signs of pregnancy disappear and later the uterus discharges a blood clot surrounding a shrivelled fetus, i.e. a carneous mole. *Septic a.* abortion associated with infection. *Therapeutic (legal) a.* one induced on medical advice because the continuance of the pregnancy would involve risk to the life of the pregnant woman, or of injury to the physical or mental health of the pregnant woman or any existing children of her family, greater than if the pregnancy were terminated or because there is a substantial risk that if the child were born it would suffer from such physical or mental abnormalities as to be seriously handicapped (1976 Abortion Act). *Threatened a.* the appearance of signs of premature expulsion of the fetus; bleeding is slight, the cervix is closed. *Tubal a.* the termination of a tubal pregnancy caused by rupture of the uterine tube.

abrachia (ə'brayki·ə) congenital absence of arms.

abrasion (ə'brayzhən) a superficial injury, where the skin or mucous membrane is rubbed or torn. *Corneal a.* this can occur when the surface of the cornea has been removed, e.g. by a scratch or other injury.

abreaction (,abri'akshən) the reliving of a past painful experience, with the release of repressed emotion.

abruptio placentae (ə,brupshioh plə'sentee, -tioh) premature detachment of the placenta, causing maternal shock.

abscess ('abses) a collection of pus in a cavity. Caused by the disintegration and replacement of tissue damaged by mechanical, chemical or bacterial injury. *Alveolar a.* an abscess in a tooth socket. *Brodie's a.* a bone abscess, usually on the head of the tibia. *Cold a.* the result of chronic tubercular infection and so called because there are few, if any, signs of inflammation. *Psoas a.* a cold abscess that has tracked down the psoas muscle from caries of the lumbar vertebrae. *Subphrenic a.* one situated under the diaphragm.

absorbent (əb'sawbənt, -'zaw-) 1. able to take in, or suck up and incorporate. 2. a tissue structure involved in absorption. 3. a substance that absorbs or promotes absorption.

absorption (ab'sawpshən,-'zaw-) 1. in physiology, the taking up by suction of fluids or other substances by the tissues of the body. 2. in psychology, great mental concentration on a single object or activity. 3. in radiology, uptake of radiation by body tissues.

abstinence ('abstinəns) a refraining from the use of or indulgence in food, stimulants or coitus. *A. syndrome* withdrawal symptoms.

abulia (ə'byooli·ə) loss of willpower.

abuse (ə'byoos) misuse, maltreatment, or excessive use. *Child a.* the non-accidental use of physical force or the non-accidental act of omission by a parent or other custodian responsible for the care of a child. *Drug a.* use of illegal drugs or misuse of prescribed drugs. *Solvent a.* the deliberate inhalation of volatile chemicals with the aim of inducing intoxication.

acanthoma (,akən'thohma) a tumour originating in the prickle cell layer of the epidermis. Usually applied to benign epithelial tumours.

acanthosis (,akən'thohsis) hyperplasia of the prickle cell layer of the epidermis, as seen in psoriasis.

acapnia (ay'kapni·ə) a deficiency of carbon dioxide in the blood.

acaricide (a'karisied) an agent which destroys mites.

Acarus ('akə·rəs) a genus of small mites. *A. scabiei* (*Sarcoptes scabiei*) the cause of scabies.

acatalepsy (,ay'katə,lepsee) lack of understanding.

acataphasia (,aykatə'fayzi·ə) loss of the ability to express connected thought, resulting from a cerebral lesion.

accessory (ak'sesə·ri,'ək-) supplementary. *A. nerve* the 11th

cranial nerve. It is made up of two portions, the cranial and the spinal.

accident form ('aksidənt ,fawm) a form which provides a record of any accident to any person on Health Authority premises. Health Authorities require that the form is completed as soon after the accident as possible.

accommodation (ə,komə'dayshən) adjustment. In ophthalmology, the term refers specifically to adjustment of the ciliary muscle, which controls the shape of the lens. In *negative a.* the ciliary muscle relaxes and the lens becomes less convex, giving long-distance vision; in *positive a.* the ciliary muscle contracts and the lens becomes more convex, giving near vision.

accouchement (ə'kooshmonh) childbirth.

accountable (ə'kowntəb'l) liable to be held responsible for a course of action. A qualified nurse has a duty to care according to law; in nursing being accountable refers to the responsibility the qualified nurse takes for prescribing and initiating nursing care. Nurses are accountable to their patients, their peers and their employing authority according to the professional code of conduct.

accretion (ə'kreeshən) growth. The accumulation of deposits, e.g. of salts to form a calculus in the bladder. In dentistry, the growth of tartar on the teeth.

accumulator (ə'kyoomyuh,laytə) an apparatus for the collection and storage of electricity. A battery that can be recharged.

ACE inhibitors (ays in'hibitəz) a group of drugs used in the treatment of hypertension. Their name, angiotensin converting enzyme inhibitors, explains part of their mode of action, though it is thought that some of their other actions may also be important in reducing blood pressure.

acephalic (ˌaykə'falik,-sə-) without a head.

acetabuloplasty (ˌasi'tabyuhloh-ˌplastee) an operation performed to improve the depth and shape of the hip socket in correcting congenital dislocation of the hip or in treating osteoarthritis of the hip.

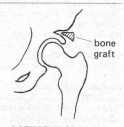

bone graft

ACETABULOPLASTY

acetabulum (ˌasi'tabyuhləm) the cup-like socket in the innominate bone, in which the head of the femur moves.

acetate ('asi,tayt) a salt of acetic acid.

acetazolamide (ə,setə'zoləmied) a sulphonamide compound which is an oral diuretic and is used in the treatment of congestive heart failure and of glaucoma.

Acetest ('asi,test) trade name for reagent tablets containing sodium nitroprusside, aminoacetic acid, disodium phosphate, and lactose. A drop of urine is placed on a tablet on a sheet of white paper; if significant quantities of acetone are present the tablet changes from a purple tint (1+), to lavender (2+), to moderate purple (3+), or to deep purple (4+).

acetic acid (ə'seetik) the acid of vinegar. It may be used as an antidote to alkaline poisons.

acetoacetic acid (ˌasitoh-ə'seetik, ə,see-) diacetic acid. A product of fat metabolism. It occurs in excessive amounts in diabetes and starvation, giving rise to acetone bodies in the urine.

acetonaemia (ˌasitə'neemi-ə,ə,see-) the presence of acetone bodies in the blood.

acetone ('asi,tohn) a colourless inflammable liquid with a characteristic odour. Traces are found in the blood and in normal urine. *A. bodies* ketones found in the blood and urine of uncontrolled diabetic patients and also in acute starvation as a result of the incomplete breakdown of fatty and amino acids.

acetonuria (ˌasitə'nyooə·ri-ə,ə,see-) the presence of an excess quantity of acetone bodies in the urine which gives it a peculiar sweet smell.

acetylcholine (ˌasitiel'kohleen, ˌasitil-) a chemical transmitter that is released by some nerve endings at the synapse between one neurone and the next or between a nerve ending and the effector organ it supplies. These nerves are said to be cholinergic, e.g. the parasympathetic nerves and the lower motor neurones to skeletal muscles. It is rapidly destroyed in the body by cholinesterase.

acetylcoenzyme A (ˌasitielkoh-'enziem, ˌasitil-) active form of acetic acid, to which carbohydrates, fats and amino acids not needed for protein synthesis are converted.

acetylsalicylic acid ('asitiel-ˌsalis-ilik, ˌasitil) aspirin. An analgesic, antipyretic and antirheumatic drug. It is available in its pure form or in combination with other drugs.

achalasia (akə'layzi-ə) failure of relaxation of a muscle sphincter causing dilatation of the part above, e.g. of the oesophagus above the cardiac sphincter.

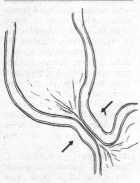

ACHALASIA

ache (ayk) a dull continuous pain.
Achilles (ə'kileez) Greek mytho-

logical hero who could be wounded only in the heel. *A. tendon* tendocalcaneus, connecting the soleus and gastrocnemius muscles of the calf to the heel bone (os calcis). Tapping the Achilles tendon normally produces the Achilles reflex or ankle jerk.

achillorrhaphy (ˌaki'lo·rəfee) repair of the Achilles tendon after it has been torn.

achillotomy (ˌaki'lotəmee) the subcutaneous division of the Achilles tendon, performed in order to lengthen it.

achlorhydria (ˌayklor'hiedri·ə) the absence of free hydrochloric acid in the stomach. May be found in pernicious anaemia, pellagra and gastric cancer.

acholia (ay'kohli·ə) a lack of secretion of bile.

acholuria (ˌaykə'lyooə·ri·ə) deficiency or lack of bile from the urine.

acholuric (ˌaykə'lyooə·rik) pertaining to acholuria. *A. jaundice* jaundice without bile in the urine.

achondroplasia (ay,kondroh'play-zi·ə) an inherited condition in which there is early union of the epiphysis and diaphysis of long bones. Growth is arrested and dwarfism is the result.

achromasia (ˌaykroh'mayzi·ə) 1. lack of colour in the skin. 2. absence of normal reaction to staining in a tissue or cell.

achromatopsia (ˌaykrohmə'top-si·ə) complete colour blindness caused by disease or trauma. It may be congenital.

achylia (ay'kieli·ə) absence of hydrochloric acid and enzymes in the gastric secretions. *A. gastrica* a condition in which gastric secretion is reduced or absent.

acid ('asid) 1. sour or sharp in taste. 2. a substance which, when combined with an alkali, will form a salt. Any acid substance will turn blue litmus red. Individual acids are given under their specific names. *A.–alcohol-fast* descriptive of stained bacteria that are resistant to decolorization by both acid and alcohol. *A.–base balance* the normal ratio between the acid ions and the basic or alkaline ions required to maintain the pH of the blood and body fluids.

acidaemia (,asi'deemi·ə) abnormal acidity of the blood, which contains an excess of hydrogen ions.

acidity (ə'siditee) 1. sourness or sharpness of taste. 2. the state of being acid.

acidosis (,asi'dohsis) a condition in which the relation of alkalinity to acidity of the blood is disturbed, with an increase in the hydrogen ion concentration. It is characterized by vomiting, drowsiness, hyperpnoea, acetone odour of breath (of 'new-mown hay') and acetone bodies in the urine. It may occur in diabetes mellitus owing to incomplete metabolism of fat. *See also* KETOSIS.

acidotic (,asi'dotik) 1. pertaining to acidosis. 2. one suffering from acidosis.

aciduria (,asi'dyooə·ri·ə) a condition in which acid urine is excreted.

acinus ('asinəs) a minute saccule or alveolus of a compound gland,

lined by secreting cells. The secreting portion of the mammary gland consists of acini.

acme ('akmee) 1. the highest point. 2. the crisis of a fever when the symptoms are fully developed.

acne ('aknee) an inflammatory condition of the sebaceous glands in which blackheads (comedones) are usually present together with papules and pustules. *A. keratitis* inflammation of the cornea associated with acne rosacea. *A. rosacea* a redness of the forehead, nose and cheeks due to chronic dilatation of the subcutaneous capillaries, which becomes permanent with the formation of pustules in the affected areas. *A. vulgaris* form that occurs commonly in adolescents and young adults, affecting the face, chest and back.

acneiform (ak'nee·i,fawm) resembling acne.

acousma (ə'koosmə) the hearing of imaginary sounds.

acoustic (ə'koostik) relating to sound or the sense of hearing.

acquired (ə'kwieəd) pertaining to disease, habits or immunity developed after birth; not inherited.

acquired immune deficiency syndrome abbreviated AIDS. *See* AIDS.

acrid ('akrid) bitter; pungent; irritating.

acriflavine (,akri'flayvin, '-veen) an antiseptic dye derived from coal tar and used in an aqueous solution for topical application.

acroarthritis (,akroh·ah'thrietis) arthritis in the joints of the hands or feet.

acrocentric (,akroh'sentrik) descriptive of chromosomes which have the centromere near to one end.

acrocephalia (,akrohke'fayli·ə, -se-) malformation of the head, in which the top is pointed. Oxycephaly.

acrocyanosis (,akroh,sieə'nohsis) persistent cyanosis, coldness of the hands and feet and profuse sweating of the digits, often associated with a vasomotor defect.

acrodynia (,akroh'dini·ə) an allergic reaction to mercury in children causing pain and erythema in the fingers and toes. Pink disease.

acromegaly (,akroh'megalee) a chronic condition producing gradual enlargement of the hands, feet and bones of the head and chest. Associated with overactivity of the anterior lobe of the pituitary gland in adults.

acromioclavicular (ə,krohmioh-,klə'vikyuhlə) pertaining to the joint between the acromion process of the scapula and the lateral aspect of the clavicle.

acromion (ə'krohmi·ən) the outward projection of the spine of the scapula, forming the point of the shoulder.

acronyx ('akrəniks) a toe- or finger-nail which becomes ingrown.

acroparaesthesia (,akroh,paris-'theezi·ə) condition in which pressure on the nerves of the brachial plexus causes numbness, pain and tingling of the hand and forearm.

acrophobia (,akroh'fohbi·ə) morbid terror of being at a height.

acrosclerosis (,akrohsklə'rohsis) a type of scleroderma which affects the hands, feet, face or chest.

acrosome ('akrə,sohm) part of the head of a spermatozoon.

acrylics (ə'kriliks) synthetic plastic materials derived from acrylic acid, from which dental and medical prostheses may be made. Used in ophthalmology for making artificial eyes, implants and lenses.

ACTH adrenocorticotrophic hormone; corticotrophin.

actin ('aktin) the protein of myofibrils responsible for contraction and relaxation of muscles.

actinism ('akti,nizəm) the ability of rays of light to produce chemical changes.

actinodermatitis (,aktinoh,dərmə'tietis) inflammation of the skin, due to the action of ultraviolet or X-rays.

Actinomyces (,aktinoh'mieseez) a genus of branching, spore-forming, vegetable parasites, which may give rise to actinomycosis and from which many antibiotic drugs are produced, e.g. streptomycin.

actinomycin (,aktinoh'miesin) a group of cytotoxic drugs used in the treatment of malignant disease.

actinomycosis (,aktinohmie'kohsis) a chronic infective disease of cattle which is also found in man. Granulated tumours occur, chiefly on the tongue and jaws.

actinotherapy (,aktinoh'therəpee) treatment of disease by rays of light, e.g. artificial sunlight.

action ('akshən) the accomplishment of an effect, whether mechanical or chemical, or the effect so produced. *Cumulative a.* the sudden and markedly increased action of a drug after administration of several doses. *Reflex a.* an involuntary response to a stimulus conveyed to the nervous system and reflected to the periphery, passing below the level of consciousness (*see also* REFLEX).

activator (ˌaktiˈvaytə) a substance, hormone or enzyme that stimulates a chemical change though it may not take part in the change. In chemistry, a catalyst. For example, yeast is the activator in the process by which sugar is converted into alcohol; the digestive secretions are activated by hormones to carry out normal digestion.

active (ˈaktiv) causing change; energetic. *A. immunity* an immunity in which the individual has been stimulated to produce his or her own antibodies. *A. movements* movements made by the patient as distinct from passive movements. *A. principle* the ingredient in a drug which is primarily responsible for its therapeutic action.

activities of daily living (akˈtivitiz əv ˌdaylee ˌliving) abbreviated ADL. Those activities usually performed in the course of a person's normal daily routine, such as eating, cleaning teeth, washing and dressing.

actomyosin (ˌaktohˈmieəsin) muscle protein complex; the myosin component acts as an enzyme which causes the release of energy.

acuity (əˈkyooitee) sharpness. *A.

of hearing an acute perception of sound. *A. of vision* clear focusing ability.

acupuncture (ˈakyuhˌpungchə) a system, which originated in China, in which the insertion of special needles into specific points along the 'meridians' of the body, is used for the production of anaesthesia, the relief of pain and the treatment of certain conditions.

acus (ˈakəs) [L.] *a needle.*

acute (əˈkyoot) a term applied to a disease in which the attack is sudden, severe and of short duration.

acyclic (ayˈsieklik) occurring independently of a natural cycle of events (such as the menstrual cycle).

acyclovir (ayˈsieklohviə) an antiviral agent used to treat herpes viruses. Uses include the treatment of varicella-zoster and herpes simplex. It is only active if started at the onset of the infection. May also be used as prophylaxis in the immunocompromised and for prevention of recurrence. It is available as a cream, ophthalmic ointment, suspension, tablets and an intravenous infusion.

acystia (ayˈsisti·ə) absence of the bladder.

adactylia (ˌaydakˈtili·ə) congenital absence of fingers or toes.

Adam's apple (ˈadəmz) the laryngeal prominence, a protrusion of the front of the neck formed by the thyroid cartilage.

adamantine (ˌadəˈmanteen, -tien) pertaining to the enamel of the teeth.

adaptation (ˌadapˈtayshən) 1. the

process of modification which a living organism undergoes when adjusting itself to new surroundings or circumstances. 2. the process of overcoming difficulties and adjusting to changing circumstances. Neuroses and psychoses are often associated with failure of adaptation. 3. used in ophthalmology to mean the adjustment of visual function according to the ambient illumination. *Colour a.* 1. changes in visual perception of colour with prolonged stimulation. 2. adjustment of vision to degree of brightness or colour tone of illumination. *Dark a.* adaptation of the eye to vision in reduced illumination. *Light a.* adaptation of the eye to vision in bright illumination (photopia), with reduction in the concentration of the photosensitive pigments of the eye.

addict ('adikt) a person exhibiting addiction.

addiction (ə'dikshən) the taking of drugs or alcohol leading to physiological and psychological dependence with a tendency to increase its use. *See* DEPENDENCE and DRUG ADDICTION.

Addison's anaemia (adisnz) *T. Addison, British physician, 1793–1860.* Pernicious anaemia.

Addison's disease deficiency disease of the suprarenal cortex; often tuberculous. There is wasting, brown pigmentation of the skin and extreme debility.

adducent (ə'dyoos'nt) leading towards the midline. *A. muscle* the medial rectus muscle of the eye which turns it inward.

adductor (ə'duktə) a muscle which draws a limb towards the midline of the body. The opposite of abductor.

adenectomy (,adə'nektəmee) excision of a gland.

adenine ('adə,neen) one of the purine bases found in deoxyribonucleic acid.

adenitis (,adə'nietis) inflammation of a gland.

adenocarcinoma (,adənoh,kahsi-'nohmə) a malignant new growth of glandular epithelial tissue.

adenofibroma (,adənohfie'brohmə) a benign tumour of connective tissue which contains glandular structures.

adenoid ('adə,noyd) resembling a gland. Generally applied to abnormal lymphoid growth in the nasopharynx.

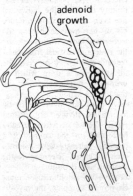

adenoid growth

ADENOID GROWTH

adenoidectomy (,adənoy'dektəmee) the surgical removal of adenoid tissue from the nasopharynx.

adenoma (,adə'nohmə) a non-malignant tumour of glandular tissue.

adenomatome (,adə'nohmə,tohm) an instrument for the removal of adenoids.

adenomyoma (,adənohmie'ohmə) an innocent new growth involving both endometrium and muscle tissue; found in the uterus or uterine ligaments.

adenopathy (,adə'nopəthee) enlargement of any gland, especially those of the lymphatic system.

adenosarcoma (,adənohsah'kohmə) a malignant tumour of connective and glandular tissue. *Embryonal a.* nephroblastoma.

adenosclerosis (,adənohsklə'rohsis) hardening of a gland. Usually the result of calcification.

adenosine (a'denoh,seen) a nucleoside consisting of adenine and D-ribose (a pentose sugar). *A. triphosphate* abbreviated ATP. A compound containing three phosphoric acids. It is present in all cells and serves as a store for energy.

adenovirus (,adənoh'vierəs) a virus of the Adenoviridae family. Many types have been isolated, some of which cause respiratory tract infections, while others are associated with conjunctivitis, epidemic keratoconjunctivitis or gastrointestinal infection.

adeps ('adeps) [L.] lard, a foundation fat for ointments. *A. lanae hydrosus* lanolin.

ADH antidiuretic hormone. Vasopressin.

adhesion (ad'heezhən) union between two surfaces normally separated. Usually the result of inflammation when fibrous tissue forms, e.g. peritonitis may cause adhesions between organs. A possible cause of intestinal obstruction.

adiaphoresis (ay,dieəfə'reesis) deficiency in the secretion of sweat.

adiaphoretic (ay,dieəfor'retik) an anhidrotic agent. A drug that prevents the secretion of sweat.

adipocele ('adipoh,seel) a hernia, with the sac containing fatty tissue.

adipocere ('adipoh,siə) a waxy substance formed in dead bodies when decomposing.

adipose ('adi,pohs, -z) of the nature of fat. Fatty.

adiposity (,adi'positee) the state of being too fat. Obesity.

adiposuria (,adipoh'syooə·ri·ə) the presence of fat in the urine. Lipuria.

aditus ('aditəs) an opening or passageway; often applied to that between the middle ear and the mastoid antrum.

adjustment (ə'justmənt) in psychology, the ability of a person to adapt to changing circumstances or environment.

adjuvant ('ajəvənt) 1. any treatment used in conjunction with another to enhance its efficacy. 2. a substance administered with a drug to enhance its effect.

ADL activities of daily living.

Adler's theory ('adləz) *A. Adler, Austrian psychiatrist, 1870–1937.* The theory that neuroses develop as a compensation for feelings of inferiority, either social or physical.

adnexa (ad'neksə) appendages. *Uterine a.* the ovaries and tubes.

adolescence (ˌadə'lesəns) the period between puberty and maturity. In the male, 14–25 years. In the female, 12–21 years.

adrenal (ə'dreen'l) 1. near the kidneys. 2. a triangular endocrine gland situated above each kidney.

adrenalectomy (əˈdreenə'lektə-mee) surgical excision of an adrenal gland.

adrenaline (ə'drenəlin) a hormone secreted by the medulla of the adrenal gland. Has an action similar to normal stimulation of the sympathetic nervous system: (1) causing dilatation of the bronchioles; (2) raising the blood pressure by constriction of surface vessels and stimulation of the cardiac output; (3) releasing glycogen from the liver. It is therefore used to treat such conditions as asthma, collapse and hypoglycaemia. It acts as a haemostat in local anaesthetics.

adrenergic (ˌadrə'nərjik) pertaining to nerves that release the chemical transmitter noradrenaline in order to stimulate the muscles and glands they supply.

adrenocorticotrophin (əˌdree-noh,kawtikoh'trohfin) adrenocorticotrophic hormone (ACTH); secreted by the anterior lobe of the pituitary body. Stimulates the adrenal cortex to produce cortisol. Corticotrophin.

adrenogenital (əˌdreenoh'jenit'l) relating to both the adrenal glands and the gonads. *A. syndrome* a condition of masculinization caused by overactivity of

the adrenal cortex resulting in precocious puberty in the male infant and masculinization in the female. Both sexes are liable to addisonian crises.

adrenolytic (ə'dreenoh'litik) a drug that inhibits the stimulation of the sympathetic nerves and the activity of adrenaline.

adsorbent (əd'sawbənt, -'zawb-) a substance that has the power of attracting gas or fluid to itself.

adsorption (əd'sawpshən, -'zawp-) the power of certain substances to attach other gases or substances in solution to their surface and so concentrate them there. This is made use of in chromatography.

adult (ə'dult, 'adult) mature. A mature person.

adulteration (əˈdultə'rayshən) addition of an impure, cheap, or unnecessary ingredient to cheat, cheapen, or falsify a preparation.

advancement (əd'vahnsmənt) in surgery, an operation to detach a tendon or muscle and reattach it further forward. Used in the treatment of strabismus and uterine retroversion.

adventitia (ˌadven'tishi-ə, -'tishə) the outer coat of an artery or vein.

Aëdes (ay'eedeez) a genus of mosquitoes. It includes *A. aegypti,* the intermediate host in the transmission of dengue and yellow fever.

aeration (air'rayshən) supplying with air. Used to describe the oxygenation of blood which takes place in the lungs.

aerobe ('air·rohb) an organism that can live and thrive only in the presence of oxygen.

aerogenous (air'rojənəs) Gas-producing. Applied to microorganisms that give rise to the formation of gas, usually by the fermentation of lactose or other carbohydrate.

aeropathy (air'ropəthee) bends (decompression sickness).

aerophagy (air'rofajee) the excessive swallowing of air.

aerosol ('air·rə,sol) finely divided particles or droplets. *A. sprays* used in medicine to humidify air or oxygen, or for the administration of drugs by inhalation.

Æsculapius ('eeskyuh'laypi·əs, 'es-) the god of healing in Roman mythology. The staff of Æsculapius, a rod or staff with a snake entwined around it, is a symbol of medicine.

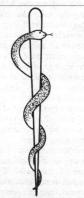

STAFF OF ÆSCULAPIUS

aetas ('eetas) [L.] *age*; abbreviated aet.

aetiology (,eeti'olajee) the science of the cause of disease.

afebrile (ay'feebriel, -'feb-) without fever.

affect (ə'fekt) in psychiatry, the feeling experienced in connection with an emotion or mood.

affection (ə'fekshən) 1. a morbid condition or disease state. 2. a warm feeling for someone or something.

affective (ə'fektiv) pertaining to the emotions or moods. *A. psychoses* major mental disorders in which there is grave disturbance of the emotions.

afferent ('afə·rənt) conveying towards the centre. *A. nerves* the sensory nerve fibres which convey impulses from the periphery towards the brain. *A. paths* or *tracts* the course of the sensory nerves up the spinal cord and through the brain. *A. vessels* arterioles entering the glomerulus of the kidney, or lymphatics entering a lymph gland. *See* EFFERENT.

affiliation (ə,fili'ayshən) the judicial decision of paternity of a child with a view to a maintenance order.

affinity (ə'finitee) in chemistry, the attraction of two substances to each other, e.g. haemoglobin and oxygen.

afibrinogenaemia (,ayfiebrinəjə'neemi·ə) absence of fibrinogen in the blood. The clotting mechanism of the blood is impaired as a result.

African tick fever ('afrikən) disease caused by a spirochaete, *Borrelia duttonii*. Transmitted by ticks. *See* RELAPSING FEVER.

afterbirth ('ahftə,bərth) a lay expression used to describe the placenta, cord and membranes expelled after childbirth.

aftercare ('ahftə,kair) social, medical or nursing care following a period of hospital treatment.

afterimage ('ahftə,imij) a visual impression that remains briefly following the cessation of sensory stimulation.

afterpain ('ahftə,payn) pain due to uterine contraction after childbirth.

afunctional (ay'fungkshənəl) lacking function.

agalactia (,aygə'lakshi·ə) absence of milk secretion after childbirth.

agammaglobulinaemia (ay,gamə,globyuhli'neemi·ə) a condition in which there is no gamma-globulin in the blood. The patients are therefore susceptible to infections because of an inability to form antibodies.

agar ('aygah) a gelatinous substance prepared from seaweed. Used as a culture medium for bacteria and as a laxative because it absorbs liquid from the digestive tract and swells, so stimulating peristalsis.

ageing ('ayjing) the structural changes that take place in time that are not caused by accident or disease.

agenesis (ay'jenəsis) failure of a structure to develop properly.

agent ('ayjənt) any substance of force capable of producing a physical, chemical or biological effect. *Alkylating a.* a cytotoxic preparation. *Chelating a.* a chemical compound which binds metal ions. *Wetting a.* a substance which lowers the surface tension of water and promotes wetting.

agglutination (ə,glooti'nayshən) the collecting into clumps, particularly of cells suspended in a fluid and of bacteria affected by specific immune serum. *Cross a.* a simple test to decide the group to which a given blood belongs (*see* BLOOD GROUP). A drop of serum of known classification is put on a microscope slide, and to this is added a drop of the blood to be tested. An even admixture indicates compatibility. A flaky spotted appearance shows incompatibility as the corpuscles have clumped together. *A. test* a means of aiding diagnosis and identification of bacteria. If serum containing known agglutinins comes into contact with the specific bacteria, clumping will take place (*see* WIDAL REACTION).

agglutinative (ə'glootinə,tiv) 1. adherent or gluing together. 2. serum which causes clumping of bacteria, e.g. in Widal reaction.

agglutinin (ə'glootinin) any substance causing agglutination (clumping together) of cells, particularly a specific antibody formed in the blood in response to the presence of an invading agent. Agglutinins are proteins (IMMUNOGLOBULINS) and function as part of the immune mechanism of the body. When the invading agents that bring about the production of agglutinins are bacteria, the agglutinins produced bring about agglutination of the bacterial cells.

agglutinogen (,agluh'tinəjən) any

substance that, when present in the bloodstream, can cause the production of specific antibodies or agglutinins.

aggregation (ˌagri'gayshən) the massing together of materials, as in clumping. *Familial a.* the increased incidence of cases of a disease in a family compared with that in control families. *Platelet a.* the clumping together of platelets which may be induced by a number of agents such as thrombin and collagen.

aggressin (ə'gresin) a substance said to be produced by some bacteria which increases their effect upon the host.

aggression (ə'greshən) animosity or hostility shown towards another person or object, as a response to opposition or frustration.

agitation (ˌaji'tayshən) 1. shaking. 2. mental distress causing extreme restlessness.

aglossia (ay'glosi·ə) absence of the tongue.

aglutition (ˌaygloo'tishən) difficulty in the act of swallowing. Dysphagia.

agnathia (ag'naythi·ə) absence or defective development of the jaw.

agnosia (ag'nohzi·ə) an inability to recognize objects as the sensory stimulus cannot be interpreted in spite of the presence of a normal sense organ.

agonist ('agənist) the prime mover. A muscle opposed in action by another (the antagonist).

agony ('agənee) extreme suffering, either mental or physical.

agoraphobia (ˌagə·rə'fohbi·ə) a fear of open spaces.

agranulocyte (ay'granyuhloh,siet) a white blood cell without granules in the cytoplasm. Includes monocytes and lymphocytes.

agranulocytosis (ay,granyuhloh-sie'tohsis) a condition in which there is a marked decrease or complete absence of granular leukocytes in the blood, leaving the body defenceless against bacterial invasion. May result from: (1) the use of drugs, e.g. gold salts, sulphonamides, thiouracil and benzol preparations; (2) irradiation. Characterized by a sore throat, ulceration of the mouth and pyrexia. It may result in severe prostration and death.

agraphia (ay'grafi·ə) absence of the power of expressing thought in writing. It arises from a lack of muscular coordination or from a cerebral lesion.

ague (ˌaygoo) malaria.

AHF antihaemophilic factor (clotting factor VIII).

AHG antihaemophilic globulin (clotting factor VIII).

AID artificial insemination of a woman with donor semen.

AIDS (aydz) acquired immune deficiency syndrome. It is the extreme end of the spectrum of disease caused by human immunodeficiency virus (HIV) infection, and impairs the body's cellular immune system. This may result in infection by organisms of normally no or low pathogenicity (opportunistic infections), principally *Pneumocystis carinii* pneumonia (PCP), or the development of unusual tumours, namely Kaposi's sarcoma (KS). *AIDS-related complex* (ARC) recurrent symptoms such as lymphaden-opathy, night sweats, diarrhoea, weight loss, malaise and chest infections. Examination of the blood may show abnormally low platelet and neutrophil counts as well as low lymphocyte counts. *See* Appendix 6.

AIH artificial insemination of a woman by her husband's semen.

ailment ('ailmənt) any minor dis-order of the body.

air (air) a mixture of gases that make up the earth's atmosphere. It consists of: non-active nitrogen 79_1; oxygen 21_1; which supports life and combustion; traces of neon, argon, hydrogen, etc.; and carbon dioxide 0.03, except in expired air, when 6_1 is exhaled, due to diffusion which has taken place in the lungs. Air has weight and exerts pressure which aids in syphonage from body cavities. *A.-bed* a rubber mattress inflated with air. *Complemental a.* additional air which can be inhaled with inspiratory effort. *A. embolism* an embolism caused by air entering the circulatory system. *A. encephalography* radiological examination of the brain after the injection of air into the subarachnoid space. *A. hunger* a form of dyspnoea in which there are deep sighing res-pirations, characteristic of severe haemorrhage or acidosis. *Resi-dual a.* air remaining in the lungs after deep expiration. *Stationary a.* that retained in the lungs after normal expiration. *Supplemental a.* the extra air for-ced out of the lungs with expira-tory effort. *Tidal a.* that which

passes in and out of the lungs in normal respiratory action.

airway ('air,way) 1. the passage by which the air enters and leaves the lungs. 2. a mechanical device (tube) used for securing unob-structed respiration during gen-eral anaesthesia or other occasions when the patient is not ventilating or exchanging gases properly. It may be passed through the mouth or nose. The tube prevents a flaccid tongue from resting against the posterior pharyngeal wall and causing obstruction of the airway.

akinesia (,ayki'neezi·ə) loss of muscle power. This may be the result of a brain or spinal cord lesion or temporarily due to anaesthesia.

akinetic (,ayki'netik) relating to states or conditions where there is lack of movement.

Al symbol for *aluminium*.

alacrima (ay'lakrimə) a deficiency or absence of secretion of tears.

alalia (ə'layli·ə) loss or impair-ment of the power of speech due to muscle paralysis or cerebral lesion.

alanine ('alə,neen, -nien) an amino acid formed by the ingestion of dietary protein.

Albers-Schönberg's disease (,al-bairz'shərnbərg) *H. E. Albers-Schönberg, German radiologist, 1865–1921.* Osteopetrosis.

albinism ('albi,nizəm) a condition in which there is congenital absence of pigment in the skin, hair and eyes. It may be partial or complete.

albino (al'beenoh) a person affec-ted with albinism.

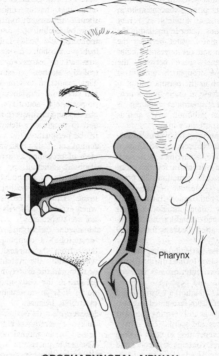

Pharynx

OROPHARYNGEAL AIRWAY

Albright's syndrome ('awlbriets) *F. Albright, American physician, 1900–1969.* Condition in which there is abnormal development of bone, excessive pigmentation of the skin and, in females, precocious sexual development.

albumin ('albyuhmin) 1. any protein that is soluble in water and moderately concentrated salt solutions and is coagulable by heat, e.g. egg white. 2. serum albumin; a plasma protein, formed principally in the liver and constituting about four-sevenths of the 6 to 8 per cent protein concentration in the plasma. Albumin is a very important factor in regulating the exchange of water between the plasma and the interstitial compartment (space between the cells). A drop in the amount of albumin in the plasma results in an increase in tissue fluid which, if severe, becomes apparent as oedema. Albumin serves also as a transport protein.

albuminuria (al,byoomi'nyooə-·ri·ə) the presence of albumin in the urine, occurring e.g. in renal disease, in most feverish conditions and sometimes in pregnancy. *Orthostatic* or *postural a.* a non-pathological form which affects some individuals after prolonged standing but disappears after bedrest for a few hours.

albumose ('albyuh,mohs, -,mohz) a substance formed during gastric digestion, intermediate between albumin and peptone.

alcohol ('alka,hol) a volatile liquid distilled from fermented saccharine liquids and forming the basis of wines and spirits. The official (BP) preparation of ethyl alcohol (ethanol) contains 95, alcohol and 5, water. Used: (1) as an antiseptic; (2) in the preparation of tinctures; (3) as a preservative for anatomical specimens. Taken internally, it acts as a temporary heart stimulant, and in large quantities as a depressant poison. It has some value as a food, 30 ml brandy producing about 400 J. *Absolute a.* that which contains not more than 1, by weight of

water. *A.-fast* pertaining to bacteria that having once been stained are resistant to decolorization by alcohol.

alcoholic (,alka'holik) 1. pertaining to alcohol. 2. a person addicted to excessive, uncontrolled alcohol consumption. This results in loss of appetite and vitamin B deficiency, leading to peripheral neuritis with eye changes and cirrhosis of the liver and to progressive deterioration in the personality.

alcoholism ('alka,holizəm) the state of poisoning as a result of alcoholic addiction.

alcoholuria (,alkəho'lyooə·ri·ə) the presence of alcohol in the urine. This may be estimated when excess blood levels of alcohol are suspected.

aldosterone (,aldoh'stiə·rohn, al-'dostə,rohn) a compound, isolated from the adrenal cortex, which aids the retention of sodium and the excretion of potassium in the body and by so doing aids in maintaining the electrolyte balance.

aldosteronism (al'dostə·rə,nizem) an excess secretion of aldosterone caused by an adrenal neoplasm. The serum potassium is low and the patient has hypertension and severe muscular weakness.

aleukaemia (,ayloo'keemi·ə) an acute condition in which there is an absence or deficiency of white cells in the blood.

alexia (ə'leksi·ə, ay-) a form of aphasia, when there is inability to recognize written or printed words. Word blindness.

algae ('aljee, -gee) simple forms

of plant life. These form a slimy film on sand filter beds and aid purification of water.

algesia (al'jeezi·ə) excessive sensitiveness to pain.

algesimetry (ˌalji'simətree) measurement of sensitiveness to pain.

algor ('algor) chill or rigor; coldness.

alienation (ˌayli·ə'nayshən) a feeling of estrangement or separation from others or from self. A symptom of schizophrenia where the sufferer feels that his thoughts are under the control of someone else. Depersonalization.

alignment (ə'lienmənt) the state of being arranged in a line, i.e. in correct anatomical position.

aliment ('alimənt) food or nourishment.

alimentary (ˌali'mentə·ree, -tree) relating to the system of nutrition. *A. canal* or *tract* the passage through which the food passes, from mouth to anus. *A. system* the alimentary tract together with the liver and other organs concerned in digestion and absorption.

alimentation (ˌalimen'tayshən) giving or receiving of nourishment. The process of supplying the patient's need for nutrition.

aliquot ('aliˌkwot) one of a number of equal parts forming a compound or solution.

alkalaemia (ˌalkə'leemi·ə) an increase in the alkali content of the blood. The pH is above 7.4. Alkalosis.

alkali ('alkəˌlie) a substance capable of uniting with acids to form salts, and with fats and fatty acids to form soaps. Alkaline solutions turn red litmus paper blue. *A. reserve* the ability of the combined buffer systems of the blood to neutralize acid. The pH of the blood normally is slightly on the alkaline side, between 7.35 and 7.45. The principal buffer in the blood is bicarbonate; the alkali reserve is essentially represented by the plasma bicarbonate concentration.

alkaline ('alkəˌlien) having the reactions of an alkali. *A. phosphatase* an enzyme localized on cell membranes that hydrolyses phosphate esters, liberating inorganic phosphate, and has an optimal pH of about 10.0. Serum alkaline phosphatase activity is elevated in obstructive jaundice and bone disease.

alkalinity (ˌalkə'linitee) 1. the quality of being alkaline. 2. the combining power of a base, expressed as the maximum number of equivalents of acid with which it reacts to form a salt.

alkaloid ('alkəˌloyd) one of a group of active nitrogenous compounds that are alkaline in solution. They are usually bitter in taste and are characterized by powerful physiological activity. Examples are morphine, cocaine, atropine, quinine, nicotine, and caffeine. The term is also applied to synthetic substances that have structures similar to plant alkaloids, such as procaine.

alkalosis (ˌalkə'lohsis) an increase in the alkali reserve in the blood. It may be confirmed by estimation of the blood carbon dioxide content and treated by giving normal saline or ammonium

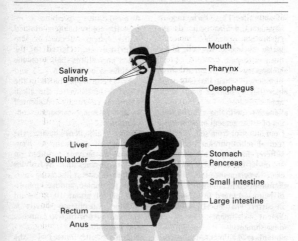

Mouth

Pharynx

Salivary glands

Oesophagus

Liver

Stomach

Gallbladder

Pancreas

Small intestine

Large intestine

Rectum

Anus

ALIMENTARY CANAL

chloride intravenously to encourage the excretion of bicarbonate by the kidneys.

alkapton (al'kapton) an abnormal product of protein metabolism, from the amino acid, tyrosine.

Homogentisic acid.

alkaptonuria (al,kaptə'nyooo·ri·ə) the excretion of alkapton in the urine. On exposure to air, oxidation takes place, giving a dark-brown colour to the urine.

alkylating agent ('alki,layting) a drug that damages the deoxyribonucleic acid (DNA) molecule of the nucleus of the cell. Many are nitrogen mustard preparations and may be termed chromosome poisons; they are used in cancer chemotherapy.

all-or-none law (,awlor'nun) principle that states that in individual cardiac and skeletal muscle fibres there are only two possible reactions to a stimulus: either there is no reaction at all or there is a full reaction, with no gradation of response according to the strength of the stimulus. Whole muscles can grade their response by increasing or decreasing the *number* of fibres involved.

allantois (ə'lantoh·is) a membranous sac projecting from the ventral surface of the fetus in its early stages. It eventually helps to form the placenta.

allele ('aleel, ə'leel) allelomorph. One of a pair of genes which occupy the same relative positions on homologous chromosomes and produce different effects on the same process of development.

allelomorph (ə'leeloh,mawf) allele.

allergen ('alə,jen) a substance that can produce an allergy or manifestation of an immune response.

allergy ('aləjee) a hypersensitivity to some foreign substances which are normally harmless but which produce a violent reaction in the patient. Asthma, hay fever, angioneurotic oedema, migraine, and some types of urticaria and eczema are allergic states. *See*

ANAPHYLAXIS.

alloaesthesia (,aloh·is'theezi·ə) allocheiria. A response or sensation felt on (referred to) the opposite side from that to which a stimulus is applied.

allocate ('alə,kayt) to assign for a particular purpose.

allocation (,alə'kayshən) the act of allocating. *Clinical a.* a period of time spent in ward/department/unit where there are patients/clients. *Patient a.* one nurse is designated as responsible for the care of one patient or a group of patients for a spell of duty. *Task a.* patient care in a ward/unit is provided by a group of nurses. Each nurse is allocated a specific nursing activity (task), e.g. one nurse in the clinical area will be responsible for bed baths whilst another will be taking and recording vital signs for the same group of patients.

allocheiria (,aloh'kieri·ə) alloaesthesia.

allograft ('alloh,grahft) tissue transplanted from one person to another. *Non-viable a.* skin taken from a cadaver which cannot regenerate. *Viable a.* living tissue transplanted.

allokeratoplasty (,aloh'kerətoh,plastee) repair of the cornea, using a material foreign to the human body, e.g. a plastic substance.

allopurinol (,aloh'pyooɔ·ri,nol) a drug which reduces the serum and urinary levels of uric acid. Used in the long-term treatment of gout to lessen the frequency and severity of attacks.

alloy ('aloy) a mixture of two or

more metals.

aloes ('alohz) a drug made from the leaves of the aloe. An irritant purgative likely to cause griping. It is contraindicated in pregnancy.

alopecia (ˌaləˈpeeshi·ə) baldness. Loss of hair. The cause of simple baldness is not yet fully understood, although it is known that the tendency to become bald is limited almost entirely to males, runs in certain families and is more common in certain racial groups than in others. Baldness is often associated with ageing. *A. areata* hair loss in sharply defined areas, usually the scalp or beard. *Cicatricial a., a. cicatrisata* irreversible loss of hair associated with scarring, usually on the scalp. *Male-pattern a.* loss of scalp hair genetically determined and androgen-dependent, beginning with frontal recession and progressing symmetrically to leave ultimately only a sparse peripheral rim of hair.

alpha ('alfə) the first letter of the Greek alphabet, α. *A. cells* cells found in the islet of Langerhans in the pancreas. They produce the hormone, glucagon. *A. receptors* tissue receptors associated with the stimulation (contraction) of smooth muscle. *A. fetoprotein* abbreviated AFP. A plasma protein originating in the fetal liver and gastrointestinal tract. The serum AFP level is used to monitor the effectiveness of cancer treatment, and the amniotic fluid AFP level is used in the prenatal diagnosis of neural tube defects.

Alport's syndrome ('awlpawts) *A.*

C. Alport, South African Physician, 1880–1959. A hereditary disorder marked by progressive nerve deafness, progressive pyelonephritis or glomerulonephritis, and occasionally ocular defects.

alternating current ('awltə,nayting) an electrical current that runs alternately from the negative and positive poles.

altitude sickness (ˌalti,tyood) condition caused by hypoxia which occurs as a result of lowered oxygen pressure at high altitudes.

alum ('aləm) a powerful astringent and styptic, composed of aluminium and potassium or ammonium sulphate. Used as a styptic or haemostatic and for its astringent properties as a mouth wash. *A. precipitated toxoid* abbreviated ATP. A preparation used for diphtheria immunization.

aluminium (ˌalyəˈmini·əm, ˌalə-) *symbol* Al. A silver-white metal with a low specific gravity, compounds of which are astringent and antiseptic. *A. hydroxide* compound used as an antacid in the treatment of gastric conditions. *A. silicate* kaolin; used as a dusting powder or as a poultice. Refined kaolin may be given orally to check diarrhoea.

alveolar (ˌalvi'ohlə) concerning an alveolus. *A. air* air found in the alveoli or air sacs of the lungs.

alveolitis (ˌalvioh'lietis) inflammation of the alveoli. *Extrinsic allergic a.* inflammation of the alveoli of the lung caused by inhalation of an antigen such as pollen.

Alzheimer's cells ('alts·hiemərz) *A. Alzheimer, German neurologist, 1864–1915.* 1. giant astrocytes with large prominent nuclei found in the brain in hepatolenticular degeneration and hepatic comas. 2. degenerated astrocytes.

Alzheimer's disease a progressive form of neuronal degeneration in the brain and the commonest cause of dementia in people of all ages. It is commoner in older than younger people and is not a just a form of presenile dementia as was originally thought. The degeneration of neurones is accompanied by changes in the brain's biochemistry. At the moment this condition is irreversible and there is no effective treatment.

amalgam (ə'malgəm) a compound of mercury and other metals. *Dental a.* used for filling teeth.

amantadine (ə'mantə,deen) an antiviral agent used against the influenza A virus, and also used as an antidyskinetic in the treatment of Parkinson's disease.

amastia (ay'masti·ə) congenital absence of breast tissue.

amaurosis (,amaw'rohsis) loss of vision, sometimes following excessive blood loss; especially after prolonged bleeding, e.g. haematuria. The visual loss may be partial or complete, temporary or permanent.

amaurotic (,amaw'rotik) pertaining to amaurosis. *A. family idiocy* Tay–Sachs disease. A familial metabolic disorder commencing in infancy or childhood. Characterized by progressive mental deterioration, blindness and spastic paralysis.

ambidextrous (,ambi'dekstrəs) equally skilful with either hand.

ambivalence (am'bivələns) the existence of contradictory emotional feelings towards an object, commonly of love and hate for another person. If these feelings occur to a marked degree they lead to psychological disturbance.

amblyopia (,ambli'ohpi·ə) dimness of vision without any apparent lesion of the eye. Uncorrectable by optical means.

amblyoscope ('amblioh,skohp) an instrument used in orthoptic treatment to aid the correction of strabismus and develop binocular vision.

ambulant ('ambyuhlənt) able to walk.

ambulatory (,ambyuh'laytə·ree) having the capacity to walk. *A. treatment* or *care* health services provided on an outpatient basis.

amelia (ay'meeli·ə) congenital absence of a limb or limbs.

amelioration (ə,meelyə'rayshən) improvement of symptoms; a lessening of the severity of a disease.

amenorrhoea (a,menə'reeə, ay-,men-) absence of menstruation. *Primary a.* the non-occurrence of the menses. *Secondary a.* the cessation of the menses after they have been established owing to disease or pregnancy.

amentia (ay'menshi·ə) mental subnormality. May be due to hereditary factors, failure of development of the embryo or birth trauma.

amethocaine ('amethoh,kayn) a local anaesthetic for mucous membranes. *A. pastille* a lozenge that, when dissolved slowly in the mouth, will aid the passage of a bronchoscope or gastroscope.

ametria (ay'meetri·ə) congenital absence of the uterus.

ametropia (,ayme'trohpi·ə) defective vision. A general word applied to incorrect refraction.

amikacin (,ami'kaysin) a semisynthetic aminoglycoside antibiotic derived from kanamycin, used in the treatment of a wide range of infections due to susceptible organisms.

amiloride (ə'milor·ried) a weak but potassium-retaining diuretic drug.

amino acid (ə'meenoh) a chemical compound containing both NH_2 and $COOH$ groups. The end-product of protein digestion. *Essential a. a.* one required for replacement and growth, which cannot be synthesized in the body in sufficient amounts and must be obtained in the diet. *Non-essential a. a.* one necessary for proper growth but which can be synthesized in the body and is not specifically required in the diet.

aminoacidopathy (ə'meenoh,asi-'dopəthee, ə,mienoh-, ə,minoh-) any inborn error of amino acid metabolism producing a metabolic block that results in accumulation of one or more amino acids in the blood (aminoacidaemia) or excess excretion in the urine (aminoaciduria) or both.

aminoglutethimide (,ameenoh-

1	Threonine
2	Lysine
3	Methionine
4	Valine
5	Phenylalanine
6	Leucine
7	Tryptophan
8	Isoleucine
9	Histidine
10	Arginine

ESSENTIAL AMINO ACIDS

gloo'tethə,mied) drug which inhibits adrenal hormone synthesis. Its use is sometimes referred to as 'medical adrenalectomy'. The effects are reversible when the drug is discontinued. Used to treat metastatic breast and prostate cancers.

aminoglycoside (ə,meenoh'glie-kə,sied) any of a group of bacterial antibiotics derived from various species of *Streptomyces* that interfere with the function of bacterial ribosomes. The aminoglycosides include gentamicin, netilmicin, streptomycin, tobramycin, amikacin, kanamycin, and neomycin. They are used to treat infections caused by Gram-negative organisms and are classified as bactericidal agents because of their interference with bacterial replication. All the aminoglycoside antibiotics are highly toxic, requiring monitoring of blood serum levels and careful observation of the patient for early signs of toxicity, particularly ototoxicity and nephrotoxicity.

aminophylline (,ami'nofa,lin) an alkaloid from camellia, it relaxes plain muscle spasm of the bronchioles and coronary arteries. It may be given by mouth, intravenously or as a suppository, and is useful in treating asthma and heart failure.

aminosalicylic acid (,aminoh,sali-'silik) *See* PARA-AMINOSALICYLIC ACID.

Aminosol (ə'meenə,sol-) trade name for an amino acid preparation for intravenous or oral use.

amitosis (,ami'tohsis) multiplication of cells by simple division or fission.

amitriptyline (,ami'triptə,leen) an antidepressant drug that is chemically related to imipramine. It is useful in relieving tension and anxiety but may cause dizziness and hypotension.

ammonia (ə'mohni·ə) NH_3. A colourless pungent gas. 'In solution, used as a cardiac stimulant.

ammonium (ə'mohni·əm) NH^4. A chemical group that combines to form salts similar to those of the alkaline metals. *A. chloride* used as a mild diuretic and to render the urine acid. Widely used in mixtures as an expectorant.

amnesia (am'neezi·ə) partial or complete loss of memory. *Anterograde a.* loss for memory of events that have taken place since an injury or illness. *Retrograde a.* loss of memory for events prior to an injury. It often applies to the time immediately preceding an accident.

amniocentesis (,amniohsen'teesis) the withdrawal of fluid from the uterus through the abdominal wall by means of a syringe and needle. It is used in the diagnosis of chromosome disorders in the fetus and in cases of hydramnios.

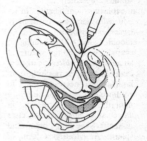

AMNIOCENTESIS

amniography (,amni'ogrəfee) radiography of the gravid uterus.

amnion ('amni·ən) the innermost membrane enveloping the fetus and enclosing the liquor amnii, or amniotic fluid.

amnioscope ('amni·ə,skohp) instrument for examining the fetus and the amniotic fluid by means of a tube passing through the abdominal wall.

amnioscopy (,amni,oskəpee) inspection of the amniotic sac using an amnioscope.

amniotic (,amni'otik) pertaining to the amnion. *A. fluid* the albuminous fluid contained in the amniotic sac. Liquor amnii.

amniotomy (,amni'otəmee) the surgical rupture of the fetal membranes to induce labour.

amoeba (ə'meebə) a minute uni-cellular protozoon. It is able to move by pushing out parts of itself (called pseudopodia). Capable of reproduction by amitotic fission. Infection of the intestines by *Entamoeba histolytica* causes 'amoebic dysentery'.

amoebiasis (,ami'bieəsis) infection with amoeba, particularly *Entamoeba histolytica*.

amoebic (ə'meebik) pertaining to, caused by, or of the nature of an amoeba. *A. abscess* an abscess cavity of the liver resulting from liquefaction necrosis due to entrance of *Entamoeba histolytica* into the portal circulation in amoebiasis; amoebic abscesses may affect the lung, brain, and spleen. *A. dysentery* a form of dysentery caused by *Entamoeba histolytica* and spread by contaminated food, water, and flies; called also amoebiasis. Amoebic dysentery is mainly a tropical disease, but many cases occur in temperate countries. Symptoms are diarrhoea, fatigue, and intestinal bleeding. Complications include involvement of the liver, liver abscess, and pulmonary abscess. For treatment several drugs are available, for example, emetine hydrochloride and chloroquine, which may be used singly or in combination.

amoeboid (ə'meeboyd) resembling an amoeba in structure or movement.

amorphous (ə'mawfəs) without definite shape. The term may be applied to fine powdery particles, as opposed to crystals.

Amoxil (ə'moksil) trade name for a preparation of amoxycillin, an antibiotic.

amoxycillin (ə,moksi'silin) a penicillin analogue similar in action to ampicillin but more efficiently absorbed from the gastrointestinal tract and therefore requiring less frequent dosage and not as likely to cause diarrhoea. It also penetrates sputum more readily than ampicillin.

ampere ('ampair) *symbol* A. The unit of intensity of an electrical current.

amphetamine (am,fetə,meen, -min) a synthetic drug which stimulates the central nervous system. It is addictive and is now seldom used except in the treatment of narcolepsy.

amphiarthrosis (,amfiah'throhsis) a form of joint in which the bones are joined together by fibrocartilage, e.g. the junctions of the vertebrae.

amphibian (am'fibi·ən) capable of living both on land and in water.

amphoric (am'for·rik) pertaining to a bottle. Used to describe the sound sometimes heard on auscultation over cavities in the lungs, which resembles that produced by blowing across the mouth of a bottle.

amphotericin (,amfə'terisin) an antifungal drug which is not absorbed by the gut. The only polyene antibiotic which may be given parenterally. Active against most yeasts and other fungi. Side-effects of fever, nausea and vomiting are common when the drug is given parenterally.

ampicillin (,ampi'silin) a broad-spectrum penicillin of synthetic origin, used in treatment of a number of infections, and available in oral preparations as well as for intramuscular injection. It is active against many of the Gram-negative pathogens, in addition to the usual Gram-positive ones that are sensitive to penicillin.

ampoule ('ampyool) a small glass or plastic phial in which sterile drugs of specified dose for injection are sealed.

ampulla (am'puhlə) the flask-like dilatation of a canal, e.g. of a uterine tube.

amputation (,ampyuh'tayshən) surgical removal of a limb or other part of the body, e.g. the breast.

amputee (,ampyuh'tee) a person who has had one or more limbs amputated.

amyl ('amil) the radical C_5H_{11}. *A. nitrite* vasodilator and heart stimulant, prescribed for inhalation in cases of angina pectoris. Capsules can be broken into a handkerchief and the fumes inhaled.

amylase ('ami,layz) an enzyme that reduces starch to maltose. Found in saliva (ptyalin) and pancreatic juice (amylopsin).

amylobarbitone (ə,mieloh'bahbi-tohn) one of the barbiturates, used as a short-acting hypnotic and sedative. Effects develop rapidly and the drug is eliminated more quickly than other barbiturates. Regular use may lead to habituation, and overdosage can produce narcosis and death. Classified as a controlled drug.

amyloid ('ami,loyd) 1. pertaining to starch. 2. a waxy starch that forms in certain tissues. *A. degeneration* amyloidosis.

amyloidosis (,amiloy'dohsis) degenerative changes in the tissues in which amyloid deposits are formed. Notably affects the kidneys, spleen, liver and heart.

amylopsin (,ami'lopsin) an enzyme found in the pancreas. Amylase.

amylum ('amiləm) [L.] *starch.*

amyotonia (ay,mieoh'tohni-ə) atonic condition of the muscles. *A. congenita* any of several rare congenital diseases marked by general hypotonia of the muscles; called also Oppenheim's disease or floppy baby syndrome.

anabolic (,anə'bolik) relating to anabolism. *A. compound* a substance that aids in the repair of body tissue, particularly protein. Androgens may be used in this way.

anabolism (ə'nabə,lizəm) the building up or synthesis of cell structure from digested food materials. *See* METABOLISM.

anacidity (,anə'siditee) decrease in normal acidity.

anaclisis (,anə'klisis) generally reclining or leaning; typically an emotional dependence on others.

anaclitic (,anə'klitik) denoting the dependence of the infant on the mother or mother substitute for his sense of well-being. *A. choice* a psychoanalytical term for the adult selection of a loved one who closely resembles one's mother (or another adult on whom one depended as a child). *A. depression* severe and progressive depression found in children who have lost their mothers and have not found a suitable substitute.

anacrotic (ˌanəˈkrotik) displaying anacrotism. *A. curve* an abnormal curve in the ascending line of a pulse tracing by sphygmograph. Typical of aortic stenosis.

anacrotism (əˈnakrəˌtizəm) an abnormal pulse wave embodying a secondary expansion.

anaemia (əˈneemi·ə) deficiency in either quality or quantity of red corpuscles in the blood, giving rise especially to symptoms of anoxaemia. There is pallor, breathlessness on exertion with palpitations, slight oedema of ankles, lassitude, headache, giddiness, albuminuria, indigestion, constipation and amenorrhoea. Anaemia may be due to many different causes. *Aplastic a.* the bone marrow is unable to produce red blood corpuscles. A rare condition of unknown cause in most cases, but it may arise from the administration of certain drugs. *Deficiency a.* any type which is due to the lack of the necessary factors for cell formation, e.g. hormones or vitamins. *Haemolytic a.* a variety in which there is excessive destruction of red blood corpuscles caused by antibody formation in the blood (*see* RHESUS FACTOR) by drugs or by severe toxaemia, as in extensive burns. *Iron-deficiency a.* the commonest type of anaemia, due to a lack of absorbable iron in the diet. It may also be due to excessive or chronic blood loss, or to poor absorption of dietary iron. *Macrocytic a.* a type in which the cells are larger than normal; present in pernicious anaemia. *Microcytic a.* a variety in which the cells are smaller than normal, as in iron deficiency. *Pernicious a.* a variety which is due to the inability of the stomach to secrete the intrinsic factor necessary for the absorption of vitamin B_{12} from the diet. *Sickle-cell a.* a hereditary haemolytic anaemia seen most commonly in black people living in or originating from the Caribbean islands, Africa, Asia, the Middle East and the Mediterranean. The red blood cells are sickle shaped. *Splenic a.* a congenital, familial disease in which the red blood cells are fragile and easily broken down. Increasingly, with the advent of electronic cell counters, anaemia is now classified according to the morphological characteristics of the erythrocytes.

anaerobe (anˈair·rohb, ˈanəˌrohb) a microorganism which can live and thrive in the absence of free oxygen. These organisms are found in body cavities or wounds where the oxygen tension is very low. Examples are the bacilli of tetanus and gas gangrene. *Facultative a.* a microorganism that can live and grow with or without molecular oxygen. *Obligate a.* an organism that can grow only in the complete absence of molecular oxygen.

anaesthesia (ˌanəsˈtheezi·ə) loss of feeling or sensation in a part or in the whole of the body, usually induced by drugs. *Basal a.* basal narcosis. Loss of consciousness, although supplemental drugs have to be given to ensure complete anaesthesia. *Epidural a.* injection into the extradural space between the vertebral spines and beneath the ligamentum flavum. *General a.* unconsciousness produced by inhalation or injection of a drug. *Hysterical a.* a common symptom in hysteria, in which the insensibility to touch or pain has a local distribution unrelated to the nerve supply. *Inhalation a.* the drugs or gas used are administered by a face mask or endotracheal tube to cause general anaesthesia. *Intravenous a.* unconsciousness is produced by the introduction of a drug, e.g. hexobarbitone, into a vein. *Local a.* local analgesia. Nerve conduction is blocked by injection of a local anaesthetic, or by freezing with ethyl chloride or by topical application. *Spinal a.* injection of anaesthetic agent into the spinal subarachnoid space.

anaesthetic (ˌanəs'thetik) a drug causing anaesthesia.

anaesthetist (ə'neesthətist) a person who is medically qualified to administer an anaesthetic.

anal ('ayn'l) pertaining to the anus. *A. eroticism.* sexual pleasure derived from anal functions. *A. fissure see* FISSURE. *A. fistula see* FISTULA.

analeptic (ˌanə'leptik) a drug that stimulates the central nervous system.

analgesia (ˌan'l'jeezi-ə) insensibility to pain, especially the relief of pain without causing unconsciousness. *Patient-controlled a.* a preset dose of analgesic which the patient controls according to need. In-built safety measures prevent accidental overdose.

analgesic (ˌan'l'jeezik, -sik) 1. relating to analgesia. 2. a remedy which relieves pain. *A. cocktail* an individualized mixture of drugs used to control pain.

analogue ('anə,log) 1. an organ with different structure and origin but the same function as another one. 2. a compound with similar structure to another but differing in respect of a particular element.

analysis (ə'nalisis) 1. the act of determining the component parts of a substance. 2. in psychiatry, the method of trying to determine the reasons for an individual's behaviour by understanding his complex mental processes, experiences and relationships with other individuals or groups of individuals.

anaphase ('anə,fayz) part of the process of mitosis or meiosis.

anaphylaxis (ˌanəfi'laksis) anaphylactic shock. A severe reaction, often fatal, occurring when a second injection of a particular foreign protein is given, e.g. horse serum. The symptoms are severe dyspnoea, rapid pulse, profuse sweating and collapse. The condition may be avoided by giving a test dose before all serum injections. If the patient has any reaction, he may be desensitized by giving repeated small doses.

anaplasia (ˌanə'playzi-ə) a change in the character of cells, seen in tumour tissue.

anarthria (an'ahthri·ə) inability to articulate speech sounds owing to a brain lesion or damage to peripheral nerves innervating articulatory muscles.

anastomosis (ə,nastə'mohsis) in surgery, any artificial connection of two hollow structures, e.g. gastroenterostomy. In anatomy, the joining of the branches of two blood vessels.

anatomy (ə'natəmee) the science of the structure of the body.

Ancylostoma (,ansi'lostəmə) a genus of nematode roundworms which may inhabit the duodenum and cause extreme anaemia. *A. duodenale* a hookworm, very widespread in tropical and subtropical areas.

androgen ('andrə,jen) one of a group of hormones secreted by the testes and adrenal cortex. They are steroids which can be synthesized and produce the secondary male characteristics and the building up of protein tissue.

android ('androyd) resembling a man. *A. pelvis* a female pelvis shaped like a male pelvis, with a wedge-shaped entrance and narrow anterior segment.

anencephaly (,anən'kefəlee, -'sef-) congenital absence of the cranial vault, with the cerebral hemispheres completely missing or reduced to small masses.

anergic (a'nərjik) sluggish, inactive.

aneurine ('anyuh,reen) thiamine. An essential vitamin involved in carbohydrate metabolism. The main sources are unrefined cereals and pork. Vitamin B_1.

aneurysm ('anyə,rizəm) a local dilatation of a blood vessel, usually an artery. Atherosclerosis is responsible for most arterial aneurysms; any injury to the arterial wall can predispose to the formation of a sac. Other diseases that can lead to an aneurysm include syphilis, certain nonspecific inflammations, and congenital defect in the artery. The pressure of blood causes it to increase in size and rupture is likely. Sometimes excision of the aneurysm or ligation of the artery is possible. *Dissecting a.* a condition in which a tear occurs in the aortic lining where the middle coat is necrosed and blood gets between the layers, stripping them apart. *Fusiform a.* a spindle-shaped arterial aneurysm. *Saccular a.* a dilatation of only a part of the circumference of an artery.

angiitis (,anji'ietis) inflammation of a blood or lymph vessel.

angina (an'jienə, 'anjienə) 1. a tight strangling sensation or pain. 2. an inflammation of the throat causing pain on swallowing. *A. cruris* intermittent claudication. Severe pain in the leg after walking. *Ludwig's a.* acute pharyngitis with swelling and abscess formation. *A. pectoris* cardiac pain which occurs on exertion owing to insufficient blood supply to the heart muscle. *Vincent's a.* infection and ulceration of the tonsils by a spirochaete, *Borrelia vincenti*, and a bacillus, *Fusiformis fusiformis*.

angiocardiography (,anjioh,kahdi'ogrəfee) radiological examination of the heart and large blood vessels by means of cardiac

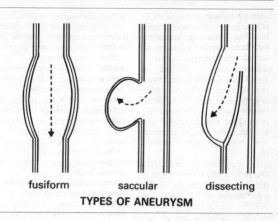

fusiform   saccular   dissecting
TYPES OF ANEURYSM

catheterization and an opaque contrast medium.

angioectasis (͵anjioh'ektəsis) abnormal enlargement of capillaries.

angiography (͵anji'ogrəfee) radiological examination of the blood vessels using an opaque contrast medium.

angioma (͵anji'ohmə) an innocent tumour composed of dilated blood vessels.

angioneurosis (͵anjiohnyuh'rohsis) a neurosis affecting the blood vessels, which may produce paralysis.

angioneurotic (͵anjiohnyuh'rotik) pertaining to angioneurosis. *A. oedema see* OEDEMA.

angioplasty (͵anjioh͵plastee) plastic surgery of blood vessels.

angiosarcoma (͵anjiohsah'kohmə) a malignant vascular growth.

angiospasm ('anjiospazəm) a spasmodic contraction of an artery, causing cramping of the muscles.

angiotensin (͵anjio'tensin) a substance that raises the blood pressure. It is a polypeptide produced by the action of renin on plasma globulins. Hypertensin.

ångström unit ('angstrom) *A.J. Ångström, Swedish physicist, 1814–1874. Symbol* Å. A non-SI unit of wavelengths of light equal to 10^{-10} metre or 0.1 nanometre.

anhidrosis (͵anhi'drohsis) marked deficiency in the secretion of sweat.

anhidrotic (͵anhi'drotik) an agent that decreases perspiration. An adiaphoretic.

anhydraemia (͵anhie'dreemi·ə) deficiency of water in the blood.

anhydrous (an'hiedrəs) containing no water.

aniline ('ani͵leen, -lin) a chemical compound derived from coal tar, used for making antiseptic dyes. It is an important cause of serious industrial poisoning associated with bone marrow depression as well as methaemoglobinaemia.

anima ('animə) 1. the soul. 2. Jung's term for the unconscious, or inner being, of the individual, as opposed to the personality he presents to the world (persona). In jungian psychoanalysis, the more feminine soul or feminine component of a man's personality.

anion ('an,ieən) a negatively charged ion which travels against the current towards the anode, e.g. chloride (Cl⁻), carbonate (CO_3^{2-}). *See* CATION.

aniridia (,ani'ridi·ə) lack of part or the whole of the iris.

anisocoria (an,iesoh'koh·ri·ə) inequality of diameter of the pupils of the two eyes.

anisocytosis (an,iesohsie'tohsis) inequality in the size of the red blood cells.

anisomelia (an,iesoh'meeli·ə) a congenital condition in which one of a pair of limbs is longer than the other.

anisometropia (an,iesohme-'trohpi·ə) a marked difference in the refractive power of the two eyes.

ankle ('angk'l) the joint between the leg and the foot formed by the tibia and fibula articulating with the talus.

ankyloblepharon (,angkiloh'blef-ə·ron) adhesions and scar tissue on the ciliary borders of the eyelids, giving the eye a distorted appearance.

ankylosis (,angki'lohsis) consolidation, immobility and stiffness of a joint as a result of disease.

Annelida (ə'nelidə) a phylum of metazoa, the segmented worms, including the leeches.

annular ('anyuhlə) ring-shaped.

anoci-association (a,nohsee·ə-,sohsi'ayshan, -,sohshi-) the exclusion of pain, fear and shock in surgical operations, brought about by means of local anaesthesia and basal narcosis.

anode ('anohd) the positive pole of an electric battery. *See* CATHODE.

anodyne ('anə,dien) a drug which relieves pain.

anomaly (ə'noməlee) considerable variation from the normal.

anomie ('anohmee) a feeling of hopelessness and lack of purpose.

anonychia (,anə'niki·ə) congenital absence of nails.

Anopheles (ə'nofi,leez) a genus of mosquito. Many are carriers of the malarial parasite and by their bite infect humans. Other species transmit filariasis.

anophthalmia (,anof'thalmi·ə) congenital absence of a seeing eye. Some portion of the eye, e.g. the conjunctiva, is always present.

anorchism (an'awkizəm) a condition in which the testicles have failed to develop or to descend.

anorexia (,anə'reksi·ə) loss of appetite for food. *A. nervosa* a condition in which there is complete lack of appetite, with extreme emaciation. It is generally due to psychological causes and usually occurs in young women.

anosmia (an'ozmi·ə) loss of the sense of smell.

anovular (an'ohvyuhlə) applied to the absence of ovulation. Usually refers to uterine bleeding when there has been no ovulation, the result of taking contraceptive pills.

anoxaemia (,anok'seemi·ə) complete lack of oxygen in the blood.

anoxia (an'oksi·ə) lack of oxygen to an organ or tissue.

Antabuse ('antə,byooz) trade name for a preparation of disulfiram, used in the treatment of alcoholism.

antacid (ant'asid) a substance neutralizing acidity, particularly of the gastric juices.

antagonist (an'tagənist) 1. a muscle that has an opposite action to another, e.g. the biceps to the triceps. 2. in pharmacology, a drug which inhibits the action of another drug or enzyme, e.g. methotrexate is a folic acid antagonist. 3. in dentistry, a tooth in one jaw opposing one in the other jaw.

anteflexion (,anti'flekshən) a bending forward, as of the body of the uterus. See RETROFLEXION.

antenatal (,anti'nayt'l) before birth.

Antepar ('anti,pah) trade name for preparations of piperazine citrate and piperazine phosphate, anthelmintics.

antepartum shortly before birth, i.e. in the last three months of pregnancy. *A. haemorrhage* bleeding occurring before birth. See PLACENTA PRAEVIA.

anterior (an'tiə·ri·ə) situated at or facing towards the front. The opposite of 'posterior'. *A. capsule*

the anterior covering of the lens of the eye. *A. chamber of eye* the space between the cornea in front and the iris and lens behind.

anterograde ('antə·roh,grayd) extending or moving forward.

anteversion (,anti'vərzhən) the forward tilting of an organ, e.g. the normal position of the uterus. *See* RETROVERSION.

anthelminthic (**anthelmintic**) (,ant·hel'mintik, ,anthel-) 1. destructive to worms. 2. an agent destructive to worms.

anthracosis (,anthrə'kohsis) a disease of the lungs, caused by inhalation of coal dust. A form of pneumoconiosis. 'Miner's lung'.

anthrax ('anthraks) an acute, notifiable, infectious disease due to *Bacillus anthracis*, acquired through contact with infected animals or their byproducts, such as carcasses, bones or skin, usually by occupational exposure. The incubation period is 2–5 days. A worldwide zoonosis, anthrax is now very uncommon in the UK.

anthropoid ('anthrə,poyd) resembling man. *A. pelvis* female pelvis in which the anteroposterior diameter exceeds the transverse diameter.

anthropology (,anthrə'poləjee) the science that concerns man, his origins, historical and cultural development, and races. *Cultural a.* that branch of anthropology that concerns man in relation to his fellows and to his environment. *Medical a.* biocultural discipline concerned with both the biological and sociocultural aspects of human behaviour, and the ways in which the two interact to influence health and diseases. *Physical a.* that branch of anthropology which concerns the physical and evolutionary characteristics of man.

anthropometric (,anthrəpə-'metrik) pertaining to anthropometry.

anthropometry (,anthrə-'pomə-tree) the science which deals with the comparative measurement of parts of the human body, such as height, weight, body fat, etc.

antibacterial (,antibak'tiə·ri·əl) a substance which destroys or suppresses the growth of bacteria.

antibiotic (,antibie'otik) substances (e.g. penicillin) produced by certain bacteria and fungi, which prevent the growth of, or destroy, other bacteria.

antibody ('anti,bodee) a specific form of blood protein produced in the lymphoid tissue and able to counteract the effects of bacterial antigens or toxins.

anticholinergic (,anti,kohlin'əjik) a drug that inhibits the action of acetylcholine.

anticholinesterase (,anti,kohli-'nestə,rayz) an enzyme that will inhibit the action of acetylcholinesterase thereby potentiating the action of acetycholine at post-synaptic receptors in the para-sympathetic nervous system, thus allowing return of normal muscle contraction.

anticoagulant (,antikoh'agyuh-lənt) a susbtance which prevents blood from clotting, e.g. heparin.

anticonvulsant (,antikən'vulsant) a substance which will arrest or prevent convulsions. Anticon-

vulsant drugs such as phenytoin are used in the treatment of epilepsy and other conditions in which convulsions occur.

anti-D gamma globulin (,anti'dee) anti-rhesus antibody which is given to a rhesus-negative woman within 36 h of delivery of her infant or following termination of pregnancy to prevent her forming her own antibodies. *See* RHESUS FACTOR.

antidepressant (,antidi'prəs'nt) one of a group of drugs which elevate mood, often diminish anxiety and increase coping behaviour. Tricyclic antidepressants are the most commonly used in treatment of depression. Monoamine oxidase inhibitors (MAOI) are less commonly used because of the dietary restriction necessary and toxic side-effects.

antidiuresis (,anti,dieyuh'reesis) a reduction in the formation of urine

antidiuretic (,anti,dieyuh'retik) a substance that reduces the volume of urine excreted. *A. hormone* abbreviated ADH. A hormone which is secreted by the posterior pituitary gland. Vasopressin.

antidote ('anti,doht) an agent which counteracts the effect of a poison.

antiembolic (,anti·em'bolik) against embolism. Antiembolic hose/stockings are worn to prevent the formation or decrease the risk of deep vein thrombosis, especially in patients after surgery or those confined to bed.

antiemetic (,anti·i'metik) a drug that prevents or overcomes nausea and vomiting.

antigen ('anti,jen, -jən) any substance, bacterial or otherwise, which in suitable conditions can stimulate the production of antibodies.

antihaemophilic (,anti,heemoh-'filik) 1. effective against the bleeding tendency in haemophilia. 2. an agent that counteracts the bleeding tendency in haemophilia. *A. factor* abbreviated AHF. One of the clotting factors, deficiency of which causes classic, sex-linked haemophilia; called also factor VIII and antihaemophilic globulin. It is available in a preparation for preventive and therapeutic use.

antihistamine (,anti'histə,meen, -min) any one of a group of drugs which block the tissue receptors for histamine. They are used to treat allergic conditions, e.g. drug rashes, hay fever and serum sickness. They include promethazine and mepyramine.

antihypertensive (,anti,hiepə-'tensiv) 1. effective against hypertension. 2. an agent that reduces high blood pressure.

antimetabolite (,antime'tabəliet) one of a group of chemical compounds which prevent the effective utilization of the corresponding metabolite, and interfere with normal growth or cell mitosis if the process requires that metabolite.

antimycotic (,antimie'kotik) a preparation effective in treating fungal infections.

antineoplastic (,anti,neeoh'plastik) effective against the multiplication of malignant cells.

antiperistalsis (,anti,peri'stalsis) contrary contractions which propel the contents of the intestines backwards and upwards.

antipruritic (,anti,prooə'ritik) an external application or drug that relieves itching.

antipyretic (,antipie'retik) an agent which reduces fever.

anti-rhesus serum (,anti'reesəs) a substance containing rhesus agglutinins produced in the blood of those who are rhesus-negative if the rhesus-positive antigen obtains access to it, e.g. by blood transfusion. Haemolysis and jaundice are the result. See RHESUS FACTOR.

antisepsis (,anti'sepsis) the prevention of infection by destroying or arresting the growth of harmful microorganisms.

antiseptic (,anti'septik) 1. preventing sepsis. 2. any substance that inhibits the growth of bacteria, in contrast to a germicide, which kills bacteria outright.

antiserum (,anti'siə·rəm) a serum prepared against a specific disease by immunizing an animal so that antibodies are formed. These can then be used to create a passive immunity or to treat the infection in man.

antisocial (,anti'sohshəl) against society. *A. behaviour* in psychiatry, the refusal of an individual to accept the normal obligations and restraints imposed by the community upon its members.

antispasmodic (,antispaz'modik) any measure used to prevent or relieve the occurrence of muscle spasm.

antistatic (ˌanti'statik) relating to measures taken to prevent the build-up of static electricity.

antitoxin (ˌanti'toksin) a substance produced by the body cells as a reaction to invasion by bacteria, which neutralizes their toxins. Serum from immunized animals contains these antitoxins, and is used in the treatment of specific diseases such as diphtheria, tetanus, etc. *See* IMMUNITY.

antitussive (ˌanti'tusiv) 1. effective against cough. 2. an agent that suppresses coughing.

antivenin (ˌanti'venin) an antitoxic serum to neutralize the poison injected by the bite of a snake or insect.

antrectomy (an'trektəmee) excision of an antrum.

antrostomy (an'trostəmee) surgical opening of an antrum, particularly the maxillary antrum, for drainage purposes.

antrum ('antrəm) a cavity in bone. *Mastoid a.* the tympanic antrum, which is an air-containing cavity in the mastoid portion of the temporal bone. *Maxillary a.* antrum of Highmore. The air sinus in the upper jaw bone.

anuria (ə'nyooə·ri·ə) cessation of the secretion of urine.

anus ('aynəs) the extremity of the alimentary canal, through which the faeces are discharged. *Imperforate a.* one where there is no opening because of a congenital defect.

anxiety (ang'zieətee) a chronic state of tension which affects both mind and body. *A. neurosis see* NEUROSIS.

anxiolytic (ˌangzieoh'litik) a substance, such as diazepam, used for relief of anxiety. Anxiolytics may quickly cause dependence and are not suitable for long-term administration. Called also antianxiety agent and minor tranquillizer.

aorta (ay'awtə) the large artery rising out of the left ventricle of the heart and supplying blood to all the body. *Abdominal a.* that part of the artery lying in the abdomen. *Arch of the a.* the curve of the artery over the heart. *Thoracic a.* that part which passes through the chest.

aortic (ay'awtik) pertaining to the aorta. *A. incompetence* owing to previous inflammation of the aortic valve has become fibrosed and is unable to close completely, thus allowing backward flow of blood (*a. regurgitation*) into the left ventricle during diastole. *A. stenosis* a narrowing of the aortic valve. *A. valve* the valve between the left ventricle of the heart and the ascending aorta, which prevents the backward flow of blood through the artery.

aortitis (ˌay·aw'tietis) inflammation of the aorta.

aortography (ay·aw'togrəfee) radiographic examination of the aorta. A radio-opaque contrast medium is injected into the blood to render visible lesions of the aorta or its main branches.

apathy ('apəthee) an appearance of indifference, with no response to stimuli or display of emotion.

aperient (ə'piəri·ənt) a drug which produces an action of the bowels. A laxative.

aperistalsis (ˌayperi'stalsis) lack of

peristaltic movement of the intestines.

Apert's syndrome (a'pairz) *E. Apert, French paediatrician, 1868–1940.* A congenital abnormality in which there is fusion at birth of all the cranial sutures in addition to syndactyly (webbed fingers).

apex ('aypeks) the top or pointed end of a cone-shaped structure. *A. beat* the beat of the heart against the chest wall which can be felt during systole. *A. of the heart* the end enclosing the left ventricle. *A. of the lung* the extreme upper part of the organ.

Apgar score ('apgah) *V. Apgar, American anaesthetist, 1909–1974.* A system used in the assessment of the newborn: reflex irritability and colour. The Apgar score is assessed 1 min after birth and again at 5 min. Most healthy infants score 9 at birth. A score below 7 would indicate cause for concern.

APH antepartum haemorrhage.

aphagia (ə'fayji·ə, ay-) loss of the power to swallow.

aphakia (ay-, ə'fayki·ə, -'fak-) absence of the lens of the eye. Aphacia.

aphasia (ə'fayzi·ə, ay-) a communication disorder due to brain damage; characterized by complete or partial disturbance of language comprehension, formulation or expression. Partial disturbance is also called dysphasia. *Broca's a.* disorder in which verbal output is impaired, and in which verbal comprehension may be affected as well. Speech is

APGAR SCORE

Sign		Score	
	0	1	2
Colour	Blue, pale	Body pink, limbs blue	Completely pink
Respiratory effort	Absent	Slow, irregular, weak cry	Strong cry
Heart rate	Absent	Slow, less than 100 bpm	Over 100 bpm
Muscle tone	Limp	Some flexion of limbs	Active movement
Reflex response to flicking foot	Absent	Facial grimace	Cry

slow and laboured and writing is often impaired. *Developmental a.* a childhood failure to acquire normal language when deafness, learning difficulties, motor disability or severe emotional disturbance are not causes.

aphonia (ə'fohni·ə, ay-) inability to produce sound. The cause may be organic disease of the larynx or may be purely functional.

aphrodisiac (,afrə'diziak) a drug which excites sexual desire.

aphthae ('apthee) small ulcers surrounded by erythema on the inside of the mouth (aphthous stomatitis).

apical ('aypik'l) pertaining to the apex of a structure.

apicectomy ('aypi'sektəmee) excision of the root of a tooth. Root resection.

aplasia (ə'playzi·ə, ay-) incomplete development of an organ or tissue or absence of growth.

aplastic (ay'plastik) without power of development. *A. anaemia see* ANAEMIA.

apnoea ('apni·ə, ap'neeə) cessation of respiration. *Cardiac a.* the temporary cessation of breathing caused by a reduction of the carbon dioxide tension in the blood, as seen in Cheyne–Stokes respiration. *A. of the newborn* apnoeic periods occurring in the respiration of newborn infants in whom the respiratory centre is immature or depressed; *A. monitors* are all designed to give an audible signal when a certain period of apnoea has occurred. *Sleep a.* transient attacks of failure of autonomic control of respiration, becoming more pronounced during sleep.

apocrine ('apəkrien, -krin) pertaining to modified sweat glands that develop in hair follicles, such as are mainly found in the axillary, pubic and perineal areas.

apomorphine (,apoh'mawfeen) a derivative of morphine which produces vomiting.

aponeurosis (a,ponyuh'rohsis) a sheet of tendon-like tissue which connects some muscles to the parts which they move.

apophysis (ə'pofisis) a prominence or excrescence, usually of a bone.

apoplexy ('apə,pleksee) a sudden fit of insensibility, usually caused by rupture of a cerebral blood vessel or its occlusion by a blood clot. The symptoms are coma, accompanied by stertorous breathing, and a varying degree of paralysis of the opposite side of the body to the lesion.

apparition (,apə'rishən) a hallucinatory vision, usually the phantom appearance of a person. A spectre.

appendectomy (,apən'dektəmee) appendicectomy.

appendicectomy (ə,pendi'sektəmee) removal of the vermiform appendix.

appendicitis (ə,pendi'sietis) inflammation of the vermiform appendix.

appendix (ə'pendiks) a supplementary or dependent part. *A. epiploicae* small tag-like structures of peritoneum containing fat which are scattered over the surface of the large intestine, especially the transverse colon. *Vermiform a.* a worm-like tube with a blind end, projecting from the caecum in the right iliac region. It may be from 2.5 to 15 cm long.

apperception (,apə'sepshən) conscious reception and recognition of a sensory stimulus.

appetite ('api,tiet) the desire for food. It is stimulated by the sight, smell or thought of food, and accompanied by the flow of saliva in the mouth and gastric juice in the stomach. The stomach wall also receives an extra blood supply in preparation for its digestive activity. Appetite is psychological, dependent on memory and associations, as compared with hunger, which is physiologically aroused by the body's need for food. Appetite can be discouraged by unattractive food, surroundings or company, and by emotional states such as anxiety, irritation, anger, and fear.

appliance (ə'plieəns) a device used for performing a particular function.

applicator ('apli,kaytə) any device used to apply medication or treatment to a particular part of the body.

apposition (,apə'zishən) the bringing into contact of two structures, e.g. fragments of bone in setting a fracture.

apprehension (,apri'henshən) a feeling of dread or fear.

apraxia (ə'praksi·ə) the inability to perform correct movements because of a brain lesion and not because of sensory impairment or loss of muscle power in the limbs. *Oral a.* inability to perform vol-itional movements of the tongue and lips in the absence of paralysis or paresis. Involuntary movements may be observed however; e.g. the patient may purse lips in order to blow out a match.

APT alum precipitated toxoid.

aptitude ('apti,tyood) the natural ability or capacity to acquire mental and physical skills.

apyrexia (,aypie'reksi·ə) the absence of fever.

aqua ('akwə) [L.] *water. A. destillata* distilled water. *A. fortis* nitric acid.

aqueduct ('akwə,dukt) a canal for the passage of fluid. *A. of Sylvius* the canal connecting the third and fourth ventricles of the brain.

aqueous ('akwi·əs, 'ay-) watery. *A. humour* the fluid filling the anterior and posterior chambers of the eye.

Ar symbol for *argon.*

Arachis ('arəkis) a genus of leguminous plants. *A. oil* peanut oil; used as a substitute for olive oil.

arachnodactyly (ə,raknoh'daktilee) abnormally long and thin fingers and toes. A congenital condition.

arachnoid (ə'raknoyd) 1. resembling a spider's web. 2. a weblike membrane covering the central nervous system between the dura and pia mater.

arborization (,ahbə·rie'zayshən) the branching terminations of many nerve fibres and processes.

arbovirus (,ahboh'vierəs) one of a large group of viruses transmitted by insect vectors (arthropodborne), e.g. mosquitoes, sandflies or ticks. The diseases caused include many types of encephalitis, also yellow, dengue, sandfly and Rift Valley fevers.

ARC AIDS-related complex. *See* AIDS and Appendix 6.

arcus ('ahkəs) [L.] *bow, arch. A. senilis* an opaque circle appearing round the edge of the cornea in old age.

ARDS adult respiratory distress syndrome.

areola (ə'reeələ) 1. a space in connective tissue. 2. a ring of pigmentation, e.g. that surrounding the nipple.

argentum (ah'jentəm) [L.] *silver.*

arginase ('ahji,nayz) an enzyme of the liver that splits arginine into urea and ornithine.

arginine ('ahji,neen, -,nin) an essential amino acid produced by the digestion of protein. It forms a link in the excretion of nitrogen being hydrolysed by the enzyme arginase.

argon ('ahgon) *symbol* Ar. An inert gaseous element less than 0.1, in the atmosphere.

Argyll Robertson pupil (ah'giel 'robətsən) *D. Argyll Robertson, British ophthalmologist, 1837–1909. See* PUPIL.

Arnold–Chiari deformity (,ahn-'ldki'ahree) *J. Arnold, German pathologist, 1835–1915; H. Chiari, German pathologist, 1851–1916.* Herniation of the cerebellum and elongation of the medulla oblongata; occurs in hydrocephalus associated with spina bifida.

arousal (ə'rowz'l) a state of alertness and increased response to stimuli.

arrachment (,arash'monh) the ex-

traction of a membranous cataract via a corneal incision.

arrector pili (ə'rektə) small muscle attached to the hair follicle of the skin. When contracted causes the hair to become erect, producing the appearance known as goose-flesh.

arrest (ə'rest) a cessation or stopping. *Cardiac a.* cessation of ventricular contractions. *Developmental a.* discontinuation of a child's mental or physical development at a certain stage. *Respiratory a.* cessation of breathing.

arrhenoblastoma (ə'reenohbla-'stohmə) a rare ovarian tumour which causes masculinization in the woman, with male distribution of hair and coarsening of the skin.

arrhythmia (ə'ridhmi·ə, ay-) variation from the normal rhythm, e.g. in the heart's action. *Sinus a.* an abnormal pulse rhythm due to disturbance of the sinoatrial node, causing quickening of the heart on inspiration and slowing on expiration.

arsenic ('ahsnik) *symbol* As. A metallic element, organic preparations of which have been widely used in medicine. These have been replaced for the most part by antibiotics, which are less toxic.

artefact ('ahti,fakt) something that is man-made or introduced artificially.

arteriectomy (ah,tiə·ri'ektəmee) the removal of a portion of artery wall, usually followed by anastomosis or a replacement graft. *See* ARTERIOPLASTY.

arteriography (ah'tiə·ri'ografee)

radiography of arteries after the injection of a radio-opaque contrast medium.

arteriole (ah'tiǝ·ri,ohl) a small artery.

arterioplasty (ah'tiǝ·rioh,plastee) the reconstruction of an artery by means of replacement surgery.

arteriorrhaphy (ah'tiǝ·ri'o·rǝfee) ligature of an artery.

arteriosclerosis (ah,tiǝ·riohsklǝ·'rohsis) a gradual loss of elasticity in the walls of arteries due to thickening and calcification. It is accompanied by high blood pressure, and precedes the degeneration of internal organs associated with old age or chronic disease.

arteriotomy (ah,tiǝ·ri'otǝmee) an incision into an artery.

arteriovenous (ah,tiǝ·rioh'vennǝs) both arterial and venous; pertaining to both artery and vein, e.g. an arteriovenous aneurysm, fistula, or shunt for haemodialysis.

arteritis (,ahtǝ'rietis) inflammation of an artery. *Giant cell a.* a variety of polyarteritis resulting in partial or complete occlusion of a number of arteries. The carotid arteries are often involved. *Temporal a.* occlusion of the extracranial arteries, particularly the carotid arteries.

artery ('ahtǝ·ree) a tube of muscle and elastic fibres lined with endothelium which distributes blood from the heart to the capillaries throughout the body.

arthralgia (ah'thralji·ǝ) neuralgic pains in a joint.

arthrectomy (ah'threktǝmee) excision of a joint.

arthritis (ah'thrietis) inflammation of one or more joints. Movement in the joint is restricted, with pain and swelling. Arthritis and the rheumatic diseases in general constitute the major cause of chronic disability in the United Kingdom, where it is estimated that 20 million persons have a rheumatic disease, of whom between 6 and 8 million are severely affected. *Acute rheumatic a.* rheumatic fever. *Osteo-a.* a degenerative condition attacking the articular cartilage and aggravated by an impaired blood supply, previous injury or overweight, mainly affecting weight-bearing joints and causing pain. *Rheumatoid a.* a chronic inflammation, usually of unknown origin. The disease is progressive and incapacitating, owing to the resulting ankylosis and deformity of the bones. Usually affects the elderly. A juvenile form is known as STILL'S DISEASE.

arthroclasia (,ahthrǝ'klayzi·ǝ) the breaking down of adhesions in a joint to produce freer movement.

arthrodesis (,ahthrǝ'deesis) the fixation of a movable joint by surgical operation.

arthrodynia (,ahthrǝ'dini·ǝ) painful joints. Arthralgia.

arthrography (ah'throgrǝfee) the examination of a joint by means of X-rays. An opaque contrast medium may be used.

arthrogryposis (,ahthrohgrie·'pohsis) 1. a congenital abnormality in which fibrous ankylosis of some or all of the joints in the limbs occurs. 2. a tetanus spasm.

arthrology (ah'throlǝjee) scientific study or description of the joints.

arthroplasty ('ahthrə,plastee) plastic surgery for the reorganization of a joint. *Cup a.* reconstruction of the articular surface, which is then covered by a vitallium cup. *Excision a.* excision of the joint surfaces affected, so that the gap thus formed then fills with fibrous tissue or muscle. *Girdlestone a.* an excision arthroplasty of the hip. *McKee Farrar a.* replacement of both the head and the socket of the femur; *Charnley's a.* is similar. *Replacement a.* partial removal of the head of the femur and its replacement by a metal prosthesis.

arthroscope ('ahthrə,skohp) an endoscope for examining the interior of a joint.

arthrotomy (ah'throtəmee) an incision into a joint.

articular (ah'tikyuhlə) pertaining to a joint.

articulation (ah'tikyuh'layshən) 1. a junction point of two or more bones. 2. the enunciation of words.

artificial (,ahti'fishəl) not natural. *A. feeding* the giving of food other than by placing it directly in the mouth. It may be provided via the mouth, using an *oesophageal* (Ryle's) tube; the food may be introduced into the stomach through a fine tube via the nostril (the nasal route). An opening through the abdominal wall into the stomach (i.e. a gastrostomy) may allow direct introduction; or food may be injected intravenously (see PARENTERAL). *A. insemination* the insertion of sperm into the uterus by means of syringe and cannula instead of by coitus. Husband's (AIH) or donor (AID) semen may be used. *A. respiration* a means of resuscitation from asphyxia.

arytenoid (,ari'teenoyd) resembling the mouth of a pitcher. *A. cartilages* two cartilages of the larynx; their function is to regulate the tension of the vocal cords attached to them.

As symbol for *arsenic*.

asbestos (as'bestos, -təs) a fibrous non-combustible silicate of magnesium and calcium, which is a good non-conductor of heat.

asbestosis (,asbes'tohsis) a form of pneumoconiosis caused by the inhalation of asbestos dust.

ascariasis (,askə'rieəsis) the condition in which roundworms are found in the gastrointestinal tract.

Ascaris ('askə·ris) a genus of roundworm. Some types may infest the human intestine.

Aschoff's nodules or **bodies** ('ashofs) *K.A.L. Aschoff, German pathologist, 1866–1942.* The nodules present in heart muscle in rheumatic myocarditis.

ascites (ə'sieteez) free fluid in the peritoneal cavity. It may be the result of local inflammation, of venous obstruction, or part of a generalized oedema.

ascorbic acid (əs'kawbik) vitamin C. This acid is found in many vegetables and fruits and is an essential dietary constituent for man. Vitamin C is destroyed by heat and deteriorates during storage. It is necessary for connective tissue and collagen fibre synthesis and promotes the healing of wounds. Deficiency causes scurvy.

asemia (ay'seemi·ə) inability to understand or to use speech or signs, due to a cerebral lesion. Aphasia.

asepsis (ay'sepsis) freedom from pathogenic microorganisms.

aseptic (ay'septik) free from sepsis. *A. technique* a method of carrying out sterile procedures so that there is the minimum risk of introducing infection. Achieved by the sterility of equipment and a non-touch technique.

asexual (ay'seksyooəl, a'sek-) without sex. *A. reproduction* the production of new individuals without sexual union, e.g. by cell division or budding.

Asilone ('asilohn) trade name for a proprietary compound antacid mixture.

asparaginase (ə'sparəji,nayz) an enzyme that catalyses the deamination of asparagine; used as an antineoplastic agent against cancers, e.g. acute lymphocytic leukaemia, in which the malignant cells require exogenous asparagine for protein synthesis.

aspartame (ə,spahtaym) a synthetic compound of two amino acids (L-aspartyl-L-phenylalanine methyl ester) used as a low-calorie sweetener. It is 180 times as sweet as sucrose (table sugar); the amount equal in sweetness to a teaspoon of sugar contains 0.1 calorie. Aspartame does not promote the formation of dental caries. The amount of phenylalanine in aspartame must be taken into account in the low-phenylalanine diet for patients with phenylketo-

nuria.

aspect ('aspekt) that part of a surface facing in a particular direction. *Dorsal a.* that facing and seen from the back. *Ventral a.* that facing and seen from the front.

aspergillosis (,aspəji'lohsis) a bronchopulmonary disease in which the mucous membrane is attacked by the fungus, *Aspergillus*.

Aspergillus (,aspə'jiləs) a genus of fungi. *A. fumigatus*, found in soil and manure, is a common cause of aspergillosis.

aspermia (ay'spərmi·ə) absence of sperm.

asphyxia (as'fiksi·ə) a deficiency of oxygen in the blood and an increase in carbon dioxide in the blood and tissues. Symptoms include irregular and disturbed respirations, or a complete absence of breathing, and pallor or cyanosis. Asphyxia may occur whenever there is an interruption in the normal exchange of oxygen and carbon dioxide between the lungs and the outside air. Common causes are drowning, electric shock, lodging of a foreign body in the air passages, inhalation of smoke and poisonous gases, and trauma to or disease of the lungs or air passages. Treatment includes immediate remedy of the situation by ARTIFICIAL RESPIRATION and removal of the underlying cause whenever possible.

aspiration (,aspi'rayshən) 1. the act of inhaling. 2. the drawing off of fluid from a cavity by means of suction.

aspirator ('aspi,raytə) any apparatus for withdrawing fluid or gases from a cavity of the body by means of suction.

aspirin ('asprin) acetylsalicylic acid. It reduces temperature and relieves pain. *Soluble a.* a combination of aspirin with citric acid and calcium carbonate, which is less irritating to the gastric mucosa.

assay ('asay, ə'say) a quantitative examination to determine the amount of a particular constituent of a mixture, or of the biological or pharmacological potency of a drug.

assertiveness (ə'sərtivnəs) a form of behaviour characterized by a confident declaration or affirmation of a statement without need of proof. To assert oneself is to compel recognition of one's rights or position without either aggressively transgressing the rights of another and assuming a position of dominance or submissively permitting another to deny one's rights or rightful position. *A. training* instruction and practice in techniques for dealing with interpersonal conflicts and threatening situations in an assertive manner, avoiding the extremes of aggressive and submissive behaviour.

assessment (ə'sesmənt) the critical analysis and valuation or judgement of the status or quality of a particular condition, situation or other subject of appraisal. In the NURSING PROCESS, assessment involves the gathering of information about the health status of the patient/

client, analysis and synthesis of that data, and the making of a clinical nursing judgement. The outcome of the nursing assessment is the establishment of a nursing DIAGNOSIS, the identification of the nursing problems.

assimilation (ə,simi'layshən) the process of transforming food, so that it can be absorbed and utilized as nourishment by the tissues of the body.

association (ə,sohsi'ayshən, -,sohshi-) coordination of function of similar parts. *Free a.* a method employed in psychoanalysis in which the patient is encouraged to express freely whatever comes into his mind. By this method material that is in the unconscious can be recalled. *A. fibres* nerve fibres linking different areas of the brain. *A. of ideas* a mental impression in which a thought or any sensory impulse will call to mind another object or idea connected in some way with the former.

associative play (ə,sohsi·ətiv) a form of play in which a group of children participate in similar activities without formal organization or direction.

astasia (a'stayzi·ə) inability to stand or walk normally, due to incoordination of muscles.

asteatosis (,aystiə'tohsis) lack of sebaceous secretion. There is a dry and scaly skin in which fissures may occur.

astereognosis (ay,stiə·ri·əg'nohsis) inability to recognize the shape of objects by feeling or touch.

asthenia (as'theeni·ə) want of

strength. Debility. Loss of tone.

asthenic (as'thenik) description of a type of body build: a pale, lean, narrowly built person with poor muscle development.

asthenopia (ˌasthe'nohpi·ə) eye strain giving rise to an aching, burning sensation and headache. Likely to arise in long-sighted people when continual effort of accommodation is required for close work.

asthma ('asmə) paroxysmal dyspnoea characterized by wheezing and difficulty in expiration. *Bronchial a.* attacks of dyspnoea in which there is wheezing and difficulty in expiration due to muscular spasm of the bronchi. The attacks may be precipitated by hypersensitivity to foreign substances or associated with emotional upsets. There is often a family history of asthma or other allergic condition. Attacks may accompany chronic bronchitis. *Cardiac a.* attacks of dyspnoea and palpitation arising most often at night, associated with left-sided heart failure and pulmonary congestion. *Renal a.* dyspnoea occurring in kidney disease, which may be a sign of developing uraemia. It is unrelated to true asthma.

astigmatism (ə'stigmə,tizəm) inequality of the refractive power of an eye, due to defective curvature of its corneal meridians. The curve across the front of the eye from side to side is not quite the same as the curve from above downwards. The focus on the retina is then not a point, but a diffuse and indistinct area. May be congenital or acquired.

astringent (ə'strinjənt) an agent causing contraction of organic tissues, thereby checking secretions, e.g. silver nitrate, tannic acid.

astrocytoma (ˌastrohsie'tohmə) a malignant tumour of the brain or spinal cord. It is slow-growing. A glioma.

Astrup machine ('astrup mə-,sheen) an apparatus for ascertaining the pH value of arterial blood.

asymmetry (ay'simitree, a-) inequality in size or shape of two normally similar structures or of two halves of a structure normally the same.

asymptomatic (ˌaysimptə'matik, a-) without symptoms.

asynergy (ay'sinə,jee) lack of coordination of structures which normally act in harmony.

asystole (ay'sistəlee) absence of heartbeat. Cardiac arrest.

'at risk' register (ˌat 'risk) a register of children considered to be at risk of NON-ACCIDENTAL INJURY (NAI). *See also* OBSERVATION REGISTER.

ataractic (aytə'raktik) 1. pertaining to or characterized by ataraxia. 2. an agent that induces antaraxia; a tranquillizer.

ataraxia (ˌatə'raksi·ə) a state of detached serenity with depression of mental faculties or impairment of consciousness.

atavism ('atə,vizəm) the reappearance of some hereditary peculiarity which has missed a few generations.

ataxia, ataxy (ə'taksi·ə) failure of muscle coordination resulting in irregular and jerky movements. *Hereditary a.* Friedrich's ataxia. *Locomotor a.* or *tabes dorsalis* a degenerative disease of the spinal cord; a manifestation of tertiary syphilis. Among signs and symptoms are: incoordinated movements of the legs in walking, absence of reflexes, and loss of sphincter control. The disease is chronic and progressive, but can be controlled by antisyphilitic treatment.

atelectasis (,atə'lektəsis) a collapsed or airless state of the lung, which may be acute or chronic, and may involve all or part of the lung. 1. from imperfect expansion of pulmonary alveoli at birth (*congenital a.*). 2. as the result of disease or injury.

atheroma (,athə'rohmə) an abnormal mass of fatty or lipid material with a fibrous covering, existing as a discrete, raised plaque within the intima of an artery.

atherosclerosis (,athə·rohsklə-'rohsis) a condition in which the fatty degenerative plaques of atheroma are accompanied by arteriosclerosis, a narrowing and hardening of the vessels.

athetosis (,athi'tohsis) a recurring series of slow, writhing movements of the hands, usually due to a cerebral lesion.

athlete's foot ('athleets) a fungal infection between the toes which is easily transmitted to others. Tinea pedis.

atlas ('atlas) the first cervical vertebra, articulating with the occipital bone of the skull.

atmosphere ('atmǝs,fiǝ) 1. the gases that surround the earth

extending to an altitude of 10 miles. 2. the air or climate of a particular place, e.g. a smoky atmosphere. 3. mental or moral environment, tone or mood.

atmospheric pressure (,atmes-'ferik) pressure exerted by the air in all directions. At sea level it is about 100 kPa (15 lb/in²).

atom ('atǝm) the smallest particle of an element that retains all the properties of that element. It is made up of a central positively charged nucleus and, moving around it in orbit, negatively charged electrons.

atomizer ('atǝ,miezǝ) an instrument by which a liquid is divided to form a fine spray or vapour (nebulizer).

atony ('atǝnee) lack of tone, e.g. in a muscle.

atopen ('atǝ,pen) an antigen responsible for causing atopy.

atopy ('atǝpee) a state of hypersensitivity to certain antigens. There is an inherited tendency which includes asthma, eczema and hayfever.

ATP adenosine triphosphate.

atracurium (,atrǝ'kyooǝ·ri·ǝm) a neuromuscular blocking agent of the non-depolarizing type spontaneously broken down in the blood by the Hofmann reaction. It has a relatively short duration of action and is particularly useful for providing muscle relaxation in patients with kidney or liver disease undergoing surgery.

atresia (ǝ'treezi·ǝ) absence of a natural opening or tubular structure, e.g. of the anus or vagina, usually a congenital malformation.

atrial ('aytri·əl) relating to the atrium. *A. fibrillation* overstimulation of the atrial walls so that many areas of excitation arise and the atrioventricular node is bombarded with impulses, many of which it cannot transmit, resulting in a highly irregular pulse. *A. flutter* rapid regular action of the atria. The atrioventricular node transmits alternate impulses or one in three or four. The atrial rate is usually about 300 beats per minute. *A. septal defect* the non-closure of the foramen ovale at the time of birth giving rise to a congenital heart defect.

atrioventricular (ˌaytriohven-'trikyuhlə) pertaining to the atrium and ventricle. *A. bundle see* BUNDLE OF HIS. *A. node* a node of neurogenic tissue situated between the two and transmitting impulses. *A. valves* the bicuspid and tricuspid valve on the left and right sides of the heart respectively.

atrium ('aytri'əm) *pl.* atria. 1. a cavity, entrance or passage. 2. one of the two upper chambers of the heart. Formerly called auricle.

atrophy ('atrəfee) wasting of any part of the body, due to degeneration of the cells, from disuse, lack of nourishment, or of nerve supply. *Acute yellow a.* massive necrosis of liver cells. A rare condition that may follow acute hepatitis or eclampsia or be precipitated by certain drugs. *Progressive muscular a.* (motor neurone disease) degeneration of the motor neurones with wasting

of muscle tissue.

atropine ('atrə,peen, -pin) the active principle of belladonna. An alkaloid which inhibits respiratory and gastric secretions, relaxes muscle spasm and dilates the pupil.

ATS anti-tetanus serum. *See* TETANUS.

attack (ə'tak) an episode or onset of illness. *A. rate* number of cases of a disease in a particular group, e.g. a school, over a given period related to the population of that group. *Transient ischaemic a's* brief attacks (a few hours or less) of cerebral dysfunction of vascular origin, without lasting neurological deficit.

attention deficit syndrome (ə-'tenshən) a disorder of childhood characterized by marked failure of attention, impulsiveness and increased motor activity.

attenuation (ə'tenyoo'ayshən) a bacteriological process by which organisms are rendered less virulent by culture in artificial media through many generations, exposure to light, air, etc. Used for vaccine preparations.

attitude ('ati,tyood) 1. a posture or position of the body; in obstetrics, the relation of the various parts of the fetal body to one another. 2. a pattern of mental views established by cumulative prior experience.

atypical (ay'tipik'l) irregular; not conforming to type.

Au symbol for gold (L. *aurum*).

audiogram ('awdioh,gram) a graph produced by an audiometer.

audiologist (ˌawdi'olə'jist) an allied

health professional specializing in audiology, who provides services that include: (1) evaluation of hearing function to detect hearing impairment and, if there is a hearing disorder, to determine the anatomical site involved and the cause of the disorder, (2) selection of appropriate hearing aids, and (3) training in lip reading, hearing aid use and maintenance of normal speech.

audiology (,awdi'olǝjee) the science concerned with the sense of hearing, especially the evaluation and measurement of impaired hearing and the rehabilitation of those with impaired hearing.

audiometer (,awdi'omitǝ) an instrument for testing hearing, whereby the threshold of the patients' hearing can be measured.

audit ('awdit) systematic review and evaluation of records and other data to determine the quality of the services or products provided in a given situation. *A. monitor* an adaptation for the UK of the USA Rush Medicus system of assessing quality of nursing care. It consists of 'checklists' for quality leading to a scoring system. *Nursing a.* an evaluation of structure, process, and outcome as a measurement of the quality of nursing care. *Concurrent a's* are conducted at the time the care is being provided to clients/patients. They may be conducted by means of observation and interview of clients/patients, review of open charts, or conferences with groups of consumers and providers of nurs-

ing care. *Retrospective a's* are conducted after the patient's discharge. Methods include the study of closed patients' charts and nursing care plans, questionnaires, interviews, and surveys of patients and families.

aura ('or·rǝ) the premonition, peculiar to an individual, which often precedes an epileptic fit.

aural ('or·rǝl) referring to the ear.

auricle ('or·rik'l) 1. the external portion of the ear. 2. obsolete term for the atrium.

auriscope ('or·ri,skohp) an instrument for examining the drum of the ear. An otoscope.

aurum ('or·rǝm) [L.] *gold.*

auscultation (,awskǝl'tayshǝn) examining the internal organs by listening to the sounds which they give out. In *direct* or *immediate a.* the ear is placed directly against the body. In *mediate a.* a stethoscope is used.

Australia antigen (o'strayli·ǝ) hepatitis B surface antigen found in the blood of a patient with serum hepatitis or who is a carrier of the virus. Dilute concentrations of the antigen can cause the disease and health care personnel must take adequate precautions to avoid inoculation accidents. Blood banks routinely screen for the antigen to exclude infected blood donations.

Australian lift (o'strayli·ǝn) a shoulder lift for moving a heavy or immobile patient. The lift is carried out by two people, one on either side of the patient. The lifters press their nearest shoulders under the patient's adjacent axillae, whilst simultaneously grasping each others' hands under the patient's thighs. By extending their knees and hips, the lifters smoothly transfer their weight on to their forward legs.

autism ('awtizəm) self-absorption. Abnormal dislike of the society of others. *Infantile a.* failure of a child to relate to people and situations, leading to complete withdrawal into a world of private fantasies.

autistic (aw'tistik) pertaining to autism.

autoagglutination ('awtoh·ə‚glooti‚nayshən) 1. clumping or agglutination of an individual's cells by his own serum, as in autohaemagglutination. Autoagglutination occurring at low temperatures is called cold agglutination. 2. agglutination of particulate antigens, e.g. bacteria, in the absence of specific antigens.

autoantibody ('awtoh'anti'bodee) an antibody formed in response to, and reacting against, an antigenic constituent of the individual's own tissues.

autoantigen (‚awtoh'antijən) a tissue constituent that stimulates production of autoantibodies in the organism in which it occurs.

autoclave ('awtə‚klayv) a steam-heated sterilizing apparatus in which the temperature is raised by reducing the air pressure inside it and then injecting steam under pressure, so bringing about efficient sterilization.

autodigestion (‚awtohdie'jeschən, -di-) dissolution of tissue by its own secretions.

autoeroticism ('awtoh·i'roti‚siz-

əm) sexual pleasure derived from self-stimulation of erogenous zones (the mouth, the anus, the genitals and the skin).

autogenous (aw'tojənəs) generated within the body and not acquired from external sources.

autograft ('awtə‚grahft) the transfer of skin or other tissue from one part of the body to another to repair some deficiency.

autoimmune disease (‚awtoh·i-'myoon) condition in which the body develops antibodies to its own tissues, as in e.g. autoimmune thyroiditis (Hashimoto's disease).

autoimmunization (‚awtoh'imyuh-nie'zayshən) the formation of antibodies against the individual's own tissue.

autoinfection (‚awtoh·in'fekshən) self-infection, transferred from one part of the body to another by fingers, towels, etc.

autoinoculation (‚awtoh·i‚nok-yuh'layshən) inoculation with a microorganism from the body itself.

autointoxication (‚awtoh·in‚toksi-'kayshən) poisoning by toxins generated within the body itself.

autologous (aw'toləgəs) related to self; belonging to the same organism. *A. blood transfusion* abbreviated ABT. The patient donates blood prior to elective surgery for transfusion postoperatively. ABT may also be obtained as a blood salvage procedure during operation or postoperatively. Avoids cross-matching, compatibility and transfusion infection problems.

autolysis (aw'tolisis) a breaking

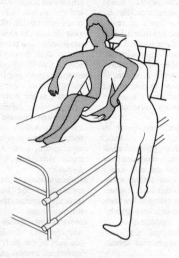

AUSTRALIAN LIFT

up of living tissues as may occur, e.g. if pancreatic ferments escape into surrounding tissues. It also occurs after death.

automatic (,awtə'matik) performed without the influence of the will.

automatism (aw'tomə,tizəm) performance of non-reflex acts without apparent volition, and of which the patient may have no memory afterwards, as in somnambulism. *Post-epileptic a.* automatic acts following an epileptic fit.

autonomic (,awtə'nomik) self-

governing. *A. nervous system* the sympathetic and parasympathetic nerves which control involuntary muscles and glandular secretion over which there is no conscious control.

autoplasty ('awtoh,plastee) 1. replacement of missing tissue by grafting a healthy section from another part of the body. 2. in psychoanalysis, instinctive modification within the psychic systems in adaptation to reality.

autopsy (aw'topsee, 'awtəp-) post-mortem examination of a body to determine the cause of death.

autosome ('awtoh,sohm) any chromosome other than the sex chromosomes. In man there are 22 pairs of autosomes and 1 pair of sex chromosomes.

autosuggestion (,awtohsə'jeschən) suggestion arising in one's self. Uncritical acceptance of ideas arising in the individual's own mind.

autotransfusion (,awtohtrans-'fyoozhən, -trahns-) reinfusion of a patient's own blood.

autotransplantation (,awtoh-,transplahn'tayshən) transfer of tissue from one part of the body to another part.

avascular (ay'vaskyuhlə) not vascular. Bloodless. *A. necrosis* death of bone owing to deficient blood supply, usually following an injury.

aversion (ə'vərshən) intense dislike. *A. therapy* a method of treating addictions by associating the craving for what is addictive with painful or unpleasant stimuli.

avitaminosis (ay,vitəmi'nohsis) a condition resulting from an insufficiency of vitamins in the diet. A deficiency disease.

avulsion (ə'vulshən) the tearing away of one part from another.

Phrenic a. a tearing away of the phrenic nerve. It paralyses the diaphragm on the affected side.

axilla (ak'silə) an armpit.

axis ('aksis) 1. a line through the centre of a structure. 2. the second cervical vertebra.

axon ('akson) the process of a nerve cell along which electrical impulses travel. The nerve fibre.

axonotmesis (,aksonət'meesis) nerve injury characterized by disruption of the axon and myelin sheath but with preservation of the connective tissue fragments, resulting in degeneration of the axon distal to the injury site; regeneration of the axon is spontaneous.

azathioprine (,azə'thieə,preen) an immunosuppressive drug widely used for transplant recipients and also as treatment for autoimmune conditions.

azoospermia (,ayzoh·oh'spərmi·ə) absence of spermatozoa in the semen.

azygos ('azi,gos, a'zie-) something that is unpaired. *A. vein* an unpaired vein that ascends the posterior mediastinum and enters the superior vena cava.

B

Ba symbol for *barium*.

Babinski's reflex or **sign** (bə-'binskee)*J.F.F. Babinski,French neurologist,1857–1932.* On stroking the sole of the foot, the great toe bends upwards instead of downwards (*dorsal* instead of *plantar* flexion). Present in disease or injury to the upper motor neurone. Babies who have not walked react in the same way, but normal flexion develops later.

baby ('baybee) an infant as yet unable to walk. *Battered b.* one suffering from the result of continued violence; extensive bruising, fractures of limbs, rib and skull, and internal trauma may be found. *Blue b.* one suffering from cyanosis at birth due to atelectasis or congenital heart malformation.

bacillaemia (,basi'leemi·ə) the presence of bacilli in the blood.

bacilluria (,basi'lyooə·ri·ə) the presence of bacilli in the urine.

Bacillus (bə'siləs) a genus of aerobic, spore-bearing Gram-positive bacteria. *B. anthracis* the causative agent of ANTHRAX.

bacillus (bə'siləs) loosely, the cause of any bacterial infection by a rod-shaped microorganism, e.g. *Escherichia coli*, the colon bacillus.

back (bak) dorsum. Posterior trunk from neck to pelvis.

B. bone the vertebral column. *Hunch b.* kyphosis. *B. slab* plaster or plastic splint in which a limb is supported.

backache ('bak,ayk) any pain in the back, usually the lower part. The pain is often dull and continuous, but sometimes sharp and throbbing. Backache, or lumbago, is one of the commonest ailments and can be caused by a variety of disorders. Nurses are at particular risk and one in six are thought to experience back pain.

baclofen ('bakloh,fen) a muscle relaxant used in the treatment of multiple sclerosis.

bacteraemia (,baktə'reemi·ə) the presence of bacteria in the bloodstream.

bacterial (bak'tiə·ri·əl) pertaining to bacteria.

bactericidal (bak,tiə·ri'sied'l) capable of killing bacteria, e.g. disinfectants, great heat, intense cold or sunlight.

bactericide (bak'tiə·ri,sied) an agent that kills bacteria.

bacteriologist (bak,tiə·ri'oləjist) one who is qualified in the science of bacteriology.

bacteriology (bak,tiə·ri'oləjee) the scientific study of bacteria.

bacteriolysin (bak,tiə·ri'olisin, -rioh'liesin) an antibody produced in the blood to assist in the destruction of bacteria. The action is specific.

bacteriolysis (bak,tiə·ri'olisis) the dissolution of bacteria by a bacteriolytic agent.

bacteriolytic (bak,tiə'rioh'litik) capable of destroying or dissolving bacteria.

bacteriophage (bak'tiə·ri·ə,fayj, -fahzh) a virus which only infects bacteria. Many strains exist, some of which are used for identifying types of staphylococci and salmonellae.

bacteriostat (bak,tiə·rioh'stat) an agent which inhibits the growth of bacteria.

bacteriostatic (bak,tiə·rioh'static) inhibiting the growth of bacteria.

bacterium (bak'tiə·ri·əm) a general name given to a minute vegetable organism which may live on organic matter. There are many varieties, only some of which are pathogenic to man, animals and plants. Each bacterium consists of a single cell and, given favourable conditions, multiplies by subdivision. Bacteria are classified according to their shape into: (1) *bacilli*, rod-shaped; (2) *cocci*, spherical; (a) streptococci, in chains; (b) staphylococci, in groups; (c) diplococci, in pairs; (3) *spirilla*, *spirochaetes*, spiral-shaped. *Pathogenic b.* one whose growth in the body gives rise to disease, either by destruction of tissue, or by formation of toxins which circulate in the blood. Pathogenic bacteria thrive on organic matter in the presence of warmth and moisture.

bacteriuria (bak,tiə·ri'yooə·ri·ə)

the presence of bacteria in the urine.

bag (bag) a sac or pouch. *Colostomy b.* a receptacle worn over the stoma by a COLOSTOMY patient, to receive the faecal discharge. *Douglas b.* a receptacle for the collection of expired air, permitting measurement of respiratory gases. *Ice b.* a rubber or plastic bag half-filled with pieces of ice and applied near or to a part of the body. *Ileostomy b.* any of various plastic or latex pouches attached to the stoma for the collection of faecal material following ILEOSTOMY. *Politzer b.* a soft bag of rubber for inflating the pharyngotympanic tube. *Urine b.* a receptacle used for urine by ambulatory patients with urinary incontinence. *B. of waters* the membranes enclosing the AMNIOTIC FLUID and the developing fetus in utero.

Bainbridge reflex ('baynbrij) *F.A. Bainbridge, British physiologist, 1874–1921.* An increase in the heart rate caused by an increase in right atrial pressure.

BAL British antilewisite. *See* DIMERCAPROL.

balanitis (,balə'nietis) inflammation of the glans penis and of the prepuce, usually associated with phimosis. Balanoposthitis.

balantidiasis (,balanti'dieəsis) a rare form of colitis or dysentery caused by intestinal infestation by *Balantidium coli*, a protozoon.

baldness ('bawldnəs) absence of hair, especially from the scalp, Alopecia.

Balkan frame ('bawlkən) a framework fitted over a bed to carry

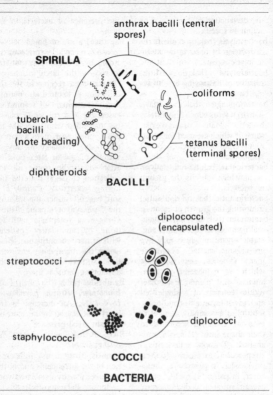

anthrax bacilli (central spores)

SPIRILLA

coliforms

tubercle bacilli (note beading)

tetanus bacilli (terminal spores)

diphtheroids

BACILLI

diplococci (encapsulated)

streptococci

diplococci

staphylococci

COCCI

BACTERIA

pulleys and slings or splints for the support of a limb undergoing surgical treatment. Used chiefly in the treatment of fractures.

ballotement (bə'lotmənt) [Fr.] a method of testing for a floating object, e.g. abdominal palpation of the uterus when testing for pregnancy. The uterus is pushed upward by a finger in the vagina, and if a fetus is present it will fall back again like a heavy body in water.

balsam ('bawlsəm) an aromatic

vegetable juice. *Friar's b.* a compound containing tincture of benzoin. Used for steam inhalations. *Peru b.* used externally as an antiseptic ointment and in *tulle gras*. *Tolu b.* used as an expectorant. A constituent of friar's balsam.

bandage ('bandij) 1. a strip or roll of gauze or other material for wrapping or binding any part of the body. 2. to cover by wrapping with such material. Bandages may be used to stop the flow of blood, to provide a safeguard against contamination, or to hold a dressing in place. They may also be used to hold a splint in position or otherwise immobilize an injured part of the body to prevent further injury and to facilitate healing.

banding ('banding) placing a band round a blood vessel to restrict the flow from it. *Pulmonary arterial b.* a palliative operation used in treating infants with ventricular septal defects.

bank (bank) an institution offering services, or a store of donated human tissues for use in the future by other individuals. e.g. *blood b.*, *human-milk b.*, *sperm b.* *Nurse b.* a group of nurses who are known to the employing authority and available for employment on an on-call basis.

Bankhart's operation ('bangkhahts) *A.S.B. Bankhart, British orthopaedic surgeon, 1879–1951.* An operation to repair a defect in the glenoid cavity causing repeated dislocation of the shoulder joint.

Banti's disease ('banteez) *G.*

Banti, Italian pathologist, 1852–1925. A clinical syndrome characterized by splenomegaly, cirrhosis of the liver, anaemia, leukopenia and gastrointestinal bleeding.

Barbados leg (bah'baydəs, -dos, -dohs) swelling and enlargement of the leg. A form of elephantiasis.

barbiturates (bah'bityuh·rəts, -'rayts) a large group of sedative and hypnotic drugs derived from barbituric acid, e.g. phenobarbitone, amylobarbitone. Prolonged use may lead to addiction.

barbotage (,bahbə'tahzh) [Fr.] a method of spinal anaesthesia by which some of the anaesthetic is injected, followed by partial withdrawal and then reinjection with more of the drug. This process is repeated until the full amount has been given, allowing dilution and mixing with the cerebrospinal fluid.

barium ('bair·ri·əm) *symbol* Ba. A soft silvery metallic element. *B. sulphate* a heavy mineral salt that is comparatively impermeable to X-rays and can therefore be used as contrast medium given as a meal or as an enema. Used to demonstrate abnormality in the stomach or intestines, and to show peristaltic movement. *B. sulphide* the chief constituent of depilatory preparations, i.e. those which remove hair.

baroreceptors (,barohri'septəz) the sensory branches of the glossopharyngeal and vagus nerves that influence the blood pressure. The receptors are situated in the walls of the carotid sinus and aortic arch.

barotrauma (ˌbaroh'trawmə) injury due to pressure, such as to structures of the ear owing to differences between atmospheric and intratympanic pressures.

Barr body (bah) *M.L. Barr, Canadian anatomist, b. 1908.* Small dark-staining area underneath the nuclear membrane of female cells. Represents an inactive X chromosome.

Barré–Guillain syndrome (ˌbaray'giyanh) *J.A. Barré, French neurologist, b. 1880; G. Guillain, French neurologist, 1876–1961.* Acute febrile polyneuritis. Called also Guillain–Barré syndrome.

barrier ('bari·ə) an obstruction. *Blood–brain b.* the selective barrier which separates the circulating blood from the cerebrospinal fluid. *B. contraceptive.* a mechanical barrier preventing the sperm entering the cervical canal, e.g. diaphragm, sheath. *B. nursing* precautions taken by nurses to prevent infection from a patient spreading to other patients and/or staff. This normally involves nursing the patient in a separate room or cubicle. *Placental b.* semi-permeable membrane between maternal and fetal blood. *Protective b.* radiation-absorbing shield, e.g. lead, concrete, to protect the body against ionizing radiations. *Reverse b. nursing* a technique used by nurses to prevent the transmission of infection to the patient who may be especially vulnerable, e.g. the immunosuppressed patient.

Bartholin's glands ('bahtəlinz)

C.T. Bartholin, Danish anatomist, 1655–1738. Two glands situated in the labia majora, with ducts opening inside the vulva.

basal ('bays'l) 1. fundamental. 2. referring to a base. *B. ganglia.* the collections of nerve cells or grey matter in the base of the cerebrum. They consist of the caudate nucleus and putamen, forming the corpus striatum, and the globus pallidus. Such cells are concerned with modifying and coordinating voluntary muscle movements. *B. metabolic rate* abbreviated BMR. An indirect method of estimating the rate of metabolism in the body by measuring the oxygen intake and carbon dioxide output on breathing. The age, sex, weight and size of the patient have to be taken into account.

base (bays) 1. the lowest part or foundation. 2. the main constituent of a compound. 3. an alkali or other substance which can unite with an acid to form a salt.

basement membrane ('baysmənt) a thin layer of modified connective tissue supporting layers of cells, found at the base of the epidermis and underlying mucous membranes.

basilar ('basilə) situated at the base. *B. artery* midline artery at the base of the skull, formed by the junction of the vertebral arteries.

basilic (bə'silik) prominent. *B. vein.* a large vein on the inner side of the arm.

basophil ('baysəˌfil) adj. *basophilic.* 1. any structure, cell, or histological element staining readily with basic dyes. 2. a granular leukocyte with an irregularly shaped, relatively pale-staining nucleus that is partially constricted into two lobes, and with cytoplasm containing coarse bluish-black granules of variable size. 3. a beta cell of the adenohypophysis.

basophilia (ˌbaysəˈfiliˑə) 1. an affinity of cells or tissues for basic dyes. 2. the reaction of relatively immature erythrocytes to basic dyes whereby the stained cells appear blue, grey, or greyish-blue, or bluish granules appear. 3. abnormal increase of basophilic leukocytes in the blood. 4. basophilic leukocytosis.

Batchelor plaster ('bachələ) *J.S. Batchelor, British surgeon.* A double abduction plaster of Paris splint which is used in the correction of congenital dislocation of the hip.

bath (bahth) 1. a medium, e.g. water, vapour, sand, or mud, with which the body is washed or in which the body is wholly or partially immersed for therapeutic or cleansing purposes; application of such a medium to the body. 2. the equipment or apparatus in which a body or object may be immersed. *Bed b.* washing a patient in bed. *Emollient b.* a bath in a soothing and softening liquid, used in various skin disorders. It is prepared by adding soothing agents, such as gelatin, starch, bran, or similar substances to the bath water, for the purpose of relieving skin irritation and pruritus. The patient is dried by patting rather than

rubbing the skin. Care must be taken to avoid chilling. *Hot b.* one in water from 36 to 44°C. Care must be taken to avoid faintness. *Sponge b.* one in which the patient's body is not immersed but is wiped with a wet cloth or sponge. Sponge baths are most often employed for reduction of body temperature in the presence of a fever, in which case the water used is tepid and may contain alcohol to increase evaporation of moisture from the skin. *Tepid b.* one in water 30 to 33°C. *Warm b.* one in water 32 to 40°C. *Whirlpool b.* (Jacuzzi) one in which the water is kept in constant motion by mechanical means. It has a gentle massaging action that promotes relaxation.

BCG vaccine (ˌbeeceeˈgee) bacille Calmette–Guérin vaccine, a tuberculosis vaccine, containing live, attenuated bovine tubercle bacilli (*Mycobacterium bovis*).

Be symbol for *beryllium.*

'bearing down' (ˌbairˑringˈdown) 1. the expulsive pains in the second stage of labour. 2. a feeling of heaviness and downward strain in the pelvis present with some uterine growths or displacements.

beat (beet) pulsation of the heart or an artery. *Apex b.* pulsation of the heart felt over its apex. The beat of the heart is felt against the chest wall. *Dropped b.* the occasional loss of a ventricular beat. *Ectopic b.* one that originates somewhere other than the sinoatrial node.

Beck inventory of depression (bek) abbreviated BID. A self-

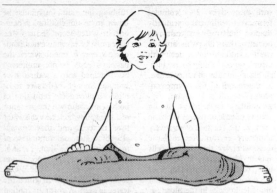

BATCHELOR PLASTER

scoring system used to determine the presence of depression.

beclomethasone dipropionate (ˌbekloh'methəzohn) a glucocorticoid administered by aerosol inhalation or spinhaler to patients who require corticosteroids for control of bronchial asthma symptoms.

becquerel (be'krel) abbreviated Bq. The SI unit of radioactivity equal to the quantity of material undergoing one disintegration per second; 3.7×10^{10} becquerels is equal to 1 curie.

bed (bed) 1. a supporting structure or tissue. 2. a couch or support for the body during sleep. *Capillary b.* the capillaries of a tissue, area or organ considered collectively, and their volume capacity. *B. cradle* a frame placed over the body of a bed patient. *See* CRADLE. *Fracture*

b. a bed for the use of patients with broken bones. *King's Fund b.* a bed fitted with jointed springs, which may be adjusted to various positions. *See also* KING'S FUND. *Nail b.* the area of modified epidermis beneath the nail over which the nail plate slides as it grows.

bed-wetting ('bed,weting) enuresis; involuntary voiding of urine. *See also* ENURESIS.

bedbug ('bed,bug) a bug of the genus *Cimex*, a flattened, oval, reddish insect that inhabits houses, furniture and neglected beds, and feeds on man, usually at night.

bedpan ('bed,pan) a shallow vessel used for defecation or urination by patients confined to bed.

bedsore ('bed,sor) an ulcerlike sore caused by prolonged pressure of the patient's body. Pressure sore is now the preferred term, as these sores are primarily due to pressure and can also occur in patients who are not confined to bed. A decubitus ulcer.

bee sting (bee sting) injury caused by the venom of a bee. Symptoms of a severe allergic reaction, such as collapse or swelling of the body, indicate ANAPHYLAXIS and require that medical help be sought.

Beer's knife (biəz) *G.J. Beer, German ophthalmologist, 1763–1821.* One with a triangular blade used in cataract operations, for incising the cornea preparatory to removal of the lens.

behaviour (bi'hayvyə) the way in which an organism reacts to an internal or external stimulus. *Incongruous b.* behaviour that is out of keeping with the person's normal reaction or has the opposite effect to that consciously desired. *B. disorders* may take many forms, such as truancy, stealing, temper-tantrums. *B. modification* an approach to correction of undesirable behaviour that focuses on changing observable actions. Modification of the behaviour is accomplished through systematic manipulation of the environmental and behavioural variables related to the specific behaviour to be changed. *B. therapy* a therapeutic approach in which the focus is on the patient's observable behaviour, rather than on conflicts and unconscious processes presumed to underlie his maladaptive behaviour. This is accomplished through systematic manipulation of the environmental and behavioural variables related to the specific behaviour to be modified; operant conditioning, systematic desensitization, token economy, aversive control, flooding and implosion are examples of techniques that may be used in behaviour therapy.

behaviourism (bi'hayvyə,rizəm) the purely objective study and observation of the behaviour of individuals.

bejel ('bayjəl) a non-venereal but infectious form of syphilis caused by a treponema indistinguishable from that causing syphilis. Occurs mainly in children of Africa and the Middle East. The primary lesion is on the mouth, spreading to the trunk, arms and legs. Treated with penicillin.

belching ('belching) the noisy expulsion of gas from the stomach through the mouth. Eructation.

belladonna (,belə'donə) a drug from the deadly nightshade plant. Used as an anti-spasmodic in colic, to check secretions, and to dilate the pupil of the eye.

Bell's palsy (belz) *Sir C. Bell, British physiologist, 1774–1842.* Facial paralysis due to oedema of the facial nerve.

belle indifference (,bel in'difə-·ronhs) [Fr.] an indication of conversion hysteria, in which the patient describes his symptoms, appearing not to be distressed by them.

Bence Jones protein (,bens 'johnz) *H. Bence Jones, British physician, 1813–1873.* See PROTEIN.

bendrofluazide (ˌbendroh'flooə-ˌzied) an oral diuretic of the thiazide group. Used primarily to treat mild hypertension and cardiac failure.

bends (bendz) a colloquial term for caisson disease. Decompression sickness.

benign (bi'nien) 1. the opposite to malignant. 2. describes a noninvasive condition or illness that is not serious even though treatment may be required for health or cosmetic reasons.

benorylate (be'nor·rilayt) an ester of paracetamol and aspirin used as an anti-inflammatory and analgesic.

benzalkonium chloride (ˌbenzal-'kohni·əm) a quaternary ammonium compound used as a surface disinfectant and detergent and as a topical antiseptic and antibiotic preservative. Incompatible with soap.

benzathine penicillin (ˌbenzətheen, peni'silin) a long-acting antibiotic. Used in treatment of Gram-positive infections. May be given orally or intramuscularly.

benzene ('benzeen) benzol. A coal-tar derivative widely used as a solvent.

benzhexol (benz'heksol) an antispasmodic drug which helps to overcome the tremors and rigidity of Parkinson's disease.

benzocaine ('benzoh,kayn) a surface anaesthetic used for the relief of pain or to anaesthetize the oropharynx or anus. Available as lozenges or ointment.

benzyl benzoate (ˌbenzil'benzoh·ayt, -ziel) an emulsion used in the treatment of scabies.

benzylpenicillin (ˌbenzil,peni-'silin, ˌbenziel-) a widely used soluble penicillin that is quickly absorbed. High blood levels can therefore be obtained.

beriberi (ˌberi'beri) a deficiency disease due to insufficiency of vitamin B_1 in the diet. The disease is more common in areas where refined rice is the main staple in the diet. It is a form of neuritis, with pain, paralysis and oedema of the extremities.

berylliosis (bəˌrili'ohsis) an industrial lung disease due to the inhaling of beryllium. Interstitial fibrosis arises, impairing lung function.

beryllium (bəˌrili·əm) *symbol* Be. A metallic element which is used in the manufacture of some aluminium alloys.

Besnier's prurigo (ˌbezni·əz proo-ə'riegoh) *E. Besnier, French dermatologist, 1831–1909.* Diathetic prurigo, a flexural neurodermatitis, is seen in young children.

beta ('beetə) the second letter in the Greek alphabet, β. *B. blockers* drugs used to block the action of adrenaline on beta-adrenergic receptors in cardiac muscle, thus decreasing the workload of the heart. *B. cells* insulin-producing cells found in the islets of Langerhans in the pancreas. *B. rays* electrons used therapeutically for treatment of lesions of the cornea and iris. *B. receptors* receptors associated with the inhibition (relaxation) of smooth muscle. They also bring an increase in the force of contraction and rate of the heart.

Betadine ('betə,deen, -din) trade name for preparations of povidone–iodine, which have a longer antiseptic action than most iodine solutions.

betamethasone (,beetə'methə,zohn) a synthetic glucocorticoid which is the most active of the anti-inflammatory steroids.

betatron ('beetə,tron) an apparatus used to accelerate a stream of electrons into a beam for use in radiotherapy.

bethanechol (bə'thani,kol) a derivative of a choline-like substance, used in the treatment of abdominal distension and urinary retention. Hypotension and dyspnoea may occur as side-effects.

bethanidine (bə'thani,deen) an adrenergic blocking agent used in the treatment of hypertension.

Betnovate ('betnəvayt) trade name for preparations containing betamethasone. Used in the treatment of severe inflammatory skin disorders unresponsive to less potent corticosteroids.

Betz cells (bets) *V.A. Betz, Russian anatomist, 1834–1894.* The pyramidal cells in the precentral area of the cerebrum.

bezoar ('beezor) a mass of hair, fruit or vegetable fibres sometimes found in the stomach or intestines.

Bi symbol for *bismuth.*

bicarbonate (bie'kaybə,nayt, -nət) any salt containing the HCO_3^- anion. *Blood b., plasma b.* the bicarbonate of the blood plasma, an important parameter of ACID–BASE BALANCE measured in BLOOD GAS ANALYSIS.

bicellular (bie'selyuhla) composed of two cells.

biceps ('bieseps) a muscle with two heads; a flexor of the arm; one of the hamstring muscles of the thigh.

biconcave (bie'konkayv) pertaining to a lens or other structure with a hollow or depression on each surface.

biconvex (bie'konvex) pertaining to a lens or other structure that protrudes on both surfaces.

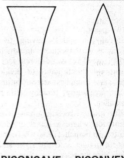

BICONCAVE BICONVEX

bicornuate (bie'kawnyooayt) having two horns. *B. uterus* a congenital malformation in which there is a partial or complete vertical division into two parts of the body of the uterus.

bicuspid (bie'kuspid) having two cusps or projections. *B. teeth* the premolars. *B. valve* the mitral valve of the heart between the left atrium and ventricle.

bidet ('beeday) a low narrow basin on a stand for washing the perineum and genitalia.

bifid ('biefid) divided or cleft into

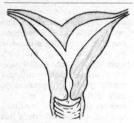

BICORNUATE UTERUS

two parts.

bifocal (bie'fohk'l) having two foci, as with spectacles in which the lenses have two different foci.

bifurcate (bie'fərkayt) to divide into two branches; arteries bifurcate frequently, thereby getting smaller.

bifurcation (,biefə'kayshən) the junction where a vessel divides into two branches, e.g. where the aorta divides into the right and left iliac vessels.

bigeminal (bie'jemin'l) double. *B. pulse* two pulse beats which occur together, regular in time and force. A regular irregularity.

biguanides (bie'gwahniedz) oral hypoglycaemic agents for treating diabetes. They exert their effect by decreasing gluconeogenesis in muscle tissue. Only effective in those diabetics with functioning islet of Langerhans cells. Most commonly used in non-insulin dependent diabetics, especially those who are overweight.

bilateral (bie'latə·ral) pertaining to both sides.

bile (biel) a secretion of the liver, greenish-yellow to brown in colour. It is concentrated in the gall-bladder and passes into the small intestine, where it assists digestion by emulsifying fats and stimulates peristalsis. *B. ducts* the canals or passageways that conduct bile. The hepatic and cystic ducts join to form the common bile duct. *B. pigments* bilirubin and biliverdin, produced by haemolysis in the spleen. Normally these colour the faeces only, but in jaundice the skin and urine may also become coloured. *B. salts* sodium taurocholate and sodium glycocholate, which cause the emulsification of fats.

Bilharzia (bil'hahtsi·ə) *T.M. Bilharz, German physician, 1825–1862.* A genus of blood fluke now known as *Schistosoma*.

bilharziasis (,bilhah'tsieəsis) schistosomiasis.

biliary ('bilyə·ree) pertaining to bile. *B. colic* spasm of muscle walls of the bile duct causing excruciating pain when gallstones are blocking the tube. Pain is in the right upper quadrant of the abdomen and referred to the shoulder. *B. fistula* an abnormal opening between the gallbladder and the surface of the body.

biliousness ('biliəs,nəs) a symptom complex comprising nausea, abdominal discomfort, headache, and constipation.

bilirubin (,bili'roobin) an orange bile pigment produced by the breakdown of haem and reduction of biliverdin; it normally circulates in plasma and is taken up by liver cells and conjugated to form bilirubin diglucuronide, the water-soluble pigment excreted in the bile. Bilirubin may be classified as indirect ('free' or unconjugated) while en route to the liver from its site of formation by reticuloendothelial cells, and direct (bilirubin diglucuronide) after its conjugation in the liver with glucuronic acid. Normally the body produces a total of about 260 mg of bilirubin per day. Almost 99 per cent of this is excreted in the faeces; the remaining 1 per cent is excreted in the urine as UROBILINOGEN. The typical yellowness of jaundice is caused by the accumulation of bilirubin in the blood and body tissues.

bilirubinaemia (ˌbiliˌroobi'neemi·ə) the presence of bilirubin in the blood.

biliuria (ˌbili'yooə·ri·ə) bile or bile salts in the urine.

biliverdin (ˌbili'vərdin) a green bile pigment, the oxidized form of bilirubin.

Billings method ('bilingz) a method of contraception. Ovulation time is estimated by observing changes in the cervical mucus that occur during the menstrual cycle.

Billroth's operation ('bilrohts) *C.A.T. Billroth, Austrian surgeon, 1829–1894. See* GASTRECTOMY.

bimanual (bie'manyooəl) using both hands. *B. examination* examination with both hands. Used chiefly in gynaecology, when the internal genital organs are examined between one hand on the abdomen, and the other hand or a finger within the vagina.

binary ('bienə·ree) made up of two parts. *B. fission* the multiplication of cells by division into two equal parts. *B. scale* one used in calculating, in which only two digits, 0 and 1, are used. Digital computers use this scale.

binaural (bie'nor·rəl) pertaining to both ears. *B. stethoscope. See* STETHOSCOPE.

Binet's test ('beenayz) *A. Binet, French physiologist, 1857–1911.* A method of ascertaining the mental age of children or young persons by using a series of questions standardized on the capacity of normal children at various ages.

Bing test (bing) *A. Bing, German otologist, 1844–1922.* A vibrating tuning fork is held to the mastoid process and the auditory meatus is alternately occluded and left open; an increase and decrease in loudness (positive Bing) is perceived by the normal ear and in sensorineural hearing impairment, but in conductive hearing impairment no difference in loudness is perceived (negative Bing).

binocular (bi'nokyuhlə, bie-) relating to both eyes.

binovular (bi'novyuhlə) derived from two ova. *B. twins* twins, which may or may not be of different sexes.

bioassay (ˌbieoh'asay) biological assay. The use of animals or an isolated organ preparation to determine the effect of the active power of a sample of a drug. Comparison is made with the effect of a standard preparation.

biochemistry (ˌbieoh'kemistree) the chemistry of living matter.

biofeedback (ˌbieoh'feed,bak) visual or auditory evidence provided to an individual of the satisfactory performance of an autonomic body function, e.g. sounding a tone when blood pressure is at a satisfactory level, so that, through conditioning, the patient may assert control over that function.

biogenesis (ˌbieoh'jenəsis) 1. the origin of life. 2. the theory that living organisms can originate only from those already living and cannot be artificially produced.

biohazard ('bieoh,hazəd) any hazard arising from inadvertent human biological processes, e.g. accidental inoculation, needle stick injury.

biology (bie'olojee) the science of living organisms, dealing with their structure, function and their relations with one another.

biometrics, biometry (ˌbieə'metriks; bie'omətree) 1. anthropometry. 2. the use of statistics in biological science.

biomicroscopy (ˌbieohmie'kroskəpee) a microscopic examination of living tissues, e.g. of the structures of the anterior of the eye during life. *See* SLIT LAMP.

bioplasm ('bieoh,plazəm) protoplasm. The active principle in matter which produces living organisms.

biopsy ('bieopsee) the removal of some tissue or organ from the living body, e.g. a lymph gland, for examination to establish a diagnosis. *Aspiration b.* biopsy in which the tissue is obtained by suction through a needle and syringe. *Cone b.* biopsy in which an inverted cone of tissue is excised, as from the uterine cervix. *Excisional b.* removal of an entire lesion and significant portion of normal-looking tissue for examination. *Needle b.* tissue obtained by the puncture of a lesion with a needle. Rotation of the needle removes tissue within the lumen of the needle. *Punch b.* tissue obtained by a punch.

biorhythm ('bieoh,ridhəm) any cyclic, biological event, e.g. sleep cycle and menstrual cycle, affecting daily life.

biosensors ('bieoh,sensəz) noninvasive instruments which measure the result of biological processes, e.g. body temperature.

biostatistics (ˌbieohstə'tistiks) that branch of biometry which deals with the data and laws of human mortality, morbidity, natality, and demography; called also vital statistics.

biosynthesis (ˌbieoh'sinthəsis) the creation of a compound within a living organism.

biotin ('bieətin) formerly termed vitamin H, now part of vitamin B complex and present in all normal diets.

biparietal (biepə'rieət'l) pertaining to both parietal eminences or bones.

biparous (bie'parəs) giving birth to two infants at a time.

bipolar (bie'pohlə) with two poles. *B. nerve cells* cells having two nerve fibres, e.g. ganglionic cells.

birth (bərth) the act of being born. *B. control* limiting the size of the family by abstention or the use or contraceptives. *B. mark* a naevus present from birth. *B. notification* a person present, or in attendance, at the birth or within 6 h afterwards, must notify the district medical officer within 36 h (Public Health Act 1936). This responsibility is accepted by the midwife when in attendance. *Premature b.* one taking place after 28 weeks of pregnancy but before term. *B. registration* either parent must register the birth within 42 days at the registrar's office in the district in which the birth took place. Failure to do so incurs a fine. The responsibility rests with the midwife if the parents default.

birthing chair ('bərthing) an especially designed chair for use in labour and delivery to promote greater mobility for the mother.

bisacodyl (,bisə'kohdil) a laxative that acts directly on the rectum. Given as tablets or in the form of suppositories.

bisexual (bie'seksyooəl) 1. having gonads of both sexes. 2. hermaphrodite. 3. having both active and passive sexual interests or characteristics. 4. capable of the function of both sexes. 5. both heterosexual and homosexual. 6. an individual who is both heterosexual and homosexual. 7. of, relating to, or involving both sexes, as bisexual reproduction.

bismuth ('bizməth) *symbol* Bi. A greyish metallic element. Certain of its salts are used as gastric sedatives and in the treatment of syphilis.

bistoury ('bistə·ree) a slender surgical knife, sometimes curved.

bite (biet) 1. to seize with the teeth. 2. a wound made by biting. 3. an impression made by the teeth on a thin sheet of malleable material such as wax.

Bitot's spots ('beetohz) *P.A. Bitot, French physician, 1822–1888.* Collections of dried epithelium, microorganisms, etc., forming shiny, greyish spots on the cornea. A sign of vitamin A deficiency.

bivalve (bie,valv) 1. having two valves, as the shells of molluscs such as oysters. 2. to cut a plaster cast into an anterior and a posterior section. *B. speculum* a vaginal speculum having two blades that can be adjusted for easy insertion.

blackhead ('blak,hed) a comedo.

blackout ('blakowt) momentary failure of vision and unconsciousness due to cerebral circulatory insufficiency.

blackwater fever ('blak,wawta) a form of malignant malaria in which severe haemolysis causes a dark discoloration of the urine.

bladder ('bladə) a membranous sac for holding fluid or gas. *Atonic b.* a condition in which there is lack of tone in the bladder wall, which may be the result of incomplete emptying over a long period. *Gall-b.* the reservoir for bile. *Irritable b.* a condition in which there is frequent desire to micturate. *Urinary b.* the reservoir for urine. *B. worm* a cysticercus.

Blalock–Taussig operation (,blaylok'tawsig) *A. Blalock, American surgeon, 1899–1964; H.B. Taussig, American paediatrician, b.1898.* Operation in which the subclavian artery is anastomosed to the pulmonary artery. Performed in cases of Fallot's tetralogy.

bland (bland) non-stimulating. *B. fluids* mild and non-irritating fluids such as barley water and milk.

blast (blahst) 1. an immature cell. 2. a wave of high air pressure caused by an explosion.

blastocyst ('blastoh,sist) blastula.

blastocyte ('blastoh,siet) an embryonic cell that has not yet become differentiated into its specific type.

blastoderm ('blastoh,derm) the germinal cells of the embryo consisting of three layers, the ectoderm, mesoderm and entoderm.

blastolysis (bla'stolisis, ,blastoh-'liesis) the destruction of germ substance.

blastomycosis (,blastohmie'koh-sis) a fungal infection which, after invasion of the skin, may cause granulomatous lesions in the mouth, pharynx and lungs.

blastula ('blastyuhlə) blastocyst. An early stage in the development of the fertilized ovum. This stage precedes the gastrula.

bleb (bleb) a blister.

bleeder ('bleedə) 1. a popular name for one who suffers from haemophilia. 2. a vessel which is difficult to seal at operation.

bleeding ('bleeding) 1. escape of blood from an injured vessel. 2. venesection. *Functional b.* bleeding from the uterus when no organic lesion is present. *B. time* the time taken for oozing to cease from a sharp prick of the finger or ear lobe. The normal is 1–3 min.

blennorrhagia (,blenə'rayji·ə) 1. an excessive discharge of mucus, e.g. leukorrhoea. 2. gonorrhoea.

blennorrhoea (,blenə'reeə) blennorrhagia.

bleomycin (,blioh'miesin) an antitumour antibiotic drug especially effective against squamous cell carcinomas.

blepharitis (,blefə'rietis) inflammation of the eyelids. *Allergic b.* that associated with response to drugs or cosmetics applied to the eye or eyelids. *Squamous b.* that associated with dandruff on the scalp.

blepharon ('blefə·ron) the eyelid.

blepharophimosis (,blefə·rohfie-'mohsis) abnormal narrowing of the aperture between the eyelids. Usually congenital but may arise from chronic inflammation.

blepharoptosis (,blefə·rop'tohsis) drooping of the upper eyelid.

blepharospasm (,blefə·roh,spaz-əm) prolonged spasm of the orbicular muscles of the eyelids.

blind (bliend) without sight. *B. spot* the point where the optic nerve leaves the retina, which is insensitive to light. Punctum caecum.

blind loop syndrome (bliend 'loop) a condition of stasis in the small intestine which aids bacterial multiplication leading to diarrhoea and salt deficiencies. The cause may be intestinal obstruction or surgical anastomosis.

blindness ('bliendnəs) lack or loss of ability to see; lack of perception of visual stimuli. Legally, blindness is defined as less than

6/60 vision with glasses (vision of 6/60 is the ability to see only at 6 metres what the normal eye can see at 60 metres).

blister (blis'tə) a bleb or vesicle. A collection of serum between the epidermis and the true skin. *Blood b.* a blister containing blood, usually caused by a pinch or bruise.

block (blok) a stoppage or obstruction. The term is used to describe (1) various forms of regional anaesthesia, e.g. epidural block; (2) obstruction to the passage of a nervous impulse due to disease, e.g. heart block (*see* HEART); (3) an interruption of mental function.

blood (blud) the fluid that circulates through the heart and blood vessels supplying nutritive material to all parts of the body, and carrying away waste products. Blood is a red viscid fluid and consists of plasma in which are suspended erythrocytes (red blood cells), leukocytes (white corpuscles) and lymphocytes, and platelets or thrombocytes. (1) The red corpuscles or ERYTHRO-CYTES contain haemoglobin which combines with oxygen in passing through the lungs. This oxygen is released into the tissues from the capillaries and oxidation takes place. (2) The white corpuscles or LEUKOCYTES defend against invading microorganisms, which they have power to destroy. (3) Blood platelets or thrombocytes are concerned with the clotting of blood. Plasma also contains many other specialized substances which have important

roles to play in immunity and the clotting of blood.

blood bank 1. a place of storage for blood. 2. an organization that collects, processes, stores and transfuses blood. In most hospitals the blood bank is located in the pathology laboratory.

blood–brain barrier abbreviated BBB. The membranous barrier separating the blood from the brain. It is permeable to water, oxygen, carbon dioxide, glucose, alcohol, general anaesthetics and some drugs.

blood casts casts of coagulated red blood cells formed in the renal tubles and found in the urine.

blood clotting, coagulation the formation of a jelly-like substance over the ends or within the walls of a blood vessel, with resultant stoppage of the blood flow. Clotting is one of the natural defence mechanisms of the body when injury occurs. A clot will usually form within 5 min after a blood vessel wall has been damaged. The exact process of clotting is not known; however, it is believed that the mechanism is triggered by the platelets, which disintegrate as they pass over rough places in the injured surface. If normal amounts of calcium, platelets and tissue factors are present (*see* diagram), pro-thrombin will be converted to thrombin. Thrombin then acts as a catalyst for the change of fibrinogen into a mesh of insoluble fibrin, in which are embedded erythrocytes and leukocytes and small amounts of fluid

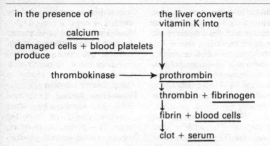

in the presence of

<u>calcium</u>

damaged cells + <u>blood platelets</u>
produce

thrombokinase ——→ <u>prothrombin</u>

the liver converts
vitamin K into

↓

thrombin + <u>fibrinogen</u>

↓

fibrin + <u>blood cells</u>

↓

clot + <u>serum</u>

CLOTTING OF BLOOD
Underlined substances are normally present in blood

Group	Antigen present in red cell	Antibody present in plasma
AB	A and B	—
A	A	Anti-B (β)
B	B	Anti-A (α)
O	—	Anti-A and Anti-B (α and β)

ABO SYSTEM

(serum). Plasma coagulation factors are:

I Fibrinogen
II Prothrombin
III Tissue thromboplastin
IV Calcium ions
VII Factor VII
VIII Antihaemophilic factor (AFH)
IX Christmas factor
X Stuart factor (Power factor)
XI Plasma thromboplastin antecedent (PTA)
XII Hageman factor
XIII Fibrin stabilizing factor

blood count the number of blood cells in a given sample of blood, usually expressed as the number of cells per litre of blood (as the red blood cell, white blood cell or platelet count). A differential white cell count determines the number of various types of leukocytes in a sample of blood. For range of normal values see Appendix 15.

blood group ABO system. In

clinical practice there are four main blood types: A, B, O and AB. In addition to this major grouping there is a rhesus (Rh) system that is important in the prevention of haemolytic disease of the newborn resulting from incompatibility of blood groups in mother and fetus. In determining blood group, a sample of blood is taken and mixed with specially prepared sera. One serum, anti-A agglutinin, causes blood of group A to agglutinate; another serum, anti-B agglutinin, causes blood of group B to agglutinate. Thus, if anti-A serum alone causes clumping, the blood is group A; if anti-B serum alone causes clumping, the blood group is B. If both cause clumping, the blood group is AB, and if it is not clumped by either, it is identified as group O. Transfusion with an incompatible ABO group will cause severe haemolytic reaction and death may occur.

blood pressure abbreviated BP. The pressure exerted on the artery walls by the blood as it flows through them. It can be measured in milligrams of mercury using a sphygmomanometer. Two readings are made. Arterial pressure fluctuates with each heart beat and one measure records the pressure whilst the heart is in systole (when the heart is ejecting blood into the arteries) and is the higher or systolic pressure. The other records while the heart is in diastole (when the aortic and pulmonary valves are closed and the heart is relaxed)

and is the lower or diastolic pressure. The range of normal blood pressure recording varies according to age and body size, but in the normal young adult is approximately: 100–120/70–80 mmHg.

blood sugar the amount of glucose present in the blood. The normal range is 2.5–4.7 mmol/litre. When the amount exceeds 10 mmol/litre, glucose is excreted in the urine, as in diabetes mellitus.

blood transfusion introduction of blood from the vein of one person (donor) or from a blood bank into the vein of another (recipient) in cases of severe loss of blood, trauma, septicaemia, etc. It is used to supplement the volume of blood and also to introduce constituents, such as clotting factors or antibodies, which are deficient in the patient. Clotting must be prevented in the transition stage. This is usually done by admixture with sodium citrate (1 g to 459 ml of blood). Too much sodium citrate tends to produce a reaction, and rigor and shock may occur.

blood urea excretory product of protein present in the blood. The normal range is 3–7 mmol/litre; this increases in renal failure when the kidneys cease to function normally.

'blue baby' (bloo) a child born with a very blue colour. The colour may be due to atelectasis or to a defect in the heart, in consequence of which arterial and venous blood become mixed. *See* FALLOT'S TETRALOGY.

blush (blush) growing redness of

the face, usually a reaction to emotion or heat.

BMR basal metabolic rate.

Bobath technique ('bohbahth, -bath) an approach to the treatment of neurological conditions developed by Dr and Mrs Bobath. It aims to facilitate movement by inhibiting abnormal tone, abnormal patterns of movement and abnormal balance reactions.

body ('bodee) 1. the trunk, or animal frame, with its organs. 2. the largest and most important part of any organ. 3. any mass or collection of material.

body image the total concept, including conscious and unconscious feelings, thoughts and perceptions, that a person has of his or her own body as an object in space, which is independent and apart from other objects.

body language the expression of thoughts or emotions by means of posture or gestures.

Boeck's disease (beks) *C.P.M. Boeck, Norwegian dermatologist, 1845–1917.* Sarcoidosis.

boil (boyl) an acute staphylococcal inflammation of the skin and subcutaneous tissues round a hair follicle. It causes a painful swelling with a central core of dead tissue (SLOUGH), which is eventually discharged. A furuncle.

bolus ('bohləs) 1. a large pill. 2. a rounded mass of masticated food immediately before being swallowed or one passing through the intestines. 3. a quantity of a drug injected directly to raise its concentration in the blood to a therapeutic level.

bonding ('bonding) the attachment process that occurs between an infant and its parents, especially the mother, during the first hours and days following birth. Bonding is a reciprocal process and is a biological need for both the future physical and emotional development of the infant.

bone (bohn) the dense connective tissue forming the skeleton. It is composed of cartilage or membrane impregnated with mineral salts, chiefly calcium phosphate and calcium carbonate. This is arranged as an outer hard compact tissue and an inner network of cells (CANCELLOUS tissue), in the spaces of which is red bone marrow. In the shaft of long bones is a medullary cavity containing yellow marrow. Microscopically, the bone tissue is perforated with minute (HAVERSIAN) canals containing blood vessels and lymphatics for the maintenance and repair of the cells. Bone is covered by a fibrous membrane, the PERIOSTEUM, containing blood vessels and by which the bone grows in girth. *B. graft* transplantation of a healthy piece of bone to replace missing or repair defective bone. *B. marrow* substance which fills the marrow cavities of bones. Basically there are two types, yellow and red marrow. The red marrow is responsible for producing the blood cells. *B. marrow transplantation* a procedure used to treat aplastic anaemia, acute leukaemia and some rare congenital disorders with varying success.

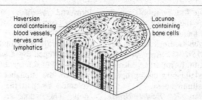

Haversian canal containing blood vessels, nerves and lymphatics

Lacunae containing bone cells

STRUCTURE OF COMPACT BONE

Healthy bone marrow is taken from the donor and infused into the blood stream of the recipient, where it 'homes' into the bone marrow where it will grow. Histocompatibility between the donor (usually a sibling) and recipient is essential.

borax ('bor·raks) a compound of soda and boric acid. Used as a mild antiseptic and as a mouthwash.

borborygmus (,bawbə'rigməs) a rumbling sound caused by gas in the intestines.

Bordetella (,bawdə'telə) a genus of bacteria. *B. pertussis* the causal agent of whooping cough.

boric acid ('bor·rik) a mild antiseptic.

Bornholm disease ('bawn,holm) an epidemic myalgia with pleural pain due to Coxsackie virus infection. It is named from the Danish island of Bornholm where there was an outbreak in 1930.

botulism ('botyuh,lizəm, 'bochə-) an extremely severe form of food poisoning due to a neurotoxin (botulin) produced by *Clostridium botulinum*, sometimes found in improperly canned or preserved foods. The symptoms include

vomiting, abdominal pain, headache, weakness, constipation, and nerve paralysis, which causes difficulty in seeing, breathing, and swallowing. Death is usually due to paralysis of the respiratory organs.

bougie ('boozhee, boo'zhee) a flexible cylindrical instrument used to dilate a stricture, as in the oesophagus or urethra. *Medicated b.* a soluble form impregnated with a medicinal substance. Used for urethral treatment.

bovine ('bohvien) relating to the cow or ox. *B. tuberculosis* that caused by infection from infected cows' milk, usually affecting glands and bones.

bowel ('bowəl) the intestine. *B. sounds* relatively high-pitched abdominal sounds caused by the propulsion of the intestinal contents through the lower alimentary tract.

bowleg ('boh,leg) deformity where there is an outward curvature of one or both legs near the knee. This results in a gap between the knees on standing. Genu varum.

Bowman's capsule ('bohmənz) *Sir W.P. Bowman, British physician, 1816–1892.* The expanded end of the kidney tubule which surrounds the glomerulus.

Boyle's anaesthetic machine (boylz) *H.E.G. Boyle, British surgeon, 1875-1941.* Apparatus by which chloroform, ether, nitrous oxide gas and now cyclopropane may be administered.

Boyle's law *R. Boyle, British physicist, 1627-1691.* Law stating that at any determined temperature a known mass of gas varies in volume inversely as the pressure.

Bq symbol for *becquerel*.

brace (brays) 1. a support used in orthopaedics to hold parts of the body in their correct positions. 2. an orthodontic appliance to correct the alignment of teeth.

brachial ('brayki·əl, 'brak-) relating to the arm. *B. artery* the continuation of the axillary artery along the inner side of the upper arm. *B. plexus* a network of nerves at the root of the neck supplying the upper limb.

brachium ('brayki·əm) the arm, especially from shoulder to elbow.

brachycephaly (,braki'kefəlee, -'sef-) the state of having a head shape in which the anteroposterior diameter is relatively short.

brachytherapy (,braki'therəpee) radiotherapy delivered into or adjacent to a tumour by means of an intracavitary or interstitial radioactive source.

bradycardia (,bradi'kahdi·ə) abnormally low rate of heart contractions and consequent slow pulse.

bradykinin (,bradi'kinin) peptide formed from the degradation of protein by enzymes. It is a powerful vasodilator which also causes contraction of smooth muscle.

braille ('brayl) a method of printing developed by *Louis Braille (1809–1852)* for the blind. Letters of the alphabet are represented by patterns of raised dots. These dots are read by passing the finger tips over them.

brain (brayn) that part of the central nervous system contained in the skull. It consists of the cerebrum, midbrain, cerebellum, medulla oblongata and pons varolii.

bran (bran) the husk of grain. The coarse outer coat of cereals. High in roughage and vitamins of the B complex. Frequently recommended as a dietary component both for those with alimentary disorders and for those in normal health.

branchial ('brangki·əl) relating to the clefts (branchia) that are present in the neck and pharynx in the developing embryo. Normally they disappear. *B. cyst.* a cystic swelling arising from a branchial remnant in the neck. *B. sinus (lateral cervical sinus)* a track leading from the posterior cervical region to open in the lower neck in front of the sternomastoid muscle.

Braun's frame ('brawnz fraym) *H.F.W. Braun, German surgeon, 1862–1934.* A metal frame which incorporates one or more pulleys and is used to elevate the lower limb and to apply skeletal traction for a compound fracture of tibia and fibula.

Braxton Hicks contractions

('brakstən 'hiks) *Braxton Hicks, British gynaecologist, 1823–1897.* Painless uterine contractions occurring during pregnancy, becoming increasingly rhythmic and intense during the third trimester. Sometimes called 'false labour'.

breast (brest) 1. the anterior or front region of the chest. 2. the mammary gland. *B. abscess* formation of pus in the mammary gland. *B. bone* the sternum. *B. cancer* the breast is the most common site of malignant tumours in women. In the United Kingdom 13 000 women a year die of this condition and although the survival rates for breast cancer continue to increase, albeit slowly, the incidence of the disease in the western world increases. Improvement in these survival rates has come from increased public awareness, breast self-examination, breast screening programmes, and improved methods of treatment. Women should train themselves to perform a simple self-examination of the breasts, described in the accompanying diagrams. The best time for this is just after menstruation when the breasts are normally soft. If any lump in the breast can be felt, a doctor should be consulted immediately. More than 90 per cent of breast cancers are discovered by the patients themselves. *B. feeding* the method of feeding a baby with milk directly from the mother's breasts. Most paediatricians agree that breast feeding is usually better for baby and mother, both physically and emotionally. *Pigeon b.* prominent sternum, a deformity resulting from rickets. *B. pump* an apparatus for removal of milk from the breast.

breath (breth) the air taken in and expelled by the expansion and contraction of the thorax.

breathing ('breedhing) the alternate inspiration and expiration of air into and out of the lungs (*see also* RESPIRATION).

breech (breech) the buttocks. *B. presentation* a position of the fetus in the uterus such that the buttocks present.

bregma ('bregmə) the anterior fontanelle. The membranous junction between the coronal and sagittal sutures.

bridge (brij) in dentistry, an irremovable prosthesis carrying false teeth that bridges gaps left when natural teeth are extracted.

Bright's disease (briets) *B. Bright, British physician, 1789–1858.* A broad description, once used for inflammation of the kidneys. Nephritis.

brilliant green ('brili·ənt) an aniline dye used as an antiseptic.

British National Formulary ('british 'nashən'l 'fawmuhlə·ree) abbreviated BNF. A publication produced twice a year by the British Medical Association and The Pharmaceutical Society of Great Britain, containing details of nearly all the drugs currently available on prescription in the United Kingdom.

British Pharmacopoeia (,british ,fahməkə'peeə) abbreviated BP. List of 'official' drugs which is

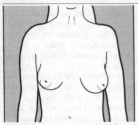

Any change in the shape and size of either breast or nipple should first be noted by looking in the mirror

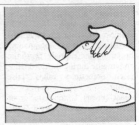

Lying down with a pillow or towel placed under the shoulder helps to spread the breast tissue for easier self examination

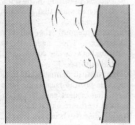

In front of the mirror, and with arms raised, view the breasts from different angles

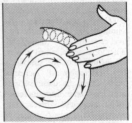

Rotate fingers in small circles and trace a spiral route around the breast to check for any lumps or unusual thickening

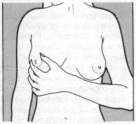

Squeeze each nipple gently, noting any discharge or bleeding

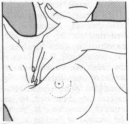

Finally, examine the armpits using the spiral technique and note any unusual findings

BREAST SELF EXAMINATION

published by HM Stationery Office. The drugs are listed on the recommendations of the Medicines Commission in accordance with the Medicines Act 1968.

broad ligaments (‚brawd) folds of peritoneum extending from the uterus to the sides of the pelvis, and supporting the blood vessels to the uterus and uterine tubes.

Broca's area of speech ('brohkəz) *P.P. Broca, French surgeon, 1824–1880.* The motor centre for speech, situated in the left cerebral hemisphere. Damage to the nerve cells contained in it can impair speech.

Brodie's abscess (‚brohdiz) *Sir B.C. Brodie, British surgeon, 1783–1862.* A chronic abscess of bone.

bromhidrosis (‚bromhi'drohsis) offensive and fetid sweat.

bromide ('brohmied) a compound of bromine. Bromides are sedatives that are strongly depressant and cumulative in action.

bromocriptine (‚brohmoh,kripteen) a dopamine agonist used in the treatment of parkinsonism in cases where levodopa is not well tolerated.

Brompton cocktail ('bromptən 'koktayl) name given to mixtures containing various combinations of morphine, diamorphine and cocaine. These mixtures often contained gin and/or chlorpromazine. They were used in the relief of pain in terminal care. They have now been replaced by a simple solution of morphine in chloroform water.

bromsulphthalein (‚bromsulf-'thayleen) a dye used in certain tests for liver function.

bronchi ('brongkee) plural of bronchus.

bronchiectasis (‚brongki'ehtəsis) chronic dilatation of the bronchi and bronchioles with secondary infection, usually involving the lower lobes of the lung. The condition may occur as a congenital malformation of the alveoli with resultant dilatation of the terminal bronchi. Most often it is an acquired disease secondary to partial obstruction of the bronchi with necrotizing infection. The symptoms include a chronic cough and purulent sputum.

bronchiole ('brongki'ohl) one of the smallest of the subdivisions of the bronchi.

bronchiolitis (‚brongkioh'lietis) inflammation of the bronchioles.

bronchitis (brong'kietis) inflammation of the bronchi. *Acute b.* a short-lived infection, common in young children and the elderly. It is a descending infection from the common cold, influenza, measles and other upper respiratory condition. *Chronic b.* a chronic infection, usually association with infection of the upper respiratory tract. It may in time lead to emphysema.

bronchoadenitis (‚brongkoh,adə-'nietis) inflammation of the bronchial glands.

bronchodilator (‚brongkohdie-'laytə) any agent that causes dilatation of the bronchi.

bronchography (brong'kogrəfee) radiography of the bronchial tree after introduction of a radio-opaque medium.

bronchomycosis (ˌbrongkohmie-
'kohsis) an industrial disease
chiefly affecting agricultural workers, stablemen, etc., and due to
inhalation of microfungi which
infect the airpassages. Causes can
be *Actinomyces* or *Aspergillus*
species. Symptoms are similar to
those of pulmonary tuberculosis.

bronchophony (brong'kofənee)
resonance of the voice as heard
in the chest over the bronchi on
auscultation.

bronchopneumonia (ˌbrongkoh-
nyoo'mohni·ə) *see* PNEUMONIA.

bronchopulmonary (ˌbrongkoh-
'pulmənə·ree, -'puhl) relating to
the lungs, bronchi and bronchioles.

bronchorrhoea (ˌbrongkə'reeə) an
excessive discharge of mucus
from the bronchi.

bronchoscope ('brongkoh,skohp)
an endoscope which enables the
operator to see inside the bronchi. It can also be used to wash
out the bronchi, to remove foreign bodies or to take a biopsy.

bronchoscopy (brong'koskə,pee)
examination of the bronchi by
means of a bronchoscope.

bronchospasm (ˌbrongkoh,spaz-
əm) difficulty in breathing caused
by the sudden constriction of
plain muscle in the walls of the
bronchi. This may arise in
asthma or chronic bronchitis.

bronchospirometer (ˌbrongkoh-
spise'romitə) an instrument used
to measure the capacity of one
lung or of one lobe of the lung,
or of each lung separately.

bronchotracheal (ˌbrongkoh-
'traki·əl, -trə'keeəl) relating to
both the trachea and the bronchi.

B. suction the removal of mucus
with the aid of suction.

bronchus (ˌbrongkəs) any of the
larger passages conveying air to
(right or left principal bronchus)
and within the lungs (lobar and
segmental bronchi).

Broviac catheter ('brohviak-
ˌkathətə) trade name for a special
catheter used to provide a central
venous line.

brow (brow) the forehead. *B. presentation* a position of the fetus
such that the forehead appears at
the cervix first.

brown fat (brown) special type
of adipose tissue found in the
newborn infant, and which is
widely distributed throughout
the body. The tissue is highly
vascular and owes its colour to
the large number of mitochondria
found in the cytoplasm of its
cells. It allows the infant to
increase its metabolic rate and
thus its heat production when
subjected to cold. At the same
time the fat itself is used up.

Brown-Séquard's syndrome
(brown 'saykahdz) *C.E. Brown-
Séquard, French physiologist,
1818–1894.* Paralysis and loss of
discriminatory and joint sensation on one side of the body
and of pain and temperature sensation on the other, due to a
lesion involving one side of the
spinal cord.

Brucella (broo'selə) a genus of
bacteria primarily pathogenic in
animals but which may affect
man.

brucellosis (ˌbroosi'lohsis) a generalized infection involving primarily the reticuloendothelial sys-

tem, marked by remittent undulant fever, malaise, headache, and anaemia. It is caused by various species of *Brucella* and is transmitted to man from domestic animals such as pigs, goats, and cattle, especially through infected milk or contact with the carcass of an infected animal. The disease is also called undulant fever because one of the major symptoms in man is a fever that fluctuates widely at regular intervals. Prevention is best accomplished by the pasteurization of milk and a programme of testing, vaccination, and elimination of infected animals. Called also Malta fever, abortus fever and Mediterranean fever.

Brudzinski's sign (broo'jinskiz) *J. Brudzinski, Polish physician, 1874–1917.* 1. passive flexion of one thigh causing spontaneous flexion of the opposite thigh. 2. flexion of the neck causing bilateral flexion of the hips and knees. These signs are indicative of meningeal irritation.

bruise (brooz) a superficial injury to tissues produced by sudden impact in which the skin is unbroken. A contusion.

bruit ('brooee) [Fr.] an abnormal sound or murmur heard on auscultation of the heart and large vessels.

Brunner's glands ('bruhnəz) *J.C. Brunner, Swiss anatomist, 1653–1727.* Small compound tubular glands in the mucous membrane of the duodenum.

Brunus edwardii the urban, companion animal bear, much admired for its low food require-ments and excellent house training, a high emotional output and complete freedom from disease. Called also *Ursus theodorus* (USA) and Pooh, Paddington or Brideshead bear (UK).

bruxism ('brooksizəm) teeth clenching, particularly during sleep. This occurs in persons under tension and may cause headaches due to muscle fatigue.

bubo ('byooboh) inflammation of the lymphatic glands of the axilla or groin. Typical of bubonic plague (*see* PLAGUE) and venereal infections.

bubonocele (byoo'boinə,seel) an inguinal hernia in the groin, resembling a bubo.

buccal ('buk'l) pertaining to the cheek or to the mouth.

buccinator ('buksi,naytə) a muscle of the cheek, between the mandible and the maxilla.

Budd–Chiari syndrome (,budki-'ahri) *G. Budd, British physician, 1808–1882; H. Chiari, Austrian pathologist, 1851–1916.* A condition in which thrombosis of the hepatic vein causes vomiting, jaundice, enlargement of the liver and ascites.

Buerger's disease ('bərgəz) *L. Buerger, American physician, 1879–1943.* Thromboangiitis obliterans.

buffer ('bufə) 1. a physical or physiological system which tends to oppose change within that system, e.g. the reflexes involved in blood pressure homeostasis. 2. a chemical system that acts to prevent change in the concentration of another chemical substance. Sodium bicarbonate is the chief buffer of the blood and tissue fluids. 3. anything that is used to reduce shock or jarring upon contact.

buggery ('bugǝ·ree) anal intercourse, either heterosexual or homosexual. In law the term also includes sexual contact with an animal.

bulbar ('bulbǝ) pertaining to the medulla oblongata. *B. paralysis see* PARALYSIS.

bulbourethral (,bulbohyuh'reethrǝl) relating to the bulb of the urethra (bulb of the penis). *B. glands* small glands opening into the male urethra. Cowper's glands.

bulimia (byoo'limi·ǝ) abnormal increase in the sensation of hunger. *B. nervosa* a pattern of 'binge eating', or episodes of uncontrolled and compulsive overeating occurring in response to stress. Bulimic 'binges' often occur in anorexia nervosa.

bulla ('buhlǝ) a large, fluid-containing blister.

bumetanide (byoo'metǝ,nied) a diuretic drug which prevents the resorption of urine from Henle's loop in the renal tubule.

bundle ('bund'l) a collection of nerve fibres all running in the same direction. *B. branch block* the delay in conduction along either branch of the atrioventricular bundle of the heart. The abnormality is detected by an ECG recording.

bundle of His ('bund'l ǝ 'his) L. *His Jr, German physiologist, 1863–1934.* The band of neuromuscular fibres which, passing through the septum of the heart,

divides at the apex into two parts, these being distributed into the wall of the ventricles. The impulse of contraction is conducted through the structure. Atrioventricular bundle.

bunion ('bunyǝn) a prominence of the head of the metatarsal bone at its junction with the great toe, caused by inflammation and swelling of the bursa at that joint. Usually due to shoes which distort the natural shape of the foot.

buphthalmos (buf'thalmǝs) abnormal enlargement of the eyes in congenital GLAUCOMA.

Burkitt's tumour (bǝrkits) *D.P. Burkitt, Irish surgeon, b. 1911.* African lymphoma. A lymphosarcoma, frequently of the jaw, occurring almost exclusively in children living in low-lying moist areas. Occurs in New Guinea and central Africa. The Epstein–Barr virus (EB virus), a herpesvirus, has been isolated from Burkitt's lymphoma cells in culture, and has been implicated as a causative agent.

burn (bǝrn) an injury to tissues caused by: (1) physical agents, the sun, excess heat or cold, friction, nuclear radiations; (2) chemical agents, acids or caustic alkalis; (3) electrical current. Burns are described as being partial thickness (involving only the epidermis) or full thickness (involving the dermis and underlying structures). Clinically, emphasis is placed on the percentage of the body area affected by the burn. The treatment of shock and prevention of infection and malnutrition need special attention.

burn out a term used to describe the result of chronic stress on members of the helping professions. Burn out is characterized by chronic low energy, defensiveness and emergence of manoeuvres designed to create distance between helper and patient/client. Dissatisfaction and tension may be carried over from the work situation into the personal one and self-esteem and confidence may suffer badly.

burr (bər) a bit for a surgical drill, used for cutting bone or teeth. *B. hole* a circular hole drilled in the cranium to permit access to the brain or to release raised intercranial pressure.

bursa ('bərsə) a small sac of fibrous tissue, lined with synovial membrane and containing synovial fluid. It is situated between parts that move upon one another at a joint to reduce friction.

bursitis (bər'sitis) inflammation of the bursa. It produces pain and may impede movement of the joint. *Prepatellar b.* housemaid's knee.

Buscopan ('buskəpan) trade name for a preparation of hyoscine butylbromide. An anti-spasmodic which relaxes smooth muscle in the gastrointestinal tract.

busulphan (byoo'sulfan) a cytotoxic drug that depresses the bone marrow and may be used to treat myeloid leukaemia.

butobarbitone (,byootoh'bahbi,tohn) an intermediate-acting barbiturate, formerly much used as a sedative. Now used only in severe insomnia.

buttock ('butək) either of the two prominences formed by the flesh-covered gluteal muscles at either side of the lower spine.

butyrophenone (,byootiroh'fee-nohn) a chemical class of major tranquillizers especially useful in the treatment of manic and moderate to severe agitated states and in the control of the vocal utterances and tics of GILLES DE LA TOURETTE'S SYNDROME.

bypass ('bie,pahs) diversion of flow. Formation of a shunt. *Aortocoronary b.* diversion of flow from the aorta to the coronary arteries via a saphenous vein or artificial graft. *Femoropopliteal b.* diversion of flow from the femoral to the popliteal artery to overcome an occlusion.

byssinosis (,bisi'nohsis) an industrial disease caused by inhalation of cotton or linen dust in factories. A type of pneumoconiosis.

C

C symbol for carbon, centigrade or celsius, and cytosine.

Ca symbol for *calcium*.

cachectic (kə'kektik) pertaining to cachexia.

cachet (ka'shay, 'ka-) [Fr.] two pieces of wafer, joined in the form of a capsule to contain an unpalatable medicine.

cachexia (kə'keksi·ə) a condition of extreme debility. The patient is emaciated, the skin being loose and wrinkled from rapid wasting, but shiny and tense over bone. The eyes are sunken, the skin yellowish, and there is a grey 'muddy' complexion. The mucous membranes are pale and anaemia is extreme. The condition is typical of the late stages of chronic diseases.

cadaver (kə'davə, -'day-) a corpse. The dead body used for dissection.

cadmium ('kadmi·əm) symbol Cd. A metallic element. Inhalation of fumes from the molten metal can cause lung irritation and, in the long term, renal impairment.

caecostomy (see'kostəmee) the making of a surgical fistula into the caecum by incision through the abdominal wall.

caecum ('seekəm) the blind pouch forming the beginning of the large intestine. The vermiform appendix is attached to it.

caesarean section (si'zairi·ən) delivery of a fetus by an incision through the abdominal wall and uterus. Should not be done before the 28th week of gestation. Performed for the safety of either the mother or the infant. Tradition has it that Julius Caesar was born in this way.

caesium ('seezi·əm) symbol Cs. A metallic element. *C.-137* radioactive caesium; a fission product from uranium. Sealed in a suitable container it can be used instead of cobalt for beam therapy; or sealed in needles, tubes or applicators it can be used for local application.

café-au-lait spot ('kafay oh 'lay) pigmented macules of a distinctive light brown colour, like coffee with milk, as in neurofibromatosis and Albright's syndrome.

caffeine ('kafeen, 'kafi,een) an alkaloid of tea and coffee which acts as a nerve stimulant and diuretic. Mixed with aspirin and codeine, it is often used as an analgesic.

caffeinism (kaf,ee·inizəm) an agitated state due to the excessive ingestion of caffeine.

caisson disease ('kays'n) decompression sickness.

calamine ('kalə,mien) preparation of zinc carbonate or zinc oxide coloured pink with ferric oxide. It is an astringent and antipruritic used in lotion or ointment form for skin diseases.

calcaneum (kal'kayni·əm) the heel bone. Calcaneus.

calcareous (kal'kair·ri·əs) chalky. Containing lime.

calciferol (kal'sifə·rol) the chemical name for vitamin D.

calcification (,kalsifi'kayshən) 1. the deposit of lime in any tissue, e.g. in the formation of callus. 2. the deposit of lime salts in cartilage as part of the normal process of bone formation. *Dystrophic c.* the deposition of calcium in abnormal tissue, such as scar tissue or atherosclerotic plaques, without abnormalities of blood calcium.

calcitonin (,kalsi'tohnin) a polypeptide hormone produced by the parafollicular or C cells of the thyroid gland which regulates blood calcium levels.

calcium ('kalsi·əm) *symbol* Ca. A metallic element necessary for the normal development and functioning of the body. Calcium is the most abundant mineral in the body; it is a constituent of bones and teeth. Deficiency or excess of serum calcium causes nerve and muscle dysfunctions and abnormalities in blood clotting. The correct concentration is regulated by hormones. *C. carbonate* chalk; *C. gluconate* used as an antacid. A compound that is easily absorbed and can be given by intramuscular or intravenous route to raise the blood calcium. *C. lactate* a compound that increases the coagulability of

blood; used orally as a calcium supplement.

calculus ('kalkyuhləs) a stony concretion which may be formed in any of the secreting organs of the body or their ducts. *Arthritic c.* gouty deposits in or near joints. *Biliary c.* gallstone. *Coral c.* a large stone in the kidney, with branches resembling coral. *Mulberry c.* a gallstone made of calcium oxalate and shaped like a mulberry. *Renal c.* one formed in the kidney. *Salivary c.* stone in a salivary duct. *Staghorn c.* a many-branched stone sometimes found in the renal pelvis. *Urinary c.* one found anywhere in the urinary tract. *Vesical c.* stone formed in the urinary bladder.

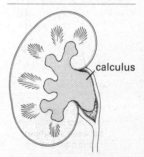

calculus

STAGHORN CALCULUS

Caldwell–Luc operation (,kawld-wel'look) *G.W. Caldwell, American otolaryngologist, 1834–1918; H. Luc, French laryngologist, 1855–1925.* An antrostomy operation to drain the maxillary sinus.

calibrator (,kali,braytə) 1. an

instrument for measuring the size of openings. 2. an instrument used to dilate a tube, e.g. in urethral stricture.

caliper ('kalipə) a two-pronged instrument that may be used to exert traction on a part. *Walking c.* an appliance fitted to a boot or shoe to give support to the lower limb. It may be used when the muscles are paralysed or in the repair stage of fractures.

ceps muscle, is pinched away from the underlying muscle using the thumb and forefinger.

callisthenics (ˌkalis'theniks) mild gymnastics for developing the muscles and producing a graceful carriage.

callosity (kə'lositee) the plaques of thickened skin often seen on the soles of the feet or the palms of the hand.

callous ('kaləs) hard and thicken-

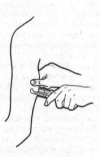

Triceps skinfold is measured at midpoint between acromion and olecranon

Skin is pinched and calipers are placed over skinfold

SKINFOLD CALIPERS

calipers ('kalipəz) compasses for measuring diameters and curved surfaces *Skinfold c.* an instrument used in nutritional assessment for determining the amount of body fat. A fold of skin and subcutaneous tissue, usually over the tri-

ed.

callus ('kaləs) 1. a callosity. 2. the tissue which grows round fractured ends of bone and develops into new bone to repair the injury.

Calmette–Guérin bacillus (ˌkalmet ge,ranh bə'siləs) *A.L.C. Cal-mette, French bacteriologist, 1863–1933; C. Guérin, French bacteriologist, 1872–1961.* A deactivated tuberculosis bacillus from which the antituberculosis vaccine, BCG vaccine, is made.

calor ('kalə) [L.] *heat;* one of the signs of inflammation.

caloric (ka'lor·rik, 'kalə·rik) pertaining to heat or calories.

calorie ('kalə·ree) *symbol* cal. A unit of heat. Used to denote physiological values of various food substances, estimated according to the amount of heat they produce on being oxidized in the body. *See* OXIDATION. A calorie (or kilocalorie) represents the heat required in raising 1 kg (1000 g or 2.2 lb) of water by 1°C. A small calorie equals the heat produced in raising 1 g of water by 1°C. In the SI system the calorie is replaced by the joule (1 cal = 4.18 kJ).

calorific (,kalə'rifik) heat-producing.

calorimeter (,kalə'rimitə) an apparatus for measuring the heat that is produced or lost during a chemical or physical change.

calvaria (kal'vair·ri·ə) the upper, dome-like part of the skull.

calvities (kal'vishi,eez) baldness.

calx (kalks) calcium oxide or lime. The basis of slaked lime, bleaching powder and quick-lime.

calyx ('kayliks, 'kal-) any cup-shaped vessel or part. *C. of kidney* the cup-like terminations of the ureter in the renal pelvis surrounding the pyramids of the kidney.

camphor ('kamfə) a crystalline substance prepared from the camphor laurel. It is used internally as a carminative. *Camphor-ated oil* is 1 part camphor to 4 parts of oil prepared for external application as a rubefacient.

Campylobacter ('kampiloh,baktə) a genus of bacteria, family Spirill-laceae, made up of Gram-negative, non-spore-forming, motile, spirally curved rods. Causes an acute intestinal illness lasting several days. Usually associated with unpasteurized milk, partially cooked meat and poultry.

canal (kə'nal) a tubular passage. *Alimentary c.* the passage along which the food passes on its way through the body. *Cervical c.* that through the cervix of the uterus. *Haversian c.* one of the minute channels that are present in bone. *C. of Schlemm* that which drains the aqueous humour. *Semicircular c.* one of the three canals in the middle ear responsible for maintenance of balance.

canaliculus (,kanə'likyuhləs) a small channel or canal.

cancellous ('kansələs) being porous or spongy. Applied to the honeycomb type of bone tissue in the ends of long bones and in flat and irregular bones.

cancer ('kansə) a general term to describe malignant growths in tissue, of which CARCINOMA is of epithelial and SARCOMA of connective tissue origin, as in bone and muscle. A cancerous growth is one which is not encapsulated, but infiltrates into surrounding tissues, the cells of which it replaces by its own. It is spread by the lymph and blood vessels and causes metastases in other parts of the body. Death is caused by destruction of organs to a degree incompatible with life, to extreme debility and anaemia, or to haemorrhage.

cancroid ('kangkroid) 1. resembling cancer. 2. a skin tumour of moderate degree of malignancy.

cancrum oris (,kangkrəm'or·ris) gangrenous stomatitis. An ulceration of the mouth which is a rare complication of measles in debilitated children. Noma.

candela (kan'deelə, -'daylə) 1. SI unit of luminous intensity; *symbol* cd. 2. a medicinal candle used in fumigation.

Candida ('kandidə) a genus of small fungi, formerly called *Monilia. C. albicans* the variety which causes candidiasis.

candidiasis (,kandi'dieəsis) infection, by the *Candida* fungus. Occurs particularly in moist areas such as mouth, vagina, skin folds. Popularly known as thrush. Candidiasis can occur as a result of a debilitating illness or immunosuppressive therapy and/or cytotoxic drugs. The infection may also occur as a result of disturbed intestinal flora and in pregnancy. Oral infection may be due to poor hygiene, carious teeth or badly fitting dentures.

canine ('kaynien) 1. pertaining to a dog. 2. an 'eye tooth'. There are two in each jaw between the incisors and the molars.

cannabis ('kanəbis) an illegal drug which may be swallowed or smoked and produces hallucinations and a temporary sense of well-being, followed by extreme lethargy. Slang terms for cannabis include marijuana, hashish, hash, grass, pot, the weed, ganga, kaya, kif, and bhang.

cannula ('kanyuhlə) a hollow tube for insertion into the body by which fluids are introduced or removed. Usually a trocar is fitted into it to facilitate its introduction.

cantharides (kan'thari,deez, kən-) an extract from the body of the Spanish fly, applied externally as a counterirritant to raise a blister. Now rarely used.

canthus ('kanthəs) the angle formed by the junction of the upper and lower eyelids.

CAPD CONTINUOUS AMBULATORY PERITONEAL DIALYSIS.

capeline bandage ('kayplien) a caplike covering of two interwoven bandages used for protecting the head or a limb stump.

capillarity (,kapi'laritee) the action by which a liquid will rise upwards in a fibrous substance or in a fine tube. Capillary attraction.

capillary (kə'pilə·ree) 1. hair-like. 2. a minute vessel connecting an arteriole and a venule. 3. a minute vessel of the lymphatic system.

capitellum (,kapi'teləm) capitulum. 1. the small rounded head at the elbow end of the humerus. 2. the bulb of a hair.

capreomycin (,kaprioh'miesin) a polypeptide antibiotic produced by *Streptomyces capreolus*, which is active against human strains of *Myobacterium tuberculosis* and has four microbiologically active components.

capsular ('kapsyuhlə) relating to a capsule. *C. ligaments* those which completely surround a movable joint, forming a capsule which loosely encloses the bones and is lined with synovial membrane which secretes a fluid for lubrication of the articular surfaces. Called also articular capsule.

capsule ('kapsyool) 1. a fibrous or membranous sac enclosing an organ. 2. a small soluble case of gelatin in which a nauseous medicine may be enclosed. 3. the gelatinous envelope which surrounds and protects some bacteria.

capsulectomy (,kapsyuh'lektə-mee) surgical excision of a capsule.

capsulitis (,kapsyuh'lietis) inflammation of the capsule of a joint.

capsulotomy (,kapsyuh'lotəmee) the incision of a capsule, particularly that of a joint or of the lens of the eye.

caput ('kaputt) head. *C. succedaneum* a transient soft swelling on an infant's head, due to pressure during labour, which disappears within the first few days of life.

carbachol ('kahbə,kol) a drug related to and acting like acetylcholine, but more stable. It causes contraction of plain muscle and relaxation of the voluntary sphincter, so relieving postoperative retention of urine. Also used in the treatment of glaucoma.

carbamazepine (,kahbə'mazi,peen) a drug used to control epilepsy and also to relieve pain; used in the treatment of trigeminal neuralgia.

carbaminohaemoglobin (kah,ba-minoh,heemə'glohbin) a compound of carbon dioxide and haemoglobin, present in the blood.

carbenicillin ('kahbeni'silin) a synthetic penicillin which is principally used in the treatment of serious infections caused by *Pseudomonas aeruginosa* and other Gram-negative organisms. Large doses, which need to be given intravenously, are required to obtain sufficiently high concentrations in the blood and tissues to be effective.

carbenoxolone (,kahbe'noksə-,lohn) an anti-inflammatory drug used in the treatment of gastric ulcers.

carbidopa (,kahbi'dohpa) an inhibitor of the decarboxylation of levodopa (L-dopa) in peripheral tissues, which does not cross the blood–brain barrier. It is used in combination with levodopa to control the symptoms of PARKINSON'S DISEASE. In the presence of carbidopa, levodopa enters the brain in larger quantities, thus avoiding the need for excessively high doses of it.

carbimazole (kah'bimə,zohl) an antithyroid drug that is used to stabilize a patient with thyrotoxicosis.

carbo ('kahboh) charcoal. *C. ligni* medicinal wood charcoal. Used for the relief of digestive disorders and diarrhoea.

carbohydrate (,kahboh'hiedrayt) a compound of carbon, hydrogen, and oxygen. Carbohydrates are classified into mono-, di-, tri-, poly- and heterosaccharides. In food they are an important and immediate source of energy for the body; 1 g of carbohydrate yields 17 kJ (4 kcal). They are synthesized by all green plants. In the body they are absorbed immediately or stored in the form of glycogen.

carbolic acid (kah'bolik) phenol.

carbon ('kahbən) *symbol* C. A non-metallic element. *C. dioxide* a gas which, dissolved in water, forms weak carbonic acid. As a product of metabolism by the oxidation of carbon, it leaves the body by the lungs. It can be compressed till it freezes, and then forms a solid (carbon dioxide snow) used as an escharotic in various skin conditions. Also known as dry ice. Inhalations of the gas in a 5–7, mixture with oxygen are useful to stimulate the depth of respiration. *C. monoxide* a colourless gas that is very poisonous. It is a major constituent of coal gas and is usually present in the exhaust gases from petrol and diesel engines. In poisoning there is vertigo, flushed faced with very red lips, loss of consciousness, and convulsions. The blood is bright red because of the formation of carboxyhaemoglobin. *C. tetrachloride* a powerful anthelmintic used in treating hookworm and whipworm. Used also in cleaning fluids; the inhalation of its vapours in solvent abuse can depress central nervous system activity and cause degeneration of the liver and kidneys.

carbonic anhydrase (kah'bonik an'hiedrayz) an enzyme that cata-

lyses the decomposition of carbonic acid into carbon dioxide and water, facilitating transfer of carbon dioxide from tissues to blood and from blood to alveolar air.

carboxyhaemoglobin (kah'boksi-,heemə'glohbin) the combination of carbon monoxide with haemoglobin in the blood in carbon monoxide poisoning.

carbuncle ('kahbungk'l) an acute staphylococcal inflammation of subcutaneous tissues, which causes local thrombosis in the veins and death of tissue with several discharging sinuses. In appearance it resembles a collection of boils

carcinogen ('kahsinə,jen, kah-'sinəjən) any substance or agent which can produce a cancer.

carcinogenic (,kahsinoh'jenik) pertaining to substances or agents which produce or predispose to cancer. Crude oils are said to contain a *c. factor*.

carcinoid ('kahsi,noyd) a tumour of the small intestine, appendix, stomach or colon. Although potentially malignant the majority behave as benign tumours. *C. syndrome* a symptom complex associated with carcinoid tumours, marked by attacks of severe cyanotic flushing of the skin lasting from minutes to days and by diarrhoeal watery stools, bronchoconstrictive attacks, sudden drops in blood pressure, oedema, and ascites. Symptoms are caused by serotonin, prostaglandins, and other biologically active substances secreted by the tumour.

carcinoma (ˌkahsi'nohmə) a malignant growth of epithelial tissue. Microscopically the cells resemble those of the tissue in which the growth has arisen. *Adenoic c.* adenocarcinoma. *Basal cell c.* a rodent ulcer (*see* ULCER). *Epithelial c.* epithelioma. *Squamous cell c.* one arising from the squamous epithelium of the skin.

carcinomatosis (ˌkahsi,nohmə-'tohsis) the condition when a carcinoma has given rise to widespread metastases.

cardia ('kahd·ə) the cardiac orifice of the stomach.

cardiac ('kahdi,ak) 1. pertaining to the heart. 2. pertaining to the cardia. *C. arrest* the cessation of the heart beat. *C. asthma see* ASTHMA. *C. atrophy* fatty degeneration of the heart muscle. *C. bed* one which can be manipulated to form a chair shape for those who are comfortable only when sitting up. *C. catheterization* a procedure whereby a radio-opaque catheter is passed from an arm vein to the heart. Its passage through the heart can be watched on a screen. Also blood pressure readings and specimens can be taken, thus aiding diagnosis of heart abnormalities. *C. cycle* the sequence of events lasting about 0.8 s during which the heart completes one contraction. *C. massage* rhythmic compression of the heart performed in order to re-establish circulation of the blood in cardiac arrest. *See* Appendix 7. *C. monitor* (cardiator) equipment used to monitor and visually record the cardiac cycle. *C. pacemaker* an electrical device which stimu-

lates the heart muscle to maintain myocardial contractions. *See* PACEMAKER. *C. stimulant* a pharmacological agent that increases the action of the heart. Cardiac glycosides, e.g. digoxin and digitalis, increase myocardial contractions and decrease the heart rate and conduction velocity, thus allowing more time for the ventricles to relax and fill with blood.

cardialgia (ˌkahdi'alji·ə) pain in the region of the heart. Cardiodynia.

cardinal ('kahdin'l) of first importance. Fundamental. *C. ligaments* deep transverse cervical ligaments. Mackenrodt's ligaments.

cardiodynia (ˌkahdioh'dini·ə) cardialgia.

cardiogenic (ˌkahdioh'jenik) originating in the heart. *C. shock* shock caused by disease or failure of heart action.

cardiography (ˌkahdi'ogrəfee) the recording of the force and movements of the heart.

cardiologist (ˌkahdi'oləjist) a medically qualified person skilled in the diagnosis of heart disease.

cardiology (ˌkahdi'oləjee) the study of the heart: how it works, and its diseases.

cardiolysis (ˌkahdi'olisis) the breaking down of adhesions between the pericardium and chest wall by operation.

cardiomyopathy (ˌkahdiohmie-'opəthee) a chronic disorder of the heart muscle not resulting from atherosclerosis.

cardiopathy (ˌkahdi'opathee) any disease of the heart.

cardiopulmonary (,kahdioh'pulmənə·ree) relating to the heart and lungs. *C. bypass* the use of the heart–lung machine to oxygenate and pump the blood round the body while the surgeon operates on the heart.

cardioscope ('kahdioh,skohp) a flexible instrument with a lens and illumination attachment; used for examining the inside of the heart.

cardiospasm ('kahdioh,spazəm) spasm of the sphincter muscle at the cardiac end of the stomach. It may result in dilatation of the oesophagus, difficulty in swallowing solids and liquids, and regurgitation of undigested food. Achalasia.

cardiothoracic (,kahdiohthor'rasik) pertaining to the heart and thoracic cavity. A specialized branch of surgery.

cardiotocography (,kahdiohtə-'kografee) the simultaneous recording of the fetal heart rate, fetal movements and the uterine contractions in order to discover possible lack of oxygen (hypoxia) to the fetus. Fetal monitoring.

cardiotomy (,kahdi'otəmee) surgical incision into the heart or the cardia. *C. syndrome* an inflammatory reaction following heart surgery. There is pyrexia, pericarditis and pleural effusion.

cardiotoxic (,kahdioh'toksik) anything which has a deleterious or poisonous effect on the heart.

cardiovascular (,kahdioh'vaskyulə) concerning the heart and blood vessels. *C. system* the heart together with the two chief networks of blood vessels, the systemic circulation and the pulmonary circulation.

cardioversion (,kahdioh'vərshən) a method of restoring an abnormal heart rhythm to normal (as in atrial fibrillation) by means of an electric shock.

carditis (kah'dietis) inflammation of the heart.

care plans (kair) *see* NURSING CARE PLANS.

caries ('kair·reez) suppuration and subsequent decay of bone, corresponding to ulceration in soft tissues. In caries, the bone dissolves; in necrosis it separates in large pieces and is thrown off. *Dental c.* decay of the teeth due to penetration of bacteria through the enamel to the dentine. *Spinal c.* tuberculosis of the spine. Pott's disease.

carina (kə'rienə, -'reenə) a keel-like structure. Usually applied to the bifurcation of the trachea into the bronchi as the terminal cartilage is keel-shaped.

carminative (kah'minətiv) an aromatic drug which relieves flatulence and associated colic. Cloves, ginger, cardamon and peppermint are examples.

carneous ('kahni·əs) fleshy. *C. mole* a tumour of organized blood clot surrounding a dead fetus in the uterus. *See* ABORTION.

carotene ('karə,teen) the colouring matter in carrots, tomatoes and other yellow foods and fats. It is a provitamin capable of conversion into vitamin A in the liver.

carotid (ka'rotid) the principal artery on each side of the neck. *C. bodies* chemoreceptors in the bifurcation of both carotid arteries that monitor the oxygen content of the blood. *C. sinuses* dilated portions of the internal carotids containing the baroreceptors which monitor blood pressure.

carpal ('kahp'l) relating to the carpus or wrist. *C. tunnel syndrome* compression of the median nerve at the wrist causing numbing and tingling in the fingers.

carphology (kah'folǝjee) constant picking at bedclothes, occurring in cases of serious illness, especially typhoid.

carpopedal (,kahpoh'ped'l) relating to the wrist and foot. *C. spasm* spasm of the hands and feet such as occurs in tetany.

carpus ('kahpǝs) the eight bones forming the wrist and arranged in two rows: (1) scaphoid, lunate, triquetral, pisiform; (2) trapezium, trapezoid, capitate, hamate.

carrier ('kari·ǝ) 1. a person who harbours the microorganisms of an infectious disease, but is not necessarily affected by it, although he may infect others. 2. one who carries and passes on a hereditary abnormality.

cartilage ('kahtilij) a specialized, fibrous connective tissue present in adults, and forming most of the temporary skeleton in the embryo. The three most important types are hyaline cartilage elastic cartilage and fibrocartilage. Also, a general term for a mass of such tissue in a particular site in the body. *Elastic c.* cartilage containing elastic fibres and forming the pinna of the ear, the epiglottis and part of the nasal septum. *Fibro-c.* cartilage in which bundles of white fibres predominate, forming the intervertebral discs and costal cartilages. *Hyaline c.* flexible, somewhat elastic, semitransparent cartilage with an opalescent bluish tint, composed of a basophilic fibril-containing substance with cavities in which the chondrocytes occur.

cartilaginous ('kahti'lajinǝs) of the nature of cartilage.

caruncle ('karǝngk'l) a small fleshy swelling. *Lacrimal c.* a small reddish body situated at the medial junction of the eyelids. *Urethral c.* a small fleshy growth occurring at the urinary orifice in females, and giving rise to great pain on micturition.

cascara (kas'kahrǝ) a laxative prepared from the bark of the Californian buckthorn. It may be prepared as an elixir or tablets.

case (kays) a particular instance of disease; as a case of leukaemia; sometimes used incorrectly to designate the patient with the disease. *C. conference* a meeting of professionals involved in the care of a particular person (often a child), to agree patterns of action and to monitor progress. *C. control study* an epidemiological study in which the characteristics of cases of disease are compared with a matched control group of persons without the disease. Called also *retrospective study, case referent study. C. fatality rate* the number of persons dying of a particular disease expressed as a proportion of the

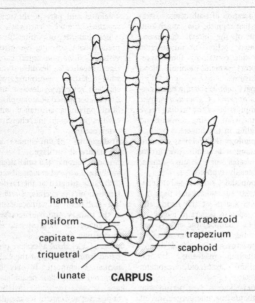

hamate
pisiform
capitate
triquetral
lunate
trapezoid
trapezium
scaphoid

CARPUS

total contracting the disease and usually expressed as a percentage. *C. history* the collected data concerning an individual, his family and environment, including his medical history and any other information that may be useful in analysing and diagnosing his case or for instructional or research purposes.

caseation (ˌkaysi'ayshən) degeneration of diseased tissue into a cheesy mass.

casein ('kaysi·in, -seen) the chief protein of milk. It forms a curd from which cheese is made. *C.*

hydrolysate a predigested concentrated protein; a useful supplement for a high protein diet.

caseinogen (ˌkaysi'inəjen, kay-'seenə-) a phosphate present in milk and precipitated when milk goes sour. The precursor of casein; activated by rennin.

cast (kahst) 1. a positive copy of an object, e.g., a mould of a hollow organ (a renal tubule, bronchiole, etc.), formed of effused plastic matter and extruded from the body, as a urinary cast; named according to constituents, as epithelial, fatty, waxy, etc. 2. a positive copy of the tissues of the jaws, made in an impression, over which denture bases or other restorations may be fabricated. 3. to form an object in a mould. 4. a stiff dressing or casing, usually made of plaster of Paris, used to immobilize body parts. 5. strabismus.

castor oil ('kahstə) a vegetable oil. Internally it is a purgative. Externally it is protective and soothing and may be used in ointments or in eye drops.

castration (ka'strayshən) removal or destruction of the testicles or, in a female, the ovaries.

CAT computerized axial tomography. *See* COMPUTED TOMOGRAPHY.

cat cry syndrome ('kat,krie) a rare disorder recognized at birth and characterized by a kitten-like mew or cry. Caused by a laryngeal anomaly associated with a defect in chromosome 5. Mental handicap and other defects are also observed. Known also as cri-du-chat syndrome.

cat-scratch disease (fever) ('kat-skratch) a benign, subacute, regional lymphadenitis resulting from a scratch or bite of a cat or a scratch from a surface contaminated by a cat. No specific causative agent has been isolated, but a viral aetiology is suspected.

catabolism (kə'tabə,lizəm) the chemical breakdown of complex substances in the body to form simpler ones, with a release of energy. *See* METABOLISM.

catalase (,katə,layz) an enzyme found in body cells including red blood cells and liver cells.

catalyst ('katə,list) a substance which hastens or brings about a chemical change without itself undergoing alteration. For example, enzymes act as catalysts in the process of digestion.

catamenia (,katə'meeni·ə) menstruation.

cataplasm ('katə,plazəm) a poultice. It acts as a counter-irritant. Materials of which it can be made are: linseed, bread and bran. Kaolin is more frequently used.

cataplexy ('katə,pleksee) sudden recurrent loss of muscle power without unconsciousness, often associated with narcolepsy. It may be produced by any strong emotion.

cataract ('katə,rakt) opacity of the crystalline lens of the eye causing partial or complete blindness. It may be congenital, or may be due to senility, injury or diabetes.

catarrh (kə'tah) chronic inflammation of a mucous membrane accompanied by an excessive discharge of mucus.

catatonia (,katə'tohni·ə) a syndrome of motor abnormalities occurring in schizophrenia, but less commonly in organic cerebral disease, characterized by stupor and the adoption of strange postures, or outbursts of excitement and hyperactivity. The patient may change suddenly from one of these states to the other.

catchment area ('kachmənt) a specific geographical area for which a district general hospital or health centre is responsible for providing the health care services.

catecholamines (ˌkatikoləˈmeenz) a group of compounds that have the effect of sympathetic nerve stimulation. They have an aromatic and an amine portion and include dopamine, adrenaline and noradrenaline.

catgut ('kat,gut) a substance prepared from the intestines of sheep and used in surgery for sutures and ligatures. It becomes gradually absorbed in the body at a variable rate, according to the preparation.

catharsis (kəˈthahsis) 1. a cleansing or purgation. 2. the bringing into consciousness and the emotional reliving of a forgotten (repressed) painful experience as a means of releasing anxiety and tension.

cathartic (kəˈthahtik) a purgative drug.

catheter ('kathitə) a tubular, flexible instrument, passed through body channels for withdrawal of fluids from (or introduction of fluids into) a body cavity. Catheters are made of a variety of materials including plastic, metal, rubber and gum-elastic. *Angiographic c.* one through which a contrast medium is injected for visualization of the vascular system of an organ. *Arterial c.* one inserted into an artery and utilized as part of a catheter–transducer–monitor system to continuously observe the BLOOD PRESSURE of critically ill patients. An arterial catheter also may be inserted for radiological studies of the arterial system and for delivery of chemotherapeutic agents directly into the arterial supply of malignant tumours. *Cardiac c.* a long, fine catheter especially designed for passage, usually through a peripheral blood vessel, into the chambers of the heart under fluoroscopic control. *Central venous c.* a long, fine catheter inserted into a vein for the purpose of administering through a large blood vessel parenteral fluids (as in parenteral NUTRITION), antibiotics and other therapeutic agents. This type of catheter is also used in the measurement of CENTRAL VENOUS PRESSURE. *Eustachian c.* a silver catheter used to open up the pharyngotympanic tube. *Self-retaining c.* a catheter made in such a way that after introduction the blind end expands so that it can remain in the bladder. Useful for continuous or intermittent drainage or where frequent specimens are required. *Ureteric c.* a fine gum-elastic catheter passed up the ureter to the renal pelvis and used to insert a dye in retrograde urography.

catheterization (ˌkathitəˌrieˈzayshən) the insertion of a catheter into a body cavity.

cathode ('kathohd) 1. the negative electrode or pole of an electric current. 2. the negative pole of a battery. *See* ANODE.

cation ('katie-ən) a positively charged ion which moves towards the cathode when an electric current is passed through an electrolytic solution, e.g. hydrogen (H^+), sodium (Na^+). *See* ANION.

cauda ('kawdah) a tail-like appendage. *C. equina* the bundle of coccygeal, sacral and lumbar nerves with which the spinal cord terminates.

caudal ('kawd'l) referring to a cauda. *C. block* an anaesthetic agent injected into the sacral canal so that operations may be carried out in the perineal area without a general anaesthetic.

caul (kawl) the amnion, which occasionally does not rupture but envelops the infant's head at birth.

causalgia (kaw'zalji·ə) an intense burning pain which persists after peripheral nerve injuries.

caustic ('kostik, 'kaw-) a substance, usually a strong acid or alkali, capable of burning organic tissue. Silver nitrate (*lunar c.*), carbolic acid and carbon dioxide snow are those most commonly used.

cauterization (,kawtə·rie'zayshən) the destruction of tissue with cautery.

cautery ('kawtə·ree) 1. the application of searing heat by a hot instrument, an electric current, or other means such as a laser. 2. an agent so used. *Cold c.* cauterization by carbon dioxide, called also cryocautery.

cavernous ('kavənəs, kə'vərnəs) having caverns or hollows. *C. breathing* sounds heard on auscultation over a pulmonary cavity. *C. sinus* a venous channel lying on either side of the body of the sphenoid bone through which pass the internal carotid artery and several nerves. *C. sinus thrombosis* a serious complication of any infection of the face, the veins from the orbit draining into the sinus and carrying the infec-

tion into the cranium.

cavitation (,kavi'tayshən) the formation of cavities, e.g. in the lung in tuberculosis.

cavity ('kavitee) a confined space or hollow or potential hollow within the body or one of its organs, e.g. the abdominal cavity or a decayed hollow in a tooth.

Cd symbol for *cadmium*.

cefotaxime (,kefoh'takseem) a third generation cephalosporin antibiotic having a broad spectrum of activity, used to treat intra-abdominal infections, bone and joint infections, gonorrhoea, and other infections due to susceptible organisms, including penicillinase-producing strains.

cefoxitin (ke'foksitin) a semisynthetic cephalosporin antibiotic, especially effective against Gram-negative organisms, with strong resistance to degradation by β-lactamase.

Celevac (sele'vak) trade name for methylcellulose.

cell (sel) 1. the basic structural unit of living organisms. A microscopic mass of protoplasm, consisting of a nucleus surrounded by cytoplasm and enclosed in a cell membrane, from which all organic tissues are constructed. Each cell can reproduce itself by mitosis. 2. a small, more or less enclosed space.

cellulitis (,selyuh'lietis) a diffuse inflammation of connective tissue, especially of subcutaneous tissue, which causes a typical brawny, oedematous appearance of the part; local abscess formation is not common.

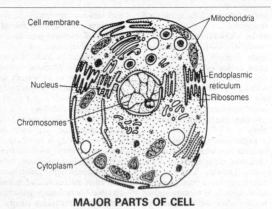

Cell membrane — Mitochondria

Nucleus —

Endoplasmic reticulum
Ribosomes

Chromosomes

Cytoplasm

MAJOR PARTS OF CELL

cellulose ('selyuh,lohs, -,lohz) a carbohydrate forming the covering of vegetable cells, i.e. vegetable fibres. Not digestible in the alimentary tract of man, but gives bulk and, as 'roughage', stimulates peristalsis.

Celsius scale ('selsi·əs) *A. Celsius, Swedish astronomer, 1701–1744.* A temperature scale with the melting point of ice set at 0° and the boiling point of water at 100°. The normal temperature of the human body is 36.9°C. Formerly known as the centigrade scale. *See* FAHRENHEIT.

cementum (si'mentəm) cement. Connective tissue with a bone-like structure which covers the root of a tooth and supports it within the socket.

censor (,sensə) 1. a member of a committee on ethics or for critical examination of a medical or other society. 2. the psychic influence which prevents unconscious thoughts and wishes coming into consciousness.

censorship ('senə,ship) in psychiatry, the process of selecting, accepting or rejecting conscious ideas, memories and impulses arising from the individual's subconscious.

census ('sensəs) enumeration of a population. The national census was first introduced in England and Wales in 1801 and has since been repeated every 10 years (except in 1941). It usually records name, address, age, sex, occupation, marital status and other social information.

Centers for Disease Control ('sentəz) abbreviated CDC. An agency of the US Department of Health and Human Services, located in Atlanta, Georgia, which serves as a centre for the control, prevention, and investigation of diseases. A similar function is performed in England and Wales by the Communicable Diseases Surveillance Centre and in Scotland by the Communicable Diseases (Scotland) Unit.

centigrade ('senti,grayd) *see* CELSIUS SCALE.

central ('sentrəl) pertaining to the centre or mid-point. *C. nervous system* abbreviated CNS. The brain and spinal cord. *C. venous pressure* the pressure recorded by the introduction of a catheter into the right atrium, in order to monitor the condition of a patient after major operative procedures such as heart surgery.

centifugal (sentri'fyoog'l) conveying away from a centre such as from the brain to the periphery. Efferent.

centrifuge ('sentri,fyooj) an apparatus that rotates at high speed. If a test tube, for example, is filled with a fluid such as blood or urine, and this is rotated in a centrifuge, any bacteria, cells, or other solids in it are precipitated.

centripetal (sen'tripit'l, 'sentri-,peet'l) the reverse of centrifugal. Conveying from the periphery to the centre. Afferent.

centromere ('sentroh,miə) the region(s) of the chromosomes which become(s) allied with the spindle fibres at mitosis and meiosis.

centrosome ('sentrə,sohm) a body in the cytoplasm of most animal cells, close to the nucleus. It divides during mitosis, one half migrating to each daughter cell.

centrosphere ('sentrə,sfiə) the cell centre, in an area of clear cytoplasm near the nucleus.

cephalalgia (,kefə'lalji-ə, ,sef-) pain in the head.

cephalexin (,kefə'leksin, ,sef-) cephalosporin antibiotic that may be administered orally.

cephalhaematoma (,kefəl,heemə-'tohmə, sef-) a swelling beneath the pericranium, containing blood, which may be found on the head of the newborn infant. Caused by pressure during labour. Gradually reabsorbed within the first few days of life.

cephalic (kə'falik, sə-) relating to or situated near the head.

cephalocele ('kefəloh,seel, 'sef-) cerebral hernia. *See* HERNIA.

cephalography (,kefə'logrəfee, ,sef-) radiographic examination of the contours of the head.

cephalometry (,kefə'lomətree, ,sef-) measurement of the dimensions of the head of a living person taken either directly or by radiography. *See* PELVIMETRY.

cephaloridine (,kefə'lo·rideen, ,sef-) an antibiotic that is effective against a wide range of organisms.

cephalosporin (,kefəloh'spor·rin, ,sef-) any one of a group of wide-spectrum antibiotics derived from the mould *Cephalosporium*.

cephradine ('kefrədeen, 'sef-) a cephalosporin antibiotic similar in action to cephaloridine.

cerclage (sər'klahzh) [Fr.] encircling of a part with a ring or loop, as for correction of an incompetent cervix uteri or fixation of the adjacent ends of a fractured bone. *See* SHIRODKAR'S SUTURE.

cerebellum (ˌseri'beləm) the portion of the brain below the cerebrum and above the medulla oblongata. Its functions include the coordination of fine voluntary movements and posture.

cerebral ('seribrəl) relating to the cerebrum. *C. cortex* the outer layer of the cerebrum composed of neurones. *C. haemorrhage* rupture of a cerebral blood vessel. Likely causes are aneurysm and hypertension. *See* APOPLEXY. *C. hernia see* HERNIA. *C. irritation* a condition of general nervous irritability and abnormality, often with photophobia, which may be an early sign of meningitis, tumour of the brain, etc. It is also associated with trauma. *C. palsy* a condition caused by injury to the brain during or immediately after birth. Coordination of movement is affected, and may cause the child to be flaccid or athetoid, in which condition there is constant random and uncontrolled movement. *See* SPASTIC.

cerebration (ˌseri'brayshən) mental activity.

cerebrospinal (ˌseribroh'spien'l) relating to the brain and spinal cord. *C. fluid* abbreviated CSF. The fluid made in the choroid plexus of the ventricles of the brain and circulating from them into the subarachnoid space around the brain and spinal cord.

cerebrovascular (ˌseribroh'vaskyuhlə) pertaining to the arteries and veins of the brain. *C. accident* a disorder arising from an embolus, thrombus or haemorrhage in the cerebrum. *C. disease*

any disorder of the blood vessels of the brain and its meninges.

cerebrum ('seribrəm) the largest part of the brain, occupying the greater portion of the cranium and consisting of the right and left hemispheres divided by the longitudinal fissure. Each hemisphere contains a lateral ventricle. The internal substance is white and the convoluted surface is grey. The centre of the higher functions of the brain.

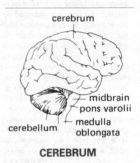

cerebrum

midbrain
pons varolii
medulla
oblongata
cerebellum

CEREBRUM

cerumen (si'roomen) a waxy substance secreted by the ceruminous glands of the auditory canal. Ear-wax.

cervical ('sərvik'l, sə'vie-) pertaining to the neck or the constricted part of an organ, e.g. uterine cervix. *C. canal* the passage through the uterine cervix. *C. cancer* cancer of the uterine cervix. *C. collar* a rigid or semirigid immobilizing support for the neck. *C. rib* a short, extra rib, often bilateral, which sometimes occurs on the seventh cervical vertebra and may cause pressure on an artery or nerve. *C. smear* a test for disorders of the cervical cells; material is scraped from the uterine cervix and examined microscopically. *C. spondylosis* a degenerative disease of the intervertebral joints and discs of the neck. *C. vertebra* one of the seven bones forming the neck portion of the spinal column.

cervicitis (ˌserviˈsietis) inflammation of the neck of the uterus.

cervix ('sərviks) a constricted portion or neck. *C. uteri* the neck of the uterus; it is about 2 cm long and projects into the vagina. Capable of wide dilatation during childbirth.

cestode ('sestohd) tapeworm.

cetrimide ('setrimied) cetyltrimethylammonium bromide (CTAB). A detergent and antiseptic widely used for preoperative skin preparation and the cleansing of wounds.

cevitamic acid (ˌseviˈtamik) ascorbic acid. Vitamin C.

chafe (chayf) irritation of the skin as caused by the friction between skin folds. Occurs particularly in moist areas.

chalazion (kəˈlaziˌən) a meibomian or tarsal cyst. A swollen sebaceous gland in the eyelid. A small, hard tumour may develop.

chalicosis (ˌkaliˈkohsis) an old term for a condition resembling silicosis, but found mainly among stone-cutters and due to the inhalation of stone dust.

chancre ('shangkə) 1. the initial lesion of syphilis developing at the site of inoculation. 2. a papular lesion occurring at the site of

entry of infection in tuberculosis or in sporotrichosis.

chancroid ('shangkroyd) soft chancre. A venereal ulceration, due to *Haemophilus ducreyi*, accompanied by inflammation and suppuration of the local glands.

charcoal ('chahkohl) carbon obtained by burning animal or vegetable tissue in a confined space. Activated charcoal, which has been treated to improve its adsorbency, is sometimes given in the form of biscuits or tablets, in cases of dyspepsia.

Charcot's disease or **joint** (shah-'kohz) *J.M. Charcot, French neurologist, 1825–1893.* A chronic progressive, degenerative disease of the stress-bearing portion of one or more joints. The disease is the result of an underlying neurological disorder, e.g. tabes dorsalis from syphilis or diabetic neuropathy or leprosy.

Charcot's triad nystagmus, intention tremor and scanning speech. A trio of signs of disseminated sclerosis.

Charnley's arthroplasty ('chahnliz) *Sir J. Charnley, British orthopaedic surgeon, 1911–1982.* The replacement of the hip joint using a plastic acetabulum and a steel femoral head. *See* ARTHROPLASTY.

chart (chaht) a record of data in graphic or tabular form. *Genealogical c.* a graph showing various descendants of a common ancestor, used to indicate those affected by genetically determined disease. *Reading c.* a chart with material printed in gradually increasing type sizes, used in testing acuity of near vision. *Reuss' c's* charts with coloured letters printed on coloured backgrounds, used in testing colour vision. *Snellen's c.* a chart printed with block letters in gradually decreasing sizes, used in testing visual acuity.

charting ('chahting) the keeping of a clinical record of the important facts about a patient and the progress of his illness. The patient's chart usually contains a medical history, a nursing history, results of physical examinations, laboratory reports, results of special diagnostic tests, and the observations of the nursing staff. Medical treatments, medications, and nursing approaches to problems are recorded on the chart, as are the patient's response to treatment. *See also* PROBLEM-ORIENTED RECORD.

cheilitis (kie'lietis) inflammation of the lip.

cheiloplasty ('kieloh,plastee) any plastic operation on the lip.

cheiloschisis (kie'loskisis) cleft lip.

cheilosis (kie'lohsis) maceration at the angles of the mouth, fissures may also occur. It may be associated with general debility or riboflavin deficiency.

cheiropompholyx (,kieroh'pompfohliks) a skin disease characterized by vesicles on the palms and soles.

cheiropractic (,kierə'praktik) *see* CHIROPRACTIC.

chelate ('keelayl-) a chemical compound in which an atom of a metal is held in a molecular ring.

chelating agent (ki'layting) a drug that has the power of combining with certain metals and so aiding excretion to prevent or overcome poisoning. *See* DIMERCAPROL and PENICILLAMINE.

chemistry ('kemistree) the science dealing with the elements and the atoms which compose them, and with the compounds that they form.

chemoreceptor (,keemohri'septə, ,kem-) a sensory nerve ending or group of cells that are sensitive to chemical stimuli in the blood.

chemosis (kee'mohsis) swelling of the conjunctiva, due to the presence of fluid; an oedema of the conjunctiva.

chemosurgery (,keemoh'sərjə-·ree, ,kem-) the destruction of tissue by chemical agents for therapeutic purposes, originally applied to chemical fixation of malignant, gangrenous, or infected tissue, with use of frozen sections to facilitate systematic microscopic control of its excision.

chemotaxis (,keemoh'taksis, ,kem-) the reaction of living cells to chemical stimuli. These are either attracted (*positive c.*) or repelled (*negative c.*) by acids, alkalis or other substances.

chemotherapy (,keemoh'therə-pee, ,kem-) the specific treatment of disease by the administration of chemical compounds.

chest (chest) the thorax. *Barrel c.* one more rounded than usual, with raised ribs and, usually, kyphosis. It is often present in emphysema. *Flail c.* one where part of the chest wall moves in opposition to respiration due to multiple fractures of the ribs. *C. leads* leads applied to the chest during the course of an electrocardiographic recording. *Pigeon c.* a chest with the sternum protruding forward.

Cheyne–Stokes respiration ('chayn'stohks) *J. Cheyne, British physician, 1776–1836; W. Stokes, British physician, 1804–1878.* Tidal respiration. A form of irregular but rhythmic breathing with temporary cessations (apnoea). It is likely to be present in cerebral tumour, in narcotic poisoning, and in advanced cases of arteriosclerosis and uraemia.

chiasma (kie,azmə) a crossing point. *Optic c.* the crossing point of the optic nerves.

chickenpox ('chikin,poks) varicella.

chilblain ('chil,blayn) a condition resulting from defective circulation when exposure to cold causes localized swelling and inflammation of the hands or feet, with severe itching and burning sensations.

child (chield) the human young, from infancy to puberty. *C. abuse* the non-accidental use of physical force or the non-accidental act of omission by a parent or other custodian responsible for the care of a child. Child abuse encompasses malnutrition and other kinds of neglect through ignorance as well as deliberate withholding from the child the necessary and basic physical care, including the medical and dental care necessary for the child to grow. Examples of physical abuse range from burns and exposure to extreme cold, to beating, poisoning, strangulation, and withholding food and water. *Deprived c.* a vague term usually implying that the child in question has been raised in a situation lacking in love, affection and consistent parenting responses from adults. Sometimes used to suggest that the child has experienced a generalized deficit of life opportunities, both interpersonal and social.

childbirth ('chield'bərth) the act or process of giving birth to a child. Parturition.

Chinese restaurant syndrome ('chineez 'restəronh) transient arterial dilatation due to ingestion of monosodium glutamate which is used in seasoning Chinese food marked by throbbing head, light headedness, tightness of the jaw, neck and shoulders, and backache.

chiropody (ki'ropədee, shi-) the study and care of the feet and the treatment of foot diseases.

chiropractic (,kierə'praktik) a system of treatment employing manipulation of the spine and other bony structures.

Chlamydia (klə'midi·ə) a genus of bacteria comprising two species: *C. trachomatis*, which causes lymphogranuloma venereum, trachoma, conjunctivitis and nongonococcal urethritis; and *C. psittaci*, which causes psittacosis (parrot fever).

chloasma (kloh'azmə) a condition in which there is brown, blotchy discoloration of the skin, appearing on the face, especially during pregnancy.

chloral ('klor·ral) an oily liquid formed by the reaction of chlorine and alcohol. Used in the production of *c. hydrate*, a drug used as a hypnotic which is well tolerated by children and old people.

chlorambucil (klor'rambyuhsil) an ankylating drug used in treating chronic leukaemia. A cytotoxic drug.

chloramphenicol (,klor·ram'fenikol) an antibiotic. It gives rise to agranulocytosis and is used only for serious infectious diseases such as typhoid fever. Used in drops and ointment for eye infections.

chlorcyclizine (klor'siekli,zeen) an antihistamine used for travel sickness.

chlordiazepoxide (,klordie,azi 'poksied) a drug that depresses the central nervous system and so relieves anxiety and tension.

chlorhexidine (klor'heksi,deen) an antibacterial compound used for surgical scrub, preoperative skin preparation, and cleansing skin wounds.

chlorine ('klor·reen, -rin) *symbol* Cl. A yellow, irritating poisonous gas. A powerful disinfectant, bleach and deodorizing agent. Used in hypochlorites for the sterilization of infant feeding bottles, etc.

chlormethiazole (,klormə'thieə,zohl) a hypnotic and sedative drug used to treat insomnia, chiefly in elderly people.

chloroacetone (,klor·roh'asi,tohn) chloracetone. Tear-gas.

chlorocresol (,klor·roh'kreesol) a coal tar product with a bactericidal action more powerful than phenol and with a lower toxicity. Used as an antiseptic and as a preservative in injection fluids.

chloroform ('klo·rə,fawm) a colourless volatile liquid administered through inhalation as a general anaesthetic. Now rarely used.

chloroma (klor'rohmə) a tumour having a greenish colour, usually found in skull bones. It is associated with myeloid leukaemia.

chlorophyll ('klo·rə,fil) the green pigment of plants which absorbs solar energy for the synthesis of complex materials from the carbon dioxide and water taken in by the plant.

chloropsia (klor'ropsi·ə) a form of colour blindness where all objects appear to have a greenish tinge.

chloroquine ('klor·roh,kween) an antimalarial drug that has a strong suppressant action and is used in the treatment of amoebic hepatitis, rheumatoid arthritis and lupus erythematosus.

chlorothiazide ('klor·roh'thieəzied) an oral diuretic used in the treatment of fluid retention and hypertension.

chlorotrianisene (,klor·rohtrie'aniseen) a long-acting oestrogen used in the treatment of menopausal symptoms and also in cancer of the prostate.

chloroxylenol (,klor·roh'zielənol) an antiseptic which is less irritating to the skin and mucous membranes than cresol and has a powerful disinfectant action.

chlorpheniramine (,klorfe,nirə,meen) an antihistamine drug used in the treatment of allergies such as hay fever and urticaria.

chlorpromazine (klor'prohmə-,zeen) a sedative anti-emetic drug widely used to treat anxiety, agitation and vomiting, particularly in the elderly, and in the management of psychiatric patients. It is also hyotensive and enhances the effect of analgesics and anaesthetics.

chlorpropamide (klor'prohpə-,mied) an oral hypoglycaemic agent used in the treatment of mild diabetes.

chlorprothixene (,klorproh'thikseen) a tranquillizer used in the treatment of schizophrenia, psychoneuroses and behaviour disorders.

chlortetracycline (,klortetrə-'siekleen) broad-spectrum antibiotic effective in treating many bacterial and protozoal infections.

chlorthalidone (klor'thali,dohn) a diuretic used in the treatment of oedema, hypertension and diabetes.

choana ('koh·anə, koh'ahnə) *pl.* choanae [L.] 1. any funnel-shaped cavity or infundibulum. 2. *choanae*, the paired openings between the nasal cavity and the nasopharynx.

cholaemia (ko'leemi·ə) the presence of bile in the blood.

cholagogue ('kohləgog) a drug which increases the flow of bile into the duodenum.

cholangiography (kə,lanji'ogrəfee) radiography of the hepatic, cystic and bile ducts after the insertion of a radio-opaque contrast medium.

cholangitis (,kohlan'jietis) inflammation of the bile ducts.

cholecystectomy (,kohlisi'stek-

təmee) excision of the gallbladder.

cholecystitis (,kohlisi'stietis) inflammation of the gallbladder.

cholecystoduodenostomy (,kohli,sistoh,dyoodi'nostəmee) an anastomosis between the gallbladder and the duodenum.

cholecystoenterostomy (,kohli,sistoh,entə'rostəmee) the formation of an artificial opening from the gallbladder into the intestine. An operation performed in cases of irremovable obstruction of the bile duct.

cholecystography (,kohlisi'stogrəfee) radiography of the gallbladder after administration of a radio-opaque contrast medium.

cholecystokinin (,kohli,sistoh-'kienin) a hormone released by the presence of fat in the duodenum which causes contraction of the gallbladder.

cholecystolithiasis (,kohli,sistohli'thieəsis) the presence of stones in the gallbladder.

cholecystotomy (,kohlisistotə-mee) an incision into the gallbladder, usually to remove gallstones.

choledochoduodenostomy (,kohli,dohkoh,dyooədi,nostəm-ee) an operation in which an anastomosis is made between the common bile duct and the duodenum.

choledocholithiasis (,kohli,dohkohli'thieəsis) the presence of stones in the bile duct.

choledocholithotomy (,kohli,dohkohli'thotəmee) incision into the bile ducts to remove stones.

choledochostomy (,kohlidoh-'kostəmee) opening and draining the common bile duct.

cholelithiasis (,kohlili'thieəsis) presence of gallstones in the gallbladder or bile ducts.

cholera ('kolə·rə) an acute, notifiable, infectious enteritis endemic and epidemic in Asia and, within the past 20 years, also in Africa. Caused by *Vibrio cholerae*, it is marked by profuse diarrhoea, muscle cramp, suppression of urine and severe prostration, and is often fatal. Travellers to areas where cholera is endemic should protect themselves by vaccination, though this only provides partial immunity. The local drinking water should be boiled and uncooked foods avoided.

cholestasis (,kohli'staysis) arrest of the flow of bile due to obstruction of the bile ducts.

cholesteatoma (,kohli,steeə'tohma) a small tumour containing cholesterol which may occur in the middle ear. Also occurs in the meninges, central nervous system and bones of the skull.

cholesterol (kə'lestə,rol) a sterol found in nervous tissue, red blood corpuscles, animal fat and bile. It is a precursor of bile acids and steroid hormones, and it occurs in the most common type of gallstone, in atheroma of the arteries, in various cysts, and in carcinomatous tissue. Most of the body's cholesterol is synthesized, but some is obtained in the diet.

cholesterolosis (kə,lestə·ro'lohsis) a chronic form of cholecystitis when the mucosa of the gallbladder is studded with deposits of cholesterol.

cholestyramine (,kohli'stierə-meen) a drug which causes the excretion of bile salts by binding with them. Given to lower blood levels of cholesterol and other fats.

choline ('kohleen) an essential amine found in the blood, cerebrospinal fluid and urine, which aids fat metabolism. Formerly classified as a vitamin of the B complex. *C. theophyllinate* an antispasmodic drug used in respiratory conditions.

cholinergic (,kohli'nərjik) pertaining to nerves that release acetylcholine at their nerve endings as the chemical stimulator. *C. drugs* drugs that inhibit cholinesterase and so prevent the destruction of acetylcholine.

cholinesterase (,kohli'nestə,rayz) an enzyme which rapidly destroys acetylcholine.

choluria (koh'lyooə·ri·ə) the presence of bile in the urine.

chondritis (kon'drietis) inflammation of cartilage.

chondroblast ('kondroh,blast) an embryonic cell which forms cartilage.

chondrocyte ('kondroh,siet) a mature cartilage cell.

chondrodynia (,kondroh'dini·ə) pain affecting a cartilage.

chondrodystrophia (,kondroh-dis,trohfi·ə) a congenital disorder of cartilage formation.

chondroma (kon'drohmə) an innocent new growth arising in cartilage.

chondromalacia (,kondrohmə'layshi·ə) a condition of abnormal softening of cartilage.

chondrosarcoma (,kondrohsah'kohmə) a malignant new growth arising from cartilaginous tissue.

chorda ('kawda) a sinew or cord.

chordee (kaw'dee) downward curvature of the penis caused by congenital anomaly (common in hypospadias) or urethral infection.

chorditis (kaw'dietis) inflammation of the vocal or spermatic cords.

chordotomy (kaw'dotəmee) an operation on the spinal cord to divide the anterolateral nerve pathways for relief of intractable pain. Cordotomy.

chorea (ko'reeə) a symptom of disease of the basal ganglia when the individual suffers from spasmodic, involuntary, rapid movements of the face, shoulders and hips. *Huntington's c.* (or Huntington's disease) a rare hereditary disorder which manifests itself in early middle age. The individual also suffers from progressive dementia, which often precedes a premature death. *Sydenham's c.* St Vitus's dance. Occurs in childhood and is associated with rheumatic fever.

choreiform (ko'ree·ifawm) resembling chorea.

choriocarcinoma (,ko·rioh,kahsi-'nohmə) formerly known as chorioepithelioma. A highly malignant NEOPLASM usually arising from the trophoblast of a HYDATIDIFORM MOLE. It may develop after an abortion or the evacuation of a hydatidiform mole or even in normal pregnancy. Metastases usually develop rapidly, but the disease normally carries a good prognosis following early treatment.

chorioepithelioma (,ko·rioh,epi-,theeli,ohmə) choriocarcinoma.

chorion ('ko·rion, 'kor·ri·ən) the outer membrane enveloping the fetus; the placenta.

chorionic (,ko·ri'onik) pertaining to the chorion. *C. gonadotrophin* human chorionic gonadotrophin (HCG). *C. villi* small protrusions on the chorion from which the placenta is formed. They are in close association with the maternal blood, and, by diffusion, interchange of nutriment, oxygen and waste matters is effected between the maternal and the fetal blood. *C. villus biopsy* tissue removed from the gestational sac early in pregnancy so that chromosome and other inherited disorders can be identified. Can be carried out at an earlier stage than amniocentesis.

chorioretinitis (,ko·rioh,reti'nietis) choroidoretinitis.

choroid ('ko·royd) the pigmented and vascular coat of the eyeball, continuous with the iris and situated between the sclera and retina. It reduces the amount of light when it falls upon the retina. *C. plexus* specialized cells in the ventricles of the brain which produce cerebrospinal fluid. There is one choroid plexus in each ventricle.

choroiditis (,ko·roy'dietis) inflammation of the choroid.

choroidocyclitis (ko,roydohsie'-klietis) inflammation of the choroid and the ciliary body.

choroidoretinitis (ko,roydoh,reti-'nietis) an inflammatory condition of both the choroid and retina of the eye.

Christmas disease ('krisməs) a hereditary bleeding disease similar to haemophilia. The name is derived from that of the first patient to be studied.

chromatography (,krohmə'togrəfee) a method of chemical analysis by which substances in solution can be separated as they percolate down a column of powdered adsorbent or ascend an absorbent paper by capillary traction. A definite pattern is produced and susbtances may be recognized by the use of appropriate colour reagents. Amino acids can be identified in this way.

chromatolysis (,krohmə'tolisis) the disintegration and disappearance of the Nissl granules of a neurone if the axon is severed.

chromatometry (,krohmə'tomətree) the measurement of colour perception.

chromatopsia (,krohmə'topsi·ə) abnormal colour vision. Partial colour-blindness.

chromic acid ('krohmik) a strong caustic sometimes used for the removal of warts.

chromicize ('krohmi,siez) to impregnate with chromic acid, e.g. chromicized catgut which is particularly strong and durable.

chromophobe (,krohmoh,fohb) a cell that is not easily stained. Applied especially to the chromophobe cells of the anterior lobe of the pituitary gland.

chromosome ('krohmə,sohm) in animal cells, a structure in the nucleus, containing a linear thread of DEOXYRIBONUCLEIC ACID (DNA), which transmits genetic information and is associated with RIBONUCLEIC ACID and histones. During cell division the material composing the chromosome is compactly coiled. Each organism of a species is normally characterized by the same number of chromosomes in its somatic cells, 46 being the number normally present in man: 22 pairs of autosomes, and the two sex chromosomes (XX or XY), which determine the sex of the organism. In the mature GAMETE (ovum or spermatozoa) the number of chromosomes is halved as a result of MEIOSIS.

chronic ('kronik) of long duration; the opposite of acute.

chrysarobin (,krisə'rohbin) a derivative of Goa powder, used in ointment form, especially in the treatment of psoriasis. It stains linen a yellow colour. See DITHRANOL.

Chvostek's sign (,vosteks) F. Chvostek, Austrian surgeon, 1835–1884. A spasm of the facial muscles which occurs in tetany. It can be elicited by tapping the facial nerve.

chyle (kiel) digested fats which, as a milky fluid, are absorbed into the lymphatic capillaries (lacteals) in the villi of the small intestine.

chylothorax (,kieloh'thor,raks) the presence of effused chyle in the pleural cavity.

chyme (kiem) the semiliquid, acid mass of food which passes from the stomach to the intestines.

chymotrypsin (,kiemoh'tripsin) an enzyme secreted by the pancreas. It is activated by trypsin and aids in the breakdown of proteins.

Ci symbol for *curie*.

cicatrix ('sikətriks) the scar of a healed wound.

cilia ('sili·ə) 1. the eyelashes. 2. microscopic filaments projecting from some epithelial cells, known as ciliated membranes, as in the bronchi, where cilia wave the secretion upwards.

ciliary ('sili·ə,ree) hair-like. *C. body* a structure just behind the corneoscleral margin composed of the ciliary muscle and processes. *C. muscle* the circular muscle surrounding the lens of the eye. *C. processes* the fringed part of the choroid coat arranged in as circle in front of the lens.

cimetidine (si'meti,deen) a histamine H_2-receptor antagonist which reduces gastric acid secretion; used in the treatment of peptic ulcers.

Cimex ('siemeks) a genus of blood-sucking bugs. *C. lectularius* the common bed-bug.

cinchocaine ('sinchohkayn) a local anaesthetic agent used mainly as a spinal anaesthetic.

cinchona (sing'kohnə) Peruvian bark, from which quinine is obtained.

cinchonism ('singkə,nizəm) poisonous effect of cinchona. Quininism.

cineangiocardiography (,sini ,anjioh,kahdi'ogrəfee) angiography using a cine-camera to show the movements of the heart and blood vessels.

cineradiography (,sini,raydi-'ogrəfee) the making of a motion picture record of successive images appearing on a fluoro-scopic screen.

cinnamon ('sinəmən) an extract from the bark of an East Indian laurel, sometimes used as a digestive and carminative.

cinnarizine (si'nari,zeen) an antihistamine drug which may also be used to treat nausea, vertigo, labyrinthine disorders and motion sickness.

circadian (sər'kaydi·ən) denoting a period of 24 h. *C. rhythm* the rhythm of certain biological activities that take place daily.

circinate (,sərsi,nayt) having a circular outline. *Tinea circinata* is ringworm.

circle of Willis (,sərk'l ə wilis) *T. Willis, British physician and anatomist, 1621–1675.* An anastomosis of arteries at the base of the brain, formed by the branches of the internal carotid and the basilar arteries.

circulation (,sərkyuh'layshən) movement in a circular course, as of the blood. *Collateral c.* enlargement of small vessels establishing adequate blood supply when the main vessel to the part has been occluded. *Coronary c.* the system of vessels which supply the heart muscle itself. *Extracorporeal c.* removal of the blood by intravenous cannulae, passing it through a machine to oxygenate it, and then pumping it back into circulation. The 'heart–lung' machine or pump respirator, used in cardiac surgery. *Lymph c.* the flow of lymph through lymph vessels and glands. *Portal c.* the passage of the blood from the alimentary tract, pancreas, and spleen, via the portal vein and its branches through the liver and into the hepatic veins. *Pulmonary c.* passage of the blood from the right ventricle via the pulmonary artery through the lungs and back to the heart by the pulmonary veins. *Systemic c.* the flow of blood throughout the body. The direction of flow is from the left atrium to the left ventricle and through the aorta with its branches and capillaries. Veins then carry it back to the right atrium, and so into the right ventricle.

circumcision (,sɜrkəm,sizhən) excision of the prepuce or foreskin of the penis. An operation performed for religious reasons, or sometimes for phimosis or paraphimosis. *Female c.* excision of the labia minora and/or labia majora, and sometimes the clitoris, still performed ritualistically in certain countries, the extent of the surgery varying from one culture to another.

circumduction (,sɜrkəm'dukshən) moving in a circle, e.g. the circular movement of the upper limb.

circumoral (,sɜrkəm'or·rəl) around the mouth. *C. pallor* a pale area around the mouth contrasting with the flushed cheeks, e.g. in scarlet fever.

circumvallate ('sɜrkəm'valyət) surrounded by a wall or raised ring. *C. papilla see* PAPILLA.

cirrhosis (si'rohsis) a degenerative change which can occur in any organ, but especially in the liver. May be due to viruses, microorganisms or toxic substances

(*portal c.*). Fibrosis results, and this interferes with the working of the organ. In the liver it causes portal obstruction, with consequent ascites. *Alcoholic c.* the result of chronic alcoholism and nutritional deficiency which affects the liver. *Cardiac c.* cirrhosis of the liver following chronic heart failure. *Post-hepatic c.* cirrhosis of the liver following hepatitis. *Pulmonary c.* cirrhosis of the lung tissue.

cisplatin ('sisplə,tin) an antineoplastic drug containing platinum which is used in the treatment of ovarian carcinomas and testicular teratomas.

cisterna (si'stɜrnə) a space or cavity containing fluid. *C. chyli* the dilated portion of the thoracic duct containing chyle. *C. magna* the subarachnoid space between the cerebellum and medulla oblongata.

cisternal (si'stɜrnəl) concerning the cisterna. *C. puncture* insertion of a hollow needle into the cisterna magna to withdraw cerebrospinal fluid.

citric acid ('sitrik) acid found in the juice of lemons, limes, etc. An antiscorbutic.

Cl symbol for *chlorine*.

clamp (klamp) a metal surgical instrument used to compress any part of the body.

clapping ('klaping) in physiotherapy, rhythmic beating with cupped hands. Frequently used over the chest to aid expectoration.

claudication (,klawdi'kayshən) lameness. *Intermittent c.* limping, accompanied by severe pain in the legs on walking, which disappears with rest. A sign of occlusive arterial disease.

claustrophobia (,klostrə'fohbi·ə, ,klaw-) fear of confined spaces such as small rooms.

clavicle ('klavik·l) the collar bone. A long bone, part of the shoulder girdle.

clavus ('klayvəs) a corn.

clawfoot (,klor'fuht) a deformity in which the longitudinal arch is abnormally raised. Pes cavus.

clawhand (,klor'hand) a deformity in which the fingers are bent and contracted, giving a claw-like appearance.

cleft (kleft) a fissure or longitudinal opening. *C. palate* a congenital defect in the roof of the mouth due to failure of the medial plates of the palate to meet. Often associated with cleft lip.

client ('klieənt) 1. a recipient of a professional service. 2. a recipient of health care, regardless of the person's state of health and where the service is delivered. 3. a patient.

climacteric (klie'maktə·rik, ,kliemək'terik) the period of the menopause in women. Also used to denote the decline in the sexual drive in men.

climax ('kliemaks) 1. the stage when a disease is at its greatest intensity. 2. the stage in sexual intercourse when orgasm occurs.

clindamycin (,klində'miesin) an antibiotic active against Gram-positive cocci and many anaerobes.

clinic ('klinik) 1. instruction of students at the bedside. 2. a department of a hospital devoted

to the treatment of a particular type of disease.

clinical ('klinik·l) relating to bedside observation and the treatment of patients. *C. nurse specialist* a qualified nurse who has acquired advanced knowledge and skills in a specific area of clinical nursing.

clip (klip) a metal device for holding the two edges of a wound together or for controlling the flow of liquid through a tube.

clitoridectomy (,klitə·ri'dektə·mee) excision of the clitoris.

clitoris ('klitə·ris, 'kliet-) a small organ, formed of erectile tissue, situated at the anterior junction of the labia minora in the female.

cloaca (kloh'ayka) 1. the common intestinal and urogenital opening present in many vertebrates. 2. opening through newly formed bone from a diseased area so that pus may escape. *See* INVOLUCRUM.

clofibrate (kloh'fiebrayt) a drug which lowers the blood cholesterol.

clomipramine (kloh'miprə,meen) an antidepressant drug used to treat patients with obsessional fears.

clonazepam (kloh'nazi,pam) an anticonvulsive drug.

clone (klohn) cells which are genetically identical to each other and have descended by asexual reproduction from the parent cell to which they are also genetically identical.

clonic ('klonik) having the character of clonus. The second stage of a grand mal fit; also referred to as a tonic–clonic seizure. *See*

EPILEPSY.

clonidine ('klohni,deen) an anti-hypertensive drug which is also used to treat migraine.

clonus ('klohnəs) muscle rigidity and relaxation which occurs spasmodically. *Ankle c.* spasmodic movements of the calf muscles when the foot is suddenly pushed upwards, the leg being extended.

Clostridium (klo'stridi·əm) a genus of anaerobic spore-forming bacteria, found as commensals of the gut of animals and man and as saprophytes of the soil. Pathogenic species include *C. botulinum* (botulism). *C. tetani* (tetanus) and *C. perfringens* (also known as *C. welchii*) (gas gangrene).

clot (klot) a semi-solid mass formed in a liquid such as blood or lymph, by coagulation.

clotrimazole (kloh'triemə,zohl) an antifungal drug.

clotting ('kloting) coagulation. The formation of a clot. *C. time* coagulation time. The length of time taken for shed blood to coagulate. Normally, this would be 4 to 15 min at 37°C.

cloxacillin (,kloksə'silin) an antibiotic drug effective against penicillin-resistant staphylococci.

clubbing ('klubing) broadening and thickening of the tips of the fingers (and toes) due to bad circulation. It occurs in chronic diseases of the heart and respiratory system, such as congenital cardiac defect and tuberculosis.

clubfoot (,klub'fuht) talipes.

clumping ('klumping) the collecting together into clumps. The reaction of bacteria and blood cells when agglutination occurs.

Clutton's joint ('klutənz) *H.H. Clutton, British surgeon, 1850–1909*. A painless synovial swelling of joints, usually the knee, associated with congenital syphilis.

Co symbol for *cobalt*.

co-trimoxazole (,kohtrie,moksə-,zohl) an antibiotic drug, taken orally and used mainly to treat urinary infections.

coagulase (koh'agyuh,layz) an enzyme formed by pathogenic staphylococci that causes coagulation of plasma. Such bacteria are termed *c. positive*.

coagulation (koh,agyuh'layshən) clotting.

coagulum (koh'agyuhləm) the mass of fibrin and cells when blood clots; the mass formed when other substances coagulate, e.g. milk curd.

coal tar (kohl tah) a by-product obtained in destructive distillation of coal; used in ointment or solution in treatment of eczema and psoriasis.

coarctation (,koh·ahk'tayshən) a condition of contraction or stricture. *C. of aorta* a congenital malformation characterized by deformity of the aorta, causing narrowing, usually severe, of the lumen of the vessel. Surgical resection of the stricture may be performed.

cobalt ('kohbawlt) *symbol* Co. A metallic element, traces of which are necessary in the diet to prevent anaemia. *Radioactive c.* cobalt-60, used as a source of gamma irradiation in radiotherapy.

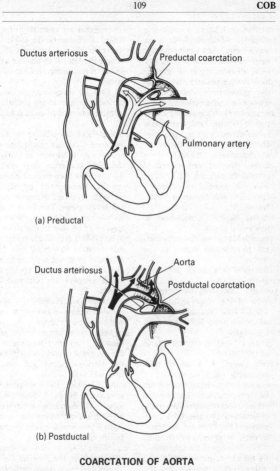

(a) Preductal

(b) Postductal

COARCTATION OF AORTA

cocaine (koh'kayn) a colourless alkaloid, obtained from coca leaves, which has a powerful but brief stimulant action. Used as a local anaesthetic. It is increasingly being replaced by less addictive preparations like procaine, lignocaine and amethocaine.

cocainism (koh'kaynizəm) addiction to cocaine. Long-term abuse is associated with a toxic psychosis similar to that caused by amphetamines. 'Crack' is a highly purified and extremely potent preparation of cocaine which is smoked or 'snorted'. Cocaine is also known as 'coke', 'snow', 'c'.

coccus ('kokəs) a bacterium of spheroidal shape.

coccydynia (,koksi'dini·ə) persistent pain in the region of the coccyx.

coccygeal (kok'siji·əl) pertaining to the coccyx.

coccyx ('koksiks) the terminal bone of the spinal column, in which four rudimentary vertebrae are fused together to form a triangle.

cochlea ('kokli·ə) the spiral canal of the internal ear.

code (kohd) 1. a set of rules governing one's conduct. 2. a system by which information can be communicated. *Genetic c.* the arrangement of nucleotides in the polynucleotide chain of a chromosome that governs the transmission of genetic information. *UKCC c.* of professional conduct for the nurse, midwife and health visitor revised periodically, this code is intended to provide definite standards of practice and conduct that are essential to the ethical discharge of the nurse's responsibility. *See* Appendix 11.

codeine ('kohdeen) an alkaloid of opium. A mild analgesic and antitussive.

cod liver oil (kod livə) purified oil from the liver of the codfish; valuable source of vitamins A and D.

coeliac ('seeli,ak) relating to the abdomen. *C. disease* gluten enteropathy. A condition of early childhood occurring soon after the child has been weaned on to cereals, characterized by steatorrhoea, distended abdomen and failure to grow. The failure of carbohydrate and fat metabolism appears to be due to the gluten in wheat and rye. The condition may continue into adult life. It is treated by giving a gluten-free diet. *C. plexus* nerve complex which supplies the abdominal organs.

coenzyme (koh'enziem) an organic molecule activator to a larger protein enzyme.

cognition (kog'nishən) action of knowing. Cognitive function of the conscious mind in contrast to the affective (feeling) and conative (willing).

coitus ('koytəs, 'koh·itəs) sexual intercourse between male and female. *C. interruptus* a method of birth control where the erect penis is removed from the vagina before ejaculation occurs.

colchicine ('kolchi,seen) a drug obtained from the seeds of *Colchicum autumnale*. Used in treating gout.

cold (kohld) 1. of low temperature. 2. a viral infection affecting the membranes of the nose and throat and the bronchial tubes. *C. sore* herpes simplex. *See* HERPES.

colectomy (koh'lektəmee) the excision of a portion or all of the colon.

colic ('kolik) acute paroxysmal abdominal pain. *Biliary c.* pain due to the presence of a gallstone in a bile duct. *Intestinal c.* severe griping spasmodic abdominal pain which may be a symptom of food poisoning or of intestinal obstruction. *Renal c.* pain due to the presence of a stone in the ureter. *Uterine c.* spasmodic pain originating in the uterus, as in dysmenorrhoea.

coliform ('kohli,fawm) resembling the bacillus *Escherichia coli.*

colistin (koh'listin) an antibiotic produced from *Bacillus polymyxa.* Used to treat gastrointestinal and other bacterial infections.

colitis (kəlietis, koh-) inflammation of the colon. It may be due to a specific organism, as in dysentery, but the term *ulcerative c.* denotes a chronic disease, often of unknown cause, in which there are attacks of diarrhoea with the passage of blood and mucus.

collagen ('kolajən) a fibrous structural protein that constitutes the protein of the white (collagenous) fibres of skin, tendon, bone cartilage, and all other connective tissues. It also occurs dispersed in a gel to provide stiffening, as in the vitreous humour of the eye. *C. diseases* a group of diseases having in common certain clinical and histological features that are

manifestations of involvement of CONNECTIVE TISSUE.

collapse (kə'laps) 1. a state of extreme prostration due to defective action of the heart, severe shock or haemorrhage. 2. falling in of a structure.

collar bone ('kolə ,bohn) the clavicle.

collateral (kə'latə-rəl) accessory to. *C. circulation* an alternative to the direct route for the blood when a primary vessel is blocked.

Colles' fracture ('koliz) *A. Colles, Irish surgeon, 1773–1843.* Fracture of the lower end of the radius at the wrist following a fall on the outstretched hand. Typically, it produces the 'dinner fork' deformity.

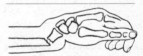

COLLES' FRACTURE

collimator ('koli,maytə) a device used in radiotherapy machines to help in determining the limits of the treatment field.

colloid ('koloyd) 1. gluelike. 2. the translucent, yellowish, gelatinous substance resulting from colloid degeneration. 3. a chemical system composed of a continuous medium of small particles, which do not settle out under the influence of gravity, and will not pass through a semipermeable membrane, as in DIALYSIS.

coloboma (,koloh'bohmə) a con-

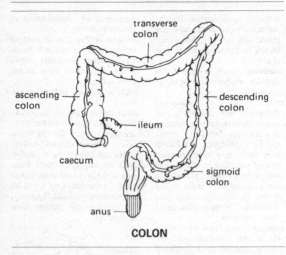

transverse colon

ascending colon

descending colon

ileum

caecum

sigmoid colon

anus

COLON

genital fissure of the eye affecting the choroid coat and the retina.

colon ('kohlon) the large intestine from the caecum to the rectum. *Ascending c.* that part arising to the right of the abdomen to in front of the liver. *Descending c.* that part running down from in front of the spleen to the sigmoid colon. *Giant c.* megacolon. *Irritable c.* IRRITABLE BOWEL SYNDROME. *Pelvic c., sigmoid c.* that part lying in the pelvis and connecting the descending colon with the rectum. *Transverse c.* that part lying across the upper abdomen connecting the ascending and descending portions.

colonic (kə'lonik) pertaining to the colon. *C. irrigation* colonic lavage (*see* LAVAGE).

colonoscope (koh'lonə,skohp) a fibreoptic instrument, passed through the anus, for examining the interior of the colon.

colony ('kolənee) a mass of bacteria formed by multiplication of cells when bacteria are incubated under favourable conditions.

colostomy (kə'lostəmee) an artificial opening (stoma) in the large intestine brought to the surface of the abdomen for the purpose of evacuating the bowel.

colostrum (kə'lostrəm) the fluid secreted by the breasts in the last few weeks of pregnancy and for the first 3 or 4 days after delivery, until lactation begins.

colour blindness ('kulə ,bliendnəs) achromatopsia.

colour index ('kulə ,indeks) an

index of the amount of haemo-globin in red blood cells. *See* BLOOD

colpitis (kol'pietis) inflammation of the vagina.

colpocele ('kolpoh,seel) a hernia of either bladder or rectum into the vagina. Vaginocele.

colpohysterectomy (,kolpoh-,histə'rektəmee) removal of the uterus through the vagina.

colpoperineorrhaphy (,kolpoh-,perini'o·rəfee) the repair by suturing of an injured vagina and torn perineum.

colpopexy ('kolpoh,peksee) su-ture of a prolapsed vagina to the abdominal wall.

colpoplasty ('kolpoh,plastee) a plastic operation on the vagina.

colporrhaphy (kol'po·rəfee) repair of the vagina. *Anterior c.* repair for cystocele. *Posterior c.* repair for rectocele.

colposcope ('kolpə,skohp) a speculum for examining the vagina and cervix by means of a magnifying lens; used for the early detection of malignant changes.

colpotomy (kol'potəmee) incision of the vaginal wall.

coma ('kohmə) a state of uncon-sciousness from which the patient cannot be aroused. Characterized by an absence both of spon-taneous eye movements and response to painful stimuli. *See* GLASGOW COMA SCALE.

comatose (,kohmə,tohs, -,tohz) in the condition of coma.

comedo (ko'meedoh) a blackhead. A plug of keratin and sebum within the dilated orifice of a hair follicle.

commensal (kə'mensəl) living on or within another organism, and deriving benefit without harming or benefiting the host individual.

comminuted ('komi,nyootid) broken into small pieces, as in a comminuted fracture. *See* FRAC-TURE.

commissure ('komis,yooə) a site of union of corresponding parts, as the angle of the lips or eyelids.

Committee on Safety of Medi-cines (kə'mittee) abbreviated CSM. An organization respon-sible for controlling the release of new drugs in the United King-dom.

communicable disease (kə'myoo-nikəb'l) a disease, the causative agents of which may pass or be carried from a person, animal or the environment to a susceptible person either directly or indirectly.

community (kə'myoonitee) a group of individuals living in an area, having a common interest, or belonging to the same organiz-ation. *C. Health Council* an organization which enables the consumer's interests to be repre-sented to those responsible at district level for the National Health Service. *C. nurse* a nurse who is based within the com-munity with a responsibility for providing nursing services within the patient's own home or environment. Community nurses have a strong commitment towards health promotion and the prevention of ill health. *Therapeutic c.* any treatment set-ting (usually psychiatric) which provides a living–learning situation through group processes emphasizing social, environmental and personal interactions.

compatibility (kəm,patə'bilitee) mutual suitability. Mixing together of two substances without chemical change or loss of power. *See* BLOOD GROUPING.

compensation (,kompən'sayshən) 1. making good a functional or structural defect. 2. mental mechanism (unconscious) by which a person covers up a weakness by exaggerating a more desirable characteristic.

complement ('komplimənt) a substance present in normal serum which combines with the antigen–antibody complex (*c. fixation*) to destroy bacteria. *C. fixation test* measurement of the amount of complement with antigen–antibody complex to destroy bacteria. Complement fixation tests are widely used to detect antibodies for infectious diseases and include the Wassermann test for syphilis.

complementary (,kompli'mentə·ree) pertaining to that which completes or makes perfect. *C. feed* feed given to infants to supplement breast feeding when the mother has insufficient milk. *C. therapies* a range of treatments, which include yoga, reflexology, homeopathy, acupuncture and others, which may be combined with traditional medicine. *See* Appendix 5.

complex ('kompleks) a grouping of various things, as of signs and symptoms, forming a syndrome. In psychology, a grouping of ideas of emotional origin which

are completely or partially repressed in the unconscious mind. *Inferiority c.* a compensation by assertiveness or aggression to cover a feeling of inadequacy. *See* ELECTRA and OEDIPUS.

complication (kompli'kayshən) an accident or second disease process arising during the course of or following the primary condition.

compos mentis ('kompəs 'mentis) [L.] *of sound mind.*

compound ('kompownd) composed of two or more parts or substances. *C. fracture* a fracture in which a wound through to the skin has also occurred.

comprehension (,kompri'henshən) mental grasp of the meaning of a situation.

compress ('kompres) folded material, e.g. lint (wet or dry), applied to a part of the body for the relief of swelling and pain.

compression (kəm'preshən) 1. the act of pressing upon or together; the state of being pressed together. 2. in embryology, the shortening or omission of certain developmental stages.

compulsion (kəm'pulshən) an overwhelming urge to perform an irrational act or ritual.

computed tomography (kəm-'pyootid tə'mogrəfee) abbreviated CT. The utilization of a computerized technique to examine a cross-section of the entire body. The CT scanner produces an image of tissue density in a complete cross-section of the part of the body being scanned.

conation (koh'nayshən) a striving in a certain direction. *See* COG-

NITION.

concave ('konkayv, kon'kayv) hollowed out. The opposite of convex.

concept ('konsept) an image or idea held in the mind.

conception (kən'sepshən) 1. the act of becoming pregnant, by the fertilization of an ovum. 2. a concept.

conceptual framework (kən'septyooal) a group of concepts that are broadly defined and organized to provide a rationale or structure for the interpretation of information.

concretion (kən'kreeshən) a calculus or other hardened material present within an organ.

concussion (kən'kushən) a violent jarring shock. *C. of the brain* temporary loss of consciousness produced by a fall or a blow on the head. There may be amnesia, slow respiration and a weak pulse.

conditioned response (kən'dishənd) a response that does not occur naturally but may be developed by regular association of some physiological function with an unrelated outside event, such as ringing of a bell or flashing of a light. Soon the physiological function starts whenever the outside event occurs. Called also conditioned reflex. *Unconditioned r.* an unlearned response, i.e. one that occurs naturally.

conditioning (kən'dishəning) a form of learning in which a response is elicited by a neutral stimulus which previously had been repeatedly presented in conjunction with the stimulus that

originally elicited the response. Called also classical and respondent conditioning. The concept had its beginnings in experimental techniques for the study of reflexes. The traditional procedure is based on the work of Ivan P. Pavlov, a Russian physiologist. In this technique the experimental subject is a dog that is harnessed in a sound-shielded room. The neutral stimulus is the sound of a metronome or bell which occurs each time the dog is presented with food, and the response is the production of saliva by the dog. Eventually the sound of the bell or metronome produces salivation, even though the stimulus that originally elicited the response (the food) is no longer presented. In the technique just described, the conditioned stimulus is the sound of the bell or metronome, and the conditioned response is the salivation that occurs when the sound is heard. The food, which was the original stimulus to salivation, is the unconditioned stimulus and the salivation that occurred when food was presented is the unconditioned response. Reinforcement is said to take place when the conditioned stimulus is appropriately followed by the unconditioned stimulus. If the unconditioned stimulus is withheld during a series of trials, the procedure is called extinction because the frequency of the conditioned response will gradually decrease when the stimulus producing the response is no longer present.

The process of extinction eventually results in a return of the preconditioning level of behaviour. *Classical c. see* CONDITIONING. *Instrumental c., operant c.* learning in which a particular response is elicited by a stimulus because that response produces desirable consequences (reward). Instrumental conditioning differs from classical conditioning in that the reinforcement takes place only after the subject performs a specific act that has been previously designated. If no unconditioned stimulus is used to bring about this act, the desired behaviour is known as an operant. Once the behaviour occurs with regularity the behaviour may be called a conditioned response. The classic example of instrumental or operant conditioning involves the use of the Skinner box, named after B.F. Skinner, an American behavioural psychologist. In this example, the subject, a rat, is kept in the box and becomes conditioned to press a bar by being rewarded with food pellets each time its early random movements caused it to press against the bar. The principles and techniques related to instrumental conditioning are used clinically in BEHAVIOUR THERAPY to help patients eliminate undesirable behaviour and substitute for it newly learned behaviour that is more appropriate and acceptable. *Respondent c. see* CONDITIONING.

condom ('kondəm) a contraceptive sheath worn by the male, affording some protection for both partners against sexually transmitted diseases.

conductor (kən'duktə) 1. a substance through which electricity, light, heat or sound can pass. 2. any part of the nervous system which conveys impulses.

condyle ('kondiel, -dil) a rounded eminence occurring at the end of some bones, and articulating with another bone.

condyloma (,kondi'lohmə) *pl.* condylomata; an elevated wart-like lesion of the skin. *Condylomata acuminata* small, pointed papillomas of viral origin, usually occurring on the skin or mucous surfaces of the external genitalia or perianal region. *Condyloma lata* wide, flat, syphilitic condylomata occurring on moist skin, especially about the genitals and anus.

cone (kohn) a solid figure with a rounded base, tapering upwards to a point. *Retinal c.* the cone-shaped end of a light-sensitive cell in the retina, used for acute vision and for distinguishing colours.

confabulation (kən,fabyuh'layshən) the production of fictitious memories, and the relating of experiences which have no relation to truth, to fill in the gaps due to loss of memory. A symptom of Korsakoff's syndrome.

confection (kən'fekshən) a preparation of sugar or honey containing drugs, e.g. senna.

confidentiality (,konfi,denshi'alitee) spoken, written or given in confidence. See ninth clause of the professional code of conduct published by the United Kingdom Central Council for Nurses, Midwives and Health Visitors (*See* Appendix 11).

conflict ('konflikt) a mental state arising when two opposing wishes or impulses cause emotional tension and often cannot be resolved without repressing one of the impulses into the unconscious. Conflict situations may be associated with an anxiety neurosis.

confluent ('konflooənt) running together.

confusion (kən'fyoozhən) disturbed orientation in regard to time, place or person, sometimes accompanied by disordered consciousness.

congenital (kən'jenit'l) present at and existing from the time of birth. *C. dislocation of hip* failure in position of the head of the femur and development of the acetabulum. *C. heart defect* a structural defect of the heart or great vessels or both; present at birth. *C. infection* an infection which takes place in utero. The most important congenital infections are rubella, cytomegalovirus, herpes simplex, human immunodeficiency virus (HIV), syphilis and toxoplasmosis.

congestion (kən'jeschən) an abnormal accumulation of blood in any part. *Pulmonary c.* congestion of the lung, as in pneumonia and congestive heart failure.

conization (,kohnie'zayshən) removal of a cone-shaped piece of tissue from the uterine cervix.

conjunctiva (,konjungk'tievə) the mucous membrane covering the front of the eyeball and lining the eyelids.

conjunctivitis (kən,jungkti'vietis) inflammation of the conjunctiva. 'Pink eye' ophthalmia. *Catarrhal c.* a mild form, usually due to cold or irritation. *Granular c.* trachoma. *Phlyctenular c.* marked by small vesicles or ulcers on the membrane. *Purulent c.* caused by virulent organisms, with discharge of pus.

Conn's syndrome ('konz) *W.J. Conn, American physician, b. 1907.* Primary hyperaldosteronism, resulting from a tumour in the adrenal cortex. *See* ALDOSTERONISM.

connective (kə'nektiv) joining together. *C. tissues* those that develop from the mesenchyme and are formed of a matrix containing fibres and cells. Areolar tissue, cartilage and bone are examples.

consanguinity (,konsang·gwinitee) blood relationship.

conscious (konshəs) the state of being awake or aware. *Levels of c.* loosely defined states of awareness of and response to stimuli, essential for the assessment of an individual's neurological status. The level of consciousness is an accurate indicator of the degree of brain (dys)function.

consent (kən'sent) in law, voluntary agreement with an action proposed by another. Consent is an act of reason; the person giving consent must be of sufficient mental capacity and be in possession of all essential information in order to give valid consent. *C. forms* in non-emergency situations, written informed consent is generally required before many clinical procedures, such as surgery (including biopsies), endoscopy and radiographic procedures involving catheterization. The doctor must explain to the patient the diagnosis, the nature of the procedure, including the risks involved and the chances of success, and the alternative methods of treatment that are available. Nurses or other members of the health care team may be involved in filling out the consent form and witnessing the signature of the patient.

conservative treatment (kən'-sərvətiv) the use of non-radical methods to restore health and preserve function.

consolidation (kən,soli'dayshən) a state of becoming solid. *C. of lung* in pneumonia the infected lobe becomes solid with exudate.

constipation (,konsti'payshən) incomplete or infrequent action of the bowels, with consequent filling of the rectum with hard faeces. *Atonic c.* constipation due to lack of muscle tone in the bowel wall. *Spastic c.* a form of constipation where spasm of part of the bowel wall narrows the canal.

consumption (kən'sumpshən) 1. the act of consuming, or the process of being consumed. 2. a wasting away of the body; once applied to pulmonary tuberculosis.

contact ('kontakt) 1. a mutual touching of two bodies or persons. 2. an individual known to have been in association with an infected person or animal or a contaminated environment which might have exposed him to infection. *C. dermatitis* a skin rash marked by itching, swelling, blistering, oozing and scaling. It is caused by direct contact between the skin and a substance to which the person is allergic or sensitive. *C. lens* a glass or plastic lens worn under the eyelids in the front of the eye. It may be worn for therapeutic or for cosmetic reasons.

contagion (kən'tayjən) 1. the communication of disease from one person to another by direct contact. 2. an infectious disease.

containment (kən'taynmənt) a term used in communicable disease control, meaning prevention of spread of disease from a focus of infection.

continuing care (kə'tinyooing) ongoing care of the physically, mentally and emotionally handicapped, and those suffering from chronic incapacitating illness.

continuing education further study after the attainment of basic qualifications. This is vital for all professional practitioners so that they may keep up to date within their field and is accomplished in the form of organized study days or courses, or by individual reading.

continuous ambulatory peritoneal dialysis abbreviated CAPD. The patient is ambulant whilst receiving peritoneal dialysis.

continuous positive airway pressure abbreviated CPAP. Medical gas is delivered to the patient at positive pressure to hold open alveoli that would normally close at the end of expiration, and thereby increase oxygenation and reduce the work of breathing.

contraception (ˌkontrə'sepshən) the prevention of conception and pregnancy.

contraceptive (ˌkontrə'septiv) an agent used to prevent conception, e.g. male sheath, cap that occludes the cervix, spermicidal pessary or cream, intrauterine device (IUD), and oral contraceptives (hormone pills).

contraction (kən'trakshən) a shortening or drawing together, especially applied to muscle action. *Uterine c's* those occurring during labour.

contracture (kən'trakchə) fibrosis causing permanent contraction. *Dupuytren's c.* contraction of the palmar fascia causing permanent bending and fixation of one or more fingers. *Volkmann's ischaemic c.* contraction resulting from impairment of the blood supply. May occur in upper or lower limbs.

contraindication (ˌkontrəˌindi-'kayshən) any condition that makes a particular line of treatment impracticable or undesirable.

contralateral (ˌkontrə'latə·rəl) occurring on the opposite side.

contrast medium ('kontrahst) a substance used in radiography to make visible or more visible certain organs.

contrecoup (ˌkontrə'koo) [Fr.] an injury occurring on the opposite side or at a distance from the site of the blow, e.g. brain damage on the opposite side of the skull to the blow.

control (kən'trohl) 1. restrain or command of objects or events. 2. a standard for testing where the procedure is identical in all respects to the experiment but the factor being studied is absent. *Birth c.* contraception.

controlled drugs (kən'trold) preparations subject to the Misuse of Drugs Act (1971), Misuse of Drugs (Notification of and Supply to Addicts) Regulations (1973) and the Misuse of Drugs Regulations (1985) which regulate the prescribing and dispensing of psychoactive drugs, including narcotics, hallucinogens, depressants and stimulants.

contusion (kan'tyoozhən) a bruise.

convalescence (ˌkonvə'les'ns) period of recovery following illness, injury or operation.

convection (kən'vekshən) a method of transmission of heat by the circulation of warmed molecules of a liquid or a gas.

conversion (kən'vərshən) 1. the act of changing into something of different form or properties. 2. the transformation of emotions into physical manifestations. 3. manipulative correction of malposition of a fetal part during labour.

convex ('konveks, kon'veks) bowing outwards. Having an outline like a segment of a sphere.

convolution ('konvə'looshən) a fold or coil, e.g. of the cerebrum or renal tubules.

convulsion (kən'vulshən) involuntary contractions of the voluntary muscles. Convulsive seizures are symptomatic of some neurological disorder; they are not in themselves a disease entity. *Clonic c.* a convulsion marked by alternative contracting and relaxing of the muscles. *Febrile c.* a convulsion occurring almost exclusively in children aged 6 months to 5 years of age, and associated with a fever of 40°C (104°F) or higher. *Tonic c.* prolonged contraction of the muscles, as a result of an epileptic discharge. *See* EPILEPSY.

Cooley's anaemia ('kooleez) *T.B. Cooley, American paediatrician, 1871–1945.* Thalassaemia.

Coombs' test (koomz) *R.R.A. Coombs, British immunologist, b. 1921.* A test to detect the presence of any antibody on the surface of the red blood cell. Used to detect rhesus incompatibility in maternal or fetal blood and in the diagnosis of haemolytic anaemia.

coordination (koh,awdi'nayshən) harmony of movement between several muscles or groups of muscle so that complicated manoeuvres can be made.

coping ('kohping) the process of contending with life difficulties in an effort to overcome or work through them. *C. mechanisms* conscious or unconscious strategies or mechanisms that a person uses to cope with stress or anxiety.

copiopia (,kopi·ə'peeə, ,kohpi·ə-) improper use of the eye or overwork leading to eyestrain. Copiopsia.

copper ('kopə) *symbol Cu.* A metallic element, traces of which are present in all human tissues.

coprolalia ('koproh'layli·ə) the uncontrolled use of obscene speech.

coprolith ('koprohlith) a faecalith.

coprostasia (,koproh'stayzi·ə) the accumulation of faecal matter in the intestines, causing obstruction.

copulation (,kopyu'layshən) coitus. Sexual intercourse between male and female.

coracoid ('ko·rə,koyd) 1. shaped like a raven's beak. 2. the coracoid process of the scapula.

cord (kawd) a long cylindrical flexible structure. *Spermatic c.* that which suspends the testicle in the scrotum, and contains the spermatic artery and vein and vas deferens. *Spinal c.* the part of the central nervous system enclosed in the spinal column. *Umbilical c.* the connection between the fetus and the placenta, through which the fetus receives nourishment. *Vocal c's* folds of mucous membrane in the larynx which vibrate to produce the voice.

cordotomy (kaw'dotəmee) *see* CHORDOTOMY.

corn (kawn) a local hardening and thickening of the skin from pressure or friction, occurring usually on the feet. Clavus.

cornea ('kawni·ə) the transparent portion of the anterior surface of the eyeball continuous with the sclerotic coat. *Conical c.* keratoconus.

corneal ('kawni·əl) pertaining to the cornea. *C. graft* a means of restoring sight by grafting healthy transparent cornea from a donor in place of diseased tissue. Keratoplasty.

corneoscleral (ˌkawnioh'skliə·rəl) relating to both the cornea and sclera. *C. junction* the point where the edge of the cornea joins the sclera. The limbus.

cornification (ˌkawnifi'kayshən) keratinization. The process whereby the skin becomes horny through the deposition of keratin.

cornu ('kawnyoo) a horn. *C. of uterus* one of the two horn-shaped projections where the uterine tubes join the uterus at the upper pole on either side.

coronal (kə'rohn'l) relating to the crown of the head. *C. suture* the junction of the frontal and parietal bones.

coronary ('ko·rənə·ree) encircling. Crown-like. *C. arteries* the vessels which supply the heart. *C. circulation see* CIRCULATION. *C. thrombosis see* THROMBOSIS.

coroner ('ko·rənə) a public official (e.g. a barrister, solicitor or doctor) who holds inquests concerning sudden, violent or suspicious deaths.

coronoid ('ko·rə,noyd) shaped like a crow's beak. *C. process* a bony process of the mandible or of the ulna.

corpse (kawps) a dead body; cadaver.

corpulent ('kawpyuhlant) obese.

corpus ('korpəs) a body. *C. albicans* the scar tissue on the surface of the ovary which replaces the corpus luteum before the recommencement of menstruation. *C. callosum* the mass of white matter which joins the two cerebral hemispheres together. *C. cavernosum* either of the two columns of erectile tissue forming the body of the clitoris or the penis. *C. luteum* the yellow body left on the surface of the ovary and formed from the remains of the graafian follicle after the discharge of the ovum. If it retrogresses, menstruation occurs, but it persists for several months if pregnancy supervenes. *C. striatum* a mass of grey and white matter in the base of each cerebral hemisphere.

corpuscle ('kawpəs'l) a small protoplasmic body or cell, as of blood or connective tissue. *See* BLOOD.

corrective (kə'rektiv) a corrigent. A drug which modifies the action of other drugs.

corrosive (kə'rohsiv, -ziv) a substance that erodes and destroys.

cortex ('kawteks) [L.] *an outer layer*, as the bark of the trunk or root of a tree, or the outer layer of an organ or other structure, as distinguished from its inner substance. *Adrenal c.* the tissue surrounding the medulla or core of the adrenal gland. *Cerebral c.* the grey matter covering the two cerebral hemispheres. *Renal c.* the outer covering of the kidney.

corticospinal (ˌkawtikoh'spien'l) relating to the cerebral cortex and the spinal cord. *C. tract* the pyramidal tract. The nerve fibres making up the main pathway for rapid voluntary movement.

corticosteroid (ˌkawtikoh'stiə·royd) any of the hormones produced by the adrenal cortex or their synthetic substitutes. Glucocorticoids are responsible for carbohydrate, fat and protein metabolism. They have powerful anti-inflammatory properties.

Mineralocorticoids, e.g. aldosterone, are responsible for salt and water regulation.

corticotrophin (ˌkawtikoh'trohfin) Adrenocorticotrophic hormone (ACTH).

cortisol ('kawti,sol) the naturally occurring hormone of the adrenal cortex. Hydrocortisone.

cortisone ('kawti,zohn, -,sohn) a naturally occurring corticosteroid. Inactive in man until converted into cortisol. *C. acetate* a synthetic preparation with anti-inflammatory and antiallergic properties.

Corynebacterium (koˌrienibak-'tie·ri·əm) a genus of slender, rod-shaped, Gram-positive and nonmotile bacteria. *C. diphtheriae* Klebs–Löffler bacillus, the causative agent of diphtheria.

coryza (kə'riezə) acute infection of the upper respiratory tract, characterized by perfuse discharge from nasal mucous membranes, sneezing and watering of the eyes.

cost effectiveness (ˌkost i'fektivnəs) a concept which relates cost to the effectiveness of a service and thus provides value for money, e.g. screening programmes to detect cervical cancer, rate of detection, cost of the service and of treatment.

costal ('kost'l) relating to the ribs. *C. cartilages* those which connect the ribs to the sternum directly or indirectly.

cot death (kot) *See* SUDDEN INFANT DEATH SYNDROME.

cotyledon (ˌkoti'leedən) A cup-shaped depression. Applied to the subdivisions of the placenta.

cough (kof) voluntary or reflex explosive expulsion of air from the lungs. Its purpose is usually to expel a foreign body or accumulations of mucus. *Dry c.* one where no expectoration occurs. *Wet c.* expectoration of mucus or foreign body occurs. *Whooping c.* infectious disease caused by *Bordetella pertussis*.

counselling ('kownsəling) a process of consultation and discussion in which one individual (the counsellor) listens and offers guidance or advice to another who is experiencing difficulties (the client). The counsellor does not direct or make decisions for the client. The general aim is to solve problems and increase awareness. The emphasis is on the client finding his own solution.

counterextension (ˌkowntə·rik-'stenshən) 1. the holding back of the upper fragment of a fractured bone while the lower is pulled into position. 2. the raising of the foot of the bed in such a way that the weight of the body counteracts the pull of the extension apparatus on the lower part of the limb. Used especially for fracture of the femur.

counterirritant (ˌkowntə·iritənt) a substance which produces mild inflammation of the skin when applied to it, but relieves pain and congestion.

countertraction (ˌkowntə,trak-shən) the reduction of fractures by traction from two opposing directions at once.

coupling ('kupling) in cardiology, the frequent occurrence of a normal heartbeat followed by an extraventricular one. May be found following digitalis overdose.

couvade (koo'vahd) the experiencing of the symptoms of pregnancy and childbirth by the father. This psychosomatic phenomenon is common in many societies.

Cowper's glands ('koopəz) *W. Cowper, British surgeon and anatomist, 1666–1709.* Bulbourethral glands.

coxa ('koksə) the hip joint. *C. valga* a deformity of the hip in which there is an increase in the angle between the neck and the shaft of the femur. *C. vara* a deformity in which the angle between the neck and the shaft of the femur is smaller than the normal.

coxalgia (kok'salji·ə) pain in the hip joint.

Coxiella (,koksi'elə) a genus of microorganisms of the order Rickettsiales. *C. burnetii* the causative agent of Q fever.

Coxsackie virus (kok'sakee) one of a group of enteroviruses that may give rise to a variety of illnesses including meningitis, pleurodynia and myocarditis.

crab louse ('krab ,lows) *Phthirus pubis.* See LOUSE.

cradle (,krayd'l) 1. a frame placed over the body or limb of a bed patient for protecting injured parts from coming in contact with the bed clothes. 2. infant's bed with protective sides and, in the past, often on rockers. 3. to support, hold, comfort in the arms. *C. cap* an oily crust sometimes seen on the scalp of nursing infants; also called milk crust (crusta lactea). Caused by excessive secretion of the sebaceous glands in the scalp.

cramp (kramp) a painful spasmodic muscular contraction which may result from fatigue. *Occupational c.* occurs in miners and stokers; it is associated with intense heat and dehydration.

cranial ('krayni·əl) relating to the cranium. *C. nerves* the 12 pairs of nerves arising directly from the brain.

craniopharyngioma (,krayniohfa-,rinji'ohmə) a cerebral tumour arising in the craniopharyngeal pouch just above the sella turcica.

craniostenosis (,krayniohstə-'nohsis) premature closure of the suture lines of the skull in an infant. Surgery may be required to relieve raised intracranial pressure.

craniosynostosis (,krayniohsi'nostəsis) premature closure of the cranial sutures.

craniotabes ('kraynioh'taybeez) a patchy thinning of the bones of the vault of the skull of an infant; associated with rickets.

craniotomy (,krayni'otəmee) a surgical opening of the skull made to relieve pressure, arrest haemorrhage or remove a tumour.

cranium ('krayni·əm) 1. the skull. 2. the bony cavity which contains the brain.

creatine ('kreeə,teen, -tin) a nitrogenous compound present in muscle. It is also found in the urine in conditions in which muscle is rapidly broken down, e.g. acute fevers and starvation. *C. phosphate* a high-energy phosphate store in muscle.

creatinine (kree'ati,neen) a normal constituent of urine; a product of protein metabolism.

creatinuria (kree,ati,nyooə·ri·ə) increased concentration of creatine in the urine.

creatorrhoea (,kreeətə'reeə) the presence of muscle fibres in the faeces. It occurs in certain diseases of the pancreas.

Credé's method ('kredayz) (*K.S.F. Credé, German gynaecologist, 1819–1892*). The expulsion of the placenta by the exertion of pressure on the uterus through the abdominal wall. Rarely used.

crenation (kri'nayshən) abnormal notching of erythrocytes, which occurs when they are exposed to hypertonic solutions such as saline, or in certain diseases, or after prolonged storage of a blood specimen.

creosote ('kreeə,soht) a mixture of phenols from wood tar; occasionally used externally as an antiseptic and internally in chronic bronchitis as an expectorant.

creosol ('kreeə,sol) one of the active constituents of creosote. Used in a wide range of disinfectants.

crepitation (,krepi'tayshən) the grating sound caused by friction of the two ends of a fractured bone.

crepitus ('krepitəs) 1. the discharge of flatus from the bowels. 2. crepitation. 3. a crepitant râle.

cretinism ('kreti,nizəm) congenital hypothyroidism. A condition caused by lack of thyroid secretion, characterized by arrested physical and mental development, dull facial expression with dry skin and lack of coordination.

Creutzfeldt–Jakob disease (,kroytsfelt'yakob) *H.G. Creutzfeldt,* German physician, 1885–1964. *A. Jakob, German physician, 1884–1931.* A rare encephalopathy due to a transmissible agent with a very long incubation period, termed a slow virus. It is manifested by confusion, dementia and ataxia, usually in persons over the age of 40 years. The only known source of infection is man.

cribriform ('kribri,fawm) perforated like a sieve. *C. plate* part of the ethmoid bone. *See* ETHMOID.

cricoid (,kriekoyd) ring-shaped. *C. cartilage* the ring-shaped cartilage at the lower end of the larynx.

cri-du-chat syndrome (,kree doo 'shah) *see* CAT CRY SYNDROME.

crisis ('kriesis) 1. a decisive point in acute disease; the turning-point towards either recovery or death. *See* LYSIS. 2. a sudden paroxysmal intensification of symptoms in the course of a disease. 3. life crisis; a period of disorganization that occurs when a person meets an obstacle to an important life goal, such as the sudden death of a family member or a difficult family conflict. *Addisonian c., adrenal c.* symptoms of fatigue, nausea and vomiting, and collapse accompanying an acute attack of adrenal failure. *Blast c.* a sudden, severe change in the course of chronic myelocytic leukaemia. The clinical picture resembles that seen in acute myelogenous leukaemia, with an increase in the proportion of myeloblasts. *Identity c.* usually occurring during adolescence, manifested by a loss of the sense of the sameness and historical continuity of one's self, and inability to accept the role the individual perceives as being expected of him by society. *C. intervention* counselling or psychotherapy for patients in a life crisis that is directed at supporting the patient through the crisis and helping the patient to cope with the stressful event that precipitated it.

criterion (krie'tiə·ri·ən) the basis on which a decision is made, e.g. for drug dosage, treatment plans, research trials, etc.

Crohn's disease (krohnz) *B.B. Crohn, American physician, b. 1884.* Regional ileitis. *See* ILEITIS.

Crosby capsule ('krozbee) *W.H. Crosby, American physician, b. 1914.* A capsule attached to the end of a flexible tube which is swallowed by the patient. When the capsule reaches the small intestine, as seen on radiological examination, a biopsy of the intestinal mucosa may be taken.

crotamiton (kroh'tamiton) an antipruritic lotion which is also used to treat scabies.

croup (kroop) a condition resulting from acute obstruction of the larynx caused by allergy, foreign body, infection, or new growth; occurs chiefly in infants and children. There is spasmodic dyspnoea, a harsh cough and stridor.

crown (krown) that part of the tooth which appears above the gum.

crowning ('krowning) the stage in labour when the top of the infant's head becomes visible at the vulva.

cruciate ('krooshiayt) resembling a cross. *C. ligament see* LIGAMENT.

crus (krus) [L.] 1. the leg, from knee to foot. 2. a leglike part.

'crush' syndrome (krush) the oedema, oliguria and other symptoms of acute renal failure that follow crushing of a part, especially a large muscle mass, causing the release of myoglobin.

crutch ('kruch) appliance to aid walking when the patient must not weight-bear (as in fractures of lower limbs) or when a lower limb is missing.

cryaesthesia (,krieis'theezi·ə) abnormal sensitiveness to cold.

cryoanalgesia (,krieoh,an'l'jeezi·ə, -si·ə) the relief of pain by application of cold by cryoprobe to peripheral nerves.

cryobank ('krieoh,bank) a facility for freezing and preserving semen at low temperatures (usually −196.5°C) for future use.

cryoextractor (,krieoh·ik'straktə) an instrument in which intense cold coagulates the lens of the eye for removal in cataract extraction.

cryoprecipitate (,krieohpri'sipi·,tayt) any precipitate that results from cooling. Of particular therapeutic value is the cryoprecipitate from fresh plasma, which is rich in factor VIII and is used to treat haemophilia.

cryopreservation (,krieoh,prezə·'vayshən) maintenance of the viability of excised tissue or organs by storing at very low temperatures.

cryosurgery (ˌkrieoh'sərjə·ree) the use of extreme cold to destroy tissue.

cryotherapy (ˌkrieoh'therəpee) therapeutic use of cold.

cryptococcosis (ˌkriptohkok'ohsis) infection caused by the fungus *Cryptococcus neoformans*, having a predilection for the brain and meninges but also invading the skin, lungs and other parts. It particularly affects persons immunocompromised by disease or therapy.

cryptogenic. (ˌkriptoh'jenik) of unknown or obscure origin.

cryptomenorrhoea (ˌkriptoh-ˌmenə'reeə) the occurrence of menstrual symptoms without external bleeding, as in imperforate hymen. Haematocolpos.

cryptorchidism (krip‚tawki‚dizəm) failure of the testicles to descend into the scrotum; cryptorchism.

crypts of Lieberkühn (ˌkrips əv 'leeə‚koon) *J.N. Lieberkühn, German anatomist, 1711–1756.* Glands, found in the mucous membrane of the small intestine, which secrete intestinal juice.

crystalline (ˌkristə‚lien) having the properties of a crystal. Transparent. *C. lens*; the lens of the eye. *See* LENS.

Cs symbol for *caesium*.

CT *see* COMPUTED TOMOGRAPHY.

Cu symbol for *copper*.

cubitus ('kyoobitəs) 1. the forearm. 2. the elbow. *C. valgus* deformity of the elbow where the palm of the hand is abducted and thus faces outwards. *C. varus* deformity where there is adduction of the forearm.

culdocentesis (ˌkuldohsen'teesis) the aspiration of fluid from the pouch of Douglas via the posterior fornix of the vagina.

culdoscope ('kuldoh‚skohp) an endoscope used in culdoscopy.

culdoscopy (kul'doskəpee) direct visual examination of the female viscera through an endoscope introduced into the pelvic cavity through the posterior vaginal fornix.

culture ('kulchə) 1. the propagation of microorganisms or of living tissue cells in special media conducive to their growth. 2. a collective noun for the symbolic and acquired aspects of human society, including convention, custom and language. 3. a singular noun for the customs and features of an ethnic (racial, religious or social) group.

cumulative ('kyoomyuhlətiv) adding to. *C. action* the toxic effects produced by prolonged use of a drug given in comparatively small doses. Usually occurs due to slow excretion of the drug.

cupping ('kuping) 1. the formation of a cup-shaped depression with the hand: (a) to produce a skin erythema, thereby improving local circulation, and (b) to loosen excessive secretions from air passages, and perhaps induce coughing. 2. the use of a cupping glass to stimulate skin blood flow.

curare (kyoo'rahree) an extract from a South American plant used to poison the tips of arrows. Used in surgery to produce complete muscle relaxation, it is given intravenously as tubocurarine.

curative ('kyooə·rətiv) anything which promotes healing by overcoming disease.

curettage ('kyooə·ri'tahzh, kyuh-'rettij) [Fr.] the scraping of a surface with a curette for therapeutic purposes or to obtain biopsy material.

curette (kyuh'ret) a spoon-shaped instrument used for the removal of unhealthy tissues by scraping.

curie ('kyooə·ree) *symbol* Ci. A unit of radioactivity. Now replaced as an SI unit by the becquerel.

curietron ('kyooə·ri,tron) an apparatus used for the treatment of cancer of the cervix and body of the uterus. The applicators are placed in the patient and the radioisotope is then moved in and out of the applicators by remote control.

Curling's ulcer ('kərlingz) an ulcer of the duodenum seen after severe burns of the body.

curvature ('kərvəchə) the curving of a line, whether normal or abnormal. *Spinal c.* abnormal deviation of the vertebral column.

Cushing's disease ('kuhshingz) *H.W. Cushing, American surgeon, 1869–1939.* A condition of oversecretion by the adrenal cortex due to an adenoma of the pituitary gland. Symptoms include obesity, abnormal distribution of hair, and atrophy of the genital organs.

cushingoid ('kushing,oyd) referring to symptoms which resemble Cushing's disease, e.g. the side-effects of steroid therapy.

cusp (kusp) a pointed or rounded projection, such as on the crown of a tooth, or a segment of a cardiac valve.

cutaneous (kyoo'tayni·əs) pertaining to the skin.

cutdown ('kut,down) an incision into a vein with insertion of a catheter for intravenous infusion. It is performed when an infusion cannot be started by venepuncture. Also used with hyperalimentation therapy when concentrated solutions need to be given into the superior vena cava.

cuticle ('kyootik'l) the narrow band of epidermis extending from the nail wall onto the nail surface; called also eponychium.

cyanide ('sieə,nied) one of the salts of hydrocyanic acid. It gives off a smell of bitter almonds and is rapidly fatal when inhaled or taken orally.

cyanocobalamin (,sieənohkoh-'baləmin) vitamin B$_{12}$ (antianaemic factor) found in liver, eggs and fish. It combines with the intrinsic factor secreted in gastric juice for absorption and is essential for erythrocyte maturation. Administered by injection in the treatment of pernicious anaemia.

cyanosis (,sieə'nohsis) a bluish appearance of the skin and mucous membranes, caused by imperfect oxygenation of the blood. It indicates circulatory failure and is common in respiratory diseases. It is also seen in 'blue babies'.

cyclamate ('sieklə,mayt, 'siklə-mayt) a non-nutritive sweetener.

cycle ('siek'l) a series of recurring events. *Cardiac c.* the events occurring between one heart beat and the next. *Menstrual c.* the changes that occur each month in the female reproductive system.

cyclic ('sieklik) pertaining to or occurring in a cycle.

cyclitis (sie'klietis) inflammation of the ciliary body of the eye.

cyclizine ('sie'kli,zeen) an antihistamine.

cyclobarbitone (,siekloh'bahbi-,tohn) a short-acting barbiturate drug administered orally in cases of insomnia. Prolonged use may lead to dependence.

cyclodialysis (,sieklohdie'alǝsis) an operation used in glaucoma to improve drainage from the anterior chamber of the eye at the corneoscleral junction.

cyclodiathermy (,siekloh,dieǝ-'thǝrmee) a treatment for glaucoma without penetration of the eyeball. Diathermy is applied to the sclera to cause fibrosis around the ciliary body, so allowing the aqueous humour to drain.

cyclopenthiazide (,sieklohpen-'thieǝ,zied) an oral diuretic.

cyclopentolate (,siekloh'pentǝ,layt) eye drops that paralyse the ciliary muscles and dilate the pupils.

cyclophosphamide (,siekloh'fosfǝ-,mied) a cytotoxic drug used in the treatment of lymphomas and leukaemia.

cycloplegia (,siekloh'pleeji·ǝ) paralysis of the ciliary muscle of the eye.

cyclopropane (,siekloh'prohpayn) a gas used for general anaesthesia. It is not irritating to the respiratory tract but is highly inflammable and is therefore potentially dangerous.

cycloserine (,siekloh'siǝ·rien) an antibiotic drug used in the treatment of tuberculosis resistant to first-line therapy.

cyclosporin (sieklohspo·rin, -spor·rin) an immunosuppressive agent which does not suppress the production of antibodies. Used as prophylaxis in graft-versus-host (GVH) disease and for the prevention of graft rejection in the field of organ and tissue transplantation.

cyclothymia ('siekloh'thiemi-ǝ) the alternation of mood seen in manic-depressive psychosis.

cyesis (sie'eesis) pregnancy. *Pseudo-c.* signs and symptoms suggestive of pregnancy arising when no fertilization has taken place. 'Phantom pregnancy'.

cyproterone (sie'prohtǝ·rohn) an antiandrogen used to treat male hypersexuality and prostatic carcinoma.

cyst (sist) 1. a cavity or sac with epithelium, containing liquid or semi-solid matter. 2. a stage in the life cycle of certain protozoan parasites when they acquire tough protective coats. *Branchial c.* one formed in the neck due to nonclosure of the branchial cleft during development. *Chocolate c.* an ovarian cyst occurring in endometriosis. *Daughter c.* a small cyst which develops from a large one. *Dermoid c.* a congenital type containing skin, hair, teeth, etc. It is due to abnormal development of embryonic tissue. *Hydatid c.* the larval cyst stage of the tapeworm, usually found in the liver. *Meibomian c.* a swelling of a meibomian gland caused by obstruction of its duct. *Multilocular c.* a cyst that is divided into compartments or locules. *Ovarian c.* a cyst of the ovary, usually non-malignant, but sometimes becoming very large and requiring surgical removal. *Retention c.* any cyst caused by blockage of a duct. *Sebaceous c.* a retention cyst caused by the blockage of a duct from a sebaceous gland so that the sebum collects. *Sublingual c.* a ranula. *Thyroglossal c.* one in the thyroglossal tract near the hyoid bone at the base of the tongue.

cystadenoma (si,stadə'nohmə) a benign neoplasm made up of cysts containing secretions.

cystalgia (si'stalji·ə) pain in the urinary bladder.

cystathioninuria (,sistə,thieohni-'nyooə·ri·ə) a hereditary disorder of cystathionine metabolism, marked by increased concentrations in the urine. May be associated with mental handicap.

cystectomy (si'stektəmee) complete or partial removal of the urinary bladder. The ureters are diverted into an isolated ileal segment (ileal conduit) or into the sigmoid colon.

cysteine ('sisti,een, sis'tayn) a sulphur-containing amino acid formed by the ingestion of dietary proteins.

cystic fibrosis ('sistik fie'brohsis) generalized hereditary disorder associated with accumulation of excessively thick and tenacious mucus and abnormal secretion of sweat and saliva; called also cystic fibrosis of the pancreas, and mucoviscidosis. The disease is inherited as a recessive trait. The severity

of cystic fibrosis varies widely. Although it is congenital, it may not manifest itself during the early weeks of life, or it may cause intestinal obstruction and perforation in the newborn. The chief cause of complications in cystic fibrosis is the extremely thick mucus predisposing to repeated infection, leading to chronic lung disease.

cysticercosis (,sistisər'kohsis) a disease caused by infestation with the cysticercus of *Taenia solium* (pork tapeworm). Has been eliminated from the UK.

cysticercus (,sisti'sərkəs) the cystic or larval form of the tapeworm.

cystine ('sisteen, -tin) an amino acid closely related to cysteine. Sometimes excreted in urine in the form of minute crystals (cystinuria).

cystinosis (,sisti'nohsis) an inherited metabolic disorder in which cystine is deposited in the tissues.

cystitis (si'stietis) inflammation of the urinary bladder.

cystitome ('sisti,tohm) a surgical knife used in cataract operations.

cystocele ('sistoh,seel) a prolapse of the bladder into the vagina.

cystodiathermy (,sistoh'dieə-,thərmee) the application of a high-frequency electric current to the bladder mucosa, usually for the removal of papillomas.

cystography (si'stogrəfee) radiography of the urinary bladder after the introduction of a radio-opaque dye. *Micturating c.* radiographic examination during the act of passing urine.

cystolithiasis (,sistohli'thieəsis)

stone or stones in the urinary bladder.

cystometer (si'stomitə) an instrument for measuring pressure inside the urinary bladder.

cystometry (si'stomətree) the study of pressure changes within the bladder and of variations in its capacity.

cystopexy ('sistoh'peksee) an operation for stress incontinence in which the bladder neck is fastened to the fascia at the back of the symphysis pubis.

cystoscope ('sistə,skohp) an endoscope for examining the interior of the urinary bladder.

cystostomy (si'stostəmee) the operation of making a temporary or permanent opening into the urinary bladder.

cystotomy (si'stotəmee) incision of the urinary bladder for removal of calculi, etc. *Supra-pubic c.* incision above the pubes.

cystourethrography (,sistoh,yooə·ri'throgrəfee) radiology of the urinary bladder and urethra.

cystourethroscope (,sistoh·yuhreethrə,skohp) an instrument for examining the urethra and bladder.

cytarabine (si'tarə,been) *see* CYTOSINE.

cytogenetics (,sietohje'netiks) the study of cells during mitosis in order to examine the chromosomes and the relationship between chromosome abnormality and disease.

cytology (sie'toləjee) the microscopic study of the form and functions of the cells of the body. *Exfoliative c.* an aid to the early diagnosis of malignant disease. Secretions or surface cells are examined for premalignant changes.

cytolysin (sie'tolisin) a substance that causes cytolysis. *See* BACTERIOLYSIN and HAEMOLYSIN.

cytolysis (sie'tolisis) the destruction of cells.

cytomegalic inclusion disease (,sietoh'megəlik in'kloozhən) an infection due to cytomegalovirus. In the congenital form, there is hepatosplenomegaly with cirrhosis, and microcephaly with mental or motor handicap. Acquired disease may cause a clinical state similar to infectious mononucleosis.

cytomegalovirus (,sietoh,megəloh'vierəs) a virus belonging to the herpes simplex group.

cytoplasm ('sietoh,plazəm) the protoplasmic part of the cell surrounding the nucleus.

cytosine ('sietoh,seen) one of the pyrimidine bases found in DEOXYRIBONUCLEIC ACID. *C. arabinoside* an antimetabolite used in the treatment of acute leukaemia. Cytarabine.

cytotoxic (,sietoh'toksik) 1. having a deleterious effect upon cells. 2. an agent that destroys cells.

cytotoxin (,sietoh'toksin) a toxin having a specific toxic action on cells of special organs.

D

D symbol for *dioptre*.

dacryoadenectomy (ˌdakriohˌadə-'nektəmee) removal of a lacrimal gland.

dacryoadenitis (ˌdakriohˌadə'nietis) inflammation of a lacrimal gland.

dacryocystitis (ˌdakriohsi'stietis) inflammation of a lacrimal sac.

dacryocystography (ˌdakriohsi-'stogrəfee) radiography of the lacrimal duct using a radio-opaque contrast medium.

dacryocystorhinostomy (ˌdakriohˌsistohrie'nostəmee) an operation to create an opening between the lacrimal sac and the nasal cavity.

dacryocystotomy (ˌdakriohsi'stotəmee) incision of a lacrimal sac.

dacryolith ('dakriohˌlith) a calculus in a lacrimal duct.

dacryoma (ˌdakri'ohmə) a benign tumour which arises from the lacrimal epithelium.

dactyl ('daktil) a finger or toe; a digit.

dactylion (dak'tili·ən) webbed fingers. *See* SYNDACTYLISM.

dactylitis (ˌdakti'lietis) inflammation of a finger or toe.

dactylology (ˌdakti'loləjee) communication between individuals by signs made with the fingers and hands.

daltonism ('dawltəˌnizəm) colour-blindness; inability to distinguish red from green.

danazol ('danəˌzol) an anterior pituitary suppressant used in the treatment of endometriosis and metastatic breast cancer. Also used for menstrual disorders, mammary dysplasia and hereditary angio-oedema.

dander ('dandə) small scales from the hair or feathers of animals, which may be a cause of allergy in sensitive persons.

dandruff ('dandruf) white scales shed from the scalp. If moist from serous exudate they have a greasy appearance.

danthron ('danthron) an orange-coloured laxative and faecal softening agent which sometimes turns the urine pink. Its use is now restricted and under review.

dapsone ('dapsohn) a sulphone drug used in the treatment of leprosy.

darwinism ('dahwiˌnizəm) *C.R. Darwin, British naturalist, 1809–1882.* The theory of the evolution of species through natural selection.

data ('daytə) *sing.* datum; a collection of facts. *Continuous d.* data which have a continuous set of values, eg. for variables such as height, weight and antibody titres in response to vaccination. *Discrete d.* data with a single value or characteristic, e.g. colour of hair. *D. processing* the storage and analysis of data to produce statistical tabulations, often by computer.

daunomycin (ˌdawnoh'miesin) a cytotoxic antibiotic; daunorubicin.

daunorubicin (ˌdawnoh'roobisin) daunomycin.

day care ('day ˌkair) a specialized service for preschool children either as a substitute for or an extension to family life.

day hospital a specialized facility that offers care, treatment and a respite service for the elderly or the mentally ill.

day patient care a service provided either in a specialized ward or in hospital ward for treatment/investigation/minor surgery. The patient is admitted and discharged in the same day.

dB symbol for *decibel*.

DDT dichlorodiphenyltrichloroethane; dicophane. A powerful insecticide.

deafness ('defnəs) the inability to hear. *Conduction* or *middle ear d.* deafness due to the sound wave failing to reach the cochlea. *Perceptive* or *nerve d.* deafness due to damage to the cochlea or auditory nerve.

deamination (deeˌami'nayshən) a process of hydrolysis taking place in the liver by which amino acids are broken down and urea is formed.

death (deth) the cessation of all physical and chemical processes that occurs in all living organisms or their cellular components. *Brain d.* the diagnosis of clinical brain stem death is governed, in the UK, by a set of guidelines ratified by the Medical Royal Colleges and their Faculties. The testing procedure is performed twice by two different doctors to eliminate any observer error. The time interval between testing is not specified. For medico-legal purposes, the time of death is that time when the second examination has been completed and the patient fulfils the criteria. Performance of the brain death criteria under the appropriate circumstances allows the patient a dignified death, reduces the agony of the relatives and releases scarce resources for other seriously ill patients. *D. certificate* certificate issued by the registrar for deaths after receipt of a preliminary certificate completed and signed by an attending doctor, indicating the date and probable cause of death. Only after issue of this certificate, indicating that the death has been registered, can the body be disposed of. *Clinical d.* the absence of heart beat (no pulse can be felt) and cessation of breathing. *Cot d.* sudden infant death syndrome (SIDS). *D. instinct* a concept introduced by Freud, proposing a self-destructive drive opposed by the sexual instinct which perpetually seeks a renewal of life. May manifest itself as a repetition COMPULSION with the aim of annihilating oneself. *D. rate* the number of deaths per stated number of persons (100 or 10,000 or 100,000) in a certain region in a certain time period.

debility (di'bilitee) a condition of weakness and lack of physical tone.

débridement (di'breedmonh, day-) [Fr.] the removal of foreign substances and injured tissues from a traumatic wound. Part of the immediate treatment to promote healing.

Debrisan ('debrizan) trade name for a preparation of dextranomer beads used to assist wound cleaning and the de-sloughing of ulcers.

debrisoquine (de'briesoh, kween) a powerful oral drug used in the treatment of resistant hypertension. It causes postural hypertension.

decalcification (dee'kalsifi'kayshən) removal of calcium salts, e.g. from bone in disorders of calcium metabolism.

decannulation (dee, kanyuh'layshən) the removal of a cannula.

decapsulation (dee, kapsyuh'layshən) removal of a fibrous capsule.

decay (di'kay) 1. the gradual decomposition of dead organic matter. 2. the process or stage of ageing of living matter. *Radioactive d.* the process by which an unstable atom loses energy by the emission of gamma rays, beta or alpha particles and is transformed to a more stable atom.

decerebrate (dee'seri, brayt) a person with brain damage whose neurological reactions are severely impaired and where cerebral functioning has ceased.

decibel ('desi, bel) *symbol* dB. A unit of intensity of sound, used particularly in estimating the degree of deafness.

decidua (di, sidyooə) the thickened lining of the uterus for the reception of the fertilized ovum to protect the developing embryo. It is shed when pregnancy terminates.

deciduoma (di, sidyoo'ohmə) an intrauterine tumour containing decidual cells. *D. malignum* chorion epithelioma.

deciduous (di'sidyooəs) falling off; subject to being shed, as deciduous teeth.

decompensation (, deekompən-'sayshən) failure to compensate. In particular, failure of the heart to overcome disability or increased work load.

decompression (, deekəm'preshən) return to normal environmental pressure after exposure to greatly increased pressure. *Cerebral d.* removal of a flap of the skull and incision of the dura mater for the purpose of relieving intracranial pressure. *D. sickness* a disorder characterized by joint pains, respiratory manifestations, skin lesions, and neurological signs, occurring as a result of rapid reduction in air pressure. Aviators flying at high altitudes and persons breathing compressed air in caissons and diving apparatus are particularly susceptible to this disorder.

decongestant (, deekən'jestənt) 1. reducing congestion or swelling. 2. an agent that reduces congestion or swelling, usually of the nasal membranes. Decongestants may be inhaled, taken as spray or nose drops, or used orally in liquid or tablet form.

decontamination (, deekən, tami-'nayshən) the freeing of a person or an object of some contaminating substance such as war gas, radioactive material, etc.

decortication (dee,kawti'kayshən) an operation to strip the outer layer of an organ, e.g. the removal of the thickened pleura in the treatment of chronic empyema.

decrudescence (,deekroo'desəns) diminution or abatement of the intensity of symptoms.

decubitus (di'kyoobitəs) the position assumed when lying down. *D. ulcer* an ulcer due to interference with the local circulation from prolonged or severe pressure on the surface body tissue resulting in tissue anoxia and cell death; called also *bedsore* and *pressure sore.*

decussation (deekə'sayshən) a crossing, particularly of nerve fibres. A chiasma. *Pyramidal d.* the crossing of the pyramidal nerve fibres in the medulla oblongata.

defaecation (,defi'kayshən) elimination of wastes and undigested food, as faeces, from the rectum.

defence (di'fens) behaviour directed to protection of the individual from injury. *Character d.* any character trait, e.g. a mannerism, attitude, or affectation, which serves as a DEFENCE MECHANISM. *Insanity d.* a legal concept that a person cannot be convicted of a crime if he lacked criminal responsibility by reason of insanity at the time of commission of the crime. *D. mechanism* in psychology, an unconscious mental process or coping pattern that lessens the anxiety associated with a situation or

internal conflict and protects the person from mental discomfort.

defervescence (,deefə'vesəns) the period of abatement of fever.

defibrillation (dee,fibri'layshən) the restoration of normal rhythm to the heart in ventricular or atrial fibrillation.

defibrillator (di'fibri,laytə) an instrument by which normal rhythm is restored in ventricular or atrial fibrillation by the application of a high-voltage electric current.

defibrination (dee,fibri'nayshən) the removal of fibrin from blood plasma to prevent clotting. Used in the preparation of sera.

deficiency disease (di'fishənsee) a condition caused by dietary or metabolic deficiency, including all diseases due to an insufficient supply of essential nutrients.

deglutition (,deegloo'tishən) the act of swallowing.

dehiscence (di'hisəns) splitting open, as of a wound.

dehydration (,deehie'drayshən) excessive loss of fluid from the body by persistent vomiting, diarrhoea or sweating, or from the lack of intake. Severe dehydration is a serious condition that may lead to fatal SHOCK, ACIDOSIS, and the accumulation of waste products in the body, as in URAEMIA.

déjà vu (,dayzhah 'voo) [Fr.] an illusion that a new experience is a repetition of a previous experience.

deleterious (,deli'tiə·ri·əs) harmful; injurious.

delinquency (di'lingkwənsee) criminal or antisocial conduct, especially among juveniles.

delirium (di'liri·əm) mental excitement. A common condition in high fever. It is marked by an irregular expenditure of nervous energy, incoherent talk, and delusions. *Traumatic d.* a possible occurrence after severe head injury. There is much confusion and disorientation. *D. tremens* an acute psychosis common in chronic alcoholism, usually following abstinence from alcohol.

delivery (di'livə·ree) childbirth; parturition.

deltoid ('deltoyd) triangular. *D. muscle* the triangular muscle of the shoulder arising from the clavicle and scapula, with insertion into the humerus.

delusion (di'loozhan) a false idea or belief held by a person which cannot be corrected by reasoning. *Depressive d.* a sense of unworthiness or sinfulness. *D. of grandeur* erroneous belief in one's own greatness, wealth or position. *D. of persecution* paranoia.

dementia (di'menshi·ə) a global and progressive deterioration of the mental faculties which is irreversible and affects memory, intellect, judgement, personality and emotional control. Dementia is the result of an organic brain syndrome. The term 'brain failure' is gradually replacing the term dementia as it conveys that brain failure is a process while the term dementia simply suggests a state associated with nihilistic views on treatment and prognosis. *Arteriosclerotic d.* dementia due to insufficient blood supply to the brain caused by arteriosclerosis. *Presenile*

d. occurring in people aged 40–60 years, it is due to early degeneration of small cerebral blood vessels. See ALZHEIMER'S DISEASE and CREUTZFELDT–JAKOB DISEASE. *Senile d.* dementia occurring in old age due to cerebral atrophy.

Demodex ('deemoh,deks) a genus of mites parasitic in the hair follicles of the host. Other species of the genus cause mange in dogs and horses.

demography (di'mografee) the social study of people viewed collectively with regard to race, occupation or conditions.

demulcent (di,mulsənt) an agent which soothes and allays irritation, especially of sensitive mucous membranes.

demyelination (di'mieəli'nayshən) destruction of the medullary or myelin sheaths of nerve fibres such as occurs in disseminated sclerosis. Demyelinization.

dendrite ('dendriet) one of the protoplasmic filaments of a nerve cell by which impulses are transmitted from one neurone to another. Dendron.

dendritic (den'dritik) 1. appertaining to a dendrite. 2. branching. *D. ulcer* a corneal ulcer caused by the virus of herpes simplex. It has a branching appearance as it spreads.

denervation (,deenər'vayshən) severance or removal of the nerve supply to a part.

dengue ('deng·gee) a painful viral disease that occurs in tropical countries throughout the world. The virus that causes the disease, one of four types of a group B arbovirus, is carried by *Aedes* mosquitoes. Because of the intense pain in the bones, dengue is also known as breakbone fever.

denial (di'nieəl) a defence mechanism in which the existence of intolerable actions, ideas, changed circumstances, terminal illness, etc. are unconsciously denied.

dentine ('denteen) the calcified substance forming the bulk of a tooth between the pulp and the enamel.

dentition (den'tishən) the process of teething. *Primary d.* cutting of the temporary or milk teeth, beginning at the age of 6 or 7 months and continuing until the end of the second year. A full set consists of eight incisors, four canines, and eight premolars: twenty in all. Deciduous dentition. *Secondary d.* cutting of the permanent teeth, beginning in the sixth or seventh year, and being complete by the twelfth to fifteenth year except for the posterior molars or 'wisdom teeth'. There are thirty-two permanent teeth—eight incisors, four canines, eight premolars or bicuspids and twelve molars. Permanent dentition.

dentoid ('dentoyd) tooth-like.

denture ('denchə) a removable dental prosthesis which may contain one tooth, several or a full set of artificial teeth.

deodorant (di'ohdə·rənt) a substance which destroys or masks an offensive odour.

deoxycortone (dee,oksi'kawtohn) a naturally occurring adrenal steroid. *D. acetate* and *d. pivalate* synthetic preparations used in the

treatment of adrenocortical insufficiency.

deoxygenated (dee'oksijə,natid) deprived of oxygen. *D. blood* that which has lost much of its oxygen in the tissues and is returning to the lungs for a fresh supply.

deoxyribonucleic acid (di,oksi ,riebohnyoo'klee·ik, -'klay-) abbreviated DNA. A nucleic acid of complex molecular structure occurring in cell nuclei as the basic structure of the genes. It is responsible for the control and passing on of hereditary characteristics, and is present in all body cells of every species, including unicellular organisms and DNA viruses. DNA molecules are linear polymers of small molecules called *nucleotides*, each of which consists of one molecule of the five-carbon sugar *deoxyribose*, bonded to a *phosphate* group and to one of the four *bases*. The four bases are two purines, *adenine* (A) and *guanine* (G), and two pyrimidines, *cytosine* (C) and *thymine* (T). The structure of DNA was described in 1953 by J.D. Watson and F.H.C. Crick.

dependence (di'pendəns) addiction; the total psychophysical state of a drug user, in which the usual or increasing doses of the drug are required to prevent the onset of WITHDRAWAL SYMPTOMS.

dependency (di'pendənsee) a state of relying on another for love, affection, mothering, comfort, security, food, warmth, shelter, protection, etc. *D. studies* the measurement of the need for care required by a patient based on

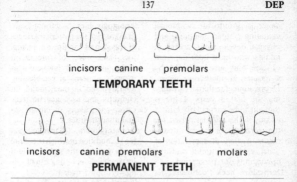

incisors   canine   premolars
TEMPORARY TEETH

incisors   canine   premolars   molars
PERMANENT TEETH

his/her level of ability to carry out self-care. The main self-care activities measured are ability to feed, carry out toilet requirements and level of mobility, including dressing. *D. studies for staffing ratios* studies undertaken to determine the number of staff required to provide the appropriate skills to care for specific types and numbers of patients (see ABERDEEN FORMULA).

depersonalization (dee,pərsənəlie-'zayshən) a condition in which the patient feels that his personality has changed so that he becomes an onlooker of his own actions. It may occur in almost any mental illness.

depilatory (di'pilətə·ree) an agent which will remove hair.

depressant (di'pres'nt) a drug which reduces functional activity of an organ. Anaesthetics, sedatives, tranquillizers and alcohol are depressants.

depression (di'preshən) 1. a hollow or depressed area. 2. a lower-ing or decrease of functional activity. 3. in psychiatry, a morbid sadness, dejection, or melancholy, distinguished from grief, which is realistic and proportionate to a personal loss. Profound depression may be symptomatic of a psychiatric disorder or it may constitute the principal manifestation of a neurosis or psychosis. *Endogenous d.* occurs sometimes without obvious cause in the course of manic-depressive psychosis. The mood change is associated with slowing of thought and action and feelings of guilt. *Reactive d.* occurs as a result of some event, such as illness, loss of money, bereavement.

deprivation (,depri'vayshən) loss or absence of parts, organs, powers, or things that are needed. *Emotional d.* deprivation of adequate and appropriate interpersonal or environmental experience in the early developmental years. *Maternal d.* syn-

drome a group of symptoms, including stunted emotional and physical development, arising in infants who have been deprived of care and love provided by a mother or mothering figure. Deprivation of maternal care during the first 3 years of life is thought to be particularly critical as this is the optimal period for the forming of social attachments. *Sensory d.* deprivation of usual external stimuli and the opportunity for perception.

Derbyshire neck ('dahbishə) *see* GOITRE.

derealization (ˌdee,riəlie'zayshən) loss of a sense of reality. Surroundings and events seem unreal.

dereism ('deeri,izəm) mental activity in which fantasy runs unhampered by logic and experience; describes autistic thinking.

dermatitis (ˌdɜrmə'tietis) inflammation of the skin. *Contact d.* that arising from touching a substance to which the person is sensitive. *Exfoliative d.* widespread scaling and itching of the skin, sometimes occurring as a reaction to treatment by certain drugs. *Industrial d., occupational d.* that caused by exposure to chemicals or other substances met with at work. *Sensitization d.* dermatitis due to an allergic reaction. *Traumatic d.* inflammation due to injury. *Varicose d.* dermatitis, usually of the lower portion of the leg, due to varicosities of the smaller veins. *X-ray d.* radiodermatitis; inflammatory reaction of the skin to radiotherapy.

dermatoglyphics (ˌdɜrmətoh'glifiks) study of the patterns of ridges of the skin of the fingers, palms, toes, and soles; of interest in anthropology and law enforcement as a means of establishing identity, and in medicine, both clinically and as a genetic indicator, particularly of chromosomal abnormalities.

dermatographia (ˌdɜrmətoh'grafi-ə) a condition in which urticarial weals occur on the skin if a blunt instrument or finger-nail is lightly drawn over it.

dermatology (ˌdɜrmə'toləjee) the science of skin diseases.

dermatome ('dɜrmə,tohm) an instrument for cutting thin slices of skin for skin grafting.

dermatomycosis (ˌdɜrmətohmie-'kohsis) a fungal infection of the skin.

dermatomyositis (ˌdɜrmətoh-ˌmieoh'sietis) a collagen disease producing inflammation of the voluntary muscles with necrosis of the muscle fibres.

dermatophyte ('dɜrmətoh,fiet) a fungus that invades the skin. There are three genera: *Epidermophyton, Microsporum* and *Trichophyton.*

dermatosis (ˌdɜrmə'tohsis) any skin disease, especially one which does not produce inflammation.

dermis ('dɜrmis) the skin, especially the layer under the epidermis.

dermoid ('dɜrmoyd) pertaining to the skin. *D. cyst see* CYST.

desensitization (dee,sensitie'zayshən) 1. the prevention or reduction of immediate hypersensitivity reactions by the administration of graded doses of allergen; hyposensitization. *See also* IMMUNOTHERAPY. 2. in behaviour therapy, the treatment of phobias and related disorders by intentionally exposing the patient, in imagination or in real life, to emotionally distressing stimuli.

desiccation (,desi'kayshən) the process of drying.

designer drug (di'zienə) drugs illicitly produced to suit the tastes of individuals but now used to describe synthetic variants (drug analogues) of potent controlled drugs (including narcotics and stimulants) but which are not themselves controlled. These substances currently circumvent existing drug legislation and many are relatively easy to synthesize from common industrial chemicals. Many designer drugs are extremely potent (some synthetic analogues of heroin are 1000 times as potent as heroin) and are consequently extremely dangerous.

desipramine (de'siprə,meen) an antidepressant.

desquamation (,deskwə'mayshən) peeling of the superficial layer of the skin, either in flakes or in powdery form.

detachment (di'tachmənt) separation. *D. of the retina* separation of the retina, or a part of it, from the choroid.

detergent (di'tərjənt) a cleansing and antiseptic agent.

deterioration (di,tiə·ri·ə'rayshən) progressive impairment of function; worsening.

detoxification (dee,toksifi'kay-

shən) the process of neutralizing toxic substances; detoxication.

detritus (di'trietəs) debris; material which has disintegrated.

detrusor (di'troozə) muscle of the urinary bladder whose action is to push down.

detumescence (,deetyuh'mesəns) 1. the subsidence of a swelling. 2. the subsidence of an erect penis after ejaculation.

development (di'veləpmənt) the process of growth and differentiation. *Cognitive d.* the development of intelligence, conscious thought and problem-solving ability that begins in infancy. *Psychosexual d.* the development of the psychological aspects of sexuality from birth to maturity. *Psychosocial d.* the development of the personality, including the acquisition of social attitudes and skills, from infancy through maturity.

developmental (di,veləp'ment'l) pertaining to development. *D. anomaly* absence, deformity, or excess of body parts as the result of faulty development of the embryo. *D. milestones* significant behaviours which are used to mark the process of development (*see* AGE achievement). Walking is a developmental milestone in locomotor development, conversation in cognitive development.

deviance ('deevi·əns) generally any pattern of behaviour which violates prevailing standards of morality or behaviour within a society. The term is usually qualified to indicate the specific form of deviance, e.g. sexual deviance.

deviation (‚deevi'ayshəh) variation from the normal. In ophthalmology, lack of coordination of the two eyes.

devitalized (dee'vietə‚liezd) devoid of vitality or life; dead.

dexamethasone (‚deksa'methə‚zohn) a powerful anti-inflammatory glucocorticoid.

dexter ('dekstə) [L.] *upon the right side.*

dextran ('dekstran) a plasma volume expander formed of large glucose molecules which, given intravenously, increases the osmotic pressure of blood.

dextrin ('dekstrin) a soluble carbohydrate which is the first product in the breakdown of starch and glycogen to sugar.

dextrocardia (‚dekstroh'kahdi·ə) location of the heart in the right side of the thorax.

dextromethorphan (‚dekstrohme-'thorfən) a synthetic morphine derivative used as an antitussive.

dextromoramide (‚dekstroh'mo·rə‚mied) a narcotic used in the treatment of chronic pain in terminal disease.

dextrose ('dekstrohz, -trohs) an old chemical name for D-glucose, an important energy source for all tissues and the sole energy source for the brain. The term dextrose continues to be used to refer to glucose solutions administered intravenously for fluid or nutrient replacement.

DF 118 trade name for preparations of dihydrocodeine.

diabetes (‚dieə'beetis, -teez) a disease characterized by excessive excretion of urine. *See* POLYURIA. *Bronze d.* haemochromatosis. *D.*

insipidus diabetes marked by an increased flow of urine of low specific gravity, accompanied by great thirst. This disease, which is due to posterior pituitary dysfunction, is treated by instilling into the nose drops containing lysine–vasopressin or the longer acting desmopressin (a synthetic form of antidiuretic hormone). *D. mellitus* a disturbance in the oxidation and utilization of glucose, which is secondary to a malfunction of the beta cells of the pancreas, whose function is the production and release of INSULIN. Because insulin is involved in the metabolism of carbohydrates, proteins, and fats, diabetes is not limited to a disturbance of glucose metabolism. Polyuria, thirst and debility are common presenting symptoms. The goal of treatment is to maintain blood glucose and lipid levels within normal limits and to prevent complications. There is strong support for the concept that microvascular sequelae of the disease can be minimized by optimal control. Good control is achieved when the following occur: fasting blood glucose is within normal limits and blood glucose is not above 10 mmol/litre 2 h after breakfast or lunch, urine is negative for glucose and before meals, the patient's weight is normal, blood lipids remain within normal limits, and the patient has a sense of health and well-being. *Diet.* A diet adjusted to individual needs is prescribed. For mild cases, there is no need to measure food intake precisely, but patients must avoid foods that have a high sugar content, and they must keep their weight within normal limits. When the disease is more severe and stricter control is required, a quantitative diet is prescribed. Such a diet will be low in animal fats and high in fibre. The total calorie intake will be set according to the patient's physical activity and the need to lose weight. *Insulin therapy.* Insulin has now been standardized at 100 units/ml. Combinations of soluble insulin with slower-acting preparations can be tailored to suit the individual patient in the 24-h control of blood sugar. All insulin has to be given by injection, usually subcutaneously. Pump systems to deliver continuous insulin under the skin are available.

diabetic (ˌdieə'betik) 1. relating to diabetes. 2. a person affected with diabetes. *D. gangrene, d. retinopathy* and *d. cataract* are complications of diabetes mellitus.

diabetogenic (ˌdieəˌbeetoh'jenik) inducing diabetes. Some drugs or physical conditions, such as pregnancy or disease, precipitate the symptoms of diabetes in those prone to the disease.

Diagnex blue test ('dieəgˌneks) a trade name for a test for the presence of hydrochloric acid secreted in the stomach. Diagnex blue tablets are given orally and cause the urine to become blue if the stomach is producing hydrochloric acid. The advantage for the patient is that a stomach tube does not need to be passed.

diagnosis (ˌdieəg'nohsis) determination of the nature of a disease. *Clinical d.* diagnosis made by the study of signs and symptoms. *Differential d.* the recognition of one disease among several presenting similar symptoms. *Nursing d.* a statement of a health care problem or the potential for one in the health status of the patient/client for which the nurse is competent to intervene and treat.

dialysate (di'aliˌsayt) the material passing through the membrane in dialysis.

dialyser ('dieəˌliezə) 1. the membrane used in dialysis. 2. the machine or 'artificial kidney' used to remove waste products from the blood in cases of renal failure.

dialysis (die'aləsis) the process by which crystalline substances will pass through a semipermeable membrane, whereas colloids will not. In medicine this process is usually employed to remove waste and toxic products from the blood in cases of renal insufficiency. *Peritoneal d.* use of the peritoneum as the semipermeable membrane. A dialysing solution is infused into the abdominal cavity and allowed to run out again when sufficient time has elapsed for dialysis to have occurred. Waste products are thus removed from the blood. *See* HAEMODIALYSIS.

diameter (die'amitə) a straight line passing through the centre of a circle to opposite points on the circumference. *Cranial d's* measurement of the skull, usually of the fetal head at term. If these

Differences between hyper- and hypoglycaemia in patients with diabetes mellitus

	Hyperglycaemia	*Hypoglycaemia*
Onset	Slow (2–3 days)	Rapid
History	Has not taken insulin/ acute infection	Taken insulin ½–4 h previously, but has not eaten/has eaten but had unusual burst of energy
Patient reactions	Thirst Nausea Abdominal pain Constipation Vomiting	Irrational Bad tempered Disorientated (may be mistaken for drunk)
Leads to	Ketoacidosis Drowsiness BP ↓ Pulse weak and rapid Skin dry Tongue dry	Respirations normal No drowsiness BP normal Pulse normal Skin moist Tongue moist
Leads to	Coma	Coma
Needs	Insulin Restoration of fluid/ balance	Glucose
Avoided by	Recognition of early symptoms and taking appropriate action	

From Faulkner, A. (1985) *Nursing: A Creative Approach*, 1st edn, Baillière Tindall, p. 232.

are abnormal delivery through the vagina may not be possible. *Pelvic d's* measurements between the bones and joints of the pelvis made in women to determine whether the fetus can pass through at the time of childbirth. **diamorphine hydrochloride** (diə-'mawfeen) a morphine derivative similar to heroin; a powerful analgesic and drug of addiction. **diapedesis** (ˌdieəpe'deesis) the passage of white blood cells through the walls of blood capillaries.

diaphoresis (,dieəfə'reesis) perspiration; particularly profuse perspiration.

diaphoretic (,dieəfor'retik) an agent which increases perspiration, eg. pilocarpine.

diaphragm ('dieə,fram) 1. the muscular dome-shaped partition separating the thorax from the abdomen. 2. any separating membrane or structure. *Contraceptive d.* a rubber cap which occludes the cervix.

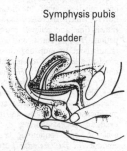

Symphysis pubis

Bladder

Uterine cervix

CONTRACEPTIVE DIAPHRAGM

diaphragmatocele (,dieəfram'atoh,seel) a herniation of the diaphragm.

diaphysis (di'afisis) the shaft of a long bone.

diarrhoea (,dieə'reeə) rapid movement of faecal matter through the intestine resulting in poor

absorption of water, nutritive elements and electrolytes, and producing abnormally frequent evacuation of watery stools. *Summer d.* gastroenteritis of infants, probably the result of a virus infection. It is highly contagious. *Tropical d.* sprue.

diarthrosis (,dieah'throhsis) a freely moving articulation, e.g. ball and socket joint. A synovial joint.

diastase ('dieə,stays, -stayz) 1. an enzyme formed during germination of seeds, which converts starch into sugar. 2. one of the pancreatic enzymes excreted in the urine and the saliva. *D. test* used to estimate the excretion of diastase and therefore pancreatic function.

diastole (die'astəlee) the phase of the cardiac cycle in which the heart relaxes between contractions; specifically, the period when the two ventricles are dilated by the blood flowing into them.

diathermy ('dieə,thərmee) production of heat in a body tissue by a high frequency electric current. *Medical d.* sufficient heat is used to warm the tissues but not to harm them. *Short-wave d.* used in physiotherapy to relieve pain or treat infection. *Surgical d.* of very high frequency; used to coagulate blood vessels or to dissect tissues. Cautery.

diathesis (die'athəsis) a constitutional predispositon to certain diseases.

diazepam (die'azi,pam) a tranquillizer with muscle relaxant and anticonvulsive properties used to relieve anxiety and in the treatment of epilepsy.

diazoxide (dieaz'oksied) a vaso-dilator given by rapid intra-venous injection in the treatment of hypertensive emergencies and orally in hypoglycaemia due to a pancreatic tumour.

dichloralphenazone (die,klor·ral-'fenə,zohn) a hypnotic drug of the chloral group well suited for children and causes fewer gastro-intestinal upsets.

dichlorphenamide (,dieklor'fenə,mied) a diuretic used to reduce intraocular pressure in glaucoma.

dichotomy (die'kotəmee) division into two parts.

dichromatic (,diekroh'matik) per-taining to colour blindness when there is ability to see only two of the three primary colours.

dicophane ('diekoh,fayn) dichloro-diphenyltrichloroethane; chloro-phenothane; DDT. An insecti-cide.

dicrotic (die'krotik) having a dou-ble beat. *D. pulse* a small wave of distension following the normal pulse beat; occurring at the clos-ure of the aortic valve.

dicyclomine (die'siekloh,meen) an anticholinergic drug used in the treatment of peptic ulcer and spastic colon.

didymitis (,didi'mietis) orchitis; inflammation of a testicle.

dienoestrol (,die-en'eestrol) a syn-thetic oestrogen used to treat symptoms of atrophic vaginitis and kraurosis vulvae.

diet ('dieət) the customary amount and kind of food and drink taken by a person from day to day; more narrowly, a diet planned to meet specific requirements of the individual, including or exclud-ing certain foods. *Bland d.* one that is free from any irritating or stimulating foods. *Elemental d.* one consisting of a well-balanced, residue-free mixture of all essen-tial and non-essential amino acids combined with simple sugars, electrolytes, trace elements and vitamins. *Elimination d.* one for diagnosis of food allergy, based on omission of foods that might cause symptoms in the patient. *High-calorie d.* one that furnishes more calories than needed to maintain weight, often more than 3500–4000 kcal/day. *High-fibre d.* one relatively high in dietary fibres, which decreases bowel transit time and relieves consti-pation. *High-protein d.* one con-taining large amounts of protein, consisting largely of meats, fish, milk, legumes and nuts. *Hospital d.* a routine diet plan provided in a hospital that includes gen-eral, soft and liquid diets and modifications of them to suit the needs of specific patients. *Keto-genic d.* one containing large amounts of fat (*see also* KETO-GENIC DIET). *Liquid d.* a diet lim-ited to liquids or to foods that can be changed to a liquid state (*see also* LIQUID DIET). *Low-calorie d.* one containing fewer calories than needed to maintain weight, e.g. less than 1200 kcal/day for an adult. *Low-fat d.* one contain-ing limited amounts of fat. *Low-residue d.* one with a minimum of cellulose and fibre and restric-tion of connective tissue found in certain cuts of meat. It is prescribed for irritations of the intestinal tract, after surgery of the large intestine, in partial intestinal obstruction, or when limited bowel movements are desirable, as in colostomy patients. Called also low-fibre diet.

dietetics (,diea'tetiks) the science of regulating diet.

diethylcarbamazine (die,ethilkah'bama,zeen) an anthelmintic drug used in the treatment of filariasis.

diethylpropion (die,ethil'prohpion) an appetite suppressant similar in action to an amphetamine drug. Dependence can occur.

dietitian (,diea'tishan) one who specializes in dietetics.

differential (,difa'renshal) making a difference. *D. blood count see* BLOOD COUNT. *D. diagnosis see* DIAGNOSIS.

differentiation (,difa,renshi'ayshan) 1. the distinguishing of one thing from another. 2. the act or process of acquiring completely individual characteristics, such as occurs in the progressive diversification of cells and tissues in the embryo. 3. increase in morphological or chemical heterogeneity.

diffuse (di'fyoos, -'fyooz) scattered or widespread, as opposed to localized.

diffusion (di'fyoozhan) 1. the spontaneous mixing of molecules of liquid or gas so that they become equally distributed. 2. dialysis.

diflunisal (die'flooni,sal) a salicylic acid derivative that, like aspirin, has analgesic and anti-inflammatory properties, but fewer side-effects than aspirin, does not affect bleeding time or function,

and has a long half-life that permits twice daily dosage.

digestion (die'jeschan, di-) 1. the act or process of converting food into chemical substances that can be absorbed into the blood and utilized by the body tissues. 2. the subjection of a substance to prolonged heat and moisture, so as to disintegrate and soften it.

digit ('dijit) a finger or toe. *Accessory d., supernumerary d.* an additional digit occurring as a congenital abnormality.

digitalis (,diji'taylis) a group of drugs used extensively for their action on the heart. They strengthen the heartbeat and slow down the conducting power of the atrioventricular bundle, thereby enabling the ventricles to beat more effectively. Particularly valuable in treating atrial fibrillation. *Digoxin* is the chief glycoside obtained from the white foxglove. The effects of digitalis are cumulative, indicated by a very slow pulse and coupling of the beats.

digitalization (,dijitalie'zayshan) the administration of digitalis in a dosage schedule designed to produce and then maintain optimal therapeutic concentrations of its cardiotonic glycosides.

dihydrocodeine (die,hiedroh-'kohdeen) a synthetic narcotic, analgesic and antitussive drug derived from codeine.

dihydroergotamine (die,hiedroh-·ar'gota,meen) a drug used in the treatment of migraine. Less effective than ergotamine, but with fewer side-effects.

dihydrotachysterol (die,hiedroh-taki'stiə·rol) a preparation closely related to vitamin D. Used in cases of vitamin D deficiency and in rickets.

dilatation, dilation (ˌdielə'tay-shən; die'layshən) 1. the act of dilating or stretching. 2. the condition, as of an orifice or tubular structure, of being dilated or stretched beyond normal dimensions. *D. and curettage* expanding of the ostium uteri to permit scraping of the walls of the uterus; also called D & C. *D. of the heart* compensatory enlargement of the cavities of the heart, with thinning of the walls.

dilator (die'laytə) 1. an instrument used for enlarging an opening or cavity such as the rectum, the male urethra or the cervix. 2. a muscle which causes dilatation. 3. a drug which causes dilatation, e.g. a vasodilator. *Hegar's d's* a series of dilators used to widen the cervical canal prior to examination of the uterus under anaesthesia.

diluent ('dilyooənt) 1. diluting. 2. an agent that dilutes or renders less potent or irritant.

dimenhydrinate (ˌdiemen'hiedri-·nayt) an antihistamine drug, useful in preventing nausea and vomiting, particularly that associated with motion sickness.

dimercaprol (ˌdiemə'kaprol) a drug which combines with heavy metals to form a stable compound, which is rapidly excreted. Used to treat poisoning by antimony, gold, mercury and other metals. Previously called British antilewisite or BAL.

dimethylphthalate (die,methil-'thalayt) abbreviated DIMP. An insect repellent in liquid or ointment form that is effective for several hours when applied to the skin.

diodone ('dieə,dohn) a contrast medium containing iodine which is similar to iodoxyl. Used in radiology of the urinary tract.

Diogenes syndrome (die'oji,nez) gross self-neglect, usually in the elderly.

dioptre (die'optə) *symbol* D. The unit used in measuring lenses for spectacles. When parallel light enters a lens and focuses at a distance of 1 m, the refractive power of the lens is 1 dioptre, and from this basis abnormalities are reckoned.

diphtheria (dif'thiə·ri·ə, dip-) a severe, notifiable, infectious disease, usually of children, characterized by the formation of membranes in the throat and nose and rarely the skin, following an open wound, and toxic neurological and cardiac complications; caused by the bacillus *Corynebacterium diphtheriae*. Primary prevention is provided by the routine immunization of the population in childhood. In the UK diphtheria toxoid is given in combination with tetanus toxoid and pertussis vaccine as 'triple-antigen' at 3 months, 4½–5 months and 8½–11 months of age. A reinforcing dose of diphtheria–tetanus toxoid is given at school entry at the age of about 5 years.

diphtheroid ('difthə,royd) resembling diphtheria. A general term applied to organisms or membranes similar to true diphtheria types.

Diphyllobothrium (die‚filoh'bothri·əm) a genus of large tapeworm. *D. latum*, the broad or fish tapeworm, grows up to 10 m long and may infest man, following the eating of uncooked infected fish.

dipipanone (die'pipə‚nohn) a potent analgesic used for the relief of severe pain.

diplegia (die'pleeji·ə) paralysis of similar parts on either side of the body.

diplococcus (‚diploh'kokəs) 1. any of the spherical, lanceolate or coffee-bean-shaped bacteria occurring, usually in pairs, as a result of incomplete separation after cell division in a single plane. 2. any organism of the genus *Diplococcus*.

diploë ('diploh·ee) the cancellous tissue between the outer and inner surfaces of the skull.

diploid ('diployd) 1. having a pair of each chromosome characteristic of a species (in man, 46). 2. a diploid individual or cell.

diplopia (di'plohpi·ə) double vision in which two images are seen in place of one, due to lack of coordination of the external muscles of the eye.

diprophylline (die'prohfileen) a theophylline derivative used in the treatment of bronchospasm or bronchial asthma associated with chronic bronchitis or asthma.

dipsomania (‚dipsoh'mayni·ə) a morbid craving for alcohol which occurs in bouts.

disability (‚disə'bilitee) any restriction or lack (resulting from an impairment) of ability to perform an activity in the manner or within the range considered normal for a human being. *Developmental d.* a substantial handicap of indefinite duration, with onset before the age of 18 years, and attributable to mental handicap, autism, cerebral palsy, epilepsy, or other neuropathy.

disaccharide (die'sakə‚ried) any of a class of sugars, e.g. maltose, lactose, each molecule of which yields two molecules of monosaccharide on hydrolysis. *D. intolerance* the inability to absorb disaccharides owing to an enzyme deficiency.

disarticulation (‚disah‚tikyuh'layshən) separation; amputation at a joint.

disc (disk) a flattened circular structure. *Intervertebral d.* a fibrocartilaginous pad that separates the bodies of two adjacent vertebrae. *Optic d.* a white spot in the retina. It is the point of entrance of the optic nerve.

discharge ('dischahj) 1. a setting free, or liberation; used for the release of a patient from hospital, clinic or therapy programme. 2. material or force set free. 3. an excretion or substance evacuated. *D. planning* the preparation required leading to the return of a patient to their usual life at home.

discission (di'sishən) the cutting into the capsule of the lens. The lens is then absorbed by the surrounding ocular fluid in the condition of a soft cataract. Called also needling.

disclosing solution (dis'klohzing) a topically applied preparation which reveals plaque and other deposits on teeth by staining them.

discography (dis'kogrəfee) radiographic examination following the injection of a radio-opaque contrast medium into an intervertebral disc.

discrete (di,skreet) composed of separate parts that do not become blended.

disease (di'zeez) a definite pathological process having a characteristic set of signs and symptoms. It may affect the whole body or any of its parts, and its aetiology, pathology, and prognosis may be known or unknown. (For separate diseases, see under individual names.)

disimpaction (,disim'pakshən) reduction of an impacted fracture.

disinfect (,disin'fekt) to destroy microorganisms, but not usually bacterial spores, reducing the number of microorganisms to a level which is not harmful to health.

disinfectant (,disin'fektənt) an agent that destroys infection-producing organisms. Heat and certain other physical agents, such as live steam, can be disinfectants, but in common usage the term is reserved for chemical substances such as glutaraldehyde, sodium hypochlorite or phenol. Disinfectants are usually applied to inanimate objects since they are too strong to be used on living tissues. Chemical disinfectants are not always effective against spore-forming bacteria.

disinfection (disin'fekshən) the act of disinfecting. *Terminal d.* disinfection of a sick room and its contents at the termination of a disease.

disinfestation (,disinfe'stayshən) destruction of insects, rodents, or pests present on the person or his clothes or in his surroundings, and which may transmit disease.

dislocation (,dislə'kayshən) the displacement of a bone from its natural position upon another at a joint; luxation.

dismemberment (dis'membəmənt) the amputation of a limb or a part of it.

disopyramide (,diesoh'pirə,mied) a drug given orally or by slow intravenous injection to treat ventricular arrhythmia.

disorientation (dis,or·rien'tayshən) the loss of proper bearings, or a state of mental confusion as to time, place, or identity.

dispensary (di'spensə·ree) any place where drugs or medicines are actually dispensed.

displacement (dis'playsmənt) removal to an abnormal location or position; in psychology, unconscious transference of an emotion from its original object on to a more acceptable substitute.

disposition (,dispə'zishən) a tendency to suffer from certain diseases.

dissect (die'sekt, di-) 1. to cut carefully in the study of anatomy. 2. during operation, to separate according to natural lines of structure.

disseminated (di'semi,naytid) widely scattered or dispersed. *D.*

intravascular coagulation abbreviated DIC. Widespread formation of thromboses in the capillaries. It is a secondary complication of a diverse group of obstetric, surgical, haemolytic and neoplastic disorders.

dissociation (di,sohsi'ayshən, -'sohshi-) separation. 1. the splitting up of molecules of matter into their component parts, e.g. by heat or electrolysis. 2. in psychology, the separation of ideas, emotions or experiences from the rest of the mind, giving rise to a lack of unity of which the patient is not aware.

distal ('dist'l) situated away from the centre of the body or point of origin. The opposite of *proximal*.

Distalgesic (,distal'jeezik) a proprietary analgesic composed of dextropropoxyphene and paracetamol.

distension (dis'tenshən) enlargement. *Abdominal d.* enlargement of the abdomen by gas in the intestines or fluid in the abdominal cavity.

distichia, distichiasis (di'stiki-ə; ,disti'kieəsis) the presence of a double row of eyelashes, one or both of which are turned against the eyeball causing irritation.

disulfiram (die'sulfi,ram) a drug used in aversion therapy in alcoholism. Antabuse is a proprietary preparation.

dithranol ('dithrə,nol) a synthetic preparation used in the treatment of psoriasis and eczema.

diuresis (,dieyuh'reesis) increased excretion of urine.

diuretic (,dieyuh'retik) 1. increasing urine excretion or the amount of urine. 2. an agent that promotes urine secretion. Diuretic drugs are classified by chemical structure and pharmacological action, although a diuretic medication may contain drugs from one or more groups, e.g. loop diuretics, osmotic and potassium-sparing diuretics, and thiazides.

diurnal (die'ərnəl) occurring during daytime or period of light. Diurnal animals have one period of rest and one of activity in 24 h.

diverticulitis (,dievə'tikyuh'lietis) inflammation of a diverticulum. It is commonest in the colon; lower abdominal pain with colic and constipation may occur. Intestinal obstruction or abscesses may develop as a result of collections of bacteria and irritating agents being trapped in small blind pouches formed in the intestinal walls.

diverticulosis (,dievə,tikyuh'lohsis) the presence of diverticula in the colon without inflammation.

diverticulum (dievə'tikyuhləm) a pouch or pocket in the lining of a hollow organ, as in the bladder, oesophagus or large intestine. *Meckel's d.* a small sac occurring in the ileum as a congenital abnormality.

dizygotic, dizygous (,diezie'gotik; die'ziegəs) pertaining to or derived from two separate zygotes (fertilized ova); said of twins.

dizziness ('dizinəs) a feeling of unsteadiness or haziness, accompanied by anxiety.

DNA deoxyribonucleic acid.

dobutamine (doh'byootə,meen) a heart muscle stimulant administered parenterally in short-term treatment of adults with cardiac decompensation either from organic heart disease or from cardiac surgical procedures.

Döderlein's bacillus ('dardə-,lienz) *A.S.G. Döderlein, German obstetrician and gynaecologist, 1860–1941.* A lactobacillus occurring normally in vaginal secretions.

dolor (,dolə, 'dohlə) [L.] *pain.*

dominant ('dominənt) in genetics, capable of expression when carried by only one of a pair of homologous chromosomes. *D. gene* one which will produce its characteristics when it is present in either a hetero- or homozygous state, i.e. it may be inherited from one parent only.

'domino' booking ('dominoh) a plan of maternity care whereby a mother has her baby in a consultant unit, cared for by the community midwife. They return home any time after 6 h following delivery. The name derives from *dom*iciliary midwife *in* and *out*.

donor ('dohnə) 1. an organism that supplies living tissue to be used in another body, as a person who furnishes blood for transfusion, or an organ for transplantation. 2. a substance or compound that contributes part of itself to another substance (acceptor). *Universal d.* a person with group O blood; such blood is sometimes used in emergency transfusion. Transfusion of blood cells rather than whole blood is preferred.

dopa ('dohpə) the precursor of dopamine and an intermediate

product in the biosynthesis of noradrenaline and adrenaline. It is used in PARKINSON'S DISEASE and manganese poisoning. Called also L-dopa and levodopa.

dopamine ('dohpə,meen) a substance allied to noradrenaline and used in the treatment of cardiogenic shock. Also occurs naturally in the adrenal medulla and the brain where it functions as a transmitter of nervous impulses.

Doppler effect ('doplə) the relationship of the apparent frequency of waves, as of sound, light, and radio waves, to the relative motion of the source of the waves and the observer.

Doppler ultrasound flowmeter a device for measuring blood flow that transmits sound at a frequency of several megahertz along a blood vessel. Rapid pulsatile changes in flow as well as steady flow can be recorded; hence, it is helpful in assessing intermittent claudication, thrombus obstruction of deep veins, and other abnormalities of blood flow in the major arteries and veins.

dorsal ('daws'l) relating to the back or posterior part of an organ.

dorsiflexion (,dawsi'flekshən) bending backwards of the fingers or toes, i.e. upwards.

dorsum ('dawsəm) 1. the back. 2. the upper or posterior surface.

dosimeter (doh'simitə) an instrument used to detect and measure exposure to radiation; worn by personnel near to radiation sources.

dothiepin (doh'thieəpin) a tricyclic antidepressant and sedative drug.

douche (doosh) a stream of fluid directed to flush out a cavity of the body.

Douglas's pouch ('dugləs) *J. Douglas, British anatomist, 1675–1742.* Rectouterine pouch.

Down's syndrome (downz) *J.L.H. Down, British physician, 1828–1896.* a congenital condition characterized by physical malformations and some degree of mental handicap. The disorder was formerly known as mongolism. It is also called trisomy 21 syndrome because the disorder is concerned with a defect in CHROMOSOME 21. The causes of Down's syndrome are not known. There is a relatively high incidence in children of mothers who are in the older childbearing age. A particular type of Down's syndrome that occurs in children of younger mothers tends to occur in certain families. The term trisomy refers to the presence of three representative chromosomes in a cell instead of the usual pair. In Down's syndrome the twenty-first chromosome pair fails to separate when the germ cell (usually the ovum) is being formed. Thus the ovum contains 24 chromosomes, and when it is fertilized by a normal sperm carrying 23 chromosomes, the child is born with an extra chromosome (or total of 47) per cell.

doxapram ('doksə'pram) a respiratory stimulant used in carbon monoxide poisoning.

doxepin ('doksipin) a tricyclic ANTIDEPRESSANT used for treatment of depression.

dracontiasis (,drakon'tieəsis) a tropical disease caused by infestation with the guinea-worm; acquired by drinking contaminated water.

Dracunculus (dra'kungkyuhləs) a genus of round worms which includes the guinea-worm.

drain (drayn) 1. to withdraw liquid gradually. 2. any device by which a channel or open area may be established for exit of fluids or purulent material from a cavity, wound, or infected area.

drawsheet ('dror,sheet) a narrow sheet placed across the bed under a patient to prevent soiling of the main sheet. The sheet is twice the width of the bed to enable a clean piece to be drawn under the patient without the whole sheet being changed.

dressing ('dresing) material applied to cover a wound or a diseased surface of the body.

drip (drip) a colloquial term used to denote intravenous infusion of fluid (blood, saline, glucose) into the body.

drive (driev) in psychology, an urge or motivating force.

droperidol (droh'peri,dol) a major tranquillizer used to control behavioural disturbances.

droplet infection ('droplət) infection due to inhalation of respiratory pathogens suspended on liquid particles exhaled from someone already infected.

dropsy ('dropsee) an old-fashioned term used to describe excess fluid in the tissues (oedema).

drug (drug) 1. any medicinal

substance. 2. a narcotic. 3. to administer a drug. *D. abuse* the use of drugs for purposes other than those for which they are prescribed or recommended. The major groups of drugs and medicines generally considered to be most commonly misused are stimulants ('uppers') depressants ('downers'), psychedelics and narcotics. *D. addiction* a state of periodic or chronic intoxication produced by the repeated consumption of a drug, characterized by (1) an overwhelming desire or need (compulsion) to continue use of the drug and to obtain it by any means, (2) a tendency to increase the dosage, (3) a psychological and usually a physical dependence on its effects, and (4) a detrimental effect on the individual and on society. *D. interaction* modification of the potency of one drug by another (or others) taken concurrently or sequentially. Some drug interactions are harmful and some may have therapeutic benefits. Present knowledge of drug interactions is limited. Drugs may also interact with various foods. In general, these interactions fall into three categories: (1) food malabsorption; (2) nutritional status; and (3) alteration of drug response by nutrients. In teaching patients self-care in the taking of prescribed medications, one should explain the need for meticulously following directions related to the intake of food and drink while the medication regimen is being followed.

Duchenne dystrophy (doo,shen)

G.B.A. Duchenne, French neurologist, 1806–1875. Progressive muscular dystrophy occurring in childhood. *See* DYSTROPHY.

Ducrey's bacillus (doo'krayz) *A. Ducrey, Italian dermatologist, 1860–1940. Haemophilus ducreyi,* the organism causing soft chancre. *See* CHANCROID.

duct (dukt) a tube or channel for the passage of fluid, particularly one conveying the secretion of a gland.

ductless (,duktləs) without an excretory duct. *D. glands* endocrine glands. *See* ENDOCRINE.

ductus ('duktəs) a duct. *D. arteriosus* a passage connecting the pulmonary artery and aorta in intrauterine life, which normally closes at birth. When it remains open it is called persistent ductus arteriosus. *See also* PATENT DUCTUS ARTERIOSUS.

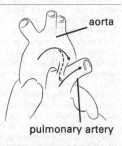

DUCTUS ARTERIOSUS

dumping ('dumping) the rapid evacuation of the contents of an organ. *D. syndrome* a feeling of fullness, weakness, sweating and dizziness which may occur after meals following a partial gastrectomy.

duodenal (,dyooə'deenəl) pertaining to the duodenum. *D. intubation* the use of a special tube which is passed via the mouth and stomach into the duodenum. Used for withdrawal of duodenal contents for pathological examination. *D. ulcer* a peptic ulcer occurring in the duodenum near the pylorus.

duodenopancreatectomy (,dyooə,deenoh,pangkri·ə'tektəmee) pancreatoduodenectomy. Surgical removal of the duodenum and much of the pancreas. Usually accompanied by anastomosis of the bile ducts and the tail of the pancreas to the jejunum.

duodenostomy (,dyooə·di'nostəmee) the formation of an artificial opening into the duodenum, through the abdominal wall, for purposes of feeding in cases of gastric disease.

duodenum (,dyooə'deenəm) the first 20–25 cm of the small intestine, from the pyloric opening of the stomach to the jejunum. The pancreatic and common bile ducts open into it.

Dupuytren's contraction or **contracture** (,duhpwi'trenz) *Baron G. Dupuytren, French surgeon, 1777–1835.* Contracture of the palmar fascia, causing permanent bending and fixation of one or more fingers.

dura mater ('dyooə·rə mahtə, -maytə) a strong fibrous membrane forming the outer covering of the brain and spinal cord.

dwarf (dwawf) an abnormally

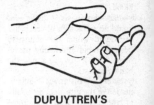

DUPUYTREN'S CONTRACTURE

undersized person.

dwarfism ('dwawfizəm) the state of being a dwarf. Arrest of growth and development, e.g. due to renal rickets, cretinism or deficient pituitary function.

dynamometer (,dienə'momitə) an instrument for measuring the force of muscular contracture.

dysaesthesia (,disis'theezi·ə) abnormal or impaired touch sensation.

dysarthrosis (,disah'throhsis) a deformed, dislocated or false joint.

dyschezia (dis'keezi·ə) difficult or painful defecation.

dyschondroplasia (,diskondroh-'playzi·ə) a condition in which cartilage is deposited in the shaft of some bones. The affected bones become shortened and deformed.

dyschromatopsia (,diskrohmə-'topsi·ə) partial loss of colour vision.

dyscrasia (dis'krayzi·ə) a morbid condition, usually referring to an imbalance of component elements. *Blood d.* any abnormal or pathological condition of the blood.

dysdiadochokinesis (,disdie,adə-kohki'neesis) a sign of cerebellar disease in which the ability to perform rapid alternating movements, such as rotating the hands, is lost.

dysentery ('dis'ntree) inflammation of the intestine, especially of the colon, with abdominal pain, tenesmus, and frequent stools often containing blood and mucus. The causative agent may be chemical irritants, bacteria, protozoa, viruses or parasitic worms. *Amoebic d.* common in tropical countries; caused by the protozoon *Entamoeba histolytica*. Spread is decreased in places with high standards of hygiene and sanitation. A notifiable disease in the UK. Called also amoebiasis. *Bacillary d.* the most common and acute form of the disease, caused by bacteria of the genus *Shigella*; *S. soِnei* is the most frequent cause in the UK. A notifiable disease. Called also shigellosis.

dysfunction (dis'fungkshən) impairment of function.

dysgammaglobulinaemia (dis-,gamə,globyuhli'neemi·ə) an immunological deficiency state marked by selective deficiencies of one or more, but not all, classes of immunoglobulins, resulting in heightened susceptibility to infectious diseases.

dysgenesis (dis'jenəsis) defective development.

dysgerminoma (,disjərmi'nohmə) a malignant tumour derived from germinal cells that have not been differentiated to either sex, occur-ring in either the ovary or the testicle.

dyshidrosis (dis·hi'drohsis) a disturbance of the sweat mechanism, in which an itching vesicular rash may be present.

dyskinesia (,diski'neezi·ə) impairment of voluntary movement.

dyslalia (dis'layli·ə) impairment of speech, caused by a physical disorder.

dyslexia (dis'leksi·ə) difficulty in reading or learning to read; accompanied by difficulty in writing and spelling correctly.

dysmaturity (,dismə'tyuoo·ritee) the condition of being small or immature for gestational age; said of fetuses that are the product of a pregnancy involving placental insufficiency or dysfunction. Called also small for dates, or light for gestational age.

dysmelia (dis'meeli·ə) malformation in the development of the limbs. *See* AMELIA.

dysmenorrhoea (dis,menə'reeə) painful menstruation. *Primary (spasmodic) d.* painful menstruation occurring without apparent cause. The onset is usually shortly following puberty and occurs with each subsequent period. May be helped by hormonal therapy. *Secondary (congestive) d.* painful menstruation occurring in a woman who has previously had normal periods for some years. Often due to endometritis. The condition tends to worsen as the local congestion increases.

dysostosis (,diso'stohsis) abnormal development of bone.

dyspareunia ('dispa'rooni·ə) painful or difficult coitus for women.

dyspepsia (dis'pepsi·ə) indigestion. There may be abdominal discomfort, flatulence, nausea and sometimes vomiting. *Nervous d.* dyspepsia in which anxiety and tension aggravate the symptoms.

dysphagia (dis'fayji·ə) difficulty in swallowing.

dysphasia (dis'fayzi·ə) difficulty in speaking, due to a brain lesion. There is a lack of coordination and an inability to arrange words in their correct order.

dysplasia (dis'playzi·ə) abnormal development of tissue.

dyspnoea (disp'neeə) difficult or laboured breathing. *Expiratory d.* difficulty in expelling air. *Inspiratory d.* difficulty in intake of air.

dyspraxia (dis'praksi·ə) partial loss of ability to perform coordinated movements.

dysrhythmia (dis'ridhmi·ə) disturbance of a regularly occurring pattern. Often applied to an abnormality of rhythm of the brain waves as shown in an electroencephalogram.

dystaxia (dis'taksi·ə) difficulty in controlling voluntary movements.

dystocia (dis'tohsi·ə) difficult or slow labour. *Maternal d.* difficult labour when the cause is with the mother, e.g. contracted pelvis. *Fetal d.* difficult labour due to abnormal size or position of the child.

dystonia (dis'tohni·ə) a lack of tonicity in a tissue, often referring to the muscles.

dystrophia (dis'trohfi·ə) dystrophy. *D. myotonica* a rare hereditary disease of early adult life in which there is progressive muscle wasting and gonadal atrophy.

dystrophy ('distrəfee) a disorder of an organ or tissue caused by faulty nutrition of the affected part. Dystrophia. *Muscular d.* a group of hereditary diseases in which there is progressive muscular weakness and wasting.

dysuria (dis'yooə·ri·ə) difficult or painful micturition.

E

ear (iə) the organ of hearing and of equilibrium. It consists of three parts: (1) the *external e.*, made up of the expanded portion, or pinna, and the auditory canal separated from the middle ear by the drum, or tympanum; (2) the *middle e.*, an irregular cavity containing three small bones of the ear (incus, malleus and stapes) which link the tympanic membrane to the internal ear; it also communicates with the pharyngotympanic tube and the mastoid cells; (3) the *internal e.*, which consists of a bony and a membranous labyrinth (the cochlea and semicircular canals).

EBM expressed breast milk.

Ebola virus disease (ee'bohlə) a central African viral haemorrhagic fever with acute onset and characteristic morbilliform rash. The incubation period is 2–21 days. Outbreaks have been reported in Sudan and Zaire. It has no known source, although it is probably a zoonosis. Person-to-person spread in hospitals and laboratories by accidental inoculation of blood and tissue fluids has occurred.

ecchondroma (,ekon'drohmə) a benign cartilaginous tumour arising as an outgrowth to cartilage or bone.

ecchymosis (,eki'mohsis) a bruise; an effusion of blood under the skin causing discoloration.

eccrine ('ekrien, -rin) secreting externally. Applied particularly to the sweat glands that are generally distributed over the body. *See* APOCRINE.

ECG electrocardiogram.

Echinococcus (e,kienoh'kokəs) a genus of tapeworms. *E. granulosus* infests dogs and may also infect man. The larval form develops into cysts (hydatids), which occur in the liver, lung, brain and other organs.

echocardiography (,ekoh,kahdi-'ografee) a method of studying the movements of the heart by the use of ultrasound.

echoencephalography (,ekoh·en,kefə'logrəfee, -,sef-) a method of brain investigation by ultrasonic echoes.

echolalia (,ekoh'layli·ə) the pathological involuntary repetition of phrases or words spoken by another person.

echophony (e,kofənee) the echo of the voice heard in the chest on auscultation.

echopraxia (,ekoh'praksi·ə) the automatic repetition of the movements of others.

echovirus ('ekoh,vierəs) a group of viruses (enteroviruses), the name of which was derived from

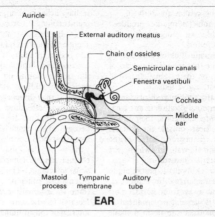

Auricle

External auditory meatus

Chain of ossicles

Semicircular canals

Fenestra vestibuli

Cochlea

Middle ear

Mastoid process   Tympanic membrane   Auditory tube

EAR

the first letters of the description 'enteric cytopathogenic human orphan'. At the time of the isolation of the viruses the diseases they caused were not known, hence the term 'orphan'. It is now known that these viruses produce many types of human disease, especially aseptic meningitis, diarrhoea and respiratory diseases.

eclampsia (i'klampsi·ə) a severe condition in which convulsions may occur as a result of an acute toxaemia of pregnancy.

ecmnesia (ek'neezi·ə) forgetfulness of recent events with remembrance of more remote ones.

ecology (ikoləjee, ee-) the study of the relationship between living organisms and the environment.

economy (i'konəmee) the management of money or domestic

affairs. *Token e.* in behaviour therapy, a programme of treatment in which the patient earns tokens, exchangeable for tangible rewards, by engaging in appropriate personal and social behaviour, and loses tokens for antisocial behaviour.

ecstasy ('ekstə,see) a feeling of exaltation. It may be accompanied by sensory impairment and lack of activity but with an expression of rapture.

ECT electroconvulsive therapy.

ectasia (ek'tayzi·ə) dilatation of a canal or organ. Ectasis.

ecthyma (ek'thiemə) a form of impetigo with an eruption of pustules usually with a hardened base. A pigmented scar remains after healing takes place.

ectoderm (,ektoh,dərm) the outer germinal layer of the developing embryo from which the skin and nervous system are derived.

ectogenous (ek'tojənəs) produced outside an organism. *See* ENDOGENOUS.

ectoparasite (,ektoh'parə,siet) a parasite that spends all or part of its life on the external surface of its host, e.g. a louse.

ectopia (ek'tohpi·ə) displacement or abnormal position of any part. *E. cordis* congenital malposition of the heart outside the thoracic cavity. *E. vesicae* a defect of the abdominal wall in which the bladder is exposed.

ectopic (ek'topik) 1. pertaining to or characterized by ectopy. 2. located away from normal position. 3. arising or produced at an abnormal site or in a tissue where it is not normally found. *E. pregnancy* pregnancy in which the fertilized ovum becomes implanted outside the uterus instead of in the wall of the uterus. Called also extrauterine pregnancy.

ectopy ('ektə,pee) displacement or malposition, especially if congenital.

ectrodactylia (,ektrohdak'tili·ə) congenital absence of one or more fingers or toes or parts of them.

ectropion (ek'trohpi·ən) eversion of an eyelid, often due to contraction of the skin or to paralysis. It causes epiphora and hypertrophy of exposed conjunctiva.

eczema ('eksimə, 'eksmə) 1. a general term for any superficial inflammatory process involving primarily the epidermis, marked early by redness, itching, minute papules and vesicles, weeping, oozing and crusting, and later by scaling, lichenification, and often pigmentation. 2. atopic dermatitis. Eczema is a common allergic reaction in children but it also occurs in adults. Childhood eczema often begins in infancy, the rash appearing on the face, neck, and folds of elbows and knees. It may disappear by itself when an offending food is removed from the diet, or it may become more extensive and in some instances cover the entire surface of the body. Severe eczema can be complicated by skin infections. The cause of eczema can either be exogenous (due to external or traumatic factors) or endogenous (due to internal or constitutional factors).

edentulous (ee'dentyuhləs, -'dench-) without natural teeth.

EDTA ethylenediamine tetraacetic acid.

EEG electroencephalogram.

effacement (i'faysmənt) taking up of the cervix. The process by which the internal os dilates, so opening out the cervical canal and leaving only a circular orifice, the external os. This process precedes cervical dilatation, particularly in a primigravida, whilst both occur simultaneously in a multigravida during labour.

effector (i'fektor) a motor or sensory nerve ending in a muscle, gland or organ.

efferent ('efə-rənt) conveying from the centre to the periphery. *E. nerves* motor nerves coming from the brain to supply the muscles and glands.

effervescent (,efə'ves'nt) foaming or giving off gas bubbles.

effleurage (‚eflə'rahzh) [Fr.] stroking movement in massage. In
NATURAL CHILDBIRTH, a light circular stroke of the lower abdomen, done in rhythm to control
breathing, to aid in relaxation of
the abdominal muscles, and to
increase concentration during a
uterine contraction. The stroking
is accomplished by moving the
wrist only.

effort syndrome a condition characterized by breathlessness, palpitations, chest pain and fatigue,
caused by an abnormal anxiety
about the condition of the heart.

effusion (i'fyoozhən) the escape
of blood, serum or other fluid
into surrounding tissues or cavities.

ego ('eegoh, 'eg-) in psychoanalytical theory, that part of the
mind which the individual
experiences as his 'self'. The ego
is concerned with satisfying the
unconscious primitive demands
of the 'id' in a socially acceptable
form.

eidetic (ie'detik) the ability to visualize exactly objects or events
which have previously been seen.
A photographic memory.

Eisenmenger's complex ('iez'n-
‚mengəz) *V. Eisenmenger, German
physician, 1864–1932.* A congenital heart defect in which a ventricular septal defect is associated
with increased pulmonary vascular resistance.

ejaculation (i‚jakyuh'layshən) the
act of ejecting semen, a reflex
action that occurs as the result of
sexual stimulation.

elastic (i'lastik) capable of stretching. *E. bandage* one that will

stretch and will exert continuous
pressure on the part bandaged.
E. stocking a woven rubber stocking sometimes worn for varicose
veins. *E. tissue* connective tissue
containing yellow elastic fibres.

elation (i'layshən) in psychiatry,
a feeling of well-being or a state
of excitement. It occurs in
marked degree in hypomania and
in intense degree in mania. *See*
EUPHORIA.

elbow ('elboh) the joint between
the upper arm and the forearm.
It is formed by the humerus
above and the radius and ulna
below.

elective (i'lektiv) that which is
chosen by the patient or physician, as opposed to an emergency procedure.

Electra complex (i'lektrə) libidin-
ous fixation of a daughter toward
her father. The female version of
the Oedipus complex.

electrocardiogram (i'lektroh'kah-
dioh‚gram) abbreviated ECG. A
tracing made of the various
phases of the heart's action by
means of an electrocardiograph.
The normal electrocardiogram is
composed of a P wave, Q, R,
and S waves known as the QRS
COMPLEX, or QRS wave, and a T
wave. The P wave occurs at the
beginning of each contraction of
the atria. The QRS wave occurs
at the beginning of each contraction of the ventricles. The T wave
seen in a normal electrocardiogram occurs as the ventricles
recover electrically and prepare
for the next contraction. There
is a refractory period between
these waves.

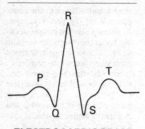

ELECTROCARDIOGRAM

electrocardiograph (i,lektroh-'kahdioh,grahf, -,graf) a machine that records electrical potential of the heart from electrodes on the chest and limbs.

electrocardiophonograph (i,lektroh,kahdioh'fohnǝ,grahf,-,i,graf) an electrical machine for recording the heart sounds graphically.

electrocautery (i'lektroh'kawtǝ·ree) an instrument for the destruction of tissue by means of an electrically heated needle or wire loop.

electrocoagulation (i,lektrohkoh-,agyuh'layshǝn) a method of coagulation using a high-frequency current. A form of surgical diathermy.

electroconvulsive therapy (i,lektrohkǝn'vulsiv) abbreviated ECT. Electroplexy. The passage of an electric current through the frontal lobes of the brain, which causes a convulsion. It is used in the treatment of depression and sometimes of schizophrenia. A general anaesthetic and muscle relaxant are given prior to treatment.

electrocorticography (i,lektroh-,kawti'kogrǝfee) electroencephalography with the electrodes applied directly to the cortex of the brain during surgery to locate a small lesion, e.g. a scar.

electrode (i'lektrohd) the terminal of a conducting system or cell of a battery, through which electricity enters or leaves the body.

electroencephalogram (i,lektroh·en'kǝfǝlǝ,gram, -'sef-) abbreviated EEG. A tracing of the electrical activity of the brain. Abnormal rhythm is an aid to diagnosis in epilepsy and cerebral tumour.

electroencephalograph (i,lektroh·en'kefǝlǝ,grahf, -graf, -sef-) a machine for recording the electrical activity of the cortex of the brain. The electrodes are applied to the scalp.

electrolysis (,ilek'trolisis, ,elek-) 1. chemical decomposition by means of electricity, e.g. an electric current passed through water decomposes it into oxygen and hydrogen. 2. the destruction of tissue by means of electricity, e.g. the removal of surplus hair.

electrolyte (i,lektrǝ,liet) a compound which, when dissolved in a solution, will dissociate into ions. These ions are electrically charged particles and will thus conduct electricity. *E. balance* the maintenance of the correct balance between the different elements in the body tissues and fluids.

electromyography (i,lektrohmie-'ogrǝfee) recording of electrical currents generated in active muscle.

electron (i'lektron) a negatively charged particle revolving round the nucleus of an atom. *See* ATOM. *E. microscope* a type of microscope employing a beam of electrons rather than a beam of light, which allows very small particles such as viruses to be identified.

electro-oculography *see* ELECTRO-RETINOGRAPHY.

electrophoresis (i,lektrohfə'reesis) a method of analysing the different proteins in blood serum by passing an electric current through the serum to separate the electrically charged particles. The particles gradually separate into bands, due to the difference in rate of movement according to the electrical charge on the particles.

electroplexy (i'lektroh,plekse, ,elek'troplek,see) electroconvulsive therapy.

electroretinogram (i,lektroh-'retinoh,gram) a record of the tracings produced by electroretinography.

electroretinography a method of examining the retina of the eye by means of electrodes and light stimulation for assessment of retinal damage.

element ('elimənt) 1. any of the primary parts or constituents of a compound. 2. in chemistry, a simple substance that cannot be decomposed by ordinary chemical means; the basic 'stuff' of which all matter is composed.

elephantiasis (,elifən'tieəsis) a chronic disease of the lymphatics producing excessive thickening of the skin and swelling of the

parts affected, usually the lower limbs. It may be due to filariasis in tropical and subtropical climates.

elevator ('eli,vaytə) an instrument used as a lever for raising bone, etc. *Periosteal e.* instrument that strips the periosteum in bone surgery.

elimination (i,limi'nayshən) the removal of waste matter, particularly from the body. Excretion.

elixir (i'liksə) a sweetened spirituous liquid, used largely as a flavouring agent to hide the unpleasant taste of some drugs.

elliptocytosis (i,liptohsie'tohsis) an hereditary disorder where the red blood cells are elliptical in shape. Increased red cell destruction leading to anaemia occurs.

emaciation (i,maysi'ayshən) excessive wasting of body tissues. Extreme thinness.

emasculation (i,maskyuh'layshən) the removal of the penis or testicles; castration.

embolectomy (,embə'lektəmee) surgical removal of an embolus, frequently arterial emboli that are cutting off the blood supply to the limbs.

embolism ('embə,lizəm) obstruction of a blood vessel by a travelling blood clot or particle of matter. *Air e.* the presence of gas or air bubbles, usually sucked into the large veins from a wound in the neck or chest. *Cerebral e.* obstruction of a vessel in the brain. *Coronary e.* the blockage of a coronary vessel with a clot. *Fat e.* globules of fat released into the blood from a fractured bone. *Infective e.* detached particles of infected blood clot from an area of inflammation which, obstructing small vessels, result in abscess formation, i.e. pyaemia. *Pulmonary e.* blocking of the pulmonary artery or one of its branches by a detached clot, usually due to thrombosis in the femoral or iliac veins. *Retinal e.* blockage, due to air or a blood clot, of the central retinal artery, resulting in loss of vision.

embolus ('embələs) a substance carried by the bloodstream until it causes obstruction by blocking a blood vessel. *See* EMBOLISM.

embrocation (,embroh'kayshən) a liquid applied to the body by rubbing to treat strains. A liniment.

embryo ('embri,oh) the fertilized ovum in its earliest stages, i.e. until it shows human characteristics during the second month. After this it is termed a fetus.

embryology (,embri'oləjee) the study of the growth and development of the embryo from the unicellular stage until birth.

embryotomy (,embri'otəmee) the cutting-up of a fetus during a difficult birth to facilitate delivery.

emesis ('eməsis) vomiting.

emetic (i'metik) an agent which can induce vomiting, e.g. salt or mustard and water by mouth, or apomorphine hypodermically.

eminence ('eminəns) a projection, usually rounded, from a surface, e.g. of a bone.

emission (i'mishən) involuntary ejection (of semen).

emmetropia (,eme'trohpi·ə) normal or perfect vision.

emollient (i'moli·ənt, -'moh-) any substance used to soothe or soften the skin.

emotion (i'mohshən) feeling or affect; a state of arousal characterized by alteration of feeling tone and by physiological behavioural changes. The physical form of emotion may be outward and evident to others, as in crying, laughing, blushing, or a variety of facial expressions. However, emotion is not always reflected in one's appearance and actions even though psychic changes are taking place. Joy, grief, fear and anger are examples of emotions.

empathy ('empəthee) the power of projecting oneself into the feelings of another person or situation.

emphysema (,emfi'seemə, -fie-) the abnormal presence of air in tissues or cavities of the body. *Pulmonary e.* a chronic disease of the lungs. Distension of alveoli causes intervening walls to be broken down and bullae to form on the lung surface. It also causes distension of the bronchioles and eventual loss of elasticity so that inspired air cannot be expired making breathing difficult. *Surgical e.* the presence of air or any other gas in the subcutaneous tissues, introduced through a wound and evidenced by crepitation on pressure.

empirical (em'pirik'l) treatment based on experience and not on scientific reasoning.

empyema (,empie'eemə) a collection of pus in a cavity, most commonly referring to the pleural cavity.

emulsion (i'mulshən) a mixture in which an oil is suspended in water, by the addition of an emulsifying agent.

en face (,onh 'fas) [Fr.] a position in which the mother's face and that of her infant are on the same plane and approximately 20 cm apart; a position usually held during breastfeeding.

enamel (i'naməl) the hard outer covering of the crown of a tooth.

enarthrosis (,enah'throhsis) a freely moving joint, e.g. ball and socket joint.

ENB English National Board for Nursing, Midwifery and Health Visiting.

encanthis (en'kanthis) a small fleshy growth at the inner canthus of the eye which may form an abscess.

encapsulated (en'kapsyuh,laytid) enclosed in a capsule.

encephalin (enkephalin) (en'kefəlin, -'sef-) an opiate-like substance which is produced by the pituitary and has analgesic effects. This substance may also be produced synthetically. *See* ENDORPHIN.

encephalitis (en'kefə'lietis, -sef-) inflammation of the brain. There are many types of encephalitis, depending on the causative agent and the structures involved. The symptoms may be mild, with headache, general malaise and muscle ache similar to that associated with influenza. The more acute and serious symptoms may include fever, delirium, convulsions and coma, and in a significant number of patients result in death.

encephalocele (en'kefəloh,seel, -'sef-) herniation of the brain through the skull.

encephalography (en'kefə'logrə-fee, -,sef-) radiographic examination of the ventricles of the brain following the insertion of air or a gas through a lumbar or cisternal puncture.

encephaloma (en'kefə'lohmə, -,sef-) a tumour of the brain.

encephalomalacia (en,kefəlohmə'layshi-ə,-,sef-) softening of the brain.

encephalomyelitis (en,kefəloh,mieə'lietis, -,sef-) inflammation of the brain and spinal cord.

encephalomyelopathy (en,kefəloh,mieə'lopəthee, -,sef-) any disease condition of the brain and spinal cord.

encephalon (en'kefəlon, -'sef-) the brain with the spinal cord, constituting the central nervous system.

encephalopathy (en,kefə'lopə-thee, -,sef-) cerebral dysfunction with diffuse disease or damage of the brain. *Dialysis e.* associated with long-term use of haemodialysis marked by speech disorders and myoclonic fits progressing to global dementia. *Hepatic e.* a condition caused by liver failure, leading to dementia and then coma. *Hypertensive e.* a transient disturbance of function associated with hypertension. Disorientation, excitability, and abnormal behaviour occur, which may be reversed if the pressure is reduced. *Wernicke's e.* A complication associated with chronic alcoholism; characterized by paralysis of the eye muscles, diplopia, nystagmus, ataxia and mental changes.

enchondroma (ˌenkon'drohmə) a benign tumour of cartilage within the shaft of the bone.

encopresis (ˌenkə'preesis) incontinence of faeces, not due to organic defect or illness.

endarterectomy (ˌendahtə'rektəmee) the surgical removal of the lining of an artery, usually because of narrowing of the vessel by artheromatous plaques. *Thrombo-e.* removal of a clot with the lining.

endarteritis (ˌendahtə'rietis) inflammation of the innermost coat of an artery. *E. obliterans* a type which causes collapse and obstruction in small arteries.

endemic (en'demik) pertaining to a disease prevalent in a particular locality.

endemiology (en,deemiolǝgee) the study of all the factors pertaining to endemic disease.

endocarditis (ˌendohkah'dietis) inflammation of the endocardium characterized by vegetations on the endocardium and heart valves. Due to infection by microorganisms, fungi or *Rickettsia*, or to rheumatic fever.

endocardium (ˌendoh'kahdi·əm) the membrane lining the heart.

endocervicitis (ˌendoh,sərvi'sietis) inflammation of the membrane lining the uterine cervix.

endocrine ('endoh,krin, -,krien) secreting within. Applied to those glands whose secretions (hormones) flow directly into the blood and not outwards through a duct. The chief endocrine glands are the thyroid, para-

thyroids, suprarenals and pituitary. The pancreas, stomach, liver, ovaries and testes also produce internal secretions.

endocrinology (ˌendohkri'nolǝjee) the science of the endocrine glands and their secretions.

endocrinopathy (ˌendohkri'nopǝthee) any disease or disorder of any of the endocrine glands or their secretions.

endoderm ('endoh,dərm) entoderm.

endogenous (en'dojǝnǝs) produced within the organism. *E. depression* one in which the disease derives from internal causes.

endolymph ('endoh,limf) the fluid inside the membranous labyrinth of the ear.

endolysin (ˌendoh'liesin, en'dolisin) a factor or enzyme present in cells that can cause dissolution of the cytoplasm.

endometriosis (ˌendoh,meetri'ohsis) the presence of endometrium in an abnormal situation, e.g. in the ovaries, the intestines or the urinary bladder. The ectopic tissue undergoes the same hormonal changes as normal endometrium. As there is no outlet for bleeding when menstruation occurs, the woman suffers severe pain.

endometritis (ˌendohmi'trietis) inflammation of the endometrium.

endometrium (ˌendoh'meetri·əm) the mucous membrane lining the uterus.

endomyocarditis (ˌendoh,mieohkah'dietis) inflammation of the lining membrane and muscles of the heart.

endoparasite (ˌendoh'parǝ,siet) a

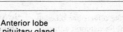

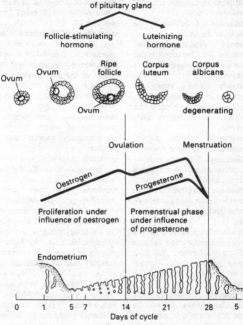

ENDOMETRIAL AND FOLLICULAR CHANGES DURING MENSTRUAL CYCLE

parasite that lives within the body of its host.

endophthalmitis (,endof'thal-'mietis) inflammation of the ocular cavity and adjacent structures.

endorphin (en'dawfin) one of a group of opiate-like peptides produced naturally by the body at neural synapses at various points in the central nervous system, where they modulate the transmission of pain perceptions. Endorphins raise the pain threshold and produce sedation and euphoria; the effects are blocked by naloxone, a narcotic antagonist.

endorrhachis (,endoh'rakis) the spinal dura mater.

endoscope ('endə,skohp) an instrument used for direct visual inspection of a hollow organ or cavity.

endosteitis (,endosti'ietis) inflammation of the endosteum.

endosteoma (en,dosti'ohma) a neoplasm in the medullary cavity of a bone.

endosteum (en'dosti·əm) the lining membrane of bone cavities.

endothelioma (,endoh,theeli'ohmə) a malignant growth originating in the endothelium.

endothelium (,endoh'theeli·əm) the membranous lining of serous, synovial and other internal surfaces.

endotoxin (,endoh'toksin) a poison produced by and retained within a bacterium, which is released only after the destruction of the bacterial cell. *See* EXOTOXIN.

endotracheal (,endohtrə'keeəl) within the trachea. *E. tube* an airway catheter which is inserted into the trachea when a patient requires ventilatory support. It also allows for the removal of secretions by suction.

enema ('enimə) 1. introduction of fluid into the rectum. 2. a solution introduced into the rectum to promote evacuation of faeces or as a means of administering nutrient or medicinal substances. 3. introduction of a radio-opaque material in a radiological examination of the colon (*barium e.*)

or via a tube inserted into the jejunum in a radiological examination of the small bowel (*small bowel e.*).

enervation (,enə'vayshən) 1. general weakness and loss of strength. 2. removal of a nerve.

engagement (in'gayjmənt) the entry of the presenting part of the fetus, normally the head, into the true pelvis. Occurs in the last stage of pregnancy.

enophthalmos (,enof'thalmos) a condition in which the eyeball is abnormally sunken into its socket.

enostosis (,eno'stohsis) a tumour or bony growth within the medullary cavity of a bone.

ensiform ('ensi,fawm) xiphoid; sword-shaped. *E. cartilage* the lowest portion of the sternum.

Entamoeba (,entə'meebə) a genus of protozoa, some of which are parasitic in man. *E. histolytica* the cause of amoebic dysentery.

enteral ('entə·ral) within the gastrointestinal tract. *E. diets* or *e. feeding* diets taken by mouth or through a nasogastric tube.

enterectomy (,entə'rektəmee) excision of a portion of the intestine.

enteric (en'terik) pertaining to the intestine. *E.-coated* a special coating applied to tablets or capsules which prevents release and absorption of their contents until they reach the intestine.

enteritis (,entə'rietis) inflammation of the small intestine.

Enterobacteriaceae (,entə·rohbaktiə·ri'aysi·ee) a family of Gramnegative, rod-shaped bacteria, many of which are normally found

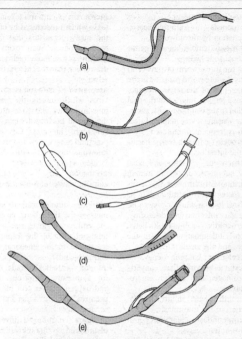

Endotracheal tubes. (a) Oxford non-kink orotracheal tube.
Requires an introducer to pass it into the trachea. (b) Magill red-
rubber orotracheal tube with inflatable cuff. (c) Nylon armoured
non-kink tube. Note the two lines on the tube. If the vocal cords
are placed between these lines then the tube will remain in the
trachea and not pass into the right bronchus. (d) Nasotracheal
tube. Thinner than an orotracheal tube, the tube to the inflatable
cuff is attached further back and is buried in the main tube to
prevent damage to the nasal mucosa. (e) Robertshaw double-
lumen tube that allows one-lung ventilation during thoracic
surgery. Note the individual inflatable cuffs for the trachea and left
bronchus

in the human intestine.

enterobiasis (ˌentə·roh'bieəsis) infestation by threadworms.

Enterobius (ˌentə'rohbi·əs) a genus of nematode worms. *E. vermicularis* the threadworm or pinworm, a small white worm parasitic in the upper part of the large intestine. Gravid females migrate to the anal region to deposit their eggs, sometimes causing severe itching. Infection is frequent in children.

enterocele (ˌentə·roh,seel) a hernia of the intestine.

enterococcus (ˌentə·roh'kokəs) any streptococcus of the human intestine. An example is *Streptococcus faecalis*, only harmful out of its normal habitat when it may cause a urinary infection or endocarditis.

enterocolitis (ˌentə·rohkə'lietis, -koh-) inflammation of both the large and the small intestine.

enterokinase (ˌentə·roh'kienayz) an intestinal enzyme that converts trypsinogen into trypsin; enteropeptidase.

enterolith ('entə·roh,lith) a concretion in the intestines.

enteropeptidase (ˌentə·roh'pepti,dayz) enterokinase.

enteropexy ('entə·roh,peksee) the surgical fixation of a part of the intestine to the abdominal wall.

enterospasm ('entə·roh,spazəm) intestinal colic.

enterostomy (ˌentə'rostəmee) the formation of an external opening into the small intestine. It may be (1) temporary, to relieve obstruction, or (2) permanent, in the form of an ileostomy in cases of total colectomy.

enterotomy (ˌentə'rotəmee) any incision of the intestine.

enterotoxin (ˌentə·roh'toksin) a toxin which is produced by one of the many organisms that cause food poisoning. Such toxins frequently prove more resistant to destruction than the bacteria themselves.

enterovirus (ˌentə·roh'vierəs) a virus which infects the gastrointestinal tract and then attacks the central nervous system. This subgroup includes Coxsackie, polio and echoviruses, and are now known, together with rhinoviruses, as picornaviruses.

enterozoon (ˌentə·roh'zoh·on) an animal parasite infesting the intestines.

entoderm ('entoh,dərm) the innermost of the three germ layers of the embryo. It gives rise to the lining of most of the respiratory tract, and to the intestinal tract and its glands.

Entonox ('entə,noks) trade name for a mixture of nitrous oxide and oxygen, 50 per cent of each, premixed in one cylinder and used as an analgesic.

entropion (en'trohpi·ən) inversion of an eyelid, so that the lashes rub against the eyeball.

enucleation (i,nyookli'ayshən) removal of an organ or other mass intact from its supporting tissues, as of the eyeball from the orbit.

enuresis (,enyuh'reesis) involuntary passing of urine, usually during sleep at night (bed-wetting).

environment (in'vierənmənt) the surroundings of an organism which influence its development and behaviour.

Environmental Health Officer (en,viə·rən'ment'l) the person employed by the local authority to improve and regulate the environment and to enforce statutory regulations. Responsibilities include housing, food hygiene, refuse collection, infestation, and air and noise pollution, etc.

enzyme ('enziem) a protein which will catalyse a biological reaction. *See* CATALYST.

eosin ('eeohsin) a red dye used to stain biological specimens. A derivative of bromine and fluorescein.

eosinophil (eeə'sinəfil) cell having an affinity for eosin. A type of white blood cell containing eosin-staining granules.

eosinophilia (,eeə,sinə'fili·ə) excessive numbers of eosinophils present in the blood.

ependyma (e'pendimə) the membrane lining the cerebral ventricles and the central canal of the spinal cord.

ependymoma (e,pendi'mohmə) a neoplasm arising from the lining cells of the ventricles or central canal of the spinal cord. It gives rise to signs of hydrocephalus and is treated by surgery and radiotherapy.

ephedrine ('efi,dreen, -drin) a drug that relieves spasm of the bronchi, having a similar action to adrenaline but can be taken orally. Widely used in asthma and chronic bronchitis.

ephidrosis (,efi'drohsis) profuse sweating; hyperhidrosis.

epiblepharon (,epi'blefə·ron) a congenital condition in which an excess of skin of the eyelid folds over the lid margin so that the eyelashes are pressed against the eyeball.

epicanthus (,epi'kanthəs) a vertical fold of skin on either side of the nose, sometimes covering the inner canthus; a normal characteristic in persons of certain races, but anomalous in others.

epicardium (,epi'kahdi·əm) the visceral layer of the pericardium.

epicondyle (,epi'kondiel) a protuberance on a long bone above its condyle.

epicritic (,epi'kritik) pertaining to sensory nerve fibres in the skin which give the appreciation of touch and temperature.

epidemic (,epi'demik) the presence in a population of disease or infection in excess of that usually expected.

epidemiology (,epi,deemi'oləjee) the study of the distribution of diseases.

epidermis (,epi'dərmis) the non-vascular outer layer or cuticle of the skin. It consists of layers of cells which protect the dermis.

epidermoid (,epi'dərmoyd) pertaining to certain tumours which have the appearance of epidermal tissue.

Epidermophyton (epi,dərmoh-'fieton) a genus of fungi which attacks skin and nails, but not hair. The cause of ringworm and athlete's foot.

epididymis (,epi'didimis) [Gr.] an elongated, cordlike structure along the posterior border of the testis, whose coiled duct provides for the storage, transport and maturation of spermatozoa.

epididymitis (,epi,didi'mietis) inflammation of the epididymis.

epididymo-orchitis (,epi,didi-moh·aw'kietis) inflammation of the epididymis and the testis.

epidural (,epi'dyooə·ral) outside the dura mater. *E. analgesia* also known as extradural or peridural anaesthesia. A form of pain relief for labour and chronic pain, obtained by the injection of a local analgesic, e.g. bupivacaine, into the epidural space in order to block the spinal nerves. It may be approached by two routes: (1) caudal, through the sacrococcygeal membrane covering the sacral hiatus, or (2) lumbar, through the intervertebral space and ligamentum flavum.

epigastrium (,epi'gastri·əm) that region of the abdomen which is situated over the stomach.

epiglottis (,epi'glotis) a cartilaginous structure which covers the opening from the pharynx into the larynx during swallowing and prevents food from passing into the trachea.

epilation (,epi'layshən) removal of hairs with their roots. It may be effected by pulling out the hairs or by electrolysis.

epilatory (e,pilatə·ree) an agent which produces epilation.

epilepsy ('epi,lepsee) convulsive attacks due to disordered electrical activity of the brain cells. In a major attack of 'grand mal' the patient falls to the ground unconscious, following an aura or unpleasant sensation. There are first tonic and then clonic contractions, from which stage the patient passes into a deep sleep. A minor attack of 'petit mal' is a momentary loss of consciousness only. Both these types

of epilepsy are idiopathic and are not caused by any damage to the brain. *Focal* or *jacksonian e.* a symptom of a cerebral lesion. The convulsive movements are often localized and close observation of the onset and course of the attack may greatly assist diagnosis. *Temporal-lobe e.* characterized by hallucinations of sight, hearing, taste and smell, paroxysmal disorders of memory and automatism. Caused by temporal or parietal lobe disease.

epileptiform (,epi'lepti,fawm) resembling an epileptic fit.

epiloia (,epi'loyə) tuberous sclerosis. A congenital disorder with areas of hardening in the cerebral cortex and other organs, characterized clinically by mental handicap and epilepsy.

epimenorrhoea (,epimenə'reeə) menstruation occurring at abnormally short intervals.

epinephrine (,epi'nefrin) adrenaline.

epineurium (,epi'nyooə·ri·əm) the sheath of tissue surrounding a nerve.

epiphora (i'pifə·rə) persistent overflow of tears, often due to obstruction in the lacrimal passages or to ectropion.

epiphysis (i'pifisis) the end of a long bone developed separately but attached by cartilage to the diaphysis (the shaft) with which it eventually unites. From the line of junction growth in length takes place.

epiplocele (i'piploh,seel) a hernia containing omentum.

epiploon (epi'ploh·on) the greater omentum.

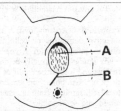

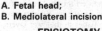

A. Fetal head;
B. Mediolateral incision

EPISIOTOMY

episcleritis (ˌepi·sklə'rietis) inflammation of the outer coat of the eyeball. It is seen as a slightly raised bluish nodule under the conjunctiva.

episiorrhaphy (ˌepi'so·rəfee) the repair of a laceration of the perineum.

episiotomy (ə'peezi'otəmee) an incision made in the perineum when it will not stretch sufficiently during the second stage of labour.

epispadias (ˌepi'spaydi·əs) a malformation in which there is an abnormal opening of the urethra on to the dorsal surface of the penis. *See* HYPOSPADIAS.

epistaxis (ˌepi'staksis) bleeding from the nose.

epithelioma (ˌepi,theeli'ohmə) any tumour originating in the epithelium.

epithelium (ˌepi'theeli·əm) the surface layer of cells either of the skin or of lining tissues.

epithelization (ˌepi,theelie'zayshən) development of epithelium. The final stage in the healing of a surface wound.

epizoon (ˌepi'zoh·on) any external animal parasite.

Epstein–Barr virus (ˌepstien'bah) *M.A. Epstein, British pathologist, b. 1921; Y. Barr.* A herpes virus that causes infectious mononucleosis. It has been isolated from cells cultured from Burkitt's lymphoma, and has been found in certain cases of nasopharyngeal cancer. Called also EB virus.

epulis (e'pyoolis) [Gr.] a fibroid tumour of the gums.

Erb's palsy (airps) *W.H. Erb, German physician, 1840–1921.* Paralysis of the arm, often due to birth injury causing pressure on the brachial plexus or lower cervical nerve roots.

erectile (i'rektiel) having the power of becoming erect. *E. tissue* vascular tissue which, under stimulus, becomes congested and swollen, causing erection of that part. The penis consists largely of erectile tissue.

erection (i'rekshən) the enlarged and rigid state of the sexually aroused penis. Erection can also occur in the clitoris and the nipples of the female.

erepsin (i'repsin) the enzyme of succus entericus, secreted by the intestinal glands, which splits peptones into amino acids.

ergometrine (ˌərgoh'metreen) an alkaloid of ergot which stimulates contraction of the uterine muscle.

ergonomics (ˌərgə'nomiks) the scientific study of man in relation to his work and the effective use of human energy.

ergosterol (ər'gostə·rol) a sterol occurring in animal and plant tissues which, on ultraviolet irradiation, becomes a potent antirachitic substance, vitamin D₂ (ergocalciferol).

ergot ('ərgot) a drug from a fungus which grows on rye. Used chiefly to contract the uterus and check haemorrhage at childbirth.

ergotamine (ər'gotə,meen) an alkaloid of ergot used in the treatment of migraine.

ergotism ('ərgə,tizəm) the effects of poisoning from ergot which may lead to gangrene of the fingers and toes.

erogenous (i'rojənəs) arousing erotic feelings. *E. zones* areas of the body stimulation of which produces erotic desire, e.g. the oral, anal and genital orifices and the nipples.

erosion (i'rohzhən) the breaking down of tissue, usually by ulceration. *Cervical e.* a covering of columnar epithelium on the vaginal part of the uterine cervix, arising from erosion of the squamous epithelium which normally covers it.

erotic (i'rotik) pertaining to sexual love or lust.

eroticism, erotism (i'roti,sizəm; 'erə,tizəm) a sexual instinct or desire; the expression of one's instinctual energy or drive, especially the sex drive.

eructation (,iruk'tayshən) belching; the escape of gas from the stomach through the mouth.

eruption (i'rupshən) a breaking out, e.g. of a skin lesion, or the cutting of teeth.

erysipelas (,eri'sipələs) a febrile disease characterized by inflammation and redness of the skin and subcutaneous tissues, and due to group A haemolytic streptococci.

erysipeloid (,eri'sipə,loyd) an infective dermatitis or cellulitis due to infection with *Erysipelothrix insidiosa*; it usually begins in a wound (often the result of a prick by a fish bone) and remains localized, rarely becoming generalized and septicaemic.

erythema (,eri'theemə) redness of the skin caused by congestion of the capillaries in its lower layers. It occurs with any skin injury, infection or inflammation. *E. induratum* a manifestation of vasculitis. *E. multiforme* an acute eruption of the skin, which may be due to an allergy or to drug sensitivity. *E. nodosum* a painful disease in which bright red, tender nodes occur below the knee or on the forearm; it may be associated with tuberculosis.

erythematous (,eri'theemətəs) characterized by erythema.

erythrasma (,eri'thrazmə) a skin disease due to infection by *Corynebacterium minutissimum*, attacking the armpits or groins. It causes no irritation, but is contagious.

erythroblast (i'rithroh,blast) originally, any nucleated erythrocyte, but now more generally used to designate the nucleated precursor from which an erythrocyte develops.

erythroblastosis (i,rithrohbla-'stohsis) the presence of erythroblasts in the blood. *E. fetalis* a severe haemolytic anaemia, with an excess of erythroblasts in the newly born. Due to rhesus incompatibility between the

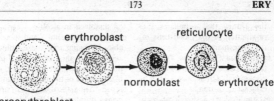

ERYTHROCYTE DEVELOPMENT IN BONE MARROW

child's and the mother's blood.

erythrocyanosis (i'rithroh,siea-'nohsis) swelling and blueness of the legs and thighs occurring mainly in young women and during cold weather.

erythrocyte (i'rithrə,siet) a mature red blood cell. The cells contain haemoglobin and serve to transport oxygen. They are developed in the red bone marrow found in the cancellous tissue of all bones. The haemopoietic factor vitamin B_{12} is essential for the change from megaloblast to normoblast, and iron, thyroxine and vitamin C are also necessary for its perfect structure. *E. sedimentation rate* abbreviated ESR. The rate at which the cells of citrated blood form a deposit in a graduated 200 mm tube (Westergren method). The normal is less than 10 mm of clear plasma in 1 h. This is much increased in severe infection and acute rheumatism.

erythrocythaemia (i,rithrohsie-'theemi·ə) increase in numbers of red blood cells due to overactivity of the bone marrow; Vazquez' disease; polycythaemia vera.

erythrocytopenia (i,rithroh,sie-toh'peeni·ə) erythropenia; deficiency in numbers of red blood cells.

erythrocytosis (i'rithrohsie'tohsis) erythrocythaemia.

erythroderma (i,rithrə'dərmə) abnormal redness of the skin, usually over a large area.

erythroedema polyneuropathy (i,rithri'deemə ,poli,nyooə'ropə-thee) a disease of infancy and early childhood. Marked by pain, swelling, and pink coloration of the fingers and toes, and by listlessness, irritability, failure to thrive, profuse perspiration, and sometimes scarlet coloration of the cheeks and tip of the nose. Called also acrodynia, pink disease.

erythromycin (i,rithroh'miesin) a broad-spectrum antibiotic produced by a strain of *Streptomyces erytreus*. It is effective against a wide variety of organisms, including Gram-negative and Gram-positive bacteria. It may be administered orally or parenterally.

erythropoiesis (i,rithrohpoy'eesis) the manufacture of red blood corpuscles.

erythropoietin (i,rithroh'poyitin, -poy'ee-) a hormone produced by the kidney that stimulates the production of red blood cells in the bone marrow.

erythropsia (,eri'thropsi·ə) a defect of vision in which all objects appear red. Often occurs after a cataract operation.

eschar ('eskar) a slough or scab which forms after the destruction of living tissue by gangrene, infection or burning.

Escherichia (,esh·ə'riki·ə) a genus of Enterobacteriaceae. *E. coli* an organism normally present in the intestines of man and other vertebrates. Although not generally pathogenic it may set up infections of the gallbladder, bile ducts and the urinary tract. It was formerly called *Bacillus coli.*

eserine ('esəreen, -in) physostigmine.

Esmarch's tourniquet ('ezmahks) *J.F.A. von Esmarch, German surgeon, 1823–1908.* A rubber bandage used in surgery to express blood from a limb and render it less vascular.

ESN educationally subnormal. Used in the context of children with learning difficulties.

esophoria (,eesoh'for·ri·ə) latent convergent strabismus. The eyes turn inwards only when one is covered up.

esotropia (,eesoh'trohpi·ə) convergent strabismus. One or other eye turns inwards, resulting in double vision.

ESR erythrocyte sedimentation rate.

ESRD end-stage renal disease. *See* RENAL.

essence ('esəns) 1. an indispensable part of anything. 2. a volatile

oil dissolved in alcohol.

essential (i'senshəl) indispensable. *E. amino acids* those amino acids which must be obtained in the diet and are necessary for the maintenance of tissue growth and repair. *See* AMINO ACID. *E. fatty acids* unsaturated fatty acids which are necessary for body growth.

ester ('estə) a compound formed by the combination of an acid and an alcohol with the elimination of water.

esterase ('estə,rayz) an enzyme that causes the hydrolysis of esters into acids and alcohol.

ethambutol (e'thambyuh,tol) a drug used in combination with other drugs in the treatment of tuberculosis.

ethanol ('ethə'nol, 'eethə-) alcohol.

ethanolamine (,ethə'nolə,meen) an intravenous sclerosing agent used to inject varicose veins.

ether ('eethə) a volatile inflammable liquid formerly used as a general anaesthetic agent.

ethics ('ethiks) a code of moral principles. *Nursing e.* the code governing a nurse's behaviour with patients and their relatives, and with colleagues. *See* Appendix 9.

ethmoid ('ethmoyd) a sieve-like bone, separating the cavity of the nose from the cranium. The olfactory nerves pass through its perforations.

ethmoidectomy (,ethmoy'dektəmee) surgical removal of a portion of the ethmoid bone.

ethnic ('ethnik) pertaining to a social group who share cultural bonds or physical (racial) characteristics. *E. minority* a social grouping of people who share cultural or racial factors but who constitute a minority within the greater culture or society.

ethnology (eth'nolǝjee) the science dealing with the races of man, their descent, relationship, etc.

ethoglucid (ˌethoh'gloosid) an antineoplastic agent which may be used to treat bladder cancers by intravesical instillations.

ethoheptazine (ˌethoh'heptǝzeen) an analgesic related to pethidine. It relieves pain and muscle spasm.

ethopropazine (ˌethoh'prohpǝzeen) an antispasmodic drug used in the treatment of parkinsonism.

ethosuximide (ˌethoh'suksiˌmied) an anticonvulsant used in the treatment of 'petit mal' epilepsy.

ethyl biscoumacetate (ˌethil,biskoomasitayt, ˌeethil-, -thiel-) an anticoagulant of the coumarin group.

ethyl chloride (ˌethil'klor·ried) a volatile liquid used as a local anaesthetic. When sprayed on intact skin it causes local insensitivity, through freezing.

ethylene oxide (ˌethileen oksied) a gas which is sporicidal and viricidal and capable of penetrating relatively inaccessible parts of an apparatus during sterilization. It is used for equipment which is too delicate to be sterilized by other methods.

ethylenediaminetetraacetic acid (ˌethileen,dieǝmeen,tetrǝ·ǝ'seetik) abbreviated EDTA. A chelating agent used in the treatment of

lead poisoning.

ethyloestrenol (ˌethil'eesterǝ,nol) an anabolic steroid that may be used to treat severe weight loss, debility and osteoporosis.

etiolation (ˌeeti·ǝ'layshǝn) paleness of the skin due to lack of exposure to sunlight.

etiology (ˌeeti'olǝjee) *see* AETIOLOGY.

eucalyptus oil (ˌyookǝ'liptǝs) an oil derived from the leaves of the eucalyptus tree; it has mild antiseptic properties and is used in the treatment of nasal catarrh.

eugenics (yoo'jeniks) the study of measures which may be taken to improve future generations both physically and mentally.

eugenol ('yooji,nol) a local anaesthetic and antiseptic, derived from oil of cloves and cinnamon, used in dentistry.

Eugynon (yoo'gienon) *E.30*, *E.50* proprietary preparations of contraceptive tablets containing oestrogen and progesterone.

Eumydrin ('yoomidrin, yoo'miedrin) trade name for atropine methonitrate, used in the treatment of pylorospasm.

eunuch ('yoonǝk) a castrated male.

euphoria (yoo'for·ri·ǝ) an exaggerated feeling of well-being often not justified by circumstances. Less than ELATION.

euplastic (yoo'plastik) capable of being transformed into healthy tissue. The term may be applied to a wound that is healing well.

eurhythmics (yoo'ridhmiks) gentle body exercises performed to music.

eusol ('yoosol) a chlorine antiseptic containing hypochlorous and boric acids. The name is derived from the initials of Edinburgh University Solution of Lime.

eustachian tube (yoo'stayshən) *B. Eustachio, Italian anatomist, 1520–1574.* The pharyngotympanic tube.

euthanasia (ˌyoothə'nayzi·ə, -zhə) 1. an easy or good death. 2. the deliberate ending of life of a person suffering from an incurable disease; this can be voluntary or involuntary.

euthyroid (yoo'thieroyd) normally functioning thyroid gland.

eutocia (yoo'tohsi·ə) easy, normal childbirth.

evacuant (i'vakyooənt) 1. promoting evacuation. 2. an agent that promotes evacuation.

evacuation (iˌvakyoo'ayshən) 1. an emptying or removal, especially the removal of any material from the body by discharge through a natural or artificial passage. 2. material discharged from the body, especially the discharge from the bowels.

evacuator (i'vakyooˌaytə) an instrument which produces evacuation, e.g. one designed to wash out small particles of stone from the bladder after lithotrity.

evaluation (iˌvalyoo'ayshən) a critical appraisal or assessment; a judgement of the value, worth, character or effectiveness of that which is being assessed. In the health care field, this includes assessment of the patient's position on the health/illness continuum, and evaluation of the effectiveness of patient care activities in bringing about a change in his position. Accepted as the fourth phase of the nursing process.

eventration (ˌeeven''trayshən) 1. the protrusion of the intestines through the abdominal wall. 2. removal of abdominal viscera.

eversion (i'vərshən) turning outwards. *E. of the eyelid* ectropion. The upper eyelid may be everted for examination of the eye or for the removal of a foreign body.

evisceration (iˌvisə'rayshən) removal of internal organs. *E. of eye* removal of the contents of the eyeball, but not the sclera.

evolution (ˌeevə'looshən) the development of living organisms which change their characteristics during succeeding generations.

evulsion (i'vulshən) extraction by force.

Ewing's tumour ('yooingz) *J. Ewing, American pathologist, 1866–1943.* A form of sarcoma usually affecting the shaft of a long bone in young adults.

exacerbation (ek'sasə'bayshən, igˌzasə-) an increase in the severity of the symptoms of a disease.

exanthem (eg'zanthəm, ek's-) an infectious disease characterized by a skin rash.

exanthematous (ˌegzan'themətəs, eks-) pertaining to any disease associated with a skin eruption.

excavation (ˌekskə'vayshən) scooping out. *Dental e.* the removal of decay from a tooth before inserting a filling.

excision (ek'sizhən) the cutting out of a part.

excitation (ˌeksie'tayshən) the act of stimulating.

excitement (ek'sietmənt) a physiological and emotional response to a stimulus.

excoriation (ek,skor·ri'ayshən) an abrasion of the skin.

excrement ('ekskrəmənt) faecal matter; waste matter from the body.

excrescence (ek'skresəns) abnormal outgrowth of tissue, e.g. a wart.

excreta (ek'skreetə) the natural discharges of the excretory system: faeces, urine and sweat.

excretion (ek'skreeshən) the discharge of waste from the body.

exenteration (eg,zentə'rayshən) evisceration; the removal of an organ. Usually performed only in cases of malignant neoplasm.

exercise ('eksə,siez) performance of physical exertion for improvement of health or correction of physical deformity. *Active e.* motion imparted to a part by voluntary contraction and relaxation of its controlling muscles. *Isometric e.* active exercise performed against stable resistance, without change in the length of the muscle. No movement occurs at any joints over which the muscle passes. *Passive e.* motion imparted to a segment of the body by another individual, machine, or other outside force, or produced by voluntary effort of another segment of the patient's own body. *Range of movement (ROM) e's* exercises that move each joint through its full range of movement, that is, to the highest degree of movement of which each joint is normally capable.

exfoliation (eks,fohli'ayshən) the splitting off from the surface of dead tissue in thin flaky layers.

exhalation (,eks·hə'layshən) 1. the giving off of a vapour. 2. the act of breathing out.

exhibitionism (,eksi'bishə,nizəm) 1. showing off; a desire to attract attention. 2. exposing the genitals to persons of the opposite sex in socially unacceptable circumstances.

exocrine ('eksoh'krin, -,krien) pertaining to those glands which discharge their secretion by means of a duct, e.g. salivary glands. *See* ENDOCRINE.

exogenous (ek'sojənəs) of external origin.

exomphalos (ek'somfələs) 1. hernia of the abdominal viscera into the umbilical cord. 2. congenital umbilical hernia.

exophoria (,eksoh'for·ri·ə) a tendency of the eyes to turn outwards.

exophthalmometer (,eksofthal'momitə) an instrument for measuring the extent of protrusion of the eyeball.

exophthalmos (,eksof'thalmos) abnormal protrusion of the eyeball which results in a marked stare. May be due to injury or disease and is often associated with thyrotoxicosis.

exostosis (,ekso'stohsis) a bony outgrowth from the surface of a bone.

exotoxin (,eksoh'toksin) a poison produced by a bacterial cell and released into the tissues surrounding it. *See* ENDOTOXIN.

exotropia (,eksoh'trohpi·ə) divergent strabismus; the eyes turn outwards.

expectorant (ek'spektə·rənt) a remedy which promotes and facilitates expectoration.

expectoration (ek,spektə'ray-shən) sputum; secretions coughed up from the air passages. Its characteristics are a valuable aid in diagnosis and note should be taken of the quantity ejected, its colour and the amount of effort required. Frothiness denotes that it comes from an air-containing cavity; fluidity indicates oedema of the lung.

expiration (,ekspi'rayshən) 1. the act of breathing out. 2. termination or death.

exploration (,eksplə'rayshən) the operation of surgically investigating any part of the body.

expression (ek'spreshən) 1. the aspect or appearance of the face as determined by the physical or emotional state. 2. the act of squeezing out or evacuating by pressure, e.g. the removal of breast milk by hand. 3. the manifestation of a heritable trait in an individual carrying the gene or genes which determine it.

exsanguination (ek,sang·gwi'nay-shən) extensive blood loss due to internal or external haemorrhage.

extension (ek'stenshən) 1. the straightening out of a flexed joint, such as the knee or elbow. 2. the application of traction to a fractured or dislocated limb by means of a weight.

extensor (ek'stensə, -sor) a muscle which extends or straightens a limb.

exterior (ek'stiə·ri·ə) on the outside.

exteriorize (ek'stiə·ri·ə,riez) 1. to bring an organ or part of one to the outside of the body by surgery. 2. in psychiatry, to turn one's interests outwards.

extirpation (,ekstər'payshən) complete removal of an organ or tissue.

extracapsular (,ekstrə'kapsyuhlə) outside the capsule. May refer to a fracture occurring at the end of the bone, but outside the joint capsule, or to cataract extraction.

extracellular (,ekstrə'selyuhlə) outside the cell. *E. fluid* tissue fluid that surrounds the cells.

extract ('ekstrakt) a concentrated preparation of a drug made by extracting its soluble principles by steeping in water or alcohol and then evaporating the fluid.

extraction (ek'strakshən) 1. the process or act of pulling or drawing out. 2. the preparation of an extract. *Breech e.* extraction of an infant from the uterus in cases of breech presentation. *Vacuum e.* removal of the uterine contents by application of a vacuum. An alternative to the forceps method of delivering a baby.

extradural (,ekstrə'dyooə·rəl) outside the dura mater. *E. haemorrhage.*

extragenital (,ekstrə'jenit'l) not related to the genitals. *E. chancre* the primary lesion of syphilis situated anywhere other than on the genital organs. *E. syphilis* syphilis spread from an extragenital lesion.

extrahepatic (,ekstrəhi'patik) outside the liver. Relating to a condition affecting the liver in which the cause is outside the liver.

extrapyramidal (,ekstrəpi'ramid'l)

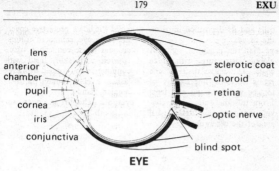

EYE

outside the pyramidal (cerebrospinal) tract. *E. system* the nerve tracts and pathways which are not within the pyramidal tracts.

extrasensory (,ekstrə'sensə-ree) outside or beyond any of the known senses. *E. perception* abbreviated ESP. Appreciation of the thoughts of others or of current or future events without any normal means of communication.

extrasystole (,ekstrə'sistəlee) premature contraction of the atria or ventricles. *See* SYSTOLE.

extrauterine (,ekstrə'yootə,rien) occurring outside the uterus. *E. pregnancy* ectopic gestation; development of a fetus outside the uterus.

extravasation (ik,stravə'sayshən) effusion or escape of fluid from its normal course into surrounding tissues. *E. of blood* a bruise.

extremity (ek'stremitee) distal part; a hand or foot.

extrinsic (ek'strinsik, -zik) originating externally. *E. factor* a

substance present in meat and other foodstuffs. Called also cyanocobalamin (vitamin B_{12}), it is necessary for the manufacture of red blood cells. The intrinsic factor produced in the stomach is necessary for the absorption of vitamin B_{12}. *E. muscle* a muscle originating away from the part which it controls, such as those controlling the movements of the eye.

extroversion (,ekstrə'vərshən) turning inside out, e.g. of the uterus, as sometimes occurs after labour.

extrovert ('ekstrə,vərt) a person who is sociable, a good mixer and interested in what goes on around him. A personality type first described by Jung. *See* INTROVERT.

extubation (,ekstyuh'bayshən) removal of a tube used in intubation.

exudation (,eksyuh'dayshən) the slow discharge of serous fluid through the walls of the blood cells and its deposition in or on the tissues.

eye (ie) the organ of sight. A globular structure with three coats. The nerve tissue of the retina receives impressions of images via the pupil and lens. From this the optic nerve conveys the impressions to the visual area of the cerebrum.

eyelid ('ie,lid) a protective covering of the eye, composed of muscle and dense connective tissue covered with skin, lined with conjunctiva and fringed with eyelashes. Eyelids contain the meibomian glands.

eyetooth (ie'tooth) an upper canine tooth.

F

F symbol for *Fahrenheit* and *fluorine*.

face (fays) the front of the head from the forehead to the chin. *F. presentation* the appearance of the face of the fetus first at the cervix during labour.

facet ('fasit) a small flat area on the surface of a bone. *F. syndrome* a slight dislocation of the small facet joints of the vertebrae giving rise to pain and muscle spasm.

facial ('fayshal) pertaining to the face or lower anterior portion of the head. *F. nerve* the seventh cranial nerve which supplies the salivary glands and superficial face muscles. A local anaesthetic may be injected into this nerve before an operation when a general anaesthetic is contraindicated. *F. paralysis see* PARALYSIS.

facies ('faysi,eez, 'fayshi-) facial expression; it often gives some indication of the patient's condition. *Adenoid f.* The open mouth and vacant expression associated with mouth breathing and nasal obstruction. *Parkinson f.* fixed expression, due to paucity of movement of facial muscles, characteristic of parkinsonism.

faecalith ('feekəlith) a hard stony mass of faecal material which may obstruct the lumen of the **appendix** and be a cause of inflammation. A coprolith.

faeces ('feeseez) waste matter excreted by the bowel, consisting of indigestible cellulose, food which has escaped digestion, bacteria (living and dead) and water.

Fahrenheit scale ('faran,hiet) *G. D. Fahrenheit, German physicist, 1686–1736.* A scale of heat measurement. It registers the freezing-point of water at 32°, the normal heat of the human body at 98.4°, and the boiling-point of water at 212°.

failure ('faylyə) inability to perform or to function properly. *Heart f.* inability of the heart to maintain a circulation sufficient to meet the body's needs. *Kidney f., renal f.* inability of the kidney to excrete metabolites at normal plasma levels under normal loading, or inability to retain electrolytes when intake is normal; in the acute form, marked by uraemia and usually by oliguria, with hyperkalaemia and pulmonary oedema. *Respiratory f., ventilatory f.* a life-threatening condition in which respiratory function is inadequate to maintain the body's needs for oxygen supply and carbon dioxide removal while at rest. *F. to thrive* retardation of normal growth and development in an infant. Causes are numerous but malnutrition or difficulty in absorbing essential nutrients are main factors, as well as those which are psychosocial in origin, e.g. maternal deprivation syndrome.

fainting ('faynting) *see* SYNCOPE.

falciform ('falsi,fawm) sickle-shaped. *F. ligament* a fold of peritoneum which separates the two main lobes of the liver, and connects it with the anterior abdominal wall and the diaphragm.

fallopian tube (fa'lohpi·ən) *G. Fallopius, Italian anatomist, 1523–1563.* Uterine tube. One of a pair of tubes about 10–14 cm long, arising out of the upper part of the uterus. The distal end of each tube is fimbriated and lies near an ovary. Their function is to conduct the ova from the ovaries to the interior of the uterus. An oviduct.

Fallot's tetralogy ('fahohz te-'tralǝjee) *E. L. A. Fallot, French physician, 1850–1911.* A congenital heart disease with four characteristic defects: (1) pulmonary artery stenosis, (2) interventricular defect of the septum, (3) overriding of the aorta, i.e. opening into both right and left ventricles, (4) hypertrophy of the right ventricle.

falx (falks) a sickle-shaped structure. *F. cerebri* the fold of dura mater which separates the two cerebral hemispheres.

familial (fǝ'mili·ǝl) occurring in or affecting members of a family more than would be expected by chance.

family ('familee) 1. a group of people related by blood or marriage, especially a husband, wife, and their children. 2. a taxonomic category below an order and above a genus. *Blended f.* a family unit composed of a married couple and their offspring including some from previous marriages. *Extended f.* a nuclear family and their close relatives, such as the children's grandparents, aunts and uncles. *Extended nuclear f.* a nuclear family who nevertheless make frequent social contacts with the extended family group despite geographical distance. *Nuclear f.* a couple and their children by birth or adoption, who are living together and are more or less isolated from their extended family. *F. planning* the arrangement, spacing and limitation of the children in a family, depending upon the wishes and social circumstances of the parents. *Single-parent f.* a lone parent and offspring living together as a family unit.

Fanconi's syndrome (fan'kohneez) *G. Fanconi, Swiss paediatrician, b. 1892.* A rare inherited disorder of metabolism in which reabsorption of phosphate, amino acids and sugar by the renal tubules is impaired. The kidneys fail to produce acid urine, and resulting features are thirst, polyuria and rickets, leading to chronic renal failure.

fang (fang) the root of a tooth.

fantasy ('fantǝsee) an imagined sequence of events or mental images that serves to satisfy unconscious wishes or to express unconscious conflicts.

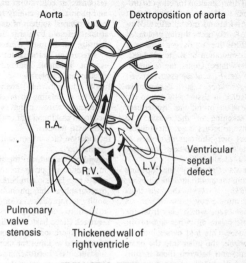

Aorta

Dextroposition of aorta

R.A.

Ventricular
septal
defect

R.V.

L.V.

Pulmonary
valve
stenosis

Thickened wall of
right ventricle

FALLOT'S TETRALOGY

farinaceous (,fari'nayshəs) starchy or containing starch. Refers to foods such as wheat, oats, barley and rice.

farmer's lung (,fahməz) a disease occurring in those in contact with mouldy hay. It is thought to be due to a hypersensitivity, with widespread reaction in the lung tissue. It causes excessive breathlessness.

FAS fetal alcohol syndrome.

fascia ('fashi-ə) a sheath of connective tissue enclosing muscles or other organs.

fasciculation (fə,sikyuh'layshən)
isolated fine muscle twitching which gives a flickering appearance.

fasciculus (fə'sikyuhləs) a small bundle of nerve or muscle fibres; a fascicle.

fastigium (fas'tiji·əm) the stage of a fever when the temperature is at its height.

fat (fat) 1. the adipose or fatty tissue of the body. 2. neutral fat; a triglyceride which is an ester of fatty acids and glycerol. *Woolf.* lanolin *see also* BROWN FAT.

fatigue (fə'teeg) a state of weariness which may range from mental disinclination for effort to profound exhaustion following great physical and mental effort. *Muscle f.* may occur during prolonged effort due to oxygen lack and accumulation of waste products.

fatty ('fatee) containing or similar to fat. *F. acid see* ESSENTIAL. *F. degeneration* a degenerative change in tissue cells due to the invasion of fat and consequent weakening of the organ. The change occurs as a result of incorrect diet, shortage of oxygen in the tissues or excessive consumption of alcohol.

fauces ('fawseez) the opening from the mouth into the pharynx. *Pillars of the f.* the two folds of muscle covered with mucous membrane which pass from the soft palate on either side of the fauces. One fold passes into the tongue, the other into the pharynx, and between them is situated the tonsil.

favism ('fayvizəm) an acute haemolytic anaemia caused by ingestion of fava beans or inhalation of the pollen of the plant, usually occurring in certain individuals as a result of a genetic abnormality with a deficiency in an enzyme, glucose-6-phosphate dehydrogenáse, in the erythrocytes. Called also fabism.

favus ('fayvəs) a type of ringworm infection rare in the UK, with formation of scabs, in appearance like a honeycomb. It usually affects the scalp and is due to a fungus infection (*Trichophyton schoenleini*).

Fe symbol for *iron* (L. *ferrum*).

fear (fiə) a normal emotional response, in contrast to anxiety and phobia, to consciously recognized external sources of danger; it is manifested by alarm, apprehension, or disquiet. *Obsessional f.* a recurring irrational fear that is not amenable to ordinary reassurance; a phobia.

febrile ('feebiel, 'feb-) characterized by or relating to fever. *F. convulsion* a convulsion which occurs in childhood and is associated with pyrexia.

fecundation (,fekan'dayshən, fee-) fertilization.

fecundity (fi'kunditee) the ability to produce offspring frequently and in large numbers. In demography, the physiological ability to reproduce, as opposed to fertility.

feedback ('feed,bak) a method of control where some of the output is returned as input for monitoring purposes. Feedback mechanisms are important in the regulation of such physiological processes as hormone and enzyme reactions. *Negative f.* a rise in the output of a substance is detected and further output is thus inhibited. *Positive f.* a rise in output causes either a direct or indirect rise in the output of another substance.

felon ('felon) an abscess of the distal phalanx of a finger; a whitlow.

Felty's syndrome ('feltiz) *A. R. Felty, American physician, b. 1895.* The triad of rheumatoid arthritis, splenomegaly and leukopenia. Often associated with anaemia, lymphadenopathy and vasculitic cutaneous ulceration.

feminization ('feminie'zayshən) 1. the normal induction or development of female sexual characteristics. 2. the induction or development of female secondary sexual characteristics in the male. *Testicular f.* a condition in which the subject is phenotypically female, but lacks nuclear sex chromatin and is of XY chromosomal sex.

femoral ('femə·rəl) pertaining to the femur. *F. artery* that of the thigh from groin to knee. *F. canal* the opening below the inguinal ligament through which the femoral artery passes from the abdomen to the thigh.

femur ('feemə) the thigh bone.

fenbufen (fen'byoofen) a non-steroidal anti-inflammatory drug (NSAID) which acts as a pro-drug. It is associated with a lower incidence of gastrointestinal haemorrhage but a higher incidence of skin rashes than other NSAIDs.

fenestra (fə'nestrə) a window-like opening. *F. ovalis* the oval opening between the middle and the internal ear.

fenestration (,feni'strayshən) an operation in which an opening is made in the bony labyrinth of the ear to assist hearing when deafness is due to otosclerosis. Now superseded by less drastic and more reliable operations.

fenfluramine (fen'flooˈrə,meen) an amphetamine-like drug used to suppress appetite in the treatment of obesity.

fenoprofen (,feenoh'prohfən) an anti-inflammatory drug used in the treatment of arthritic conditions.

fentanyl ('fentə,nil) a short-acting narcotic analgesic, widely used during anaesthesia, especially for children and the elderly.

ferritin ('feritin) a complex formed of an iron and protein molecule, one of the forms in which iron is stored in the body.

ferrous ('ferəs) containing iron. *F. fumarate, f. gluconate, f. succinate* and *f. sulphate* are iron salts which are given orally to treat iron-deficiency anaemia.

ferrule ('ferool,-rəl) a rubber cap used on the end of walking sticks, frames and crutches to prevent slipping.

fertilization (,fərtilie'zayshən) the impregnation of the female sex cell, the ovum, by a male sex cell, a spermatozoon. *In vitro f.* artificial fertilization of the ovum in laboratory conditions. The timing and conditions for implantation into a uterus have to be perfect if successful pregnancy is to ensue.

fester ('festə) to become superficially inflamed and to suppurate.

festination (,festi'nayshən) an involuntary tendency to take short accelerating steps in walking; seen in conditions such as Parkinson's disease.

fetal ('feet'l) pertaining to the fetus. *F. alcohol syndrome* abbreviated FAS. Physical and mental abnormalities due to maternal alcohol intake during pregnancy. Abnormalities may include microcephaly, growth deficiencies, mental handicap, hyperactivity, heart murmurs and skeletal malformation. The exact amount of alcohol consumption that will produce fetal damage is unknown, but the periods of gestation during which the alcohol is most likely to result in fetal damage are 3–4.5 months after conception and during the last trimester. *F. assessment* determination of the well-being of the fetus. Assessment techniques and procedures include: (1) medical and family histories and physical examination of the mother, (2) ULTRASONOGRAPHY, (3) assessment of fetal activity using the Cardiff kick chart, (4) chemical assessment of placental function, (5) assays of amniotic fluid obtained by AMNIOCENTESIS, and (6) electronic and ultrasonic fetal heart rate monitoring.

fetishism ('feti,shizm) a state in which an object is regarded with an irrational fear, or an erotic attraction which may be so strong that the object is necessary for achieving sexual excitement.

fetor ('feetə, -tor) an offensive smell.

fetoscope ('feetə,skohp) an endoscope for viewing the fetus in utero.

fetus ('feetəs) the developing baby between the 8th week and the end of pregnancy.

fever ('feevə) 1. an abnormally high body temperature; pyrexia. 2. any disease characterized by marked increase of body temperature.

fibre ('fiebə) a thread-like structure.

fibreoptics (,fiebə'roptiks) the transmission of light rays along flexible tubes by means of very fine glass or plastic fibres. Use is made of this in endoscopic instruments such as the gastroscope.

fibrescope ('fiebə,skohp) an endoscope in which fibreoptics are used.

fibrillation (,fibri'layshən, ,fie-) a quivering, vibratory movement of muscle fibres. *Atrial f.* rapid contractions of the atrium causing irregular contraction of the ventricles in both rhythm and force. *Venticular f.* fine rapid twitchings of the venticles leading to circulatory arrest. Rapidly fatal unless it can be controlled.

fibrin ('fiebrin) an insoluble protein that is essential to CLOTTING of blood, formed from fibrinogen by action of thrombin.

fibrinogen (fie'brinəjən) a soluble protein which is present in blood plasma and is converted into fibrin by the action of thrombin when the blood clots.

fibrinolysin (,fiebri'nolisin) a proteolytic enzyme that dissolves fibrin.

fibrinolysis (,fiebri'nolisis) the dissolution of fibrin by the action of fibrinolysin. The process by which clots are removed from the circulation after healing has taken place.

fibrinopenia (,fiebrinoh'peeni-ə) a deficiency of fibrinogen in the blood. There is a tendency to bleed as the coagulation time is increased.

fibroadenoma (,fiebroh,adə'nohmə) a benign tumour of glandular and fibrous tissue. *See* ADENOMA.

fibroangioma (,fiebroh,anji'ohmə)

a benign tumour containing both fibrous and vascular tissue.

fibroblast ('fiebroh,blast) a connective tissue cell.

fibrocartilage (,fiebroh'kahtilij) cartilage with fibrous tissue in it.

fibrochondritis (,fiebrohkon-'drietis) inflammation of fibrocartilage.

fibrocyst ('fiebroh,sist) a fibroma that has undergone cystic degeneration.

fibrocystic (,fiebroh'sistik) fibrous and cystic. *F. disease of the pancreas* an inherited disease affecting the mucus-secreting glands, the sweat glands and the pancreas. It is characterized by fatty stools and repeated lung infections. Mucoviscidosis; cystic fibrosis.

fibroid ('fiebroyd) 1. having a fibrous structure. 2. a fibroma or a fibromyoma, usually one occurring in the uterus.

fibroma (fie'brohmə) a benign tumour of connective tissue. *Cystic f.* fibrocyst.

fibromyoma (,fiebrohmie'ohmə) a tumour consisting of fibrous and muscle tissue; frequently found in or on the uterus.

fibroplasia (,fiebroh'playzi·ə) the formation of fibrous tissue when a wound heals. *Retrolental f.* a condition characterized by the presence of fibrous tissue behind the lens, leading to detachment of the retina and blindness, attributed to use of excessively high concentrations of oxygen in the care of preterm infants.

fibrosarcoma (,fiebrohsah'kohmə) a malignant tumour arising in fibrous tissue.

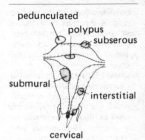

FIBROMYOMATA OF UTERUS

fibrosis (fie'brohsis) fibrous tissue formation such as occurs in scar tissue or as the result of inflammation. It is the cause of adhesions of the peritoneum or other serous membranes. *F. of lung* condition that may precede bronchiectasis and emphysema.

fibrositis (,fiebrə'sietis) inflammation of fibrous tissue. The term is loosely applied to pain and stiffness, particularly of the back muscles, for which no other cause can be found.

fibula ('fibyuhlə) the slender bone from knee to ankle, on the outer side of the leg.

field of vision (,feeld əv 'vizhən) the area within view, as for the fixed eye, a camera or in an operation. *Visual f.* the area within which stimuli will produce the sensation of sight with the eye in a straight-ahead position.

filament ('filəmənt) a small thread-like structure.

Filaria (fi'lair·ri·ə) a genus of

nematode worms which may be found in the connective tissues and lymphatics, having been transmitted to man by mosquitoes. Found mainly in the tropics and subtropics.

filariasis (ˌfiləˈrieəsis) an infection by filaria, particularly by *Wuchereria bancrofti*, resulting in blockage of the lymphatics, which causes swelling of the surrounding tissues. Elephantiasis may occur.

filiform (ˈfili,fawm, fie-) threadlike. *F. papillae* the fine threadlike processes that cover the anterior two-thirds of the tongue.

filopressure (ˈfieloh,preshə) compression of a blood vessel by a thread.

filter (ˈfiltə) a device for eliminating certain elements, as (1) particles of certain size from a solution, or (2) rays of certain wavelength from a stream of radiant energy. *Millipore f.* trade name for a device used to filter nutrient solutions as they are administered intravenously.

filtrate (ˈfiltrayt) the fluid which passes through a filter.

filtration (filˈtrayshən) 1. the removal of precipitate from a liquid by means of a filter. 2. the removal of rays of a certain wavelength from an electromagnetic beam. *F. angle* the angle of the anterior chamber of the eye through which the aqueous humour drains; blockage of this channel gives rise to glaucoma.

fimbria (ˈfimbri·ə) a fringe. *F. of the uterine tube* the thread-like projections that surround the pelvic opening of the uterine tube.

finger (ˈfing·gə) a digit of the hand. *Clubbed f.* one with enlargement of the terminal phalanx with constant osseous changes; occurs in many heart and lung diseases. *Hammer f., mallet f.* permanent flexion of the distal phalanx of a finger due to avulsion of the extensor tendon. *Trigger f.* temporary flexion of a finger which is overcome in a sudden jerk by active or passive extension of the finger. It is caused by thickening of the flexor tendon in a narrowed tendon sheath. *Webbed f's* fingers more or less united by strands of tissue; syndactyly.

first aid (fərst ayd) emergency care and treatment of an injured person before complete medical and surgical treatment can be secured.

firm (fərm) a medical or surgical hospital team usually comprising 2 house officers, a senior house officer (SHO), a registrar, and a senior registrar, directed by a consultant physician or surgeon.

fission (ˈfishən) a form of asexual reproduction by dividing into two equal parts, as in bacteria. *Binary f.* the splitting in two of the nucleus and the protoplasm of a cell, as in protozoa. *Nuclear f.* the splitting of the nucleus of an atom with the release of a great quantity of energy.

fissure (ˈfishə) a narrow slit or cleft. *Anal f.* a painful crack in the mucous membrane of the anus. *F. of Rolando* a furrow in the cortex of each cerebral hemisphere dividing the sensory from the motor area; the central sulcus.

fistula ('fistyuhlə) an abnormal passage between two epithelial surfaces usually connecting the cavity of one organ with another or a cavity with the surface of the body. *Anal f.* the result of an ischiorectal abscess where the channel is from the anus to the skin. *Biliary f.* a leakage of bile to the exterior, following operation on the gallbladder or ducts. *Blind f.* one which is open at only one end. *Faecal f.* one in which the channel is from the intestine through the wound caused by an operation on the intestines when sepsis is present. *Rectovaginal f.* fistula from the rectum to the vagina which may result from severe perineal tear following childbirth. *Tracheo-oesophageal f.* an opening from the trachea into the oesophagus; a congenital deformity. *Vesicovaginal f.* an opening from the bladder to the vagina, either from error during operation, or from ulceration as may occur in carcinoma of the cervix.

fit (fit) a commonly used term for paroxysmal motor discharges leading to sudden convulsive movements, as in epilepsy, eclampsia and hysteria. The term is sometimes applied to apoplexy.

fixation (fik'sayshən) 1. the process of rendering something immovable, such as a joint or a fractured bone. 2. in psychology, a term used to describe a failure to progress wholly or in part through the normal stages of psychological development to a fully developed personality. 3.

in ophthalmology, directing the sight straight at an object.

flaccid ('flaksid,'flasid) soft, flabby. *F. paralysis see* PARALYSIS.

flagellum (flə'jelom) the whip-like protoplasmic filament by which some bacteria and protozoa move.

Flagyl ('flagil) trade name for a preparation of metronidazole, an antibacterial and antiprotozoal.

flail (flayl) exhibiting abnormal or pathological mobility, as flail chest or flail joint. *F. chest* a loss of stability of the chest wall due to multiple rib fractures or detachment of the sternum from the ribs as a result of a severe crushing chest injury. The loose chest segment moves in a direction which is the reverse of normal. *F. joint* an unusually movable joint.

flap (flap) a mass of tissue used for grafting in plastic surgery, which is left attached to its blood supply and used to repair defects either adjacent to it or at some distance from it.

flare (flair) the response of the skin to an allergic or hypersensitivity reaction. Reddening of the skin that spreads outwards.

flatfoot ('flat,fuht) a condition due to absence or sinking of the medial longitudinal arch of the foot, caused by weakening of the ligaments and tendons. Pes planus.

flatulence ('flatyuhləns) excessive formation of gases in the stomach or intestine.

flatulent ('flatyuhlənt) suffering from flatulence. *F. distension* swelling due to gas in the stomach or intestines. It is a common complication after abdominal operations and is caused by intestinal stasis.

flatus ('flaytəs) gas in the stomach or intestine.

flea (flee) a small, wingless, blood-sucking insect parasite. The common human flea, *Pulex irritans*, rarely transmits disease. Cat and dog fleas, *Ctenocephalides*, are also relatively harmless. The rat fleas *Xenopsylla* and *Nosopsyllus* are the vectors of bubonic plague.

flexibilitas cerea (,fleksi,bilitəs 'seeə·ri·ə) waxy flexibility; a cataleptic state in which the limbs retain any position in which they are placed. A symptom of some forms of schizophrenia; also occurs occasionally in hysteria.

flexion ('flekshən) bending; moving a joint so that the two or more bones forming it draw towards each other. *Dorsi-f.* bending the fingers or toes backwards. *Plantar f.* bending the fingers or toes downwards.

Flexner's bacillus ('fleksnəz) S. Flexner, American bacteriologist, 1863–1946. One of the group of pathogenic bacteria which cause bacillary dysentery; *Shigella flexneri*.

flexor ('fleksə) any muscle causing flexion of a limb or other part of the body.

flexure ('flekshə) a bend or curve.

flight of ideas (fliet ov iediəz) the rapid movement of ideas and speech from one fragmentary topic to another that occurs in mania.

floaters ('flohtəz) wisps or strands within the eye that are visible to the patient. Usually caused by detachment and collapse of the vitreous humour and the normal ageing process.

floccillation (,floksi'layshən) involuntary picking at the bedclothes, a phenomenon often seen in delirious patients.

flocculent ('flokyuhlənt) woolly or flaky. Human milk forms a flocculent curd.

flooding ('fluding) 1. excessive loss of blood from the uterus. 2. a form of desensitization for the treatment of phobias and related disorders. The patient is repeatedly exposed, in imagination or real life, to emotionally distressing aversive stimuli of high intensity. Called also implosion.

florid ('flo·rid) a flushed facial appearance.

flowmeter ('floh,meetə) an instrument used to measure the flow of liquids or gases.

flucloxacillin (,flookloksə'silin) an antibiotic drug used in the treatment of infection by penicillin-resistant bacteria.

fluctuation (,fluktyoo'ayshən, -chyoo-) a wave-like motion felt on palpation of the abdomen.

fludrocortisone (,floodroh'kawti,sohn, -,zohn) a synthetic corticosteroid used in the treatment of adrenal disorders.

fluid ('flooid) 1. a liquid or gas; any liquid of the body. 2. composed of molecules which freely change their relative positions without separation of the mass. *Amniotic f.* the fluid within the amnion that bathes the developing fetus and protects it from mechanical injury. *Body f's* the

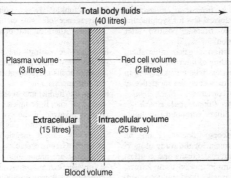

Diagrammatic representation of the body fluids, showing the extracellular fluid volume, intracellular fluid volume, blood volume and total body fluids.

TOTAL BODY FLUIDS

fluids within the body, composed of water, electrolytes, and non-electrolytes. The volume and distribution of body fluids vary with age, sex and amount of adipose tissue. *Cerebrospinal f.* the fluid contained within the ventricles of the brain, the subarachnoid space and the central canal of the spinal cord. *Interstitial f.* the extracellular fluid bathing most tissues, excluding the fluid within the lymph and blood vessels.

fluid balance a state in which the volume of body water and its solutes (electrolytes and non-electrolytes) is within normal limits and there is normal distribution of fluids within the intracellular and extracellular compartments. The total volume of

body fluids should be about 60 per cent of the body weight.

fluke (flook) one of a group of parasitic flatworms (Trematoda). Different varieties may affect the blood, the intestines, the liver or the lungs.

fluorescein (ˌflooə'resee·in) a dye used to detect corneal ulceration. When it is dropped on the eye the ulcer stains green.

fluorescence (ˌflooə'res'ns) the property of reflecting back light waves, usually of a lower frequency than that absorbed so that invisible light (e.g. ultraviolet) may become visible.

fluorescent (ˌflooə'res'nt) capable of producing fluorescence. *F. screen* a screen which becomes fluorescent when exposed to X-rays. *F. treponemal antibody test* a serological test for syphilis; the first to become positive after infection.

fluoridation (ˌflooə-riˈdayshən) the adding of fluorine to water in those areas where it is lacking in order to reduce the incidence of dental caries.

fluorine (ˈflooə-reen) *symbol* F. Any binary compound of fluorine.

fluoroscope (ˌflooə-rəˌskohp) an instrument for the study of moving internal organs and contrast medium in motion using X-rays.

fluorouracil (ˌflooə-rohˈyooə-rəsil) an antimetabolite cytotoxic drug used particularly in the treatment of solid tumours.

flupenthixol (ˌfloopenˈthiksol) a thioxanthene used in the treatment of schizophrenia.

fluphenazine (flooˈfenəˌzeen) a major tranquilliser.

flurandrenolone (ˌflooə-ranˈdrenəlohn) a topical steroid used for eczema and other inflammatory skin conditions which have not responded to weaker steroids.

flurazepam (ˌflooəˈrazipam) a hypnotic, used as the hydrochloride salt.

flurbiprofen (ˌfləˈbiˈprohfen) a non-steroidal anti-inflammatory drug.

flush (flush) a redness of the face and neck. *Hectic f.* one occurring in conditions such as septic poisoning and pulmonary tuberculosis. *Hot f.* one occurring during the menopause accompanied by a feeling of heat.

flutter (ˈflutə) an irregularity of the heartbeat.

focus (ˈfohkəs) 1. the point of convergence of light or sound waves. 2. the local seat of a disease.

focusing (ˈfohkəsing) the ability of the eye to alter its lens power so as to focus correctly at different distances.

folic acid (ˈfohlik) one of the VITAMINS of the B complex. Folic acid is involved in the synthesis of amino acids and DNA; its deficiency causes megaloblastic anaemia. Green vegetables, liver, and yeast are major sources. *F. a. antagonist.* any antimetabolite cytotoxic drug which inhibits the action of the folic acid enzyme.

folie à deux (foˈlee) [Fr.] the occurrence of identical psychoses simultaneously in two closely associated persons.

follicle (ˈfolikˈl) a very small sac or gland. *Graafian f.* a vesicular ovarian follicle. *See* GRAAFIAN FOLLICLE. *Hair f.* The sheath in which a hair grows. *F.-stimulating hormone* abbreviated FSH. A hormone produced by the anterior pituitary gland which controls the maturation of the graafian follicles in the ovary.

follicular (foˈlikyuhlə) pertaining to a follicle. *F. conjunctivitis* inflammation occurring in the lower conjunctival fornix. *F. tonsillitis* tonsillitis arising from infection of the tonsillar follicles.

folliculosis (foˌlikyuhˈlohsis) an abnormal increase in the number of lymph follicles. *Conjunctival f.* a benign non-inflammatory overgrowth of follicles of the conjunctiva of the eyelids.

fomentation (ˌfohmenˈtayshən)

treatment by warm, moist applications; also, the substance thus applied.

fomes ('fohmeez) *see* FOMITES.

fomites (fə'mieteez, 'fohmə-) [L.] *sing.* fomes; inanimate objects or material on which disease-producing agents may be conveyed.

fontanelle (,fontə'nel) a soft membranous space between the cranial bones of an infant. *Anterior f.* that between the parietal and frontal bones, which closes at about the age of 18 months. Rickets causes delay in this process. *Posterior f.* the junction of the occipital and parietal bones, at the sagittal suture, which closes within 3 months of birth.

food (food) anything which when taken into the body, serves to nourish or build up the tissues or to supply body heat. *F. poisoning* a group of notifiable acute illnesses due to ingestion of contaminated food. It may result from toxaemia from foods, such as those inherently poisonous or those contaminated by poisons; foods containing poisons formed by bacteria, or foodborne infections. Food poisoning usually causes inflammation of the gastrointestinal tract (gastroenteritis). This may occur quite suddenly, soon after the food has been eaten. The symptoms are acute, and include tenderness, pain or cramps in the abdomen, nausea, vomiting, diarrhoea, weakness and dizziness. *See* BOTULISM.

foot (fuht) the terminal part of the lower limb. *Athlete's f.* ringworm of the foot; tinea pedis. *F.*

THE FONTANELLES

drop inability to keep the foot at the correct angle owing to paralysis of the flexors of the ankle. *F. presentation* the presentation of one or both legs instead of the head during labour. *Madura f.* mycetoma of the foot; maduromycosis. *Trench f.* a condition similar to frostbite, due to prolonged standing in cold water.

foramen (fo'raymən) an opening or hole, especially in a bone. *F.*

magnum the hole in the occipital bone through which the spinal cord passes. *F. ovale* the hole between the left and right atria in the fetus. *Obturator f.* the large hole in the innominate bone. *Optic f.* the opening in the posterior part of the orbit through which the optic nerve and the ophthalmic artery pass.

forceps ('forseps) surgical instruments used for lifting or compressing an object. *Artery f. (Spencer Wells f.)* compress bleeding points during an operation. *Cheatle's f.* long forceps for lifting utensils. *Obstetric f.* of various patterns are used in difficult labour to facilitate delivery. *Vulsellum f.* have claw-like ends for exerting traction.

forensic (fə'renzik, -sik) pertaining to or applied in legal proceedings. *F. medicine* the branch that is concerned with the law and has a bearing on legal problems. It includes the investigation of unexplained death or injury.

foreskin ('for,skin) the prepuce.

formaldehyde (faw'maldi,hied) a gaseous compound with strongly disinfectant properties. It is used in solution (formol) for disinfection of excreta and utensils and also in the preparation of toxoids from toxins.

formication (,fawmi'kayshən) a sensation as of insects creeping over the body.

formula ('fawmyuhlə) [L] 1. an expression, using numbers or symbols, of the composition of, or of directions for preparing, a compound, such as a medicine, or of a procedure to follow to obtain a desired result, or of a single concept. 2. a mixture for feeding an infant, composed of milk and/or other ingredients.

formulary ('fawmyuhlə·ree) a prescriber's handbook of drugs. *See* BRITISH NATIONAL FORMULARY.

fornix ('forniks) an arch. *F. cerebri* an arched structure at the back and base of the brain. *Conjunctival f.* the reflection of the conjunctiva from the eyelids on to the eyeball. *F. of the vagina* the recesses at the top of the vagina in front (*anterior f.*), back (*posterior f.*) and sides (*lateral f.*) of the cervix uteri.

fossa ('fosə) a small depression or pit. Usually applied to fossae in bones. *Cubital f.* the triangular depression at the front of the elbow. *Iliac f.* the depression on the inner surface of the iliac bone. *Pituitary f.* the depression in the sphenoid bone. *See* SELLA TURCICA.

foster children children under the care of foster parents.

foster parents persons who undertake for reward the care of children who are not related to them within the meaning of the Children Act (1975).

Fothergill's operation ('fodha-,gilz) *W. E. Fothergill, British gynaecologist, 1865–1926.* Amputation of the cervix, with anterior and posterior colporrhaphy for prolapse of the uterus.

fourchette (fooə'shet) [Fr.] the fold of membrane at the perineal end of the vulva.

fovea ('fohvi·ə) a fossa; a small depression, particularly that of the retina which contains a large

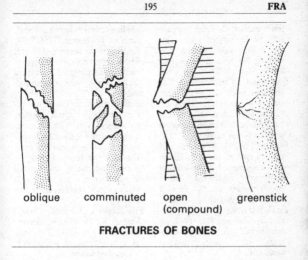

oblique   comminuted   open   greenstick
                           (compound)

FRACTURES OF BONES

number of cones, giving form and colour, and is therefore the area of most accurate vision.

fracture ('frakchə) 1. to break a part, especially a bone. 2. a break in the continuity of bone. The signs and symptoms are: pain, swelling, deformity, shortening of the limb, loss of power, abnormal mobility, and crepitus. Fractures are generally caused by trauma, either by a direct or an indirect force on the bone. Fractures may also be caused by muscle spasm or by disease that results in decalcification of the bone. The different types and classification of fractures are shown in the illustrations. *Pathological f.* one due to weakening of the bone structure by pathological processes, such as neo-

plasia, osteomalacia or osteomyelitis. *Pott's f.* a fracture dislocation of the ankle involving the lower end of the fibula and sometimes the internal malleolus of the tibia. *Spontaneous f.* one that occurs as a result of little or no violence, usually of a bone weakened by disease.

framboesia (fram'beezi·ə) yaws.

frame (fraym) a rigid supporting structure or a structure for immobilizing a part. *Balkan f.* see BALKAN FRAME. *Braun f.* a metal frame used to elevate the lower limb in fractures of the tibia and fibula. *Quadriplegic standing f.* a device for supporting in the upright position a patient whose four limbs are paralysed. *Stryker f.* one consisting of convas stretched on anterior and posterior frames, on which the patient can be rotated around his longitudinal axis. *Walking f.* a walking aid with three or four legs.

framycetin (,frami'seetin) an aminoglycoside antibiotic, very similar to neomycin. Used for topical application or to reduce bacterial population of the colon prior to bowel surgery.

freckle ('frek'l) a brown pigmented spot on the skin. *Hutchinson's melanotic f.* a non-invasive malignant melanoma which occurs mainly on the face of middle-aged women.

Frei's test (friez) *W. S. Frei, German dermatologist, 1885–1943.* An intradermal test to aid the diagnosis of lymphogranuloma venereum.

Freiberg's disease (friebərgz) *A. H. Freiberg, American surgeon, 1868–1940.* Osteochondritis of the second metatarsal bone, in which there is pain on walking and standing.

fremitus ('fremitəs) a thrill or vibration, e.g. that produced in the chest by speaking and felt on palpation.

Frenkel's exercises ('frenkəlz) *H. S. Frenkel, German neurologist, 1860–1931.* Exercises used in the treatment of tabes dorsalis to teach muscle and joint sense.

frenotomy (fri'notəmee) the cutting of the frenulum of the tongue to cure tongue-tie.

frenulum ('frenyuhləm) frenum; a fold of mucous membrane which limits the movement of an organ. *F. of the tongue* the fold under the tongue.

freudian ('froydi·ən) *S. Freud, Austrian psychiatrist, 1856–1939.* Relating to the theories of Freud, who was the originator of psychoanalysis and the psychoanalytical theory of the cause of neurosis.

friable ('frieəb'l) easily crumbled.

friction ('frikshən) the act of rubbing one object aginst another. *F. massage* a circular or transverse pressure applied by fingertip or thumb to a localized area. Used for the relief of pain. *F. murmur* the grating sound heard in auscultation when two rough surfaces rub together, as in dry pleurisy.

Friedländer's bacillus ('freedlendəz) *K. Friedländer, German pathologist, 1847–1887.* The cause of a rare form of pneumonia. *Klebsiella friedländeri.*

Friedreich's ataxia or **disease** ('freedrieks) *N. Friedriech, German physician, 1825–1882.* A rare form of hereditary ataxia.

frigidity (fri'jiditee) an absence of normal sexual desire, especially in women.

Frölich's syndrome ('frərliks) *A. Frölich, Austrian neurologist, 1871–1953.* A group of symptoms associated with disease of the pituitary body. These are: increased adiposity, atrophy of the genital organs, and development of feminine characteristics.

frontal ('frunt'l) 1. relating to the forehead. 2. relating to the front or anterior aspect of a structure.

frostbite ('frost,biet) impairment of circulation, chiefly affecting the fingers, the toes, the nose and the ears, due to exposure to severe cold. The first stage is represented by chilblains. Advanced cases show thrombosis and dry gangrene.

frottage (fro'tahzh) [Fr.] 1. a rubbing movement in massage. 2. sexual gratification by rubbing against another person's body.

frozen shoulder ('frohzən) a stiff and painful shoulder; capsulitis. Treatment is by stretching under anaesthesia combined with exercises. The cause is unknown.

fructose ('fruktohs, -tohz, 'fruhk-) Fruit sugar, a monosaccharide.

frusemide ('froozəmied) a diuretic with a rapid and powerful action used in the treatment of oedema and of acute renal failure.

FSH follicle-stimulating hormone.

fugue (fyoog) a period of altered awareness during which a person may wander for hours or days and perform purposive actions though his memory for the period may be lost. It may follow an epileptic fit or occur in hysteria or schizophrenia.

fulguration (,fulgyuh'rayshən) the destruction by diathermy of papillomata (warts), particularly inside the urinary bladder.

fulminating ('fuhlmi,nayting, 'ful-) sudden in onset and rapid in course.

fumigation (,fyoomi'gayshən) disinfection by exposure to the fumes of a vaporized germicide.

fundus ('fundəs) the base of an organ or the part farthest removed from the opening. *F. of the eye* the posterior part of the inside of the eye as shown by the ophthalmoscope. *F. of the stomach* that part above the cardiac orifice. *F. of the uterus* the top of the uterus; that part farthest from the cervix.

fungate ('fung·gayt) to grow rapidly and produce fungus-like growths. Often occurs in the late stages of malignant tumours.

fungicide ('funji,sied) a preparation that destroys fungal infection.

fungiform ('funji,fawm) shaped like a fungus or mushroom.

fungus ('fung·gəs) a low form of vegetable life which includes mushrooms and moulds. Some varieties cause disease, such as actinomycosis and ringworm.

funis ('fyoonis) the umbilical cord.

funnel chest ('fun'l) a developmental deformity in which there is a depression in the sternum and an inward curvature of the ribs and costal cartilages.

furor ('fyooə·raw) a state of intense excitement during which violent acts may be performed. This may occur following an epileptic fit.

furuncle ('fyooə·rungk'l) a boil.

furunculosis (fyuh,rungkyuh'lohsis) a staphylococcal infection represented by many, or crops of, boils.

furunculus (fyuh'rungkyuhləs) a furuncle. *F. orientalis* a protozoal infection mainly of the tropics, which causes a chronic ulceration. Cutaneous leishmaniasis.

fusidic acid (fyoo'sidik) an antibiotic used to treat penicillin-resistant staphylococci. It is usually used in combination with another antibiotic effective against staphylococci.

fusiform ('fyoozi,fawm) shaped like a spindle.

fusion ('fyoozhən) 1. the union between two adjacent structures. 2. the coordination of separate images of the same object in the two eyes into one image.

Fusobacterium (,fyoozohbak-'tiə·ri·əm) a genus of anaerobic Gram-negative bacteria found as normal flora in the mouth and large bowel, and often in necrotic tissue, probably as secondary invaders.

Fybogel ('fiebohjel) trade name for preparations of ispaghula husk, a laxative.

G

g symbol for *gram*.

G symbol for *guanine*.

Ga symbol for *gallium*.

gag (gag) 1. an instrument placed between the teeth to keep the mouth open. 2. the reflex action which occurs when the back of the throat is stimulated.

gait (gayt) manner of walking. *Ataxic g.* the foot is raised high, descends suddenly, and the whole sole strikes the ground. *Cerebellar g.* a staggering walk indicative of cerebellar disease. *Four-point g.* a method which may be adopted when using sticks or crutches, which allows maximum stability. *Spastic g.* stiff, shuffling walk, the legs being kept together.

galactagogue (gə'laktə,gog) an agent causing increased secretion of milk.

galactocele (gə'laktə,seel) 1. a milk-containing cyst in the breast. 2. a hydrocele containing a milky fluid.

galactorrhoea (,galəktə'reea) 1. an excessive flow of milk. 2. secretion of milk after breast-feeding has ceased.

galactosaemia (gə'laktə'seemi·ə) an inborn error of metabolism in which there is inability to convert galactose to glucose. The disorder becomes manifest soon after birth and is characterized by feeding problems, vomiting and diarrhoea, abdominal distension, enlargement of the liver and mental handicap. Treatment consists of exclusion from the diet of milk and all foods containing galactose or lactose.

galactose (gə'laktohz, -ohs) a monosaccharide derived from lactose. D-Galactose is found in lactose or milk sugar and cerebrosides of the brain. *G. tolerance test* a laboratory test to determine the liver's ability to convert the sugar galactose into glycogen.

gall (gawl) bile, a digestive fluid secreted by the liver and stored in the gallbladder. *G.bladder* the sac under the lower surface of the liver, which acts as a reservoir for bile. *G.stone* a concretion formed in the ballbladder or bile ducts. Gallstones are often multiple and faceted. *G.stone colic see* BILIARY COLIC.

gallamine ('galə,meen) a synthetic muscle relaxant, chemically related to curare but less potent and shorter acting.

gallipot ('gali,pot) a small receptacle for lotions.

gallium ('gali·əm) symbol Ga. A radioisotope used in detecting some soft tissue disorders.

gallop rhythm ('galəp) heart rhythm which may occur when there is ventricular overload.

galvanofaradization ('galvənoh-,farədie'zayshən) the simultaneous application of continuous and interrupted currents to a nerve or muscle.

galvanometer (,galvə'nomitə) an instrument for detecting or measuring the strength of a current of electricity.

gamete ('gameet) a sex cell which combines with another to form a zygote, from which a complete organism develops. A spermatozoon or an ovum.

gametocyte (gə'meetoh,siet) a cell that is undergoing gametogenesis.

gametogenesis (,gamitoh'jenəsis) the production of the gametes by the gonads.

gamma ('gamə) the third letter in the Greek alphabet, γ. *G.-benzene hexachloride* a drug used as a cream or lotion or as a shampoo to treat head lice. *G. camera* an apparatus for depicting a part of the body into which radioactive isotopes emitting gamma rays have been introduced. *G. encephalography* a method of localizing a brain tumour by using radioactive isotopes emitting gamma rays. *G.-globulin* a class of plasma proteins composed almost entirely of IgG, an IMMUNOGLO-BULIN protein that contains most antibody activity. *G. rays* electromagnetic rays of shorter wavelength and with greater penetration than X-rays, which are given off by certain radioactive substances and which are used in radiotherapy. Also used in the sterilization of articles which would be destroyed by the heat

and moisture required in autoclaving.

ganglion ('gang·gli·ən) 1. a collection of nerve cells and fibres, forming an independent nerve centre, as is found in the sympathetic nervous system. 2. a cystic swelling on a tendon.

ganglionectomy (,gang·gli·ə'nektəmee) excision of a ganglion.

gangrene ('gang·green) death of body tissue, generally in considerable mass, either due to loss of blood supply, or to the effects of certain infections. *Dry g.* occurs gradually and results from slow reduction of the blood flow in the arteries. There is no subsequent bacterial decomposition; the tissues become dry and shrivelled. It occurs only in the extremities, and can occur with ARTERIOSCLEROSIS and DIABETES MELLITUS. *Gas g.* results from dirty lacerated wounds infected by anaerobic bacteria, especially species of *Clostridium*. It is an acute, severe, painful condition in which muscles and subcutaneous tissues become filled with gas and a serosanguineous exudate. *Moist g.* is caused by sudden stoppage of blood, resulting from burning by heat or acid, severe freezing, physical accident that destroys the tissue, or a clot or other embolism. At first, tissue affected by moist gangrene has the colour of a bad bruise, is swollen, and often blistered. The gangrene is likely to spread with great speed. Toxins are formed in the affected tissues and absorbed.

Ganser's syndrome (state) ('ganzəz) *S. J. M. Ganser, Ger-*

man psychiatrist, 1853–1931. Amnesia, disturbance of consciousness and hallucinations, associated with senseless answers to questions, and absurd acts. Usually a transient response to a troublesome situation, e.g. prisoners on remand (prison psychosis).

gargle ('gahg'l) 1. a solution for rinsing the mouth and throat. 2. to rinse the mouth and throat by holding a solution in the open mouth and agitating it by expulsion of air from the lungs.

gargoylism ('gahgoy·lizem) mucopolysaccharidosis; an inherited condition due to a deficiency of α-L-iduronidase and transmitted as a recessive trait in which coarse features and large head are prominent. Vision is defective and there are learning difficulties. Hurler's syndrome.

gas (gas) molecules of a substance very loosely combined; a vapour. *G. and air analgesia* an authorized form of analgesia using nitrous oxide and air, by which the pains of labour are lessened without affecting uterine contractions. *G.-gangrene* the result of infection of a wound by anaerobic organisms, especially *Clostridium perfringens*. (also known as *C. welchii*). *Laughing g.* nitrous oxide. *Marsh g.* methane. *Sternutatory g.* one which causes sneezing. *Tear g.* one that is irritating to the eyes and causes excessive lacrimation.

Gasser's ganglion ('gasəz) *J. L. Gasser, Austrian anatomist, 1723–1765.* The trigeminal ganglion. The ganglion of the sen-

sory root of the fifth cranial nerve.

gasserectomy (,gasə'rektəmee) excision of the trigeminal ganglion.

gastraliga (ga'stralji·ə) pain in the stomach.

gastrectomy (ga'strektəmee) excision of part or whole of the stomach. *Partial g.* removal of a part, usually the distal portion, of the stomach. Commonly performed in the surgical treatment of peptic ulcer. *Billroth g.* removal of most of the lesser curvature and pyloric portion and joining of the duodenum to the refashioned stomach. This cuts down the production of secretin and acid. *Polya g.* removal of the first part of the duodenum and the greater part of the stomach, and anastomosis of the stomach to the jejunum. The blind portion of the duodenum supplies the bile and pancreatic and duodenal secretions.

gastric ('gastrik) pertaining to the stomach. *G. analysis* analysis of the stomach contents by microscopy and tests to determine the amount of acid present. *G. bypass* surgical creation of a small gastric pouch that empties directly into the jejunum through a gastrojejunostomy, thereby causing food to bypass the duodenum; done for the treatment of gross OBESITY. *G. flu* a popular term for what may be any of several disorders of the stomach and intestinal tract. The symptoms are nausea, diarrhoea, abdominal cramps and fever. *G. juice* the clear fluid secreted by the glands of the stomach to assist digestion. It contains an enzyme called pepsin, which acts upon proteins in the presence of weak hydrochloric acid. *G. lavage* a treatment for some types of poisoning where the stomach contents are washed out through a stomach tube. *G. ulcer* ulceration of the gastric mucosa associated with hyperacidity and often precipitated by stress.

gastrin ('gastrin) a hormone, secreted by the walls of the stomach, which excites continued secretion of digestive juice whilst food is in the stomach.

gastritis (ga'strietis) inflammation of the lining of the stomach.

gastrocnemius (,gastrok'neemi·əs) the principal muscle of the calf of the leg. It flexes both the ankle and the knee.

gastrocolic (,gastroh'kolik) pertaining to the stomach and colon. *G. reflex* following a meal, increased peristalsis causes the colon to empty into the rectum. This gives rise to a desire to defecate.

gastroduodenostomy (,gastroh-,dyooədi'nostəmee) a surgical anastomosis between the stomach and the duodenum.

gastroenteritis (,gastroh,entə'rietis) inflammation of the lining of the stomach and intestine. Psychological causes of gastroenteritis include fear, anger and other forms of emotional upset. Allergic reactions to certain foods can cause gastroenteritis, as can irritation by excessive use of alcohol. Severe gastroenteritis, with such symptoms as headache, nau-

sea, vomiting, weakness, diarrhoea and gas pains, may result from various viral and bacterial infections such as INFLUENZA.

gastroenterology (,gastroh,entə-'roləjee) the study of diseases of the gastrointestinal tract.

gastroenteropathy (,gastroh,entə-'ropəthee) any disease condition affecting both the stomach and the intestine.

gastroenterostomy (,gastroh,entə-'rostəmee) a surgical anastomosis between the stomach and small intestine.

Gastrografin (,gastroh'grafin) a proprietary oral diagnostic radio-opaque contrast medium.

gastroileac (,gastroh'iliak) pertaining to the stomach and ileum. *G. reflex* food entering the stomach sets up powerful peristalsis in the ileum and opening of the ileocaecal valve.

gastrointestinal (,gastroh·in'testin'l) pertaining to the stomach and intestine. *G. tract* the alimentary tract.

gastrojejunostomy (,gastroh,jejuh'nostəmee) a surgical anastomosis between the stomach and the jujunum.

gastromalacia (,gastrohmə'layshi·ə) an abnormal softening of the walls of the stomach.

gastro-oesophagostomy (,gastroh·i,sofə'gostəmee) a surgical anastomosis between the stomach and the oesophagus.

gastropathy (ga'stropəthee) any disease of the stomach.

gastroplasty ('gastroh,plastee) plastic repair of the stomach.

gastroptosis (,gastrop'tohsis) downward displacement of the stomach owing to weakening of supporting ligaments or of its own musculature.

gastroscope ('gastrə,skohp) an endoscope especially designed for passage into the stomach to permit examination of its interior. The gastroscope is a hollow, cylindrical tube fitted with special lenses and lights which acts by reflecting light and creating a mirror effect, making it possible to 'go around corners', and facilitating visualization of the curvature of the stomach.

gastrostomy (ga'strostəmee) the creation of an opening into the stomach. This procedure is done to provide for the administration of food and liquids when stricture of the oesophagus or other conditions make swallowing impossible. See ARTIFICIAL FEEDING.

gastrotomy (ga'strotəmee) a surgical incision of the stomach.

gastrula ('gastruhlə) an early stage in the development of the fertilized ovum.

Gaucher's disease (gho'shayz) *P. C. E. Gaucher, French physician, 1854–1918.* A rare familial disease in which fat is deposited in the reticuloendothelial cells causing an enlarged spleen and anaemia.

gauze (gawz) a thin open-meshed material used for dressing wounds.

gavage ('gavahzh) forced feeding; the giving of fluids and nourishment by oesophageal or other type of tube directly into the stomach.

Geiger counter ('giegə) *H. Geiger, German physicist, 1882–1945.* An instrument for detecting and registering radioactivity. The apparatus is sensitive to the rays emitted.

gelatin ('jelətin) an albuminoid, obtained from connective tissue or bone. Used in pharmacy for suppositories and capsules, and in bacteriology as a culture medium. In absorbable film and sponge, it is used in surgical procedures.

gender ('jendə) sex; the category to which an individual is assigned on the basis of sex. *G. identity disorder* a psychiatric label for those disorders marked by a sense of inappropriateness and attendant discomfort concerning one's sexual anatomy and sex role. This category usually includes transvestism, transsexualism and gender identity disorders in childhood.

gene (jeen) one of the biological units of heredity, self-reproducing, and located at a definite position (locus) on a particular chromosome. *Dominant g.* one that is capable of transmitting its characteristics irrespective of the genes from the other parent. *Recessive g.* one that can pass on its characteristics only if it is present with a similar recessive gene from the other parent. See MENDEL'S THEORY.

genetic (jə'netik) 1. pertaining to reproduction or to birth or origin. 2. inherited. *G. code* the arrangement of genetic material stored in the DNA molecule of the chromosome. *G. counselling* supportive service for prospective parents who can receive advice as to the likelihood of their children being born with a genetically transmitted disorder.

genetics (jə'netiks) the study of heredity and natural development.

genitalia (,jeni'tayli·ə) the organs of reproduction.

genitourinary (,jenitoh'yooə·rinə·ree) referring to both the reproductive organs and the urinary tract.

genotype ('jenoh,tiep, 'jeenoh-) the genetic characteristics of an individual.

gentamicin (,jentə'miesin) an antibiotic effective against many Gram-negative bacteria, especially *Pseudomonas* species, as well as certain Gram-positive bacteria, especially *Staphylococcus aureus*.

genu ('jenyoo) [L.] *the knee. G. valgum* knock-knee. *G. varum.* bow-leg.

genupectoral (,jenyoo'pektə·rəl) relating to the knee and chest. *G. position* the knee–chest position. *See* POSITION.

genus ('jeenəs) a classification of animals and plants, the species within a genus having characteristics common to themselves, but differing from those of other genera.

geriatrics (,jeri'atriks) the branch of medicine covering old age and the disorders arising from it.

germ (jərm) 1. a microbe. 2. that from which something may develop; a seed.

German measles ('jərmən 'meez·'lz) *see* RUBELLA.

germicide ('jərmi,sied) an agent capable of destroying pathogenic microorganisms.

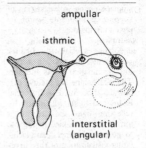

ECTOPIC GESTATION

germinoma (,jərmi'nohmə) a neoplasm of the testis or ovum.

gerontology (,jeron'toləjee) the study of old age and the ageing processes.

Gessel's developmental chart ('ges'lz) *A. Gessell, Americian psychologist*, 1880–1961. A chart which shows the expected motor, social and psychologicial development of children.

gestaltism (gə'shtaltizəm) a theory of holism in psychology which claims that ideas come as a whole and are not subdivisible.

gestation (je'stayshən) the period of development of the young in mammals, from the time of fertilization of the ovum to birth. *See also* PREGNANCY. *G. period* the duration of pregnancy; in the human female about 280 days when measured from the first day of the last menstrual period. *Ectopic g.* fetal development in some part other than the uterus – most usually the uterine tube.

Ghon focus (gon) *A. Ghon, Czechoslovakian pathologist, 1866–1936.* The primary lesion of pulmonary tuberculosis, as seen on an X-ray film, after it has healed by fibrosis and calcification.

giardiasis (ˌjiah'dieəsis) *A. Giard, French biologist, 1846–1908.* An infection with *Giardia lamblia,* a pear-shaped protozoon that causes a persistent protracted diarrhoea, often resulting in intestinal malabsorption.

gibbosity (gi'bositee) a humped back; kyphosis.

gigantism ('jiegan,tizəm, jie'gantizəm) abnormal growth of the body, often due to overactivity of the anterior lobe of the pituitary gland.

Gilles de la Tourette's syndrome (disease) (ˌzheel də lah tooə'rets) *G.A.E.B. Gilles de la Tourette, French neurologist, b. 1857.* Multiple tics, especially of the face and upper part of the body, often associated with involuntary obscene utterances. The condition usually has its onset in childhood and often becomes chronic. The cause is unknown.

Gilliam's operation ('gili-əmz) *D. T. Gilliam, American gynaecologist, 1844–1923.* The correction of retroversion of the uterus by shortening the round ligaments; ventrosuspension.

gingiva ('jinjivə, jin'jievə) the gum; connective tissue surrounding the necks of the teeth.

gingivectomy (ˌjinji'vektəmee) the surgical removal of the gum margins to get rid of pockets and improve the shape of the gums.

gingivitis (ˌjinji'vietis) inflammation of the gums.

ginglymus ('jing·gliməs) a hinge joint allowing movement in one plane only.

gladiolus (gladi'ohləs) the blade-like portion of the sternum.

gland (gland) an organ composed of cells which secrete fluid prepared from the blood, either for use in the body, or for excretion as waste material. *Ductless (endocrine) g.* one which produces an internal secretion but has no canal (duct) to carry the secretion away, e.g. the thyroid gland. *Exocrine g.* one which discharges its secretion through a duct, e.g. the parotid gland. *Lymph g. see* LYMPH NODES. *Mucous g.* one which secretes mucus.

glanders ('glandəz) a disease of horses communicable to man, and caused by the glanders bacillus, *Pseudomonas mallei.* It is marked by a purulent inflammation of the mucous membranes and an eruption of nodules on the skin.

glandular ('glandyuhlə) pertaining to a gland. *G. fever see* INFECTIOUS MONONUCLEOSIS.

glans (glanz) an acorn-shaped body, such as the rounded end of the penis or the clitoris.

Glasgow coma scale (ˌglazgoh 'kohmə ˌskayl) a standardized system for quickly evaluating the level of consciousness in the critically ill. Measures include: eye opening according to four criteria, verbal response against five criteria and motor response using six criteria. Scores of 7 or less qualify as 'coma'. Coma is defined as no response and no eye opening.

glaucoma (glaw'kohmə) raised intraocular pressure. *Primary g.* one that occurs without any previous disease. It is a common cause of blindness, partial or complete, in the elderly. *Closed-angle g.* one that occurs when there is a mechanical defect in the drainage angle and may be primary or secondary. It may be acute, when there is pain and blurring of vision, or chronic, when there may be no pain, but a gradual loss of vision. *Open-angle g.* chronic primary glaucoma in which the angle remains open but drainage becomes gradually diminished. *Secondary g.* one that occurs when some ocular disease is complicated by an increase in intraocular pressure.

gleet (gleet) chronic gonococcal urethritis marked by a transparent mucous discharge.

glenohumeral (,gleenoh'hyoomə-·rəl) referring to the shoulder joint.

glenoid ('gleenoyd) resembling a hollow. *G. cavity* the socket of the shoulder joint.

glia ('glieə) neuroglia; the connective tissue of the brain and spinal cord.

glibenclamide (glie'benklə,mied) an oral hypoglycaemic agent of the sulphonylurea group used in the treatment of diabetes mellitus.

glioblastoma (,glieohbla'stohmə) a malignant glioma arising in the cerebral hemispheres.

glioma (glie'ohmə) a malignant

tumour composed of neuroglia cells affecting the brain and spinal cord; seldom metastasizes.

Glisson's capsule ('glisənz) *F. Glisson, British physician and anatomist, 1597–1677.* The connective tissue capsule of the liver which envelops the portal vein, hepatic artery and hepatic ducts.

globin ('glohbin) a protein used in the formation of haemoglobin.

globulin ('globyuhlin) a protein constituent of the blood (*serum g.*) and cerebrospinal fluid.

globulinuria (,globyuhli'nyooə-·ri·ə) the presence of globulin in the urine.

globus ('glohbəs) a ball or globe. *G. hystericus* a symptom of hysteria when a patient feels he cannot swallow because he has a lump in his throat. *G. pallidus* the pale medial part of the lentiform nucleus of the brain.

glomerulitis (glo,meryuh'lietis) inflammation of the glomeruli of the kidney.

glomerulonephritis (glo,meryuh-lohnə'frietis) a bilateral, non-infectious inflammation of the kidneys. The cause is unknown but it is associated with immunological disturbance. It may be acute, presenting rapidly but reversibly, or it may be chronic, presenting slowly and irreversibly.

glomerulosclerosis (glo,meryuh-lohsklə'rohsis) degenerative changes in the glomerular capillaries of the renal tubule leading to renal failure.

glomerulus (glo'meryuhləs) the tuft of capillaries within the nephron, which filters urine from the blood.

glossal ('glos'l) relating to the tongue.

Glossina (glo'sienə) a genus of biting flies, the tsetse flies.

glossitis (glo'sietis) inflammation of the tongue.

glossodynia (,glosə'dini·ə) a painful sensation in the tongue when no lesion is visible.

glossolalia (,glosə'layli·ə) unintelligible speech. The patient speaks in an imaginary language.

glossopharyngeal (,glosoh,fə'rinji·əl,-,farin'jeeəl) pertaining to the tongue and pharynx. *G. nerve* the ninth cranial nerve.

glossoplegia (,glosoh'pleeji·ə) paralysis of the tongue.

glottis ('glotis) the space between the vocal cords. The term is sometimes used for that part of the larynx which is associated with voice production.

glucagon ('glookə,gon) a polypeptide produced by the pancreas. It aids glycogen breakdown in the liver and raises the blood sugar level.

glucocorticoid (,glookoh'kawti,koyd) any corticoid substance that raises the concentration of liver glycogen and blood sugar, i.e. cortisol (hydrocortisone), cortisone and corticosterone.

gluconeogenesis (,glookoh,neeoh'jenəsis) the production of glucose from the non-nitrogen portion of the amino acids after deamination. It occurs in the liver and kidneys.

glucose ('glookohs, -kohz) dextrose or grape-sugar; a simple sugar, a monosaccharide in certain foodstuffs, especially fruit,

and in normal blood; the chief source of energy for living organisms. *See also* DEXTROSE. *G.-6-phosphate dehydrogenase* a red-cell enzyme. Inherited deficiency causes a tendency to haemolytic anaemia. *See* FAVISM. *G. tolerance test* test in which a quantity of glucose is given and the concentration of glucose in the blood is estimated at intervals afterwards. Used mainly when diabetes mellitus is suspected.

glue sniffing ('gloo ,snifing) solvent abuse.

glutamic acid (gloo'tamik) one of the 22 amino acids formed by the digestion of dietary protein.

glutamic–oxaloacetic transaminase (gloo,tamik,oksəloh·ə'seetik tranz'ami,nayz) an enzyme found in cardiac muscle and the liver. Raised serum levels (SGOT) may indicate an acute myocardial infarction or the presence of liver disease.

glutamic–pyruvic transaminase (gloo,tamikpie'roovik tranz'ami,nayz) an enzyme found in the liver. Measurement of serum levels (SGPT) is used in the study and diagnosis of liver diseases.

glutaraldehyde (,glootə'raldi,hied) a disinfectant active against all viruses, fungi, vegetative bacteria and spores. Used in aqueous solution for sterilization of non-heat-resistant equipment.

gluteal ('glooti·əl, gloo'ti·əl) relating to the buttocks. *G. muscles* three muscles which form the fleshy part of the buttocks.

gluten ('glootən) the protein of wheat and other grains. *G.-induced enteropathy* coeliac dis-

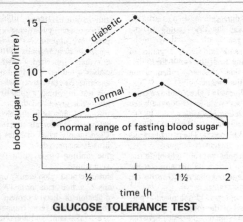

GLUCOSE TOLERANCE TEST

ease.

glycerin ('glisə,rin) a colourless syrupy substance obtained from fats and fixed oils. It has a hygroscopic action. As an emollient it is an ingredient of many skin preparations. *G. suppository* one composed of glycerin and gelatin, used as an evacuant. *G. of thymol* an antiseptic mouth wash and gargle.

glyceryl trinitrate (,glisə·ril trie-'nietrayt) nitroglycerin. Glyceryl trinitrate is a vasodilator and used to relieve certain types of pain, especially in the prophylaxis and treatment of ANGINA PECTORIS. It is administered sublingually or by transdermal patch or gel.

glycine ('glieseen) a non-essential amino acid.

glycogen ('gliekəjən) the form in which carbohydrate is stored in the liver and muscles. Animal starch. *G. storage disease* inherited disease in which there is a deficiency in the synthesis of glycogen. This accumulates in the liver causing enlargement.

glycogenesis (,gliekoh'jenəsis) the process of glycogen formation from the blood glucose.

glycogenolysis (,gliekəjə'nolisis) the breakdown of glycogen in the body so that it may be utilized.

glycoside ('gliekə,sied) a crystalline body in plants which, when acted on by acids or ferments, produces sugar. If the sugar is glucose it may be termed a glucoside. *See* DIGITALIS.

glycosuria (,gliekoh'syooə·ri·ə) an excess of glucose in the urine, a symptom of diabetes mellitus. *Renal g.* sugar in the urine in an otherwise healthy person due to an inherited inability to reabsorb glucose normally.

glymidine ('gliemi,deen) a drug of the sulphonylurea group used in the treatment of diabetes mellitus.

gnathic ('nathik) pertaining to the jaw.

gnathoplasty ('nathoh,plastee) a plastic operation on the jaw.

goblet cell ('goblit ,sel) a goblet-shaped cell, found in the intestinal epithelium, which produces mucus.

goitre ('goytə) enlargement of the thyroid gland, causing a swelling in the front part of the neck. Simple endemic goitre, sometimes referred to as Derbyshire neck, is usually caused by lack of iodine in the diet. *Colloid g.* an enlarged but soft thyroid gland with no signs of hyperthyroidism. *Exophthalmic g.* hyperthyroidism with marked protrusion of the eyeballs (exophthalmos). Graves' disease. *Intrathoracic g.* enlargement of the gland mainly in the thorax, so the swelling may not be easily visible. *Sporadic g.* a simple nontoxic enlargement. *Substernal g.* enlargement of the gland behind the sternum so that swelling in the neck may not be apparent. *Toxic g.* signs of excess of thyroxine in the blood, where the gland has not been previously enlarged. The patient complains of weight loss and is generally nervous. Exophthalmos may be present.

gold (gohld) *symbol* Au. A metallic element used in treating rheumatoid arthritis. Gold salts are among the most toxic of therapeutic agents. Toxic reactions may vary from mild to severe kidney or liver damage and blood dyscrasias. *Radioactive g.* an isotope which gives off beta and gamma rays. Used in the form of small grains or seeds it may be implanted into malignant tissues. In colloidal form it may be instilled into a serous cavity to treat malignant effusions.

Golgi apparatus or **body** ('goljee, 'golgee) *C. Golgi, Italian histologist, 1844–1926.* Specialized structures seen near the nucleus of a cell during microscopic examination.

Golgi's organ the sensory end organs in muscle tendons that are sensitive to stretch.

gonad ('gohnad,'gonad) a reproductive gland; the testicle or ovary.

gonadotrophic (,gonədoh'trohfik) having influence on the gonads. *G. hormones* gonadotrophin.

gonadotrophin (,gonədoh'trohfin) any hormone having a stimulating effect on the gonads. Two such hormones are secreted by the anterior pituitary: follicle-stimulating hormone (FSH) and luteinizing hormone (LH) both of which are active, but with differing effects, in the two sexes. *Chorionic g.* a gonad-stimulating hormone produced by cytotrophoblastic cells of the placenta; used in treatment of underdevelopment of the gonads and to induce ovulation in infertile women.

gonagra (go'nagrə) gout in the knee.

gonion ('gohni·ən) [Gr.] the midpoint of the mandible (lower jaw).

gonioscope ('gohnioh,skohp) an apparatus for examining the angle of the anterior chamber of the eye.

goniotomy (,gohni'otəmee) an operation for glaucoma; it consists in opening Schlemm's canal under direct vision.

gonococcus (,gonoh'kokəs) *Neisseria gonorrhoeae*, a diplococcus which causes gonorrhoea.

gonorrhoea (,gonə'reeə) a common venereal disease caused by *Neisseria gonorrhoeae* infecting the genital tract of either sex, causing a discharge and pain on micturition, although the disease is often asymptomatic in females. Spread by the bloodstream, it may give rise to iritis or arthritis. Scar tissue formation may bring about urethral stricture or infertility owing to occlusion of the uterine tubes. The eyes of babies may be infected at birth during passage through the birth canal of an infected mother. The condition is called OPHTHALMIA NEONATORUM (notifiable disease). In the past it was a major cause of blindness in babies.

gonorrhoeal (,gonə'reeəl) relating to gonorrhoea. *G. arthritis* intractable infection of joints causing great pain and disability.

Goodpasture's syndrome ('guhd-,pahschəz) *E. W. Goodpasture, American pathologist, 1886–1960.* A rare haemorrhagic lung disorder associated with glomerulonephritis.

gouge (gowj) a curved chisel used for scooping out diseased bone, or other hard substances.

gout (gowt) a hereditary form of

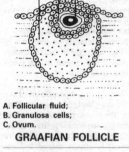

A. Follicular fluid;
B. Granulosa cells;
C. Ovum.

GRAAFIAN FOLLICLE

arthritis with an excess of uric acid in the blood. It is characterized by painful inflammation and swelling of the smaller joints, especially those of the big toe and thumb. Inflammation is accompanied by the deposit of urates around the joints.

GPI general paralysis of the insane; dementia paralytica. *See* PARALYSIS.

graafian follicle ('grahfi·ən) *R. de Graaf, Dutch physician and anatomist, 1641–1673.* A follicle which is formed in the ovary and contains an ovum. A follicle matures during each menstrual cycle, ruptures and releases the ovum (ovulation) which is then picked up by the fimbriated end of the uterine tube.

graft (grahft) 1. any tissue or organ for implantation or transplantation. 2. to implant or transplant such tissue. *Autogenous g.*

a graft taken from and given to the same individual. *Bone g.* a portion of bone transplanted to repair another bone. *Corneal g.* a portion of cornea, usually from a recently dead person, used to repair a diseased cornea. *Homologous g.* tissue obtained from the body of another animal of the same species but with a genotype differing from that of the recipient; a homograft or allograft. *Pedicle g* a skin graft, one end of which remains attached to its original site until the grafting has become established.

graft-versus-host disease (reaction) (ˌgrahftvərsiz'hohst) abbreviated GVH disease. A condition that occurs when immunologically competent cells or their precursors are transplanted into an immunologically incompetent recipient (host) that is not histocompatible with the donor. Characteristic signs include skin lesions, ulceration, alopecia, painful joints and haemolytic anaemia. GVH disease is a frequent complication of bone marrow transplants. HLA matching of the donor and recipient reduces the possibility of GVH disease.

gram (gram) *symbol* g. The fundamental SI unit of weight, equal to one thousandth of a kilogram.

Gram's stain (gramz) *H. Gram, Danish physician, 1853–1938.* A method of staining bacteria which is used to classify them into Gram-negative and Gram-positive bacteria.

grand mal (ˌgronh 'mal) [Fr.] major epilepsy. *See* EPILEPSY.

granular ('granyuhlə) containing small particles. *G. casts* the degenerated cells from the lining of renal tubules excreted in the urine in certain kidney disorders.

granulation (ˌgranyuh'layshən) 1. the division of a hard solid substance into small particles. 2. the growth of new tissue by which ulcers and wounds heal when the edges are not in apposition. It consists of new capillaries and fibroblasts which fill in the space and later form fibrous tissue. The resulting scar is often unsightly.

granule ('granyool) 1. a small particle or grain. 2. a small pill made of sucrose.

granulocyte ('granyuhlə,siet) any cell containing granules in its cytoplasm, especially polymorphonuclear leukocytes which contain granular neutrophils, basophils and eosinophils in their cytoplasm.

granulocytopenia (ˌgranyuhloh-ˌsietə'peeni-ə) a marked reduction in the number of granulocytes in the blood. The condition may precede agranulocytosis.

granuloma (ˌgranyuh'lomə) a tumour composed of granulation tissue, usually due to chronic infection or invasion by a foreign body.

granulomatosis (ˌgranyuh,lohmə-'tohsis) an infection producing granulomata. *Lipoid g.* xanthomatosis; Hand–Schüller–Christian disease. *Malignant g.* lymphadenoma; Hodgkin's disease.

gravel ('grav'l) small 'sandy' calculi formed in the kidneys and bladder, and sometimes excreted with the urine.

Graves' disease (grayvz) *R. J. Graves, Irish physician, 1796–1853.* Exophthalmic goitre; thyrotoxicosis.

gravid ('gravid) pregnant.

gravity ('gravətee) weight. *Specific g.* the weight of a substance compared with that of an equal volume of water.

gray (gray) *symbol* Gy. The SI unit used to denote the absorbed dose in radiation therapy.

grey-scale display (gray) a method to show the texture of tissue on ULTRASOUND display. The amplitude of each echo is represented by varying shades of grey. A bright white outline is seen from specular surfaces, a mottled grey from various tissue areas, and black from collections of fluid such as the bladder and amniotic sac.

griseofulvin (,grizioh'fuhlvin) an oral antifungal antibiotic that is used in the treatment of infections of the skin, hair and nails.

group therapy (groop) a form of psychotherapy in which a group of patients meets regularly with the therapist in order to discuss and share problems, anxieties and fears in a psychotherapeutic setting. The group also provides emotional support for self-revelation and a structured environment for trying out new ways of relating to people.

growing pains ('groh·ing) recurrent quasirheumatic limb pains peculiar to early youth, once believed to be caused by the growing process. It is now recognized that growth does not cause pain and that these pains can be a symptom of many different disorders.

growth (grohth) 1. the progressive development of a living thing, especially the process by which the body reaches its point of complete physical development. 2. an abnormal formation of tissue, such as a tumour. *G. hormone* a substance that stimulates growth, especially a secretion of the anterior lobe of the PITUITARY GLAND that directly influences protein, carbohydrate and lipid metabolism, and controls the rate of skeletal and visceral growth.

guanethidine (gwah'nethi,deen) a drug used in the treatment of hypertension. It is an adrenergic blocking agent.

guanine ('gwahneen) a purine base, one of the constituents of all nucleic acids.

guardian ad litem (,gahdi·ən ad 'liekem) a person, usually from the local authority social service department, who is appointed by a court to look after the interests of a child before its full Adoption Order is granted. Meanwhile the prospective adoptive parents have continuous possession of the child, and are visited and interviewed by the guardian *ad litem* to ensure that the home will be satisfactory.

Guillain–Barré syndrome (,giyanh-'baray) *G. Guillain, French neurologist, 1876–1961; A. Barré, French neurologist, b. 1880.* Acute infective polyneuritis. After an infection, usually respiratory, there is a general weakness or paralysis which frequently affects the respiratory muscles as well as the peripheral ones.

guillotine ('gilǝ,teen) a surgical instrument used for excising tonsils.

guinea-worm ('gini,wǝrm) a nematode worm, *Dracunculus medinensis*, which burrows into human tissues, particularly into the legs or feet.

gumboil ('gum,boyl) the opening on the gum of an abscess at the root of a tooth.

gumma ('gummǝ) a soft, degenerating tumour characteristic of the tertiary stage of syphilis. It may occur in any organ or tissue.

gustatory (gu'staytǝ-ree) relating to taste.

gut (gut) the intestine.

Guthrie test ('guthri ,test) a blood test carried out on a neonate between the 6th and 14th days of life to diagnose PHENYLKETO-NURIA.

gutta ('gutǝ) a drop. *G. percha* the juice of a tropical tree which, when dried, forms an elastic

semi-solid substance. Used in dentistry as a root filler.

GVH disease graft-versus-host disease.

Gy symbol for *gray*.

gynaecoid ('gienǝ,koyd) like the female. *G. pelvis* one with a round brim and shallow cavity suited to childbearing. A normal female pelvis.

gynaecologist (,gienǝ'kolǝ,jist) one who specializes in the diseases of the female genital tract.

gynaecology (,gienǝ'kolǝjee) the science of those diseases which are peculiar to the female genital tract.

gynaecomastia (,gienǝkoh'masti·ǝ) excessive growth of the male breast.

Gynovlar (,gien'ohvlah) trade name for a contraceptive tablet containing OESTROGEN and PRO-GESTERONE.

gypsum ('jipsǝm) plaster of Paris (calcium sulphate).

gyrus ('jierǝs) a convolution as of the cerebral cortex.

H

H symbol for *hydrogen*.

habit ('habit) automatic response to a specific situation acquired as a result of repetition and learning. *Drug h.* drug addiction. *H. training* a method used in psychiatric nursing whereby deteriorated patients can be rehabilitated and taught personal hygiene by constant repetition and encouragement.

habituation (hə,bityuh'ayshən, -,bichuh-) the gradual adaptation to a stimulus or to the environment. The acquisition of a habit, e.g. a condition resulting from the repeated consumption of a drug, with a desire to continue its use, but with little or no tendency to increase the dose; there may be psychic but no physical dependence on the drug.

haemangioblastoma (hee,manjiohbla'stohmə) a tumour of the brain or spinal cord consisting of proliferated blood vessel cells.

haemangioma (,heemanji'ohmə) a benign tumour formed by dilated blood vessels. *Strawberry h.* a birthmark, which may become very large, but frequently disappears in a few years.

haemarthrosis (,heemah'throsis) an effusion of blood into a joint.

haematemesis (,heemə'teməsis) vomiting of blood. If it has been in the stomach for some time and become partially digested by gastric juice, it is of a dark colour and contains particles resembling coffee grounds.

haematin ('heemətin) the iron-containing part of haemoglobin.

haematocele ('heemətoh,seel) a swelling produced by effusion of blood, e.g. in the sheath surrounding a testicle or a broad ligament.

haematocolpos (,heemətoh'kolpos) an accumulation of blood or menstrual fluid in the vagina. *See* CRYPTOMENORRHOEA.

haematocrit ('heemətoh,krit, hi-'mat-) the volume of red cells in the blood. Usually expressed as a percentage of the total blood volume.

haematology (,heemə'toləjee) the science dealing with the nature, functions and diseases of blood.

haematoma (,heemə'tohmə) a swelling containing clotted blood.

haematometra (,heemətoh'meetrə) an accumulation of blood or menstrual fluid in the uterus.

haematomyelia (,heemətohmie-'eeli-ə) an effusion of blood into the spinal cord.

haematosalpinx (,heemətoh'salpingks) an accumulation of blood in the uterine tubes; haemosalpinx.

haematuria (,heemə'tyooə·ri·ə)

the presence of blood in the urine, due to injury or disease of any of the urinary organs.

haemochromatosis (,heemoh-,krohmə'tohsis) a condition in which there is high absorption and deposition of iron leading to a high serum level, pigmentation of the skin and liver failure. Bronze diabetes.

haemoconcentration (,heemoh-,konsən'trayshən) a loss of circulating fluid from the blood resulting in an increase in the proportion of red blood cells to plasma. The viscosity of the blood is increased.

haemocytology (,heemohsie'tol-əjee) the study of the cellular contents of blood.

haemocytometer (,heemohsie-'tomitə) an apparatus for counting the blood corpuscles in a specific volume of blood.

haemodialysis (,heemohdie'aləsis) the removal of waste material from the blood of a patient with acute or chronic renal failure by means of a dialyser or artificial kidney. The apparatus is coupled to an artery and dialysis is achieved by the blood and rinsing fluid (DIALYSATE) passing through a semipermeable membrane. Blood is returned through a vein.

haemoglobin (,heemə'glohbin) the complex protein molecule contained within the red blood cells which gives them their colour and by which oxygen is transported.

haemoglobinaemia (,heemə-,glohbi'neemi-ə) the presence of haemoglobin in the blood plasma.

haemoglobinometer (,heemə-'glohbi'nomitə) an instrument for estimating the haemoglobin content of the blood.

haemoglobinopathy (,heemə-,glohbi'nopəthee) any one of a group of hereditary disorders, including sickle-cell anaemia and thalassaemia, in which there is an abnormality in the production of haemoglobin.

haemolysin (hee'molisin) a substance which destroys red blood cells. It may be an antibody, a bacterial toxin or a component of a virus.

haemolysis (hee'molisis) the disintegration of red blood cells. Excessive haemolysis, which may produce anaemia, may be caused by poisoning or by bacterial infection.

haemolytic (,heemə'litik) having the power to destroy red blood cells. *H. disease of the newborn* a condition associated with rhesus incompatibility. *See* RHESUS FACTOR.

haemophilia (,heemoh'fili-ə) a condition characterized by impaired coagulability of the blood, and a strong tendency to bleed. Over 80 per cent of all patients with haemophilia have haemophilia A (classic haemophilia), which is characterized by a deficiency of clotting factor VIII. Haemophilia B (Christmas disease), which affects about 15 per cent of all haemophiliac patients, results from a deficiency of factor IX. Inherited as an X-linked recessive trait, it is transmitted by females only, to their

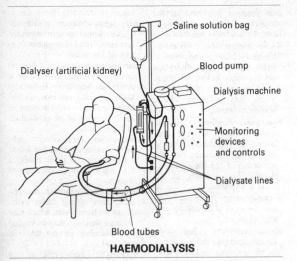

Saline solution bag

Dialyser (artificial kidney)

Blood pump

Dialysis machine

Monitoring devices and controls

Dialysate lines

Blood tubes

HAEMODIALYSIS

male offspring. In order to avoid the debilitating and crippling effects of haemophilia, treatment must raise the level of the deficient clotting factor and maintain it in order to stop local bleeding. The patient must learn to avoid trauma and to obtain prompt treatment for bleeding episodes. Before surgery or dental treatment the patient must be given an infusion of the appropriate clotting factor.

Haemophilus (hee'mofiləs) a genus of Gram-negative rod-like bacteria. *H. ducreyi* the cause of soft chancre. *H. influenzae* a species once thought to be the cause of epidemic influenza; it prod-

uces a highly fatal form of meningitis, especially in infants. *H. pertussis* the cause of whooping cough; Bordet–Gengou bacillus.

haemophthalmia (‚heemof'thal-mi·ə) bleeding into the vitreous of the eye, usually the result of trauma; haemophthalmos.

haemopneumothorax (‚heemoh-‚nyoomoh'thor·raks) the presence of blood and air in the pleural cavity, usually due to injury.

haemopoiesis (‚heemohpoy'eesis) the formation of red blood cells which takes place normally in the bone marrow and continues throughout life. *Extramedullary h.* the formation of blood cells other than in the bone marrow, e.g. in the liver or spleen.

haemopoietic (ˌheemoh poy'etik) relating to red blood cell formation. *H. factors* those necessary for the development of red blood cells, e.g. vitamin B$_{12}$ and folic acid.

haemoptysis (hee'moptisis) the coughing up of blood from the lungs or bronchi. Being aerated, it is bright red and frothy.

haemorrhage ('hemə·rij) an escape of blood from a ruptured blood vessel, externally or internally. *Arterial h.* bright red blood which escapes in rhythmic spurts, corresponding to the beats of the heart. *Venous h.* dark red blood which escapes in an even flow. Haemorrhage may also be: primary, at the time of operation or injury; reactionary or recurrent, occurring later when the blood pressure rises and a ligature slips or a vessel opens up; secondary, as a rule about 10 days after injury, and usually due to sepsis. Special types are: *Antepartum h.* that which occurs before labour starts. *See* PLACENTA PRAEVIA. *Cerebral h.* an episode of bleeding into the cerebrum; one of the three main forms of STROKE. *Concealed h.* collection of the blood in a cavity of the body. *Intracranial h.* bleeding within the cranium, which may be extradural, subdural, subarachnoid or cerebral. *Intradural h.* bleeding beneath the dura mater. It may be due to injury and causes signs of compression. The cerebrospinal fluid will be blood-stained. *Postpartum h.* that which occurs within 12–24 h of delivery, from the genital tract, which either measures 500 ml or more, or which adversely affects the woman's condition. Secondary postpartum haemorrhage is excessive bleeding more than 24 h after delivery.

haemorrhagic (ˌhemə'rajik) pertaining to or characterized by haemorrhage. *H. disease of newborn* a self-limited haemorrhagic disorder of the first days of life, caused by deficiency of vitamin K-dependent blood clotting factors II, VII, IX and X. It should be prevented by the prophylactic administration of vitamin K to all newborn babies. *Viral h. fevers* a group of notifiable virus diseases of diverse aetiology but with similar characteristics of fever, headache, myalgia, prostration and haemorrhagic symptoms. They include dengue haemorrhagic fever, Marburg disease, Ebola virus disease, Lassa fever and yellow fever.

haemorrhoid ('hemə‚royd) a 'pile' or locally dilated rectal vein. Piles may be either external or internal to the anal sphincter. Pain is caused on defecation, and bleeding may occur.

haemorrhoidectomy (ˌhemə·roy-'dektəmee) the surgical removal of haemorrhoids.

haemosalpinx (ˌheemo'salpingks) haematosalpinx.

haemosiderosis (ˌheemoh‚sidi-'rohsis) iron deposits in the tissues following excessive haemolysis of red blood cells.

haemostasis (ˌheemoh'staysis, hee'mostəsis) the arrest of bleeding or the slowing up of blood flow in a vessel.

haemostatic (,heemoh'statik) a drug or remedy for arresting haemorrhage; a styptic.

haemothorax (,heemoh'thor·raks) blood in the thoracic cavity, e.g. from injury to soft tissues as a result of fracture of a rib.

Hageman factor ('haygəmən) factor XII, which facilitates the clotting of blood (called after the first person found to be suffering from a deficiency of it).

hair (hair) a delicate keratinized epidermal filament growing out of the skin. The root of the hair

is enclosed beneath the skin in a tubular follicle.

Haldol ('haldol) trade name for a preparation of haloperidol, an antipsychotic agent.

halibut oil ('halibat, oyl) a vitamin-rich (A and D) oil derived from the liver of halibut.

halitosis (,hali'tohsis) foul-smelling breath.

hallucination (hə,loosi'nayshən) a sensory impression (sight, touch, sound, smell or taste) that has no basis in external stimulation. Hallucinations can have psychological causes, as in mental ill-

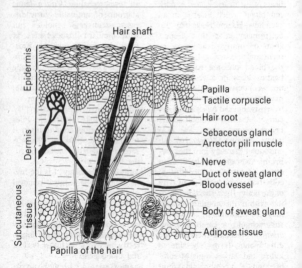

STRUCTURE OF A HAIR

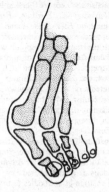

HALLUX VALGUS

ness, or they can result from drugs, alcohol, organic illnesses, such as brain tumour or senility, or exhaustion.

hallucinogen (həˈloosinə,jen) an agent that causes hallucinations, e.g. LSD and cannabis.

hallux (ˈhaləks) the big toe. *H. valgus* a deformity in which the big toe is bent towards the other toes. *H. varus* a deformity in which the big toe is bent outwards away from the other toes.

halo (ˈhayloh) a circular structure, such as a luminous circle seen surrounding an object or light. *Glaucomatous h.*, *h. glaucomatosus* a narrow light zone surrounding the optic disc in glaucoma.

halo effect a beneficial effect noted following a health care intervention, visit or research project. The halo effect cannot be attributed to the content of the interview, visit or project but is the outcome of indefinable factors as a result of the intervention.

halo splint an orthopaedic device used to immobilize the head and neck to assist in the healing of cervical injuries and postoperatively following cervical surgery.

halogen (ˈhalə,jen, -lojən) one of the non-metallic elements chlorine, iodine, bromine and fluorine.

haloperidol (,halohˈperi,dol) a sedative and tranquillizer used in the treatment of schizophrenia and other psychiatric disorders, particularly mania.

halothane (ˈhaloh,thayn) a widely used anaesthetic; used as an inhalation to induce and maintain anaesthesia.

hamamelis (,haməˈmeelis) a soothing agent prepared from witch-hazel and used in suppository form in the treatment of haemorrhoids.

hamartoma (,hamahˈtohmə) a benign nodule which is an overgrowth of mature tissue.

hammer (ˈhamə) the malleus. *H.-toe* a deformity in which the first phalanx is bent upwards, with plantar flexion of the second and third phalanx.

hamstring (ˈham,string) the flexors of the knee joint that are situated at the back of the thigh.

hand (hand) the terminal part of the arm below the wrist. *Claw h.* a paralytic condition in which the hand is flexed and the fingers contracted, caused by injury to nerves or muscles. *Cleft h.* a congenital deformity in which the cleft between the 3rd and 4th fingers extends into the palm. *H., foot and mouth disease* a mild infectious disease in children caused by Coxsackie virus which results in vesicle formation on all three sites. Not the same as foot-and-mouth disease.

Hand–Schüller–Christian disease (,hand,shoolə'krischən) *A. Hand, American paediatrician, 1868–1949; A. Schüller, Austrian neurologist, b. 1874; H.A. Christian, American physician, 1876–1951.* A disease of the reticuloendothelial system in which granulomata containing cholesterol are formed, chiefly in the skull.

handicap ('handi,kap) a disadvantage for a given individual, resulting from an impairment or a disability that limits or prevents the fulfilment of a role that is normal (depending on age, sex, and social and cultural factors) for that individual.

Hansen's disease ('hansənz) *G.H.A. Hansen, Norwegian physician, 1841–1912.* Leprosy, caused by Hansen's bacillus, *Mycobacterium leprae*.

haploid ('haployd) having one set of chromosomes after division instead of two.

harelip ('hairlip) cleft lip, a congenital fissure in the upper lip, often accompanied by cleft palate. Outdated term.

Harris's operation ('harisiz) *S. Harris, Australian surgeon, 1880–1936.* Suprapubic transvesical prostatectomy.

Harrison's groove or **sulcus** ('haris'nz) *E. Harrison, British physician, 1789–1838.* A horizontal groove along the lower border of the thorax corresponding to the costal insertion of the diaphragm; seen in rickets.

Hartnup disease ('hahtnup) an hereditary defect in amino acid metabolism which may produce learning difficulties (named after the first person found to suffer from it).

Hashimoto's disease (,hashi-'mohtohz) *H. Hashimoto, Japanese surgeon, 1881–1934.* A lymphadenoid goitre caused by the formation of antibodies to thyroglobulin. It is an autoimmune condition giving rise to hypothyroidism.

hashish ('hasheesh, -ish) Indian hemp. *See* CANNABIS.

haustration (haw'strayshən) a haustrum, or the process of forming one.

haustrum ('hawstrəm) any one of the pouches formed by the sacculations of the colon.

haversian canal (hə'vərsi·ən, -shən) *C. Havers, British physician and anatomist, 1650–1702.* One of the minute canals which permeate compact bone, containing blood and lymph vessels to maintain its nutrition. *See* BONE.

Hawthorne effect ('hawthawn) the term given to the usual beneficial effect of a study on the persons participating in the study. It was named after an industrial management study in the USA, where the effect was first identified.

hay fever (hay) an atopic ALLERGY

characterized by sneezing, itching and watery eyes, running nose and a burning sensation of the palate and throat. It is a localized anaphylactic reaction to an extrinsic allergen, most commonly pollens and the spores of moulds. When the allergen comes in contact with mast cell-bound IgE immunoglobulin in the tissues of the conjunctiva, nasal mucosa and bronchial tree, the cells release mediators of ANAPHYLAXIS and produce the characteristic symptoms of hay fever.

HCG human chorionic gonadotrophin. *See* GONADOTROPHIN.

HEA Health Education Authority.

head (hed) the anterior or superior part of a structure or organism, in vertebrates containing the brain and the organs of special sense. *H. injury* traumatic injury to the head resulting from a fall or violent blow. Such an injury may be open or closed and may involve a brain CONCUSSION, skull fracture, or contusions of the brain. All head injuries are potentially dangerous because there may be a slow leakage of blood from damaged blood vessels into the brain, or the formation of a blood clot which gradually increases pressure against brain tissue. Long-term effects of head injury may include chronic headache, disturbances in mental and motor function, and a host of other symptoms that may or may not be psychogenic. Organic brain damage and post-traumatic epilepsy resulting from scar for-

mation are possible sequels to head injury.

headache ('hed,ayk) a pain or ache in the head. One of the most common ailments of man, a symptom rather than a disorder. It accompanies many diseases and conditions, including emotional distress. *See also* MIGRAINE.

Heaf test (heef) *FG.R. Heaf, British physician, 1894–1973.* A form of tuberculin testing. A drop of tuberculin solution on the skin is injected by means of a number of very short needles mounted on a spring-loaded device (Heaf's gun).

healing ('heeling) the process of return to normal function, after a period of disease or injury. *H. by first intention* signifies union of the edges of a clean incised wound without visible granulations, and leaving only a faint linear scar. *H. by second intention* is union of the edges of an open wound by the formation of granulations from the bottom and sides. *H. by third intention* is union of a wound that is closed surgically several days after the injury.

health (helth) the World Health Organization (WHO) states that 'Health is a state of complete physical, mental and social well-being and not merely the absence of disease or infirmity.' *H. centre* a community health organization for providing ambulatory health care and coordinating the efforts of all health agencies, commonly focused around the general practitioner's services. *Holistic h.* a system of preventive medicine that takes into account the whole individual, his own responsibility for his well-being, and the total influences (social, psychological, environmental) that affect health, including nutrition, exercise, and mental relaxation. *Public h.* the field of medicine that is concerned with safeguarding and improving the health of the community as a whole. *H. services* the term is usually employed to connote the system or programme by which health care is made available to the population and financed by government or private enterprise or both. *H.. statistics* summated data on any aspect of the health of populations, for example, mortality, morbidity, use of health services, treatment outcome, costs of health care.

health care system an organized plan of health services. The term usually is employed to denote the system or programme by which health care is made available to the population and financed by government or private enterprise or both.

health education various methods of education aimed at the prevention of disease. All nurses, midwives and health visitors have particular responsibilities and opportunities to promote good health.

health visitor a registered nurse who is also either a midwife or has undertaken a 12-week obstetric course and who has completed a 52-week course leading to a health visiting certificate.

The main area of responsibility of health visitors is health education and preventive care of mothers and children under five, although some specialize in school health and preventive care of the elderly.

hearing ('hiə·ring) the reception of sound waves and their transmission onwards to the brain in the form of nerve impulses. *H. aid* an apparatus, usually electronic, to amplify sounds before they reach the inner ear.

heart (haht) a hollow, muscular organ which pumps the blood throughout the body, situated behind the sternum slightly towards the left side of the thorax. *H. attack* myocardial infarction. *H. block* impairment of conduction in heart excitation; often applied specifically to atrioventricular heart block. *H. failure* may be acute, as in coronary thrombosis, or chronic. *H.–lung machine* an apparatus used to perform the functions of both the heart and the lungs during heart surgery. *H. murmur* an abnormal sound heard in the heart, frequently caused by disease of the valves. Occurs when the blood flow through the heart exceeds a certain velocity. *H. sounds* the sounds heard when listening to the heartbeat. They are caused by the closure of the valves.

heartburn ('haht,bərn) indigestion marked by a burning sensation in the oesophagus, often with regurgitation of acid fluid. Pyrosis.

heat (heet) warmth. A form of energy, which may cause an

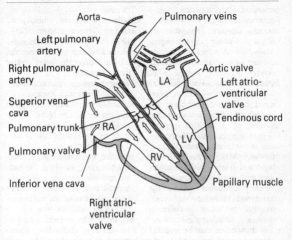

HEART

increase in temperature or a change of state, e.g. the conversion of water into steam. *H. exhaustion* a rapid pulse, anorexia, dizziness, cramps in arms, legs or abdomen and sometimes followed by sudden collapse, caused by loss of body fluids and salts under very hot conditions. *H.-stroke* a severe life-threatening condition resulting from prolonged exposure to heat. *See* SUN-STROKE. *Prickly h.* miliaria; heat rash. Acute itching caused by blocking of the ducts of the sweat glands following profuse sweating.

hebephrenia (ˌhebiˈfriːniˑə) a form of schizophrenia character-ized by thought disorder and emotional incongruity. Delusions and hallucinations are common.

Heberden's nodes (ˈhebəˌdɒnz) *W. Heberden, British physician, 1710–1801.* Bony or cartilaginous outgrowths causing deformity of the terminal finger joints in osteo-arthritis.

hebetude (ˈhebityood) emotional dullness. A common symptom in dementia and schizophrenia.

hectic (ˈhektik) occurring regularly. *H. fever* a regularly occurring increase in temperature; it is frequently observed in pulmonary tuberculosis. *H. flush* a redness of the face accompanying a sudden rise in temperature.

hedonism ('heedə‚nizəm, 'hed-) excessive devotion to pleasure.

Hegar's dilators ('haygahz) *A. Hegar, German gynaecologist, 1830–1914.* A series of graduate dilators used to dilate the uterine cervix.

Heimlich manoeuvre ('hiemlik) *H.J. Heimlich, American physician, b. 1920.* A technique for removing foreign matter from the trachea of a choking person. Wrap the arms around the person and allow their torso to hang forward. Make a fist with one hand and grasp it with the other, then with both hands against the victim's abdomen (above the navel and below the rib cage), forcefully press into the abdomen with a sharp upward thrust. The manoeuvre may be repeated several times if necessary to clear the air passages. If the victim is unconscious or prone, turn him on to his back, kneel astride his torso and with both hands use the manoeuvre as described.

Heine–Medin disease (‚hienə'-maydin) the major form of POLI-OMYELITIS.

heliotherapy (‚heelioh'therəpee) treatment of disease by exposure of the body to sunlight.

helium ('heeli·əm) *symbol* He. An inert gas sometimes used in conjunction with oxygen to facilitate respiration in obstructional types of dyspnoea and for decompressing deep-sea divers.

helix ('heeliks) 1. a spiral twist. Used to describe the configuration of certain molecules, e.g. deoxyribonucleic acid (DNA). 2. the outer rim of the auricle of the ear.

Heller's operation ('heləz) *E. Heller, German surgeon, 1877–1964.* An operation for the relief of cardiospasm by dividing the muscle coat at the lower end of the oesophagus.

helminthiasis (‚helmin'thieəsis) an infestation with worms.

hemeralopia (‚hemə·rə'lohpi·ə) day blindness. The vision is poor in a bright light but is comparatively good when the light is dim. *See* NYCTALOPIA.

hemianopia (‚hemi·ə'nohpi·ə) partial blindness, in which the patient can see only one half of the normal field of vision. It arises from disorders of the optic tract and of the occipital lobe.

hemiballismus (‚hemibə'lizməs) involuntary chorea-like movements on one side of the body only.

hemicolectomy (‚hemikoh'lektəmee) the removal of the ascending and part of the transverse colon with an ileotransverse colostomy.

hemiglossectomy (‚hemiglo'sektəmee) removal of approximately half the tongue.

hemiparesis (‚hemipə'reesis) paralysis on one side of the body; hemiplegia.

hemiplegia (‚hemi'pleeji·ə, -jə) paralysis of one half of the body, usually due to cerebral disease or injury. The lesion is on the side of the brain opposite to the side paralysed.

hemisphere ('hemi‚sfiə) a half sphere. In anatomy, one of the two halves of the cerebrum or cerebellum.

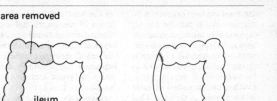

**HEMICOLECTOMY AND TRANSVERSE
ILEOCOLOSTOMY**

hemp (hemp) *see* CANNABIS.

henbane ('henbayn) *see* HYOSCY-
AMUS.

Henle's loop ('henleez) *F.G.J.
Henle, German anatomist, 1809–
1885.* The U-shaped loop of the
uriniferous tubule of the kidney.

Henoch's purpura (henokhs)
*E.H. Henoch, German paediatri-
cian, 1820–1910.* Allergic purpura. *See* PURPURA.

heparin ('hepə·rin) an anticoagulant formed in the liver and circu-
lated in the blood. Injected
intravenously it prevents the conversion of prothrombin into
thrombin, and is used in the
treatment of thrombosis.

hepatectomy (,hepə'tektəmee)
excision of a part or the whole
of the liver.

hepatic (hi'patik) relating to the
liver. *H. flexure* the angle of the
colon which is situated under the
liver.

hepaticojejunostomy (hi,patikoh-
,jejuh'nostəmee) the anastomosis
of the hepatic duct to the jejunum
usually following extensive excision for carcinoma of the pancreas.

hepaticostomy (hi,pati'kostəmee)
a surgical opening into the hepatic duct.

hepatitis (,hepə'tietis) inflammation of the liver. *Amoebic h.*
inflammation that may arise during amoebic dysentery and lead
to liver abscesses. *Anicteric h.*
viral hepatitis without jaundice,
tending to occur chiefly in infants
and young children; symptoms
include mild anorexia and gastrointestinal disturbances, slight
fever, and enlargement and tenderness of the liver. *Fulminant h.*
(acute hepatitis with coma) an
acute fulminating form of hepa-

titis resulting from extensive hepatic necrosis. It may be due to: (1) toxic liver injury, as in carbon tetrachloride poisoning or paracetamol overdosage; (2) a hypersensitivity reaction to a drug, such as halothane; or (3) viral hepatitis. Death is usually caused by acute yellow atrophy of the liver. *Viral h.* an acute, notifiable, infectious hepatitis caused by one of at least two different viral strains: hepatitis A virus (HAV) and hepatitis B virus (HBV). Type A hepatitis was formerly called infectious hepatitis, epidemic hepatitis, and acute catarrhal jaundice. Type B hepatitis was formerly called serum hepatitis and homologous serum jaundice.

hepatization (,hepətɪ'zayshən) the changing of lung tissue into a solid mass resembling liver which occurs in acute lobar pneumonia.

hepatocele ('hepətoh,seel) herniation of the liver through the abdominal wall or the diaphragm.

hepatocellular (,hepətoh'selyuhlə) referring to the cells of the liver.

hepatocirrhosis (,hepətohsɪ'rohsɪs) cirrhosis of the liver.

hepatogenous (,hepə'tojənəs) arising in the liver. Applied to jaundice where the disease arises in the parenchymal cells of the liver.

hepatolenticular ('hepətohlen-'tikyuhlə) pertaining to the liver and the lentiform nucleus. *H. degeneration* Wilson's disease; a progressive condition usually occurring between the ages of 10 and 25 years. There are tremors

of the head and limbs, pigmentation of the cornea and sometimes defective twilight vision.

hepatolithiasis (,hepətohlɪ'thiəsɪs) calculi formation in the liver.

hepatoma (,hepə'tohmə) a primary malignant tumour arising in the liver cells.

hepatomegaly (,hepətoh'megələe) an enlargement of the liver.

hepatosplenomegaly (,hepətoh-,spleenoh'megəlee) enlargement of the liver and spleen, such as may be found in kala-azar.

hepatotoxic (,hepətoh'toksik) applied to drugs and substances that cause destruction of liver cells.

herd immunity (hərd) the immunity of a population. When there is a high enough number of persons in a population immune to a particular infection, the infection fails to spread because of the absence of enough susceptibles. For example, in measles this could probably be achieved by vaccination of 90–95 per cent of the population.

hereditary (hi'reditə-ree) derived from ancestry; inherited.

heredity (hi,reditee) the transmission of both physical and mental characteristics to the offspring from the parents. Recessive characteristics may miss one or two generations and reappear later.

hermaphrodite (hər'mafrə,diet) an individual whose gonads contain both testicular and ovarian tissue. These may be combined as an ovotestis or there may be a testis on one side and an ovary on the other. The external genitalia may be indeterminate or of either sex. *Psuedo-h.* one whose gonads are histologically of one sex but in whom the genitalia have the appearance of the opposite sex. *True h.* one who possesses both male and female gonads.

hernia ('hərni·ə) a protrusion of any part of the internal organs through the structures enclosing them. *Cerebral h.* a protrusion of brain through the skull. *Diaphragmatic h.* and *hiatus h.* a protrusion of a part of the stomach through the oesophageal opening in the diaphragm. *Femoral h.* a loop of intestine protruding into the femoral canal. More common in females. *Incisional h.* a hernia occurring at the site of an old wound. *Inguinal h.* protrusion of the intestine through the inguinal canal. This may be congenital or acquired, and is commoner in males. A rupture. *Irreducible h.* a hernia that cannot be replaced by manipulation. *Reducible h.* a hernia that can be returned to its normal position by manipulative measures. *Strangulated h.* a hernia of the bowel in which the neck of the sac containing the bowel is so constricted that the venous circulation is impeded, and gangrene will result if not treated promptly. *Umbilical h.* protrusion of bowel through the umbilical ring. This may be congenital or acquired. *Vaginal h.* rectocele or cystocele.

hernioplasty ('hərnioh,plastee) a plastic repair of the abdominal wall performed after reducing a hernia.

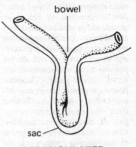

bowel

sac

STRANGULATED HERNIA

herniorrhaphy (,hərni'o·rəfee) removal of a hernial sac and repair of the abdominal wall.

herniotomy (,hərni'otəmee) an operation to remove a hernial sac.

heroin ('heroh·in) a diacetate of morphine used as an analgesic and abused illicitly for its euphoriant effects. The drug readily induces physical dependence and may be sniffed, smoked ('chasing the dragon') or injected subcutaneously or intravenously ('shooting up' or 'mainlining'). Slang terms for heroin include 'smack', 'H', and 'brown sugar'.

herpes ('hərpeez) an inflammatory skin eruption showing small vesicles caused by a herpes virus. *H. simplex* a viral infection which gives rise to localized vesicles in the skin and mucous membranes and is characterized by latency and subsequent recurrence. It is caused by herpes simplex viruses types 1 and 2. Type 1 infection is common in children and is often symptomless. Type 2 infection is common in older age groups and is associated with sexual activity. Lesions appear on the cervix, vulva, and surrounding skin in women and on the penis in men. In homosexual men rectal lesions are common. Recurrent genital herpes may follow primary infection. Type 2 virus may cause aseptic meningitis. *H. zoster* is a local manifestation of reactivation of infection of the varicella-zoster virus, the causative agent of chickenpox, characterized by a vesicular rash in the area of distribution of a sensory nerve. Called also shingles.

herpes virus ('hɜrpeez, vierəs) one of a group of DNA-containing viruses. They include the causative agents of herpes simplex, herpes zoster, chickenpox, cytomegalic inclusion disease and infective mononucleosis.

Herxheimer reaction ('hɜrks·hiemə) *K. Herxheimer, German dermatologist, 1861–1944.* An inflammatory reaction in the tissues in cases of syphilis, which can occur on starting treatment.

Hess's test ('hesiz) *A.F. Hess, American physician, 1875–1933.* A test used to diagnose purpura. An inflated blood pressure cuff causes an increase in capillary pressure and rupture of the walls, causing purpuric spots to develop.

heterochromia (,hetə·roh'krohmi·ə) a difference in colour in the irises of the two eyes or in different parts of one iris. It may be congenital or secondary due to inflammation.

heterogeneous (,hetəroh'jeeni·əs) composed of diverse constituents.

heterogenous (,hetə'rojənəs) derived from different sources.

heterophoria (,hetə·roh'for·ri·ə) a tendency to squint when fusion is interrupted. It occurs mainly when the person is tired or in poor health.

heterosexual (,hetə·roh'seksyoo·əl) 1. pertaining to, characteristic of, or directed towards the opposite sex. 2. a person with erotic interests directed towards the opposite sex.

heterotropia (,hetə·roh'trohpi·ə) a marked deviation of the eyes; strabismus or squint.

heterozygous (,hetə·roh'ziegəs) possessing dissimilar alternative genes for an inherited characteristic, one gene coming from each parent. One gene is dominant and the other is recessive.

hexachlorophane (,heksə'klor·rə'feen) a detergent and germicidal compound commonly incorporated in soaps and dermatological agents. Topical preparations have been associated with severe neurotoxicity and should not be used on children under 2 years except on medical advice. Avoid on large raw areas.

hexamine ('heksə,meen) methenamine; a urinary antiseptic which releases formaldehyde in an acid urine.

Hg symbol for *mercury* (L. *hydrargyrum*).

hiatus (hie'aytəs) a space or opening. *H. hernia* a protrusion of a part of the stomach through the oesophageal opening in the diaphragm.

hiccup ('hikup) hiccough; a spasmodic contraction of the diaphragm causing an abrupt inspiratory sound.

Hickman line ('hikmən ‚lien) trade name for a central venous line catheter.

hidrosis (hi'drohsis) the excretion of sweat.

high-altitude sickness (hie-'altityood) the condition resulting from difficulty in adjusting to diminished oxygen pressure at high altitudes. It may take the form of mountain sickness, high-altitude pulmonary oedema or cerebral oedema.

hilum ('hieləm) hilus; a recess in an organ, by which blood vessels, nerves and ducts enter and leave it.

hindbrain ('hiend‚brayn) that part of the brain consisting of the medulla oblongata, the pons and the cerebellum.

hip (hip) 1. the region of the body at the articulation of the femur and the innominate bone at the base of the lower trunk. These bones meet at the hip joint. Called also *coxa*. 2. loosely, the hip joint. *Total h. replacement* replacement of the femoral head and acetabulum with prostheses that are cemented into the bone; called also *total hip arthroplasty*. The procedure is done to replace a severely damaged arthritic hip joint.

hippus ('hipəs) alternate contraction and dilatation of the pupils. This occurs in various diseases of the nervous system, e.g. multiple sclerosis.

Hirschsprung's disease ('hərshspruhngz) *H. Hirschsprung, Danish physician, 1831–1916.* See MEGACOLON.

hirsute ('hərsyoot) hairy.

hirsutism ('hərsyoo‚tizəm) excessive hairiness.

hirudin (hi'roodin) the active principle in the secretion of the leech and certain snake venoms which prevents clotting of blood.

Hirudo (hi'roodoh) a genus of leeches. *H. medicinalis* the medical leech.

histamine ('histəmeen) an enzyme that causes local vasodilatation and increased permeability of the blood vessel walls. Readily released from body tissues, it is a factor in allergy response, greatly increases gastric secretion of hydrochloric acid and increases the heart rate. *H. test* 1. subcutaneous injection of 0.1 per cent solution of histamine to stimulate gastric secretion in order to measure maximal acid output. 2. after rapid intravenous injection of histamine phosphate, normal persons experience a brief fall in blood pressure, but in those with phaeochromocytoma, after the fall, there is a marked rise in blood pressure.

histidinaemia (‚histidi'neemi-ə) a hereditary metabolic defect marked by excessive histidine in the blood and urine due to deficient histidase activity; many affected persons show mild mental handicap and disordered speech development.

histidine ('histi‚deen) one of the 9 essential amino acids formed by the digestion of dietary protein. Histamine is derived from it.

histiocyte ('histioh,siet) a stationary macrophage of connective tissue. Derived from the reticuloendothelial cells, it acts as a scavenger, removing bacteria from the blood and tissues.

histiocytoma (,histiohsie'tohmə) a tumour containing histiocytes causing a vascular nodule.

histiocytosis (,histiohsie'tohsis) a group of diseases of bone in which granulomata containing histiocytes and eosinophil cells appear. *See* LETTERER–SIWE DISEASE and HAND–SCHÜLLER–CHRISTIAN DISEASE.

histocompatibility (,histohkəm-,patə'bilitee) the ability of cells to be accepted and to function in a new situation. Tissue typing reveals this and ensures a higher success rate in organ transplantation.

histogram ('histə,gram) a bar-chart. Statistical values are expressed as blocks on a graph.

histology (hi'stoləjee) the science dealing with the minute structure, composition and function of tissues.

histolysis (hi'stolisis) the disintegration of tissues.

histoplasmosis (,histohplaz'mohsis) infection caused by inhalation of the spores of a yeast-like fungus, *Histoplasma capsulatum*. Usually symptomless, the infection may progress and produce a condition resembling tuberculosis.

HIV human immunodeficiency virus.

hives (hievz) urticaria.

Hodge pessary (,hoj 'pesə·ree) *H.L. Hodge, American gynaecologist, 1796–1873.* A pessary which is used to maintain the position of the uterus following correction of a retroversion. *See* PESSARY.

Hodgkin's disease ('hojkinz) *T. Hodgkin, British physician, 1798–1866.* Lymphadenoma, a malignant condition of the reticuloendothelial cells. There is progressive enlargement of lymph nodes and lymph tissue all over the body. Treated by radiotherapy and cytotoxic drugs. This disease has a good prognosis.

Hofmann reaction ('hofman ri,akshə) chemical inactivation, without the activity of enzymes, of compounds that occur spontaneously in the blood.

Hogben test ('hogbən ,test, 'hohbən) a pregnancy test, rarely used since the immunological tests were introduced, in which pregnancy urine is injected into the dorsal lymph sac of the *Xenopus* toad. If gonadotrophic hormone is present in the urine, the toad will ovulate in about 8–15 hours after the injection. The test is then said to be positive for pregnancy.

holism ('hohlizəm) a philosophy in which the person is considered as a functioning whole rather than as a composite of several systems.

holistic (hoh'listik) pertaining to holism.

Homans' sign ('hohmənz) *J. Homans, American surgeon, 1877–1954.* Pain elicited in the calf when the foot is dorsiflexed.

Indicative of venous thrombosis.

homatropine (hoh'matrə,pin) a short-acting mydriatic used in ophthalmology to dilate the pupil and so allow a better view of the fundus of the eye.

home help service (,hohm 'help ,sərvis) a branch of the social services department, which provides domestic and housekeeping assistance to those in need. It is on either a short-term or long-term basis, and payment is according to means. Maternity cases are a priority.

homeopathy (,hohmi'opəthee) a system of medicine promulgated by C.F.S. Hahnemann (*German physician, 1755–1843*) and based upon the principle that 'like cures like'. Remedies are given which can produce in the patient the symptoms of the disease to be cured, but they are administered in minute doses.

homeostasis (,hohmioh'staysis, ,hom-) a tendency of biological systems to maintain stability while continually adjusting to conditions that are optimal for survival.

homicide ('homi,sied) the killing of a human being. *Culpable h.* covers murder (malice aforethought), manslaughter (without malice aforethought), causing death by reckless driving, and infanticide. *Non-culpable h.* covers justifiable homicide (e.g. lawful execution) and excusable homicide (misadventure or accident). *See* MCNAGHTEN'S RULES.

homogeneous (,homə'jeeni-əs) uniform in character. Similar in nature and characteristics.

homogenize (ho'mojə,niez) to make homogeneous. To reduce to the same consistency.

homogenous (ho'mojənəs) derived from the same source.

homograft ('homə,grahft, 'homoh-) a tissue or organ transplanted from one individual to another of the same species. An allograft.

homolateral (,homə'latə-rəl, ,hohmoh-) on the same side; ipsilateral.

homologous (hə'moləgəs) 1. in anatomy, having the same embryological origin although performing a different function. 2. in chemistry, possessing a similar structure. *H. chromosomes* those that pair during meiosis and contain an identical arrangement of genes in the DNA pattern.

homologue ('homə,log) a part or organ which has the same relative position or structure as another one.

homoplasty ('homoh,plastee, 'hohm-) surgical replacement of defective tissues with a homograft.

homosexual (,homoh'seksyooəl, ,hohm-) 1. of the same sex. 2. a person who is sexually attracted to a person of the same sex.

homosexuality (,homoh,seksyoo-'alitee, ,hohm-) sexual and emotional orientation toward persons of the same sex.

homozygous (,homoh'ziegəs) possessing an identical pair of genes for an inherited characteristic. *See* HETEROZYGOUS.

hookworm ('huhk,wərm) *see* ANCYLOSTOMA.

hordeolum (hordi'ohləm) a stye; inflammation of the sebaceous glands of the eyelashes.

hormone ('hawmohn) a chemical substance which is generated in one organ and carried by the blood to another, in which it excites activity.

Horner's syndrome ('hawnəz) *J.F. Horner, Swiss ophthalmologist, 1831–1886.* A condition in which there is a lesion on the path of sympathetic nerve fibres in the cervical region. The symptoms include enophthalmos, ptosis, a contracted pupil and a decrease in sweating.

Horton's syndrome ('hawtənz) *B.T. Horton, American physician, b. 1895.* Severe headache caused by the release of histamine in the body or by its administration. Histamine cephalalgia.

hospice ('hospis) the concept of hospice is that of a caring community of professional and non-professional people, together with the family. Emphasis is on dealing with emotional and spiritual problems as well as the medical problems of the terminally ill. Of primary concern is control of pain and other symptoms, keeping the patient at home for as long as possible or desirable, and making the remaining days as comfortable and meaningful as possible. After the patient dies, family members are given support throughout their period of bereavement.

hospital ('hospit'l) an institution for the care and treatment of the sick and injured. *H.-acquired infection* see hospital-acquired INFECTION. *H. activity analysis* abbreviated HAA. A system for collecting, on Regional Heath Authority computers, a series of data items for each patient discharged from hospital in the region, and the source of a national sample, the Hospital Inpatient Enquiry (HIPE). HAA and HIPE were superseded in 1987 by systems based on KÖRNER DATA SETS.

host (hohst) the animal, plant or tissue on which a parasite lives and multiplies. *Definitive* or *final h.* one that harbours the parasite during its adult sexual stage. *Intermediate h.* one that shelters the parasite during a non-reproductive period.

hour-glass contraction ('owə-‚glahs kən‚trakshən) a contraction near the middle of a hollow organ, such as the stomach or uterus, producing an outline resembling that shape.

housemaid's knee ('howsmaydz) prepatellar bursitis; inflammation of the prepatellar bursa, which becomes distended with serous fluid.

humidity (hyoo'miditee) the degree of moisture in the air. *H. therapy* the therapeutic use of water to prevent or correct a moisture deficit in the respiratory tract. The principal reasons for employing humidity therapy are: (1) to prevent drying and irritation of the respiratory mucosa; (2) to facilitate ventilation and diffusion of oxygen and other therapeutic gases being administered; and (3) to aid in the removal of thick and viscous secretions that obstruct the air passages. Another important use of water aerosol therapy is to aid in obtaining an induced sputum specimen.

humour ('hyoomə) any fluid of the body, such as lymph or blood. *Aqueous h.* the fluid filling the anterior chamber of the eye. *Vitreous h.* the jelly-like substance which fills the chamber of the eye between the lens and the retina.

Huntington's chorea (disease) ('huntingtənz) *G.S. Huntington, American physician, 1851–1927.* A rare, degenerative inherited disorder of the brain in which there is progressive chorea and mental deterioration (dementia).

Hurler's syndrome (,hɜrlərz) *G. Hurler, Austrian paediatrician.* An inherited disorder in which learning difficulties are caused by excess mucopolysaccharides being stored in the brain and reticuloendothelial system. Gargoylism.

Hutchinson's teeth ('hutchinsənz) *Sir J. Hutchinson, British surgeon, 1828–1913.* Typical notching of the borders of the permanent incisor teeth occurring in congenital syphilis.

hyaline ('hiə,lien) resembling glass. *H. degeneration* a form of deterioration which occurs in tumours due to deficiency of blood supply. It precedes cystic degeneration. *H. membrane disease see* RESPIRATORY DISTRESS SYNDROME.

hyaluronidase (,hiəəlyuh'roni,dayz) an enzyme which facilitates the absorption of fluids in subcu-

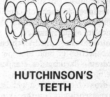

HUTCHINSON'S TEETH

taneous tissues. It is found in the testes of mammals, and a preparation of it is particularly used with subcutaneous infusions to promote absorption.

hydatid ('hiedətid) a cystic swelling containing the embryo of *Echinococcus granulosus.* It may be found in any organ of the body, e.g. in the liver. 'Daughter cysts' are produced from the original. Infection is from contaminated foods, e.g. salads. *H. disease* the result of the presence of hydatids in the lungs, liver or brain.

hydatidiform (,hiedə'tidi,fawm) resembling an hydatid cyst. *H. mole see* MOLE.

hydraemia (hie'dreemi·ə) a modification of the blood in which there is an excess of plasma in relation to the cells. A degree of this is physiological in pregnancy.

hydragogue ('hiedrə,gog) a purgative causing copious liquid evacuations, e.g. magnesium sulphate, jalap.

hydralazine (hie'dralə,zeen) a vasodilator and antihypertensive agent used to lower blood pressure.

hydramnios (hie'dramnios) an excessive amount of amniotic fluid in the uterus in the later months of pregnancy.

hydrarthrosis (,hiedrah'throhsis) a collection of fluid in a joint.

hydrate ('hiedrayt) a compound of an element with water.

hydroa (hie'droh·ə) a childhood hypersensitivity of the skin to sunlight, resulting in the formation of a vesicular eruption on the exposed parts, with intense irritation.

hydrocarbon (,hiedroh'kahbən) a compound of hydrogen and carbon. Fats are of this type.

hydrocele ('hiedrə,seel) a swelling caused by accumulation of fluid, especially in the tunica vaginalis surrounding the testicle.

hydrocephalus (,hiedroh'kefələs, -'sef-) 'water on the brain'. Enlargement of the skull due to an abnormal collection of cerebrospinal fluid around the brain or in the ventricles. It may be either congenital or acquired from inflammation of the meninges during infancy. The most effective treatment is surgical correction employing a shunting technique. It frequently accompanies spina bifida.

hydrochloric acid (,hiedrə-'klo·rik, -'klor·rik) HCl, a colourless compound of hydrogen and chlorine. In 0.2, solution it is present in gastric juice and aids digestion.

hydrochlorothiazide (,hiedrə ,klor·roh'thieə,zied) a valuable oral diuretic similar to but more potent than chlorothiazide. It is used in the treatment of oedema and hypertension.

hydrocortisone (,hiedroh'kawti,zohn) cortisol, the principal GLUCOCORTICOID secreted by the adrenal gland; it is used in the treatment of inflammations, allergies, pruritus, collagen diseases, adrenocortical insufficiency, severe status asthmaticus, shock and certain neoplasms.

hydrocyanic acid (,hiedrohsie'anik) a highly poisonous acid. In liquid or gaseous form it can be fatal within minutes. It smells of bitter almonds. Prussic acid.

hydroflumethiazide (,hiedroh,floomi'thieə,zied) an oral thiazide diuretic used in the treatment of oedema and hypertension.

hydrogen ('hiedrəjən) *symbol* H. A combustible gas, present in nearly all organic compounds which, in combination with oxygen, forms water. *H. ion concentration* the amount of hydrogen in a liquid, which is responsible for its acidity. The degree of acidity is expressed in pH values, and the higher the hydrogen ion concentration, the greater the acidity, and the lower the pH value. The concentration in the blood is of importance in acidosis. *H. peroxide*, H_2O_2, a strong disinfectant cleansing and bleaching liquid used, diluted in water, for cleansing wounds.

hydrolysis (hie'drolisis) the process of splitting up into smaller molecules by uniting with water.

hydrometer (hie'dromitə) an instrument for estimating the specific gravity of fluids, e.g. a urinometer.

hydromyelia ('hiedrohmie'eeli·ə) a dilatation of the central canal of the spinal cord caused by an accumulation of cerebrospinal fluid.

hydronephrosis (,hiedrohnə'frohsis) an accumulation of urine in the pelvis of the kidney, resulting in atrophy of the kidney structure, due to an obstruction to the flow of urine from the kidney. The condition may be: (1) congenital, due to malformation of the kidney or ureter; or (2) acquired, due to an obstruction of the ureter by tumour or stone, or to back pressure from stricture of the urethra or an enlarged prostate gland.

hydropathy (hie'dropəthee) the treatment of disease by the use of water internally and externally; hydrotherapy.

hydropericarditis (,hiedroh,perikah'dietis) inflammation of the pericardium resulting in serous fluid in the pericardial sac.

hydroperitoneum (,hiedroh,peritə'neeəm) *see* ASCITES.

hydrophobia (,hiedrə'fohbi·ə) 1. rabies. 2. irrational fear of water.

hydropneumothorax (,hiedroh,nyoomoh'thor·raks) the presence of fluid and air in the pleural space.

hydrops ('hiedrops) [L.] abnormal accumulation of serous fluid in the tissues or in a body cavity; called also dropsy. *Fetal h., h. fetalis* gross oedema of the entire body of the newborn infant, occurring in haemolytic disease of the newborn.

hydrosalpinx (,hiedroh'salpingks) distension of the uterine tubes by fluid.

hydrotherapy (,hiedroh'therəpee) the treatment of disease by means of water.

hydrothorax (,hiedroh'thor·raks) fluid in the pleural cavity due to serous effusion as in cardiac, renal and other diseases.

hydroureter ('hiedroh·yuh'reetə) an accumulation of water or urine in a ureter.

hydroxytryptamine (hie,droksi-'triptə,meen) serotonin.

hydroxyurea (hie,droksiyuh'reeə) an orally active cytotoxic agent used mainly in the treatment of melanoma, resistant chronic myelocytic leukaemia, and recurrent, metastatic or inoperable ovarian carcinoma.

hygiene ('hiejeen) 1. the science of health and its preservation. 2. a condition or practice, such as cleanliness, that is conducive to preservation of health. *Communal h.* the maintenance of the health of the community by the provision of a pure water supply, efficient sanitation, good housekeeping, etc. *Industrial h.* (occupational health) care of the health of workers in the industry. *Mental h.* the science dealing with development of healthy mental and emotional reactions and habits. *Oral h.* the proper care of the mouth and teeth. *Personal h.* individual measures taken to preserve one's own health.

hygroma (hie'grohmə) a swelling caused by fluid. *Cystic h.* a cystic lymphangioma of the neck. *Subdural h.* a collection of clear fluid in the subdural space.

hygrometer (hie'gromitə) an instrument for measuring the water vapour in the air.

hygroscopic (,hiegroh'skopik) readily absorbing moisture. An example is glycerin, which is used in suppositories as a means of aiding evacuation by moistening the faeces.

hymen ('hiemen) a fold of mucous membrane partially closing the entrance to the vagina. *Imperforate h.* a membrane which completely occludes the vaginal orifice.

hymenectomy (,hiemə,nektəmee) the surgical removal of the hymen.

hymenotomy (,hiemə'notəmee) a surgical incision of the hymen.

hyoid ('hieoyd) shaped like a U. *H. bone* a U-shaped bone above the thyroid cartilage, to which the tongue is attached.

hyoscine ('hieə,seen) scopolamine; an anticholinergic drug used as an anaesthetic premedicant, antispasmodic, and in the treatment of motion sickness. Should be avoided in the elderly because of its tendency to cause restlessness and confusion (central cholinergic syndrome).

hyoscyamus (,hieoh'sieəməs) henbane. The dried leaves have an antispasmodic action which relieves the griping pain of excessive peristalsis.

hypaesthesia (,hiepis'theezi-ə) impairment of the sense of touch.

hypalgesia (,hiepal'jeezi-ə) a decrease in sensitivity to pain.

hypamnios (hiep'amnios) a deficiency of fluid in the amniotic sac.

hyperacidity (,hiepə-rə'siditee) excessive acidity. *Gastric h.* hyperchlorhydria.

hyperactive (,hiepə'raktiv) exhibiting hyperactivity; hyperkinetic.

hyperactivity (,hiepə-rak'tivitee) abnormally increased activity. Developmental hyperactivity of children (hyperkinesia) is characterized by very restless, impulsive behaviour. These children are usually inattentive and have a poor concentration span. Other features which may be associated with hyperactivity include aggression, anxiety, poor eating and sleeping patterns, and social and learning difficulties.

hyperaemia (,hiepə'reemi-ə) excess of blood in any part.

hyperaesthesia (,hiepə-ris'theezi-ə) excessive sensitiveness to touch or to other sensations, e.g. taste or smell.

hyperalgesia (,hiepə-ral'jeezi-ə) excessive sensibility to pain.

hyperalimentation (,hiepə,rali-men'tayshən) a programme of parenteral administration of all nutrients for patients with gastrointestinal dysfunction; also called total parenteral alimentation (TPA) and total parenteral nutrition (TPN). Although the term hyperalimentation is commonly used to designate total or supplementary nutrition by intravenous feedings, it is not technically correct inasmuch as the procedure does not involve an abnormally increased or excessive amount of feeding. *See* parenteral NUTRITION.

hyperasthenia (ˌhiepə·ras'thee-ni·ə) extreme weakness.

hyperbaric (ˌhiepə'barik) at a greater pressure than normal; applied to gases under greater than atmospheric pressure. *H. oxygenation* exposure to oxygen under conditions of greatly increased pressure. The patient is placed in a sealed enclosure, called a hyperbaric chamber. Compressed air is introduced, at the same time the patient is given pure oxygen through a face mask. Patients suffering from tetanus and gas gangrene, infections caused by bacteria that are resistant to antibiotics but vulnerable to oxygen, are helped by hyperbaric oxygenation. The technique is also useful in radiotherapy for cancer. When full of oxygen, cancer cells seem more vulnerable to radiation. Carbon monoxide poisoning can be treated by hyperbaric oxygenation. Carbon monoxide molecules, displacing the oxygen in the erythrocytes, usually cause asphyxiation, but hyperbaric oxygenation can often keep the patient alive until the carbon monoxide has been eliminated from his system.

hyperbilirubinaemia (ˌhiepə,bili-ˌroobi'neemi·ə) an excess of bilirubin in the blood.

hypercalcaemia (ˌhiepəkal'seemi·ə) an excess of calcium in the blood. May be caused by overadministration of vitamin D, hyperparathyroidism, thyrotoxicosis, breakdown of bone by malignant disease, or impaired renal function.

hypercalciuria (ˌhiepəˌkalsi'yooə-

·ri·ə) a high level of calcium in the urine leading to renal stone formation.

hypercapnia (ˌhiepə'kapni·ə) an increased amount of carbon dioxide in the blood causing overstimulation of the respiratory centre. Hypercarbia.

hypercatabolism (ˌhiepəkə'tabə-ˌlizəm) an excessive rate of catabolism leading to wasting or destruction of a part or tissue.

hyperchloraemia (ˌhiepə,klo'reemi·ə) an excess of chloride in the blood.

hyperchlorhydria (ˌhiepəklor'hiedri·ə) an excess of hydrochloric acid in the gastric juice.

hypercholesteraemia, hypercholesterolaemia (ˌhiepəkəˌlestə-'reemi·ə; ˌhiepəkəˌlestə·ro'leemi·ə) excess of cholesterol in the blood. Predisposes to atheroma and gallstones.

hypercusis (ˌhiepə'kyoosis) excessive sensitivity to sound.

hyperdynamia (ˌhiepədie'nami·ə) excessive muscle activity. *H. uteri* excessive uterine contractions in labour.

hyperemesis (ˌhiepə'remɘsis) excessive vomiting. *H. gravidarum* an uncommon, serious complication of pregnancy, characterized by severe and persistent vomiting, the aetiology of which is not fully understood.

hyperextension (ˌhiepə·rek'stenshən) the forcible extension of a limb beyond the normal. It is used to correct orthopaedic deformities.

hyperflexion (ˌhiepə'flekshən) the forcible bending of a joint beyond the normal.

hypergalactia, hypergalactosis (,hiepəgə'lakti·ə; ,hiepə,galək-'tohsis) excessive secretion of milk.

hypergammaglobulinaemia (,hiepə,gamə,globyuhli'neemi·ə) increased gamma-globulins in the blood.

hyperglycaemia (,hiepəglie'seemi·ə) excess of sugar in the blood (normal 2.5–4.7 mmol/litre when fasting); a sign of diabetes mellitus.

hyperhidrosis (,hiepəhi'drohsis) excessive perspiration; hyperidrosis.

hyperinsulinism (,hiepə'insyuhli-,nizəm) 1. excessive secretion of insulin. 2. shock produced by an overdose of insulin.

hyperkalaemia (,hiepəkə'leemi·ə) an excess of potassium in the blood. If untreated, this will lead to cardiac arrest.

hyperkeratosis (,hiepə,kerə'tohsis) hypertrophy of the horny layers of the skin.

hyperkinesis (,hiepəki'neesis) a condition in which there is excessive motor activity. *See* HYPERACTIVITY.

hyperlipaemia (,hiepəli'peemi·ə) an excess of fat or lipids in the blood.

hypermastia (,hiepə'masti·ə) 1. the presence of one or more supernumerary breasts. 2. overdevelopment of one or both breasts.

hypermetropia (,hiepəme'trohpi·ə) hyperopia; long-sightedness. The light rays entering the eye converge beyond the retina. Clear vision can be obtained by the wearing of spectacles or contact lenses.

hypermotility (,hiepəmoh'tilitee) excessive movement. *Gastric h.* increased muscle action of the stomach wall, associated with increased secretion of hydrochloric acid.

hypernatraemia (,hiepənə'treemi·ə) an excess of sodium in the blood, usually diagnosed when the plasma sodium is above 150 mmol/litre. Due to loss of water and electrolytes from the body caused by diarrhoea, polyuria, excessive sweating or inadequate fluid intake. May also occur in infants if excessive salt has been added to feeds, resulting in convulsions and brain damage.

hypernephroma (,hiepəne'frohmə) a malignant tumour of the kidney; renal cell carcinoma.

hyperostosis (,hiepə·ro'stohsis) a thickening of bone; a bony outgrowth; exostosis.

hyperparathyroidism (,hiepə,parə'thieroy,dizəm) excessive activity of the parathyroid glands, causing drainage of calcium from the bones, with consequent fragility and liability to spontaneous fracture.

hyperphagia (,hiepə'fayji·ə) overeating.

hyperphasia (,hiepə'fayzi·ə) excessive talkativeness.

hyperphenylalaninaemia (,hiepə,feenie,laləni'neemi·ə) an excess of phenylalanine in the blood, as in phenylketonuria.

hyperpituitarism (,hiepəpi'tyooitə,rizəm) overactivity of the pituitary gland.

hyperplasia (,hiepə'playzi·ə) excessive formation of normal cells in a tissue or organ, which increases in size.

hyperpnoea ('hiepə'neeə, -pəp-'neeə) over-breathing; hyperventilation; an abnormal increase in the rate and depth of breathing.

hyperprolactinaemia (ˌhiepə-proh,lakti'neemi·ə) increased levels of prolactin in the blood; in women, it is associated with infertility and may lead to galactorrhoea, and it has been reported to cause impotence in men.

hyperpyrexia (ˌhiepəpie'reksi·ə) an excessively high body temperature, i.e. over 41°C.

hypersensitivity (ˌhiepə'sensi'tivitee) abnormal sensitivity, especially to a particular antigen. The reactions include allergies (such as asthma) and anaphylaxis. *Contact h.* produced by contact of the skin with a chemical substance having the properties of an antigen or hapten; it includes CONTACT DERMATITIS. *Delayed h.* a slowly developing increase in cell-mediated immune response (involving T-lymphocytes) to a specific antigen, as occurs in graft rejection, autoimmune disease, etc. *Immediate h.* antibody-mediated hypersensitivity characterized by lesions resulting from release of histamine and other mediators of hypersensitivity from reagin-sensitized mast cells, causing increased vascular permeability, oedema, and smooth muscle contraction; it includes anaphylaxis and atopy.

hypersplenism (ˌhiepə'splenizəm) overactivity of an enlarged spleen resulting in the destruction of blood cells and platelets.

hypertelorism (ˌhiepə'telə,rizəm) abnormally increased distance between two organs or parts. *Ocular h., orbital h.* increase in the interocular distance, often associated with craniofacial dysostosis and sometimes with mental handicap.

hypertension (ˌhiepə'tenshən) persistently high BLOOD PRESSURE. In adults, it is generally agreed that a blood pressure is abnormally high when the resting, supine arterial systolic pressure is equal to or greater than 140 mmHg and the diastolic pressure is equal to or greater than 90 mmHg. A diagnosis of hypertension should be based on a series of readings rather than a single measurement. *Essential h.* high blood pressure without demonstrable change in kidneys, blood vessels or heart. *Malignant h.* a form of hypertension which may develop at a comparatively early age, in which the prognosis is poor. *Portal h.* raised pressure in the portal system. *Pulmonary h.* increased pressure in the arteries of the lung, usually following emphysema or fibrosis.

hyperthermia (ˌhiepə'thərmi·ə) an exceedingly high body temperature. *Malignant h.* a serious condition sometimes arising during general anaesthesia.

hyperthymia (ˌhiepə'thiemi·ə) excessive emotionalism with a tendency for the individual to be impulsive.

hyperthyroidism (ˌhiepə'thieroy-,dizəm) excessive activity of the thyroid gland. *See* THYROTOXICOSIS.

hypertonic (,hiepə'tonik) 1. showing excessive tone or tension, as in a blood vessel or muscle. 2. describing a solution that has greater osmotic pressure than another with which it is compared. Hypertonic saline has a greater osmotic pressure than normal physiological tissue fluid.

hypertrichosis (,hiepətri'kohsis) excessive growth of hair on any part of the body.

hypertrophy (hie'pərtrəfee) an increase in the size of a tissue or a structure caused by an increase in the size of the cells that compose it (as opposed to an increase in the number of cells). *See* HYPERPLASIA.

hyperuricaemia (,hiepə,yoo·ri-'seemi·ə) an excess of uric acid in the blood. *See* GOUT.

hyperventilation (,hiepə,venti-'layshən) 1. increase of air in the lungs above the normal amount. 2. abnormally prolonged and deep breathing, usually associated with acute anxiety or emotional tension. Hyperpnoea.

hypervitaminosis (,hiepə,vitəmi-'nohsis) a condition caused by the intake of an excessive quantity of vitamins, particularly vitamins A and D.

hypervolaemia (,hiepovo'leemi·ə) abnormal increase in the volume of circulating fluid (plasma) in the body.

hyphaema (hie'feemi·ə) haemorrhage into the anterior chamber of the eye.

hypnosis (hip'nohsis) an artificially induced passive state in which there is increased amenability and responsiveness to suggestions and commands. In hypnosis, a drowsy phase is followed by a sleep. It may also be used to produce painless childbirth and tooth extraction.

hypnotherapy (,hipnoh'therəpee) treatment by hypnosis or by the induction of prolonged sleep.

hypnotic (hip'notik) an agent which causes sleep; a soporific.

hypnotism ('hipnə,tizəm) the practice of hypnosis.

hypoaesthesia (,hiepoh·is'theez-i·ə) hypaesthesia.

hypoalgesia (,hiepoh·al'jeezi·ə) hypalgesia.

hypobaric (,hiepoh'barik) at a pressure lower than normal.

hypocalcaemia (,hiepohkal'seemi·ə) a deficiency of calcium in the blood.

hypocapnia (,hiepoh'kapni·ə) a deficiency of carbon dioxide in the blood.

hypochloraemia (,hiepohklo'reemi·ə) a deficiency of chloride in the blood.

hypochlorhydria (,hiepohklor'hiedri·ə) a less than normal amount of hydrochloric acid in the gastric juice.

hypochlorite (,hiepoh'klor·riet) any salt of hypochlorous acid used in solution to yield chlorine, a disinfecting and germicidal agent. Widely used in skin care for wound and ulcer cleansing, e.g. Dakin's solution and eusol. Milton, a proprietary preparation, is used in solution for the disinfection of equipment and infant feeding utensils.

hypochondria (,hiepə'kondri·ə) a

morbid preoccupation or anxiety about one's health. The sufferer feels that first one part of his body and then another part is the seat of some serious disease.

hypochondriac (,hiepə'kondri,ak) one affected by hypochondria. *H. region* the hypochondrium.

hypochondrium (,hiepoh'kondri·əm) the upper region of the abdomen on each side of the epigastrium.

hypochromic (,hiepoh'krohmik) deficient in pigmentation or colouring.

hypodermic (,hiepə'dərmik) beneath the skin; applied to subcutaneous injections and to the syringes used for such injections.

hypofibrinogenaemia (,hiepohfie,brinəjə'neemi·ə) a lack of fibrinogen in the blood. This may occur in severe trauma or haemorrhage or as an inherited condition.

hypogammaglobulinaemia (,hiepoh,gamə,globyuhli'neemi·ə) a deficiency of gamma-globulin in the blood rendering the person susceptible to infection.

hypogastrium (,hiepoh'gastri·əm) the lower middle area of the abdomen, immediately below the umbilical region.

hypoglossal (,hiepoh'glos'l) under the tongue. *H. nerve* the twelfth cranial nerve.

hypoglycaemia (,hiepohglie'seemi·ə) a condition in which the blood-sugar level is less than normal. Usually arising in diabetic patients due to insulin overdosage, delay in eating, or a rapid combustion of carbohydrate. *See* HYPERGLYCAEMIA.

hypokalaemia (,hiepohkə'leemi·ə) a low potassium level in the blood. This is likely to be present in dehydration and with the repeated use of diuretics.

hypomania (,hiepoh'mayni·ə) a degree of elation, excitement and activity higher than normal but less severe than that present in mania.

hypomastia (,hiepoh'masti·ə) underdevelopment of the breasts.

hypometropia (,hiepohme'trohpi·ə) myopia; short-sightedness.

hypomotility (,hiepohmoh'tilitee) deficient power of movement in any part.

hyponatraemia (,hiepohnə'treemi·ə) a deficiency of sodium in the blood.

hypoparathyroidism (,hiepoh,parə'thieroy'dizəm) a lack of parathyroid secretion leading to a low blood calcium and tetany.

hypophysectomy (hie,pofi'sektəmee) excision of the pituitary gland.

hypophysis (hie'pofisis) an outgrowth. *H. cerebri* the pituitary gland.

hypopiesis (,hiepohpie'eesis) abnormally low blood pressure.

hypopituitarism (,hiepohpi'tyooitə,rizəm) deficiency of secretion from the anterior lobe of the pituitary gland, causing excessive deposit of fat in children. *See* FRÖLICH'S SYNDROME. Dwarfism may result. In adults asthenia, drowsiness and adiposity may occur, together with an impairment of sexual activity and premature senility.

hypoplasia (,hiepoh'playzi·ə) imperfect development of a part or organ.

hypopnoea (,hiepoh'neeǝ,-'pop-ni-ǝ) shallow breathing.

hypoproteinaemia (,hiepoh,proh-ti'neemi-ǝ) a deficiency of serum proteins in the blood.

hypoprothrombinaemia (,hie-pohproh,thrombi'neemi-ǝ) a deficiency of prothrombin in the blood leading to a tendency to bleed. *See* HAEMOPHILIA.

hypopyon (hie'pohpi-ǝn) an accumulation of pus in the anterior chamber of the eye.

hyposecretion (,hiepohsi'kree-shǝn) a deficiency in secretion from any glandular structure or secreting cells.

hyposensitivity (,hiepoh,sensi-'tivitee) a lack of sensitivity, especially to a particular allergen with which the patient may have been overdosed over a period.

hypospadias (,hiepǝ'spaydi-ǝs) a developmental anomaly in the male in which the urethra opens on the under side of the penis or on the perineum. *Female h.* a developmental anomaly in the female in which the urethra opens into the vagina.

hypostasis (,hie'postǝsis) 1. a sediment or deposit. 2. congestion of blood in a part, due to slowing of the circulation.

hypostatic (,hiepoh'statik) relating to hypostasis. *H. pneumonia see* PNEUMONIA.

hyposthenia (,hiepǝs'theeni-ǝ) weakness; decreased strength.

hypotension (,hiepoh'tenshǝn) abnormally low arterial blood pressure; hypopiesis. *Controlled* or *induced h.* an artificially produced lowering of the blood pres-

sure so that an operation field is rendered practically bloodless. *Orthostatic* or *postural h.* temporary hypotension when the patient stands up, producing giddiness and sometimes a faint.

hypotensive (,hiepoh'tensiv) producing a reduction in tension, especially pertaining to a drug that lowers the blood pressure.

hypothalamus (,hiepǝ'thalǝmǝs) the portion of the diencephalon lying beneath the thalamus at the base of the cerebrum, and forming the floor and part of the lateral wall of the third ventricle. It influences peripheral autonomic mechanisms, endocrine activity, and many somatic functions, e.g. a general regulation of water balance, body temperature, sleep, thirst and hunger, and the development of secondary sexual characteristics. It plays an important role in the regulation of protein, fat, and carbohydrate metabolism, body fluid volume and electrolyte content, and internal secretion of endocrine hormones.

hypothermia (,hiepoh'thǝrmi-ǝ) 1. a severe reduction in the body temperature. The condition usually arises gradually and may prove fatal if untreated. It is most common among babies and elderly people. 2. artificial cooling of the body to reduce the oxygen requirements of the tissues. *Mild h.* a reduction of the body temperature to 34°C, which may be induced by surface cooling with cold air. Generalized lowering of the body temperature is used in three main situations: (1) to control fever as in malignant hyperthermia; (2) to enable certain cardiac and neurological operations to be carried out; and (3) to protect the brain from raised intracranial pressure in patients with head injuries or following drowning.

hypothesis (hie'pothisis) a supposition that appears to explain a group of phenomena and is assumed as a basis of reasoning and experimentation.

hypothrombinaemia (,hiepoh-,thrombi'neemi·ə) a diminished amount of thrombin in the blood with a consequent tendency to bleed.

hypothyroidism (,hiepohthie-roydizəm) an insufficiency of thyroid secretion. In children it may produce cretinism. In adults it leads to myxoedema.

hypotonia (,hiepoh'tohni·ə) 1. deficient muscle tone. 2. deficient tension in the eyeball.

hypotonic (,hiepoh'tonik) describing a solution that has a lower osmotic pressure than another one. *See* HYPERTONIC.

hypoventilation (,hiepoh,venti-'layshən) hypopnoea; shallow breathing, usually at a very slow rate. It may cause a build-up of carbon dioxide in the blood.

hypovitaminosis (,hiepoh,vitəmi-'nohsis) a deficiency of vitamins due to a lack of intake or an inability to absorb them.

hypovolaemia (,hiepohvo'leemi·ə) a reduction in the circulating blood volume due to external loss of body fluids or to loss from the blood into the tissues, as in shock.

hypoxaemia (,hiepok'seemi·ə) an insufficient oxygen content in the blood.

hypoxia (hie'poksi·ə) a diminished amount of oxygen in the tissues. *Anaemic h.* low oxygen content due to deficiency of haemoglobin in the blood.

hystera (hi'sterə) [Gk.] *the uterus.*

hysteralgia (,histə'ralji·ə) pain in the uterus.

hysterectomy (,histə'rektəmee) removal of the uterus. *Abdominal h.* removal via an abdominal incision. *Subtotal h.* removal of the body of the uterus only. *Total h.* removal of the body and the cervix. *Vaginal h.* removal through the vagina. *Wertheim's h.* additional excision of the parametrium, upper vagina and lymph glands. Radical abdominal hysterectomy.

hysteria (his'tiə·ri·ə) a psychoneurosis in which the individual converts anxiety created by emotional conflict into physical symptoms, e.g. tics, mutism or paralysis of an arm or leg, that have no organic basis; called also conversion reaction or conversion hysteria. The term hysteria is also used to describe a state of tension or excitement in which there is a temporary loss of control over the emotions.

hysterical (hi'sterik'l) relating to hysteria.

hysterocele (,histə-rohseel) a hernia containing part of the uterus.

hysteromyoma (,histə-rohmie-'ohmə) a fibromyoma of the uterus.

hysteromyomectomy (,histə-roh-,mieə-

'mektəmee) excision of a hysteromyoma.

hystero-oöphorectomy (‚histə‚roh‚oh·əfə'rektəmee) excision of the uterus and the ovaries.

hysteropexy ('histə‚roh‚peksee) fixation of the uterus to the abdominal wall, to remedy displacement. Hysterorrhaphy. *See* VENTROFIXATION.

hysteroptosis (‚histərop'tohsis) prolapse of the uterus.

hysterosalpingography (‚histə‚roh‚salping'gogrəfee) radiographic examination of the uterus and uterine tubes following the injection of a radio-opaque dye. Uterosalpingography.

hysterosalpingostomy (‚histə‚roh‚salping'gostəmee) the establishment of an opening between the distal portion of the uterine tube and the uterus in an effort to overcome infertility when the medial portion is occluded or excised.

hysterotomy (‚histə'rotəmee) incision of the uterus, usually in order to remove a fetus in mid-pregnancy when it is too late to perform a therapeutic abortion. *See* CAESAREAN SECTION.

I

I symbol for *iodine*.

iatrogenic (ie,atroh'jenik) brought about by surgical or medical treatment, e.g. unwanted effects of drugs.

ibuprofen (ie,byooproh,fen) an anti-inflammatory analgesic and antipyretic drug used in the treatment of mild rheumatic and arthritic conditions.

ice (ies) water in a solid state, at or below freezing point. *I. bag* a rubber or plastic bag half-filled with pieces of ice and applied near or to a part to relieve pain or swelling. *Dry i.* carbon dioxide snow.

ichthammol ('ikthə,mol) an ammoniated coal tar product, used in ointment form for certain skin diseases.

ichthyosis (,ikthi'ohsis) a congenital abnormality of the skin in which there is dryness and roughness, the horny layer is thickened and large scales appear. These patients are liable to eczema and industrial dermatitis.

ICM International Confederation of Midwives.

ICN Infection Control Nurse; International Council of Nurses.

ICP intracranial pressure.

ICSH interstitial cell stimulating hormone.

icterus (iktə·rəs) jaundice. *I. gravis* a fatal form of jaundice occurring in pregnancy. Acute yellow atrophy. *I. gravis neonatorum* haemolytic disease of the newborn. *See* RHESUS FACTOR.

id (id) that part of the personality, containing the instinctive drives, which leads to gratification of primitive needs and which lives in the unconscious.

idea (ie'diə) a mental impression or conception. *Autochthonous i.* a strange idea that comes into the mind in some unaccountable way, but is not a hallucination. *Compulsive i.* an idea that persists despite reason and will and that drives one to action, usually inappropriate. *Dominant i.* a morbid or other impression that controls or colours every action and thought. *Fixed i.* a persistent morbid impression or belief that cannot be changed by reason. *I. of reference* the incorrect idea that the words and actions of others refer to one's self, or the projection of the causes of one's own imaginary difficulties upon someone else.

ideation (,iedi'ayshən) the formulation of ideas.

idée fixe (,eeday 'feeks) [Fr.] a *fixed idea*.

identical (ie'dentik'l) exactly alike. *I. twins* twins of the same sex developing from a single fertilized ovum.

identification (ie͵dentifiˈkayshən) a mental mechanism by which an individual adopts the attitudes and ideas of another, often admired, person.

ideomotion (͵iediohˈmohshən) the association of ideas and muscle action as in involuntary acts.

idiopathic (͵idiohˈpathik) self-originated; applied to a condition the cause of which is not known.

idiosyncrasy (͵idiohˈsingkrəsee) 1. a habit or quality of body or mind peculiar to any individual. 2. an abnormal susceptibility to an agent (e.g. a drug) that is peculiar to the individual.

idoxuridine (͵iedoksˈyooə·rideen) an iodine-containing drug used to treat infections caused by herpes virus, particularly keratitis and dendritic corneal ulcer.

ileal (ˈili·əl) referring to the ileum. *I. conduit* a surgical procedure in which the ureters are transplanted into the ileum, an isolated loop of which is then brought to the surface of the abdomen in order to allow the urine to drain into a bag.

ileitis (͵iliˈietis) inflammation of the ileum. *Regional i.* Crohn's disease. A chronic condition of the terminal portion of the ileum in which granulation and oedema may give rise to obstruction.

ileocolitis (͵iliohkəˈlietis) inflammation of the ileum and colon.

ileocolostomy (͵iliohkəˈlostəmee) the making of a permanent opening between the ileum and some part of the colon.

ileocystoplasty (͵iliohˈsistoh͵plastee) repair of the wall of the urinary bladder with an isolated segment of the ileum.

ileoproctostomy (͵iliohprokˈtostəmee) surgical anastomosis between the ileum and the rectum; ileorectal anastomosis.

ileorectal (͵iliohˈrektˈl) referring to the ileum and rectum. *I. anastomosis* ileoproctostomy.

ileosigmoidostomy (͵ilioh͵sigmoyˈdostəmee) surgical anastomosis between the ileum and the sigmoid flexure (pelvic colon).

ileostomy (͵iliˈostəmee) an artificial opening (stoma) created from the ileum and brought to the surface of the abdomen for the purpose of evacuation. Ileostomy is an inevitable part of proctocolectomy. An ileostomy may be temporary or permanent. *I. bags* disposable bags to collect the liquid faecal matter discharged from an ileostomy. The bags can be adhesive or worn on a belt.

ileum (ˈili·əm) the last part of the small intestine, terminating at the caecum.

ileus (ˈili·əs) intestinal obstruction, especially failure of peristalsis. The condition frequently accompanies peritonitis and usually results from disturbances in neural stimulation of the bowel. The principal symptoms of ileus are abdominal pain and distension, vomiting (the vomitus may contain faecal material), and constipation. If the intestinal obstruction is not relieved, the patient becomes extremely ill with SHOCK and DEHYDRATION.

iliac (ˈili͵ak) pertaining to the ilium. *I. artery* the right and left arteries form the terminal branches of the abdominal aorta and supply blood to the pelvic region and the lower limbs. *I. crest* the crest of the hip-bone. *I. fossa* the depression on the concave surface of the iliac bone. *I. vein* the right and left veins join to form the inferior vena cava and drain the blood from the lower limbs and pelvis.

ilium ('ili·əm) the haunch-bone; the upper part of the hip-bone.

illness ('ilnəs) a condition marked by pronounced deviation from the normal healthy state; sickness.

illusion (i'loozhən) a mistaken perception due to a misinterpretation of a sensory stimulus; believing something to be what it is not.

image ('imij) 1. the mental recall of a former percept. 2. the optical picture transferred to the brain cells by the optic nerve.

imago (i'maygoh, i'mahgoh) [L.] 1. in psychoanalysis, a childhood memory or fantasy of a loved person that persists in adult life. 2. the adult or definitive form of an insect.

imbalance (im'baləns) lack of balance, e.g. of endocrine secretions, between water and electrolytes, or of muscles.

imipramine (i'miprə,meen) a drug, chemically related to chlorpromazine, that may be effective in relieving depression. *See* ANTI-DEPRESSANT. Also used to treat nocturnal enuresis in children.

immature (,imə'tyooə) unripe; not fully developed, as a cataract when only a part of the lens is opaque.

immiscible (i'misəb'l) incapable of being mixed, e.g. oil and water.

immobilize (i'mohbi,liez) to render incapable of being moved, as by a plaster of Paris cast.

immune (i'myoon) protected against a particular infection or allergy. *I. reaction, i. response* 1. the reaction to and interaction with substances interpreted by the body as not-self which causes a body to reject a transplanted organ. 2. formation of a papule and areola without development of a vesicle following smallpox vaccination.

immunity (i'myoonitee) the resistance possessed by the body to infectious diseases, foreign tissues, foreign non-toxic substances and other ANTIGENS. *Acquired i.* is produced specifically in response to an ANTIGEN. It involves a change in the behaviour of cells and in the production of antibody. Antibody is produced as a primary response, and after a short while the body becomes sensitized. The secondary response is produced more quickly and is more marked. *Active i.* this may be (1) natural, i.e. from infectious diseases, or (2) artificial, i.e. from injection of living or dead organisms or their products in the form of toxins and toxoids. *Passive i.* this may be: (1) natural, e.g. maternal immunoglobulin G (IgG) via the placenta protects the infant from various infectious diseases for a few months, but undesirable antibodies such as anti-D immunoglobulin may also be transmitted to the fetus; or (2) acquired, e.g. the temporary immunity which follows the injection of antibodies of human (GAMMA-GLOBULIN) or, more rarely, animal origin. *Natural* or *innate i.* is mainly non-specific. It is provided by intact cellular barriers of epithelium and by humoral substances such as COMPLEMENT and LYSOZYME. It is affected by genetic factors, age, race and hormone levels.

immunization (,imyuhnie'zayshən) the act of creating immunity by artificial means. *I. schedule* a standard schedule for immunization against infectious diseases.

immunoassay (,imyuhnoh'asay) a quantitative estimate of the proteins contained in the blood serum.

immunodeficiency (,imyuhnohdi'fishənsee) a deficiency of the immune response, either that mediated by humoral antibody or by immune lymphoid cells, producing increased susceptibility to infectious disease.

immunoglobulin (,imyuhnoh'globyuhlin) antibody. A variety of chemical compound found mainly in GAMMA-GLOBULIN. Types are as follows: (1) immunoglobulin G (IgG) is small and crosses the placental barrier; (2) immunoglobulin M (IgM) is composed of large molecules; (3) immunoglobulin A (IgA) is produced in secretions, colostrum and breast milk. It lines the gut and, with LACTOFERRIN, promotes the growth of non-pathogenic lactobacilli and inhibits pathogens; (4) immunoglobulin D (IgD), whose function is not yet known; (5) immunoglobulin E (IgE), responsible for atopic hypersensitivity, often called allergy.

immunology (,imyuh'noləjee) the study of immunity and the body's defence mechanisms.

immunosuppression (,imyuhnohsə'preshən) inhibition of the formation of antibodies to antigens that may be present; used in transplantation procedures to prevent rejection of the transplanted organ or tissue.

immunosuppressive (,imyuhnohsə'presiv) 1. pertaining to or inducing immunosuppression. 2. an agent that induces immunosuppression.

immunotherapy (,imyuhnoh'therəpee) 1. treatment by immunization. Sometimes used in the treatment of leukaemia. 2. the establishing of passive immunity.

immunotransfusion (i,myoonohtrans'fyoozhən, -trahns-) transfusion of blood from a donor previously rendered immune to the disease affecting the patient.

Imodium (i'mohdiəm) trade name for preparations of loperamide hydrochloride, an antidiarrhoeal.

impaction (im'pakshən) a state of being wedged. *Dental i.* the condition in which a tooth, usually a molar, is unable to erupt through the gum because it is lodged in position by bone or the other teeth. *Faecal i.* a collection of putty-like or hardened faeces in the rectum or sigmoid.

impairment (im'pairmənt) any loss or abnormality of psychological, physiological, or anatomical structure or function.

IMMUNIZATION SCHEDULE

Vaccine	Age	Notes
Diphtheria/tetanus/ pertussis (D/T/P) and polio	Primary course— 1st dose: 3 months 2nd dose: 4½–5 months 3rd dose: 8½–11 months	
Measles	12–18 months	Can be given at any age over 12 months
Measles/mumps/ rubella (MMR)	12–18 months	As for measles
Diphtheria/tetanus (D/T) and polio	4–5 years	
Rubella	10–14 years	
Bacillus of Calmette–Guérin (BCG)	10–14 years	Interval of 3 weeks between BCG and rubella
Tetanus and polio	15–18 years	

Children should therefore have received the following vaccines:
By end of first year: 3 doses of D/T/P and polio, or D/T and polio.
By end of second year: measles (MMR from 1 October 1988).
By school entry: 4th D/T and polio; measles or MMR if missed earlier.
Between 10 and 14 years: BCG and rubella.
Before leaving school: 5th polio and tetanus.

Source: Immunization against Infectious Disease, DHSS, 1988.

---

impalpable (im'palpəb'l) incapable of being felt by manual examination. May apply to an organ or a tumour.

imperforate (im'pərfə·rət) without an opening. *I. anus* a congenital defect in which this opening is closed. *I. hymen* complete closure of the vaginal opening by the hymen. *See* CRYPTOMEN-ORRHOEA.

impermeable (im'pərmi·əb'l) not permitting the passage of fluid or molecules.

impetigo (,impə'tiegoh) an acute contagious inflammation of the skin marked by pustules and scabs; of streptococcal or staphylococcal origin. It occurs mainly on the face and limbs, particularly those of children.

implant (im'plahnt, 'implahnt) any substance grafted into the tissues. *Hormone i.* a pellet of deoxycortone acetate or testosterone, which may be implanted subcutaneously. *Intraocular lens i.* a plastic lens which may be implanted in the eye after lens extraction. *Plastic i.* a Silastic implant may be used in plastic surgery, e.g. to reshape the breast.

implantation (,implahn'tayshən) the act of planting or setting in. 1. the embedding of the fertilized ovum in the wall of the uterus. 2. the placing of a drug within the tissues. 3. the surgical introduction of healthy tissue to replace tissue that has been damaged.

implementation ('implioment'tayshən) the third phase of the nursing process signifying the giving of care in relation to defined nursing interventions and goals. During implementation the nursing care plan is tested for effectiveness and accuracy. Data gathering continues and plans may change on the basis of new information obtained. The implementation phase concludes with the recording of the activities performed and the response of the patient. *See* ASSESSMENT and EVALUATION.

implosion (im'plohzhən) in behaviour therapy, a form of desensitization used in the treatment of phobias and related disorders. *See* FLOODING.

impotence ('impətəns) inability in a man to carry out sexual intercourse from either psychological or physical causes.

impregnation (,impreg'nayshən) insemination; rendering pregnant.

impulse ('impuls) 1. a sudden pushing force. 2. a sudden uncontrollable act. 3. nerve impulse. *Cardiac i.* movement of the chest wall caused by the heart beat. *Nerve i.* the electrochemical process propagated along nerve fibres.

IMV intermittent mandatory ventilation.

in situ (in'sityoo) [L.] *in the original position.*

in vitro (in'veetroh, -'vit-) [L.] *in a glass.* Refers to observations made outside the body. *See* IN VIVO.

in vivo (in'veevoh) [L.] *within the living body. See* IN VIVTRO

inaccessibility (,inak,sesə'bilitee) state of unresponsiveness characteristic of certain psychiatric patients, e.g. schizophrenics.

inanition (,inə'nishən) wasting of the body from want of food.

inappetence (in'apitəns) lack of desire or appetite, usually for food.

inarticulate (,inah'tikyuhlət) 1. without joints. 2. unable to speak intelligibly.

incarcerated (in'kahsə,raytid) held fast. Applied to (1) a hernia which is immovable, and therefore only curable by operation, and (2) a pregnant uterus held under the sacral brim.

incest ('insest) sexual intercourse

between people so closely related that marriage between them is legally or culturally prohibited.

incidence ('insidəns) the number of particular new events which occur in a population in a given period of time. For example, the number of new cases of a disease such as measles expressed per 1000 of population per year.

incipient (in'sipi·ənt) beginning to exist.

incision (in'sizhən) 1. in surgery, a cut into soft tissue. 2. the act of cutting.

incisor (in'siezə) one of the four front teeth in the centre of each jaw.

inclusion (in'kloozhən) something that is enclosed or the act of enclosing. *I. bodies* particles that are temporarily enclosed in the cytoplasm of a cell. For example, in trachoma virus particles can be seen in the conjunctival epithelial cells.

incoherent (inkoh'hiə·rənt) 1. unconnected; inconsistent. 2. uttering speech that is disconnected and rambling.

incompatibility (,inkəmpatə'bil-itee) the state of two or more substances being antagonistic, or destroying the efficiency of each other. Applied to mixtures of drugs, and to blood. *See* BLOOD GROUPING.

incompetence (in'kompitəns) inefficiency. *Aortic i.* failure of the aortic valves to regulate the flow of blood. *Mitral i.* failure of the mitral valve to close properly.

incontinence (in'kontinəns) inability to control natural functions or discharges. *Faecal i.*

inability to control the movements of the bowels. *Overflow i.* that from an overfull bladder, most common in elderly men with urinary obstruction. *Paralytic i.* loss of control of anal and urethral sphincters due to injury to nerve centres. *Stress i.* that which is due to a defect in the urethral sphincters and is liable to occur when intra-abdominal pressure is increased as in coughing or lifting heavy weights; most common in women with weak pelvic muscles. *Urinary i.* inability to control the outflow of urine.

incoordination (,inkoh,awdi'nayshən) inability to adjust harmoniously various muscle movements.

incrustation (,inkru'stayshən) the formation of a crust or scab on a wound.

incubation ('ingkyuh'bayshən) the development and growth of microorganisms and animal embryos. *I. period* the period between the date of infection and the appearance of symptoms of an infectious disease.

incubator ('ingkyuh,baytə) 1. a warmed servo-controlled Perspex box for nursing ill and preterm babies. 2. an apparatus used to develop bacteria at a uniform temperature suitable to their growth.

incus ('ingkəs) the small anvil-shaped bone of the middle ear. The second auditory ossicle.

indican ('indikən) a potassium salt which is excreted in the urine following the decomposition of tryptophan in the intestines.

indicator ('indi,kaytə) 1. the index

finger, or the extensor muscle of the index finger. 2. any substance that indicates the appearance or disappearance of a chemical by a colour change or attainment of a certain pH.

indigenous (in'dijənəs) occurring naturally in a certain locality.

indigestion (,indi'jeschən) *See* DYSPEPSIA.

Indocid ('indoh,sid) trade name for indomethacin.

indole ('indohl) a product of protein decomposition in the bowel. It is excreted in the faeces, and also in the urine as indican.

indolent ('indələnt) slow growing. Reluctant to heal. Largely painless. *I. ulcer* a chronic ulcer of the skin or mucous membrane.

indomethacin (,indoh'methəsin) an anti-inflammatory analgesic used in the treatment of arthritis and of acute attacks of gout.

induction (in'dukshən) the act of initiating something. *I. of abortion* the intentional bringing about of an abortion. *I. of anaesthesia* the start of the administration of a general anaesthetic. *Electromagnetic i.* the production of an electric current in a body because of its nearness to an electrified (or magnetized) body. *I. of labour* the artificial starting of the process of childbirth.

induration (,indyuh'rayshən) the abnormal hardening of a tissue or organ.

industrial (in'dustri-əl) referring to industry. *I. diseases* those that are caused by the nature of the work. *Prescribed i. diseases* those for which sickness benefit is payable, including those that are notifiable under the Factories Act (1961).

inebriation (i,neebri'ayshən) the condition of being intoxicated by alcohol; drunkenness.

inert (i'nərt) having no action. *I. gas* a gas which does not react with other elements, e.g. neon.

inertia (i'nərshə) sluggishness; inability to move except when stimulated by an external force. *Uterine i.* lack of muscle contraction during the first and second stage of labour.

infant ('infənt) a child under 1 year of age. Educationally, a child under 7 years of age. *I. feeding* the supplying of nutrition to an infant. Breast milk is the ideal food for the baby and if breast feeding is established satisfactorily for the first few months it can aid physical and emotional development. Where it is not possible an infant food formula can be given. *Floppy i. floppy i. syndrome* a congenital myopathy of infants, marked clinically by myotonia and muscle weakness. *I. mortality rate* the number of deaths of children under 1 year of age per 1000 live births in any one year. *Premature i.* one born before the state of maturity. *See* PRETERM.

infanticide (in'fanti,sied) the killing of a child by its mother during the first year of its life.

infantile ('infən,tiel) concerning an infant; childish. *I. paralysis* poliomyelitis.

infantilism (in'fanti,lizəm) persistence of the characters of childhood into adult life, marked by underdevelopment of the reproductive organs, and often dwarfism.

infarct ('infahkt) the wedge-shaped area of necrosis in an organ produced by the blocking of a blood vessel, usually due to an embolus. *Red i.* a haemorrhage infarct. Red blood cells infiltrate the area. *White i.* an anaemic infarct. The area is suddenly deprived of blood and is pale in colour.

infarction (in'fahkshən) the formation of an infarct. *Myocardial i.* an infarct of the heart muscle following a coronary thrombosis. *Pulmonary i.* an infarct resulting from obstruction of a branch of the pulmonary artery by embolism or thrombosis.

infection (in'fekshən) 1. invasion and multiplication of microorganisms in body tissues, especially that causing local cellular injury due to competitive metabolism, toxins, intracellular replication, or antigen–antibody response. 2. an infectious disease. *Airborne i.* infection by inhalation of organisms suspended in air on water droplets, droplet nuclei or dust particles. *Anaerobic i.* infection caused by ANAEROBES. *I. control* the utilization of procedures and techniques in the surveillance, investigation and compilation of statistical data in order to reduce the spread of infection, particularly hospital-acquired infections. Practitioners in infection control are frequently nurses who are employed by Health Authorities. They have titles such as Infection Control Officer and Infection Control Nurse, and they function as liaison between staff, nurses, doctors, department heads, the infection control committee and the health authority. Such practitioners also assume some responsibility for teaching patients and their families, as well as employees of the Health Authority. *Cross i.* infection transmitted between patients infected with different pathogenic microorganisms. *Droplet i.* infection due to inhalation of respiratory pathogens suspended on liquid particles exhaled by someone already infected. *Dustborne i.* infection by inhalation of pathogens that have become affixed to particles of dust. *Hospital-acquired i's* those acquired during hospitalization; called also nosocomial infections. A prevalence survey showed that 10 per cent of patients in hospitals in England and Wales in 1982 acquired an infection whilst in hospital. The most common causative agents are *Escherichia coli, Proteus, Pseudomonas* and *Klebsiella,* among the Gram-negative organisms, and *Staphylococcus* and *Enterococcus* among the Gram-positive organisms. *See also* INFECTION CONTROL (above). *Mixed i.* infection with more than one kind of organism at the same time. *Secondary i.* infection by a pathogen following an infection by a pathogen of another kind. *Subclinical i.* infection associated with no detectable symptoms but caused by microorganisms capable of producing easily recognizable diseases, such as poliomyelitis or mumps; it is detected by the production of antibody, or by delayed hypersensitivity exhibited in a skin test reaction to such antigens as tuberculoprotein.

infectious (in'fekshəs) caused by or capable of being communicated by infection. *I. disease* disease resulting from multiplication of microorganisms in the body. Most are communicable but not all. *See also* COMMUNICABLE DISEASE. *I. mononucleosis (glandular fever)* an acute virus infection characterized by sore throat and glandular enlargement caused by the Epstein–Barr (EB) virus. Worldwide common infection particularly prevalent in older children and young adults in western countries. The source of infection is man and spread is by oropharyngeal secretions, for example, during kissing. The incubation period is 4 to 6 weeks and infectivity after the disease may be prolonged. *See* GLANDULAR FEVER.

infective (in'fektiv) infectious, capable of producing infection; pertaining to or characterized by the presence of pathogens.

inferior (in'fiə·ri·ə) lower. *I. vena cava* the lower large vein.

inferiority (in‚fiə·ri'oritee) lesser rank, stature, position or ability. *I. complex see* COMPLEX.

infertility (‚infər'tilətee) inability of a woman to conceive or of a man to bring about conception.

infestation (‚infe'stayshən) the presence of animal parasites, e.g. mites, ticks or worms, in or on the body, in clothing or in a house.

COMMON INFECTIOUS DISEASES

Disease	Incubation period (days)	Period of infectivity
Chickenpox (varicella)	10–20	2–3 days before until 10 days after onset of rash
Diphtheria	2–7	Until culture of three consecutive nose swabs proves negative
Enteric fevers		
Typhoid	6–21	Until at least 1 month after onset of disease and after six consecutive negative stools
Paratyphoid		
Measles (morbilli)	6–12	4 days before until 4 days after onset of rash
Mumps (parotitis)	12–28	48 h before onset until resolution of symptoms
Pertussis (whooping cough)	7–14	7 days before until 3 weeks after onset of cough
Rubella (German measles)	14–21	During incubation period until 2 days after resolution of symptoms

infiltration (ˌinfil'trayshən) the entrance and diffusion of some abnormal substance, either fluid or solid, into tissues or cells. *I. analgesia* the injection into tissues of a local analgesic solution.

inflammation (ˌinflə'mayshən) a localized protective response elicited by injury or destruction of tissues, which serves to destroy, dilute or wall off both the injurious agent and the injured tissue. The cardinal signs are: heat, swelling, pain and redness. *Acute i.* sudden onset of inflammation, with marked and progressive symptoms. *Catarrhal i.* inflammation in which mucous surfaces are attacked, with stimulation of exudation. *Chronic i.* inflammation that develops slowly. Granulation tissue forms and tends to localize the infection. *Diffuse i.* extensive inflammation, as in nephritis and cellulitis. *Suppurative i.* one marked by pus formation. *Traumatic i.* that which follows an injury.

influenza (ˌinfloo'enzə) an acute viral infection of the respiratory tract, occurring in isolated cases, epidemics and pandemics. Called also 'flu. Transmission is by droplet inhalation and the period of infectivity lasts from 1 day before the onset of symptoms until up to 7 days later. In the UK, most cases occur between December and May, with the peak incidence being in February. There is fever, headache, pain in the back and limbs, anorexia and sometimes nausea and vomiting. The fever subsides in 2 to 3 days, leaving a feeling of lassitude. There is no specific drug cure for influenza. But an influenza vaccine is available, the formulation of which is changed annually to include recently circulating strains of viruses on recommendation of the WHO. Annual vaccination is advised for persons with chronic heart, lung or renal disease, those with diabetes, and patients on immunosuppressive therapy. It should also be considered for residents of old people's homes.

informed consent (in'fawmd) *see* CONSENT.

infrared (ˌinfrə'red) rays of a lower wavelength than those in the visible spectrum. They can produce radiant heat which is used in the treatment of rheumatic conditions. *See* ULTRA-VIOLET.

infundibulum (ˌinfun'dibyuhləm) a funnel-shaped passage or part.

infusion (in'foozhən) 1. the process of extracting the soluble principles of substances (especially drugs) by soaking in water. 2. the solution thus produced. 3. the slow therapeutic introduction by gravity of fluid other than blood into a vein.

ingestion (in'jeschən) the taking in of food and drugs by mouth.

inguinal ('ing·gwin'l) relating to the groin. *I. canal* the channel through the abdominal wall, above Poupart's ligament, through which the spermatic cord and vessels pass to the testis in the male, and which contains the round ligament of the uterus in the female. *I. ligament* Poupart's ligament; that connecting the anterior superior spine of the ilium to the tubercle of the pubis.

inhalation (ˌinhəˈlayshən) 1. the drawing of air or other substances into the lungs. 2. any drug or solution of drugs, administered (as by means of nebulizers or aerosols) by the nasal or oral respiratory route.

inhaler (inˈhaylə) an apparatus used for administering an inhalation.

inherent (inˈhiə·rənt, -ˈher-) a characteristic that is innate or natural and essentially a part of the person.

inheritance (inˈheritəns) the acquisition of qualities and characteristics from parents and ancestors.

inhibition (ˌinhiˈbishən) arrest or restraint of a process. In psychiatry, the unconscious restraining of an instinctual drive.

injection (inˈjekshən) 1. the forcing of a liquid into a part, as into the subcutaneous tissues, the vascular tree or an organ. 2. a substance so forced or administered; in pharmacy, a solution of a medicament suitable for injection. 3. prominence of small blood vessels on the surface of an organ or tissue, frequently indicating the vascular phase of an inflammatory response. *Hypodermic i.* that made just below the skin; a subcutaneous injection. *Intramuscular i.* that made into a muscle. *Intrathecal i.* that made into the subarachnoid space of the spinal cord. *Intravenous i.* that made into a vein. *Subcutaneous i.* that made into the subcutaneous tissues; a hypodermic injection.

inlay (ˈinˌlay) material inserted to replace a defect in a tissue, for example a bone graft or a filling cast in metal to fit a hole in a tooth.

innate (iˈnayt) inborn; present in the individual at birth.

innervation (ˌinəˈvayshən) nerve supply to a part.

innocent (ˈinəsənt) as applied to a tumour, benign or non-malignant.

innocuous (iˈnokyooəs) harmless.

innominate (iˈnominət) unnamed. *I. artery* a branch of the aorta, now termed the brachiocephalic trunk. *I. bone* the hip bone, formed by the union of the ilium, ischium and pubis.

inoculation (iˌnokyuhˈlayshən) 1. introduction of pathogenic microorganisms, injected material, serum, or other substances into tissues of living organisms or into culture media. 2. introduction of a disease agent (usually a live infectious agent) into a healthy individual to produce a mild form of the disease, followed by IMMUNITY.

inorganic (ˌinawˈganik) of neither animal nor vegetable origin.

inositol (iˈnohsiˌtol) a form of muscle or plant carbohydrate that has the same formula as simple sugar but not its other properties. *I. nicotinate* a vasodilator used in peripheral vascular disease.

inotropic (ˌienəˈtrohpik, -ˈtropik) affecting the force or energy of muscular contractions, particularly the heart muscle. Beta-blocking drugs are said to be inotropic.

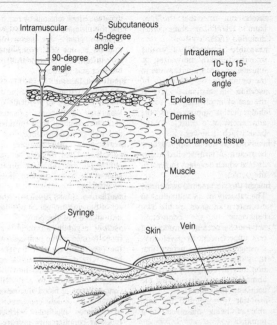

INTRAMUSCULAR, SUBCUTANEOUS, INTRADERMAL AND INTRAVENOUS INJECTIONS

inquest ('inkwest) a legal inquiry held by a coroner, with or without a jury, into the cause of sudden or unexpected death.

insanity (in'sanətee) a legal term for mental illness, roughly equivalent to PSYCHOSIS and implying inability to be responsible for one's acts.

insecticide (in'sekti,sied) one of a large group of chemical compounds that kill insect pests.

insemination (in,semi'nayshən) 1. fertilization of an ovum by a spermatozoon. 2. introduction of semen into the vagina. *Artificial i.* insemination by means other than sexual intercourse. The semen can be either the husband's (*AIH*) or some other donor's (*AID*).

insensible (in'sensəb'l) 1. unable to perceive with the senses. 2. unconscious. 3. imperceptible to the senses.

insertion (in'sərshən, -'zər-) 1. the act of implanting. 2. something that is implanted. 3. the attachment of a muscle to the bone which it moves.

insidious (in'sidi-əs) approaching by stealth. A term applied to any disease which develops imperceptibly.

insight ('in,siet) mental awareness. The capacity of an individual to estimate a situation or his own behaviour or the connection between his present attitudes and past experiences. In psychiatry, a recognition by the patient that he is ill. Insight in this connection may be complete, partial or absent, and may alter during the course of the illness.

insoluble (in'solyuhb'l) not capable of being dissolved in a liquid.

insomnia (in'somni·ə) inability to sleep.

inspiration (inspi'rayshən) the act of drawing in the breath.

inspissated (in'spisaytid) thickened, through evaporation or absorption of fluid.

instillation (,insti'layshən) the act of pouring a liquid into a cavity drop by drop, e.g. into the eye.

instinct ('instingkt) a complex of unlearned responses characteristic of a species. *Death i.* in psychoanalysis, the latent instinctive impulse towards death; the

drive to reduce tensions by reaching the ultimate tensionless state of death. *Herd i.* the instinct or urge to be one of a group and to conform to its standards of conduct and opinion.

institutionalization (insti,tyooshənəlie'zayshən) a condition of apathy occurring in residents of long stay institutions, prisons, etc., as a result of rigid routines and lack of independence.

insufficiency (,insə'fishənsee) inadequacy. Used to describe the failure of function of an organ such as the heart, stomach, liver or muscles.

insufflation (,insu'flayshən) the act of blowing air, gas or powder into a cavity of the body.

insulin ('insyuhlin) a protein hormone formed in the beta cells of the pancreatic islets of Langerhans. The major fuel-regulating hormone, it is secreted into the blood in response to a rise in concentration of blood glucose or amino acids. A deficiency results in diabetes mellitus. Various types of commercially prepared insulin are available. There are three main groups: rapid acting, intermediate acting and long acting. Diabetic patients react differently in the rate at which they absorb and utilize insulin; therefore, the duration of action varies from patient to patient. Insulin is measured in units. The concentration used now is U100. This strength allows for more accurate measurement of dosage and reduces the possibility of error in calculating an individual dose. *I. pump* a device consisting of a syringe filled with a predetermined amount of short-acting insulin, a plastic cannula and a needle, and a pump that periodically delivers the desired amount of insulin.

insulin sensitivity test a test used to determine the body's response to hypoglycaemia induced by a small intravenous dose of insulin. It is used to test anterior pituitary function, particularly the ability to secrete growth hormone.

insulinase ('insyuhli,nayz) an enzyme that destroys the action of insulin.

insulinoma (,insyuhli'nohmə) a benign adenoma of the islet cells of the pancreas, causing hypoglycaemia.

integument (in'tegyuhmənt) 1. the skin. 2. a layer of tissue covering a part or organ of the body.

intellect ('intə'lekt) the mind, thinking faculty, or understanding.

intelligence (in'telijəns) 1. the capacity to understand. 2. general mental ability. *I. quotient* abbreviated IQ. A measure of the mental development of a child. The ratio of the mental age to the chronological age expressed as a percentage. *I. test* a test designed to measure the level of intelligence, usually expressed as an IQ.

intensive care unit (in'tensiv) abbreviated ICU. A hospital unit in which is concentrated special equipment and specially trained personnel for the care of seriously ill patients requiring immediate and continuous monitoring and treatment. Called also critical care unit (CCU), intensive therapy unit.

intention (in'tenshən) a process of healing.

intercellular (,intə'selyuhlə) between the cells of a structure. May be applied to the connective tissue or to fluid bathing the cells.

intercostal (,intə'kost'l) between the ribs. *I. muscles* muscles situated between the ribs and controlling their movements during inspiration and expiration.

intercourse ('intə,kaws) 1. social exchange. 2. coitus.

intercurrent (,intə'kurənt) occurring at the same time. Describes a disease occurring during the course of another disease in the same person.

interferon (,intə'fie-ron) a protein produced by cells infected by a virus which has an inhibitory effect on the multiplication of the invading viruses.

interlobular (,intə'lobyuhlə) between lobules. *I. veins* branches of the portal vein in the liver.

intermenstrual (,intə'menstrooəl) occurring between two menstrual periods.

intermission (,intə'mishən) a temporary interruption, particularly of a feverish condition.

intermittent (,intə'mitənt) occurring at intervals. *I. claudication See* CLAUDICATION. *I. fever* one in which the temperature drops to normal or lower, at times. *I. mandatory ventilation* abbreviated IMV. A type of mechanical ventilation in which the VENTILATOR is set to deliver a prescribed tidal volume at specified intervals and a high-flow gas system permits the patient to breathe spontaneously between cycles. *I. positive airway ventilation* abbreviated IPAV. A method of assisted ventilation, in which oxygen or air is used under pressure to inflate the lungs, when the patient is unable to breathe spontaneously.

internal (in'tərn'l) situated on the inside. *I. haemorrhage* one occurring in a cavity or into the tissues. *I. secretion* one in which the hormones pass directly into the bloodstream from the secreting gland.

interphase ('intə,fayz) the period between two cells divisions during which the chromosomes are not easily visible.

intersex ('intə,seks) 1. a congenital abnormality in which anatomical features of both sexes are evident. 2. a person displaying intersexuality.

intersexuality (,intə,seksyoo'alitee) an intermingling of the characters of each sex, including phsyical form, reproductive tissue and sexual behaviour, in one individual, as a result of some flaw in embryonic development.

interstitial (,intə'stishəl) situated within the tissue spaces or between the tissues. *I. fluid* the fluid in which body cells are bathed. It acts as an intermediary between the cells and the blood. Extracellular fluid. *I. cell stimulating hormone* abbreviated ICSH. luteinizing hormone. *I. keratitis* See KERATITIS. *I. nephritis* chronic nephritis associated with fibrosis and hypertension.

intertrigo (,intə'triegoh) an irritating, eczematous skin eruption caused by chafing of two moist skin surfaces.

intervertebral (,intə'vərtibrəl) between the vertebrae. *I. disc* the pad of fibrocartilage between the bodies of the vertebrae. Protrusion of the contents of the disc may give rise to sciatica by pressing on the nerve roots.

intestinal (,inte'stienəl, in'testin'l) referring to the intestine.

intestine (in'testin) that part of the alimentary canal which extends from the stomach to the anus. *Small i.* the first 6 m (20 ft) from the pylorus to the caecum, consisting of the duodenum, the jejunum and the ileum. *Large i.* the final 2 m (6 ft), consisting of the caecum, the ascending, transverse and descending colon, and the rectum.

intima ('intimə) the innermost coat of an artery or vein.

intolerance (in'tolə·rəns) lack of power to endure. Applied to the effect of some drugs on individuals, e.g. iodine and quinine. See IDIOSYNCRASY.

intoxication (in,toksi'kayshən) 1. poisoning by drugs or harmful substances. 2. the condition produced by excessive use of alcohol.

intra-abdominal (,intrə-əb'domin'l) within the abdomen.

intra-articular (,intrəah'tikyuhlə) within a joint capsule. *I-a. injection* injection into a joint capsule, applicable to hydrocortisone, for example.

intra-atrial (,intrə'aytri·əl) within the atrium. *I-a. thrombosis* a blood clot formed in the atrium of the heart.

intracapsular (,intrə,kapsyuhlə) within a capsule, usually of a joint. *I. extraction* the removal of the whole lens with its capsule in the treatment of cataract. *I. fracture see* FRACTURE.

intracellular (,intrə'selyuhlə) within a cell. *I. fluid* the water and its dissolved salts found within the cells.

intracerebral (,intrə'seribrəl) within the brain substance. *I. haemorrhage* an escape of blood in the cerebrum, most often arising from the middle cerebral artery or from an aneurysm.

intracranial (,intrə'krayni·əl) within the skull. *I. abscess* one arising within the brain or meninges. *I. aneurysm* dilatation of one of the cerebral vessels. It may be congenital or acquired. *I. pressure* abbreviated ICP. The pressure exerted by the cerebrospinal fluid within the subarachnoid space and ventricles of the brain.

intractable (in'traktəb'l) not able to be relieved, controlled or cured.

intradermal (,intrə'dərməl) between the layers of the skin.

intradural (,intrə'dyooə·rəl) within the dura mater. *I. haemorrhage see* HAEMORRHAGE.

intragastric (,intrə'gastrik) within the stomach.

intrahepatic (,intrəhi'patik) within the liver. Referring to a condition of the liver cells or connective tissue.

intralipid (,intrə'lipid) trade name for an intravenous fat emulsion

used to prevent or correct deficiency of essential fatty acids and to provide calories in high density form during total parenteral nutrition.

intralobular (,intrə'lobyuhlə) within a lobule. *I. veins* veins which collect blood from within the lobules of the liver.

intramedullary (,intrəmə'dulə·ree) 1. within the medulla oblongata. 2. within the bone marrow. *I. nail* a metal pin used for the internal fixation of fractures.

intramuscular (,intrə'muskyuhlə) within muscle tissue.

intranasal (,intrə'nayz'l) within the nose.

intraocular (,intrə'okyuhlə) within the eyeball.

intraorbital (,intrə'awbit'l) within the orbit of the eye.

intraosseous (,intrə'osi·əs) within a bone.

intraperitoneal (,intrə,peritə'neeəl) within the peritoneal cavity.

intrathecal (,intrə'theek'l) within the meninges of the spinal cord, usually in the subarachnoid space.

intratracheal (,intrə'traki·əl, -trə'keeəl) endotracheal; within the trachea. *I. anaesthesia* inhalation anaesthesia *see* ANAESTHESIA.

intrauterine (,intrə'yootə·rien) within the uterus. *I. contraceptive device* a contraceptive device introduced into the uterine cavity. *I. douche* irrigation of the uterine cavity. A special grooved nozzle is used, so that the fluid can return and is not forced into the uterine tubes. *I. growth retardation* associated with a poor

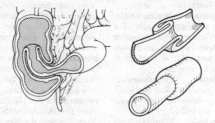

INTUSSUSCEPTION

blood supply to the placenta, or maternal disease. Other factors include infection during pregnancy, maternal smoking or drug addiction. The infant at birth 'is small for dates' and falls below the tenth percentile appropriate gestational age for infants. *I. life* fetal development in the uterus.
intravenous (,intrə'veenəs) within a vein. *I. infusion* the therapeutic introduction of a fluid, such as saline, into a vein. The infusion works by gravity in that the container of fluid is higher than the blood vessel into which the fluid is being introduced. *I. flow rate* the rate at which fluids, medications and blood products flow into the bloodstream during intravenous infusion. The flow rate is usually ordered by the doctor as total volume (ml) per total hours or, in the case of drugs, total dose per total hours. *I. urography* radiographic examination of the urinary tract after the injection of a radio-opaque contrast medium into a vein.
intraventricular (,intrəven'trik-

yuhlə) within a ventricle; may apply to a cerebral or a cardiac ventricle.
intrinsic (in'trinsik, -zik) particular to or contained within an organ. *I. factor* a glycoprotein contained in the gastric juices which is necessary for the absorption of the extrinsic factor (vitamin B$_{12}$).
introitus (in'troh·itəs) [L.] an opening or entrance into a hollow organ or cavity. *I. vaginae* the vulva.
introjection (,intrə'jekshən) a mental process by which an individual takes into himself the personal characteristics of another person, usually those of someone much loved or admired.
introspection (,intrə'spekshən) a subjective study of the mind and its processes, in which an individual studies his own reactions.
introversion (,intrə'vərshən) 1. a turning inwards within itself of a hollow organ. 2. pre-occupation with oneself, with reduction of interest in the outside world.
introvert ('intrə,vərt) a person

whose interests are turned inward upon himself. *See* EXTROVERT.

intubation (,intyuh'bayshən) the introduction of a tube into a part of the body, particularly into the air passages to allow air to enter the lungs.

intumescence (,intyuh'mesəns) a swelling or increase in bulk, as of nasal mucous membrane in catarrh.

intussusception (,intəsə'sepshən) prolapse of one part of the intestine into the lumen of an immediately adjacent part, causing INTESTINAL OBSTRUCTION.

inunction (in'ungkshən) the act of rubbing an oily or fatty preparation into the skin.

invagination (in,vaji'nayshən) 1. the folding inwards of a part, thus forming a pouch. 2. intussusception.

invasion (in'vayzhən) 1. the entry of bacteria into the body. 2. the entrance of parasites into the body of a host.

invasive (in'vaysiv, -ziv) 1. having the quality of invasiveness. 2. involving puncture or incision of the skin or insertion of an instrument or foreign material into the body; said of diagnostic techniques.

invasiveness (in'vaysivnəs) 1. the ability of microorganisms to enter the body and spread in the tissues. 2. the ability to infiltrate and actively destroy surrounding tissue, a property of malignant tumours.

inversion (in'vərshən) a turning upside down or inside out. *Sexual i.* homosexuality. *Uterine i.* the condition of the uterus after par-

turition when a part of its upper segment protrudes through the cervix.

invertase (in'vərtayz, 'in-) a ferment of intestinal juice which hydrolyses cane sugar.

invertebrate (in'vərti,brət, -brayt) 1. without a spinal column. 2. an animal without a spinal column.

involucrum (,invo'lookrəm) new bone which forms a sheath around necrosed bone, as in chronic osteomyelitis.

involuntary (in'voləntə·ree) independent of the will. *I. muscle* one that acts without conscious control, for instance the heart and stomach muscles.

involution (,invə'looshən) 1. turning inward; describes the contraction of the uterus after labour. The process whereby the uterus returns to its normal size. 2. the progressive degeneration occurring naturally with advancing age, resulting in shrivelling of organs or tissues.

iodine ('ieə,deen) *symbol* I. A non-metallic element with a distinctive odour, obtained from seaweed. Iodine is essential in nutrition, being especially prevalent in the colloid of the THYROID GLAND. It is used in the treatment of HYPOTHYROIDISM and as a topical antiseptic. It is a frequent cause of poisoning. Iodine is opaque to X-rays, and can be combined with other compounds for use as contrast media in diagnostic radiology.

iodism ('ieə,dizəm) poisoning from the prolonged use of iodine or iodine compounds causing coryza, ptyalism, frontal headache, emaciation, weakness and skin eruptions.

iodopsin (,ieə'dopsin) a violet pigment found in the retinal cones of the eye.

iodosorb (ie'ohdohzawb) tradename for a preparation of cadexomer iodide used to cleanse venous leg ulcers and pressure sores.

iodoxyl (,ieadoksil) a radio-opaque contrast/medium used in INTRAVENOUS UROGRAPHY.

ion ('ieən) an atom or group of atoms having a positive (cation) or negative (anion) electric charge by virtue of having gained or lost one or more electrons. Substances forming ions are ELECTROLYTES. *See* HYDROGEN.

ionization (,ieənie'zayshən) the breaking up of molecules into electrically charged particles or ions when an electric current is passed through an electrolyte solution.

iontophoresis (ie,ontohfə'reesis) the introduction through the skin of therapeutic ions by ionization.

ipecacuanha (,ipi,kakyoo'ahnə) the dried root of a Brazilian shrub, given in small doses as an expectorant and, in larger doses, as an emetic.

IPPV intermittent positive-pressure ventilation.

iproniazid (,ieprə'nieəzid) an antidepressant drug that belongs to the group of monoamine oxidase inhibitors.

ipsilateral (,ipsi'latə'rəl) occurring on the same side. Applied particularly to paralysis or other symptoms occurring on the same side as the cerebral lesion causing them.

IQ intelligence quotient. *See* INTELLIGENCE.

IRDS infant respiratory distress syndrome.

iridectomy (,iri'dektəmee) excision of a part of the iris, usually for the treatment of glaucoma.

iridencleisis (,iriden'kliesis) an operation to make a drain out of a part of the iris, used in the treatment of glaucoma.

iridium (i'ridi·əm) *symbol* Ir. A radioactive metal, often used in the form of wires or hairpins to treat superficial malignancies, e.g. those of the tongue, cheek or breast.

iridocele (i'ridoh,seel) herniation of a part of the iris, through a corneal wound.

iridocyclitis (,iridohsie'klietis) inflammation of the iris and ciliary body.

iridodialysis (,iridohdie'aləsis) the separation of the outer border of the iris from its ciliary attachment, often a result of trauma.

iridodonesis (,iridohdə'neesis) trembling of the iris due to lack of support from the lens in dislocation of the lens or after a cataract extraction.

iridoplegia (,iridoh'pleeji'·ə) paralysis of the iris.

iridoptosis (,iridop'tohsis) prolapse of the iris.

iridotomy (,iri'dotəmee) the making of a hole in the iris to form an artificial pupil.

iris ('ieris) the coloured part of the eye made of two layers of muscle, the contraction of which alters the size of the pupil and so controls the amount of light entering the eye. *I. bombé* a bulging forward of the iris due to pressure of the aqueous humour when its passage into the anterior chamber is obstructed.

iritis (ie'rietis) inflammation of the iris, causing pain, photophobia, contraction of the pupil and discoloration of the iris. *See* UVEITIS.

iron ('ieən) *symbol* Fe. A metallic element which is present in the body in small quantities and is essential to life. A deficiency may produce anaemia.

irradiation (i,raydi'ayshən) the treatment of disease by electromagnetic radiation.

irreducible (,iri'dyoosəb'l) incapable of being replaced in a normal position. Applied to a fracture or a hernia.

irrigation (,iri'gayshən) the washing out of a cavity or wound with a stream of lotion or water.

irritable ('iritəb'l) reacting excessively to a stimulus. *I. bowel syndrome* mucous colitis; spastic colon. The patient complains of disordered bowel function with abdominal pain, but no organic disease can be found.

irritant ('iritənt) an agent causing stimulation or excitation.

irritation (,iri'tayshən) 1. a condition of undue nervous excitement, through abnormal sensitiveness. *Cerebral i.* a stage of excitement present in many brain conditions, and typical of the recovery stage of concussion. 2. itching of the skin.

ischaemia (is'keemi·ə) a deficiency in the blood supply to a part of the body. *Myocardial i.* ischaemia of the heart muscles, which causes angina pectoris.

ischiorectal (,iskioh'rekt'l) concerning the ischium and the rectum. *I. abscess* a collection of pus in the ischiorectal connective tissue. An anal fistula may result.

ischium ('iski·əm) the lower posterior bone of the pelvic girdle.

Ishihara colour charts (,ishi-'hahrə) *S. Ishihara, Japanese ophthalmologist, 1879–1963.* Patterns of dots of the primary colours on similar backgrounds. The patterns can be seen by a normal-sighted person, but one who is colour blind will only be able to identify some of them.

Islet of Langerhans (,ielet əv 'langə,hanz) *P. Langerhans, German pathologist, 1847–1888.* One of a group of cells in the pancreas that produce insulin and glucagon; islet of the pancreas.

isocarboxazid (,iesohkah'boksə-,zid) a monoamine oxidase inhibitor used in the treatment of depressive illness.

Isogel ('iesoh,jel) proprietary, bulk forming laxative prepared from the husks of mucilaginous seeds. Used in chronic constipation.

isograft ('iesoh,grahft) a tissue graft from one identical twin to another.

isoimmunization (,iesoh,imyuh-nie'zayshən) the development of antibodies against an antigen derived from an individual of the same species, e.g. a rhesus-negative woman may immunize herself against her fetus, if it is rhesus-positive, by forming specific ANTIBODY.

isolation (,iesə'layshan) the separation of a person with an infectious disease from those noninfected. *I. period* quarantine; the length of time during which a patient with an infectious fever is considered capable of infecting others by contact.

isoleucine (ˌiesohˈlooseen) one of the 9 essential amino acids which are vital for health in the adult.

isometric (ˌiesohˈmetrik) having equal dimensions. *I. exercises* the contraction and relaxation of muscles without producing movement; used to maintain muscle tone following a fracture.

isoniazid (ˌiesohˈnieəzid) INH. A drug given orally in combination with streptomycin or para-aminosalicylic acid (PAS) which is effective in treating tuberculosis. Combined therapy reduces the risk of bacterial resistance.

isoprenaline (ˌiesohˈprenəlin) a sympathomimetic drug which has an action like adrenaline and can be used to treat asthma.

isosorbide dinitrate (ˌiesohˌsorbied dieˈnietrayt) a short-acting vasodilator similar in action to glyceryl trinitrate and used in the treatment of angina pectoris.

isotonic (ˌiesohˈtonik) having uniform tension. *I. solution* is of the same osmotic pressure as the fluid with which it is compared. Normal saline (0.9 per cent solution of salt in water) is isotonic with blood plasma.

isotope (ˈiesohˌtohp) one of the several forms of an element with the same atomic number but different atomic weights. *Radioactive i.* an unstable isotope which decays and emits alpha, beta or gamma rays. May be used in the diagnosis and treatment of malignant disease.

isthmus (ˈisməs) a narrow connection between two larger bodies or parts, e.g. the band of tissue between the two lobes of the thyroid gland.

itch (ich) a skin eruption with irritation. *Baker's i.* eczema of the hands due to the proteins of flour. *Barber's i.* sycosis; tinea barbae. *Dhobie i.* TINEA CRURIS. The name is derived from the belief in India that the spread of infection was due to washermen (dhobies) wearing their clients' clothes. *I. mite* the cause of scabies, *Sarcoptes scabiei*. *Washerwomen's i.* dermatitis of the hands due to the constant use of soda and detergents.

ITP idiopathic thrombocytopenic purpura.

IUCD intrauterine contraceptive device.

IVF in vitro fertilization. *See* FERTILIZATION.

IVP intravenous pyelography.

IVU intravenous urography.

J

J symbol for *joule*.

Jacksonian epilepsy (jak'sohni·ən) *J.H. Jackson, British neurologist, 1835–1911.* Focal motor EPILEPSY.

Jacquemier's sign ('zhahkhmi·ayz ,sien) *J.M. Jacquemier, French obstetrician, 1806–1879.* Blueness of the lining of the vagina seen from the early weeks of pregnancy.

jactitation (,jakti'tayshən) the extreme restlessness of an acutely ill patient.

Jakob–Creutzfeldt disease (yakob'kroytsfelt di,zeez) *A.M. Jakob, German psychiatrist, 1884–1931; H.G. Creutzfeldt, German psychiatrist, 1885–1964.* Pre-senile dementia due to a slow virus.

jargon ('jahgən) 1. the terminology used and generally understood only by those who have knowledge of that speciality, e.g. medical jargon, legal jargon. 2. gibberish talked by the insane.

jaundice ('jawndis) icterus; a yellow discoloration of the skin and conjunctivae, due to the presence of bile pigment in the blood. It may be: (1) *Haemolytic j.* due to excessive destruction of red blood cells, causing increase of bilirubin in the blood. The liver is not involved. *Acholuric j.* is of this type. It is characterized by increased fragility of the red blood cells. (2) *Hepatocellular j.* in which the liver cells are damaged by either infection or drugs. (3) *Obstructive j.* in which the bile is prevented from reaching the duodenum owing to obstruction by a gallstone, a growth or a stricture of the common bile duct. (4) *Phsyiological j.* (icterus neonatorum) which occurs within the first few days of life, and is caused by the breakdown of the excessive number of red blood cells present in the newborn.

jaw (jor) a bone of the face in which the teeth are embedded. *Lower j.* the mandible. *Upper j.* the two maxillae.

jejunectomy (,jejuh'nektəmee) excision of a part or the whole of the jejunum.

jejunoileostomy (ji,joonoh,ili'ostəmee) the making of an anastomosis between the jejunum and the ileum.

jejunostomy (,jejuh'nostəmee) the making of an opening into the jejunum through the abdominal wall.

jejunotomy (,jejuh'notəmee) an incision into the jejunum.

jejunum (ji'joonəm) the portion of the small intestine from the duodenum to the ileum; about 2.4 m (8 ft) in length.

jelly ('jelee) a soft, coherent, resilient substance; generally, a colloidal semisolid mass. *Contraceptive j.* a non-greasy jelly used in the vagina for prevention of conception (*see also* CONTRACEPTION). *Petroleum j.* a purified mixture of semisolid hydrocarbons obtained from petroleum (called also PETROLATUM). *Wharton's j.* the soft, jelly-like intracellular substance of the umbilical cord, which insulates the vein and arteries preventing occlusion and fetal hypoxia.

jerk (jərk) a sudden muscular contraction. *Knee j.* a kicking movement produced by tapping the tendon below the patella. Used with other jerks, such as the ankle jerk, to test the nervous reflexes.

jigger ('jigə) a sand flea found in the tropics which burrows into the soles of the feet and causes severe irritation.

joint (joynt) an articulation; the point of junction of two or more bones, particularly one which permits movement of the individual bones relative to each other.

joule (jool) *symbol* J. The SI unit of energy.

judgement ('jujmənt) the ability of an individual to estimate a situation, to arrive at reasonable conclusions and to decide on a course of action.

jugular ('jugyuhlə) relating to the neck. *J. veins* several veins in the neck which drain the blood from the head.

Jung (yuhng) *Carl Gustav, Swiss psychologist and psychiatrist, 1875–1961.*

juvenile ('joovə,niel) relating to young people.

juxta-articular (,jukstə-ah'tik-yuhlə) near a joint.

juxtaglomerular (,jukstəglo'mer-yuhlə) near to a glomerulus of the kidney. *J. cells* specialized cells found in the kidney which appear to play an important part in the control of aldosterone release.

juxtaposition (,jukstəpə'zishən) adjacent; side-by-side.

K

K symbol for *potassium*.

Kahn test (kahn) *B.L. Kahn, American bacteriologist, b. 1887.* An agglutination test for syphilis.

kala-azar (,kahlə-ə'zah) visceral leishmaniasis. A tropical disease caused by the protozoan parasite *Leishmania donovani* which is carried by the sand-fly. Symptoms include enlargement of the liver and spleen, anaemia and wasting. The disease is often fatal.

kanamycin (,kana'miesin) a broad-spectrum antibiotic for use against severe infections with Gram-negative organisms where penicillin is ineffective.

kaolin ('kayəlin) powdered clay containing aluminium silicate. It is taken orally in the treatment of diarrhoea and is also used as a dusting powder and for poultices.

Kaposi's sarcoma ('kapoh,zeez) *M.K. Kaposi, Austrian dermatologist, 1837–1902.* A multifocal, metastasizing, malignant reticulosis with angiosarcoma-like features, involving chiefly the skin. Rarely seen in the developed world until the outbreak of AIDS. Kaposi's sarcoma is a major feature of this disease, particularly in homosexuals.

Kaposi's spots a serious complication of infantile eczema occurring on exposure to herpes simplex virus infection. More commonly known as Kaposi's varicelliform eruption.

karaya (kə'rie-ə) a gum made from certain species of *Sterculia*, a genus of tropical trees and shrubs. Used as an aid to applying ostomy bags to the skin.

karyotype ('karioh,tiep) 1. the chromosomal constitution and arrangement of a cell of an individual. 2. the pattern which is seen when human chromosomes are photographed during metaphase. The pictures are then enlarged and paired according to the length of their short arm.

Kayser–Fleischer ring (,kiezə-'flieshə) *B. Kayser, German ophthalmologist, 1869–1954; B. Fleischer, German ophthalmologist, 1848–1904.* A brownish pigmented ring seen in the cornea of patients with hepatolenticular degeneration (Wilson's disease).

Kegel exercises ('kaygəl) specific exercises named after Dr Arnold H. Kegel, a gynaecologist who first developed the exercises to strengthen the pelvic-vaginal muscles as a means of controlling stress incontinence in women.

Keller's operation ('keləz) *W.L. Keller, American surgeon, 1874–1959.* An operation for correcting hallux valgus.

keloid ('keeloyd) hard, whitish scar tissue in the skin, common in people with dark skins. A type occurs in a healed wound due to overgrowth of fibrous tissue, causing the scar to be raised above the skin level. They may be removed but keloids tend to re-form in the new scar.

Kennedy's syndrome ('kenədiz) *F. Kennedy, American neurologist, 1884–1952.* Ipsilateral optic atrophy caused by a frontal lobe tumour which involves one of the optic nerves.

keratectasia (,kerətek'tayzi·ə) protrusion of the cornea following inflammation.

keratectomy (,kerə'tektəmee) excision of a portion of the cornea.

keratic (kə'ratik) 1. horny. 2. relating to the cornea. *K. precipitates* inflammatory exudates adhering to the back of the cornea; a sign of iritis and cyclitis.

keratin ('kerətin) an albuminoid substance which forms the principal constituent of all horny tissues.

keratinize (kə'rati,nayz) to make or become horny.

keratitis (,kerə'tietis) inflammation of the cornea. The causes may be physical (trauma, exposure to dust or vapours or to ultraviolet light) or due to infectious conditions such as corneal and dendritic ulcers. *Interstitial k.* deep chronic keratitis, usually arising out of congenital syphilis. *Striate k.* inflammation that appears in lines due to the folding over of the cornea after injury or operation, particularly one for cataract.

keratocele ('kerətoh,seel) descemetocele; protrusion of Descemet's membrane through the base of a corneal ulcer. A horny growth of the skin.

keratoconjunctivitis (,kerətohkən-'jungkti'vietis) inflammation of both the cornea and the conjunctiva of the eye.

keratoconus (,kerətoh'kohnəs) a conical cornea. A degenerative condition in which the cornea becomes thin and protruded into a cone-shape.

keratoiritis (,kerətoh·ie'rietis) inflammation of both the cornea and iris.

keratoma (,kerə'tohmə) keratosis.

keratomalacia (,kerətohmə'layshi·ə) ulceration and softening of the cornea due to a deficiency of vitamin A.

keratome ('kerə,tohm) a knife with a trowel-shaped blade for incising the cornea.

keratometer (kerə'tomitə) ophthalmometer. An instrument by which the amount of corneal astigmatism can be measured accurately.

keratophakia (,kerətoh'fayki·ə) keratoplasty in which a slice of donor's cornea is shaped to a desired curvature and inserted between layers of the recipient's cornea to change its curvature.

keratoplasty ('kerətoh,plastee) a plastic operation on the cornea, including corneal grafting.

keratoscope ('kerətoh,skohp) an instrument for examining the eye to detect keratoconus. Placido's disc.

keratosis (,kerə'tohsis) a skin disease marked by excessive growth of the epidermis or horny tissue.

keratotomy (,kerə,totəmee) incision of the cornea.

kerion ('keeri·ən) a complication of ringworm of the scalp, with formation of pustules.

kernicterus (kər'niktə·rəs) a condition in the newborn marked by severe neural symptoms, associated with high levels of bilirubin in the blood; it is commonly a sequela of icterus gravis neonatorum.

Kernig's sign ('kərnigz) *V.M. Kernig, Russian physician, 1840–1917.* A sign of meningitis. When the thigh is supported at right angles to the trunk, the patient is unable to straighten his leg at the knee joint.

ketamine ('ketə,meen) a rapidly acting, non-barbiturate, general anaesthetic which is given by intramuscular or intravenous injection.

ketogenic (,keetoh'jenik) forming or capable of being converted into ketone bodies. *K. diet* one containing large amounts of fat, with minimal amounts of protein and carbohydrate. The object of such a diet is to produce KETOSIS; it is occasionally used in the treatment of certain types of epilepsy in young children.

ketone ('keetohn) an organic compound containing the carbonyl group (CO) attached to two hydrocarbon groups. Ketones are produced by the metabolization of fats.

ketonuria (,keetoh'nyooə·ri·ə) the presence of ketones in urine; acetonuria.

ketosis (kee'tohsis) the condition in which ketones are formed in excess in the body and accumulate in the blood. Severe acidosis may occur.

ketosteroid (,keetoh'stiə·royd) a steroid hormone which contains a ketone group attached to a carbon atom. *17-K's* are excreted in the urine and formed from the adrenal corticosteroids, testosterone and, to a lesser extent, from oestrogens.

kick chart ('kik, chaht) a method of fetal assessment carried out by the mother. The number of kicks or movements felt during the day is counted and noted. If less than ten kicks are felt in a 12-h daytime period on two consecutive occasions, the mother is advised to contact her midwife or doctor immediately. If no movements are felt in any day, the mother is advised to contact the hospital at once. The value of this test is that it can highlight the potential case of fetal distress and alert medical attention before it is too late.

kidney ('kidnee) one of two organs situated in the lumbar region, which purify the blood and secrete urine. It secretes renin and renal erythropoietic factor. *Articial k.* the apparatus used to remove retained waste products from the blood when kidney function is impaired. *K. failure* the condition in which renal function is severely impaired and the organs are unable to maintain the fluid and electrolyte balance of the body. *Granular k.* the small fibrosed kidney of chronic nephritis. *Horseshoe k.* a congenital

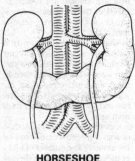

HORSESHOE KIDNEY

defect producing a fusion of the two kidneys into a horseshoe shape. *Polycystic k.* a congenital bilateral condition of multiple cysts replacing kidney tissue. *K. transplant* the surgical implantation of a kidney taken from a live donor or from one who has recently died. Used in the treatment of renal failure.

Kimmelstiel–Wilson syndrome (ˌkiməlsteel'wilsən) *P. Kimmelstiel, German pathologist, 1900–1970; C. Wilson, British physician, b.1906.* A degenerative complication of DIABETES MELLITUS, with albuminuria, oedema, hypertension, renal insufficiency and retinopathy. Called also intercapillary glomerulosclerosis.

kinaesthesia (ˌkinis'theezi·ə) the combined sensations by which position, weight and muscular position are perceived.

kinanaesthesia (ˌkinanəs'theezi·ə) an inability to perceive the sensation of movements of parts of the body.

kinase ('kienayz) an enzyme-activator; *see* ENTEROKINASE and THROMBOKINASE.

kineplasty ('kini,plastee) plastic amputation; amputation in which the stump is so formed as to be utilized for producing motion of the prosthesis.

kinetic (ki'netik) producing or pertaining to motion.

King's Fund (kingz fund) King Edward's Hospital Fund for London was founded in 1897 for the support, by the giving of grants, of voluntary hospitals in London. Since the inception of the National Health Service in 1948, it had been concerned with funding of experimental schemes, particularly relating to the management of services. *K.F. bed* a bed fitted with jointed springs which may be adjusted to various positions, developed as the result of research undertaken on behalf of and funded by the King's Fund.

kinin ('kienin) a polypeptide which occurs naturally and is a powerful vasodilator.

kinship ('kin·ship) relationship. *K. studies* (anthropological term) the study of kin (relatives) and their patterns of marriage, descent, inheritance, habitation, social values and economics.

Kirschner wire ('kiəshnə) *M. Kirschner, German surgeon, 1879–1942.* A thin wire that may be passed through a bone to apply skeletal traction.

kiss of life (‚kis əv 'lief) the expired air method of artificial respiration, by either mouth-to-nose or mouth-to-mouth breathing.

Klebsiella (‚klebsi'elə) a genus of Gram-negative bacteria (family Enterobacteriaceae).

Klebs–Löffler bacillus (‚klebz-'lərflə) *T.A.E. Klebs, German bacteriologist, 1834–1913; F.A.J. Löffler, German bacteriologist, 1852–1915. Corynebacterium diphtheriae,* the causative agent of diphtheria.

Kleihauer test ('kliehowə) a microscopic test to detect fetal cells in the maternal circulation, usually done immediately after delivery so that, if the mother is rhesus-negative and the fetus rhesus-positive, anti-D immunoglobulin may be given to prevent isoimmunization.

kleptomania (‚kleptəmayni·ə) an irresistible urge to steal when there is often no need and no particular desire for the objects. Often associated with depression.

Klinefelter's syndrome ('klien-feltəz) *H.F. Klinefelter, American physician, b. 1912.* A congenital chromosome abnormality in which each cell has three sex chromosomes, XXY, rather than the usual XX or XY, making a total of 47 (normal is 46). Affected men have female breast development and small testes and are infertile.

Klippel–Feil syndrome (‚klip'l-'fiel) *M. Klippel, French neurologist, 1858–1942; A. Feil, French physician, b. 1884.* A congenital abnormality in which the neck is very short due to absence or fusion of several vertebrae in the cervical region.

Klumpke's paralysis ('kloomp-kəz) *A. Déjerine-Klumpke, French neurologist, 1859–1927.* A palsy affecting the hand and arm, usually caused by a birth injury to the brachial plexus.

knee (nee) the joint between the femur and the tibia. *K. cap* the patella. *K. jerk* an upward jerk of the leg obtained by striking the patellar tendon when the knee is passively flexed. *Housemaid's k.* prepatellar bursitis. *Knock-k.* a condition in which the knees turn inwards towards each other; genu valgum.

Koch's bacillus (‚koks bə'siləs) *R. Koch, German bacteriologist, 1843–1910. Mycobacterium tuberculosis,* the causative organism of tuberculosis.

Köhler's disease ('kərləz) *A. Köhler, German physician and radiologist, 1874–1947.* Osteochondritis of the navicular bone of the foot, occurring in children.

koilonychia (‚koylə'niki·ə) the development of brittle, spoon-shaped nails which may occur in iron-deficiency anaemia.

Koplik's spots ('kopliks) *H. Koplik, American paediatrician, 1858–1927.* Small white spots that sometimes appear on the mucous membranes inside the mouth in measles on the second day of onset, before the general rash.

Korotkoff's method (ko'rotkofs) *N.S. Korotkoff, Russian physician, 1874–1920.* A method of finding the systolic and diastolic blood pressure by listening to the sounds produced in an artery while the pressure in a previously inflated cuff is gradually reduced.

Korsakoff's syndrome or psychosis ('kawsəkofs) *S.S. Korsakoff, Russian neurologist, 1854–1900.* A chronic condition in which there is impaired memory, particularly for recent events, and the patient is disorientated for time and place. It may be present in psychosis of infective, toxic or metabolic origin, or in chronic alcoholism.

Krabbe's disease ('krabeez) *K.H. Krabbe, Danish neurologist, 1885–1961.* A familial form of mental subnormality due to degenerative disease of the white matter of the brain resulting in learning difficulties; leukodystrophy.

kraurosis (kror'rohsis) dryness and shrinking of a part of the body. *K. vulvae* a degenerative condition of the vulva. May be treated by giving oestrin preparations.

Kreb's cycle (krebz) *Sir H.A. Krebs, German–British biochemist, 1900–1981.* A series of reactions during which the aerobic oxidation of pyruvic acid takes place. This is part of carbohydrate metabolism. *K. urea c.* the way in which urea is formed in the liver.

Krukenberg's tumour ('krookenbərgz) *G.P.H. Krukenberg, German gynaecologist, 1871–1946.* A large secondary malignant growth in an ovary. The primary one is usually in the stomach and is small.

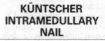

KÜNTSCHER INTRAMEDULLARY NAIL

Küntscher nail ('koontshə) *G. Küntscher, German orthopaedic surgeon, 1902–1972.* An intramedullary nail used in treating fractures of long bones, especially the shaft of the femur.

Kupffer's cells ('kuhpfəz) *K.W. von Kupffer, German anatomist, 1829–1902.* Phagocytic reticuloendothelial cells of the liver that form bile from haemoglobin released by disintegrated erythrocytes.

kuru ('kuhroo) a progressive, fatal central nervous system disorder thought to be due to a slow virus and transmissible to subhuman primates; seen only in the peoples of New Guinea.

Kveim test ('kvaym) *M.A. Kveim, Norwegian physician, b. 1892.* A test for sarcoidosis where antigen from the lymph nodes or spleen of a sarcoidosis patient is injected intradermally.

kawashiorkor (ˌkwshi'awkə) a condition of protein malnutrition occurring in children in under-privileged populations. Fatty infiltration of the liver arises and may cause cirrhosis.

kymograph ('kieməˌgrahf, -ˌgraf) an instrument for recording variations or undulations, arterial or other.

kyphoscoliosis (ˌkiefohˌskohli-'ohsis) an abnormal curvature of the spine in which there is forward and sideways displacement.

kyphosis (kie'fohsis) posterior curvature of the spine; humpback.

L

l symbol for litre.

labetalol (lə'beetəlol) an alpha- and beta-adrenergic receptor blocker used in the treatment of hypertension.

labial ('laybi·əl) pertaining to the lips or labia.

labile ('laybiel) unstable. Applied to those chemicals that are subject to change or readily altered by heat.

lability (lə'bilətee) instability. *L. of mood* the tendency to sudden changes of mood of short duration.

labioglossopharyngeal (,laybioh- ,glosohfə'rinji·əl, -,farin'jeeəl) concerning the lips, tongue and pharynx. *L. paralysis* bulbar paralysis. *See* PARALYSIS.

labium ('laybi·əm) a lip. *L. majus pudendi* the large fold of flesh surrounding the vulva. *L. minus pudendi* the lesser fold within the labium majus.

labour ('laybə) parturition or childbirth, which takes place in three stages: (1) dilatation of the cervix uteri; (2) passage of the child through the birth canal; and (3) expulsion of the placenta. *Induced l.* labour brought on by artificial means before term, as in cases of contracted pelvis or if overdue. *Obstructed l.* labour in which there is a mechanical hindrance. *Precipitate l.* labour in which the baby is delivered extremely rapidly. *Premature l.* labour which occurs before term. *Spurious l.* ineffective labour pains which sometimes precede true labour pains.

labyrinth ('labə'rinth) the structures forming the internal ear, i.e. the cochlea and semicircular canals. *Bony l.* the bony canals of the internal ear. *Membranous l.* the soft structure inside the bony canals.

labyrinthectomy (,labə·rin'thektəmee) excision of the labyrinth.

labyrinthitis (,labə·rin'thietis) inflammation of the labyrinth, causing vertigo.

laceration (,lasə'rayshən) a wound with torn and ragged edges.

lacrimal ('lakriməl) relating to tears. *L. apparatus* the structures secreting the tears and draining the fluid from the conjunctival sac. *L. gland* a gland that secretes tears, which drain through two small openings in the eyelids (*l. puncta*) into a pair of ducts (*l. canaliculi*) into the sac and finally into the nasal cavity through the nasolacrimal duct. Situated in the outer and upper corner of the orbit.

lacrimation (,lakri'mayshən) an excessive secretion of tears.

lacrimator ('lakri,maytə) a substance which causes excessive

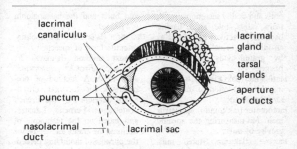

LACRIMAL APPARATUS

secretion of tears, e.g. tear-gas.

lactagogue ('laktə,gog) galactagogue.

lactalbumin (lak'talbyuhmin) an albumin of milk.

lactase ('laktayz) an enzyme produced in the small intestine which converts lactose into glucose and galactose.

lactate ('laktayt) 1. any substance given to promote lactation. 2. any salt of lactic acid. 3. to secrete milk. *L. dehydrogenase* abbreviated LD, LDH. An enzyme that catalyses the interconversion of lactate and pyruvate. Widespread in tissues and particularly abundant in kidney, skeletal muscle, liver and myocardium. It has five isoenzymes denoted LD_1 to LD_5. The 'flipped' pattern in which the serum LD_1 level is greater than the LD_2 level is indicative of an acute myocardial infarction. This pattern occurs within 12–24 h after the attack.

lactation (lak'tayshən) 1. the period during which the infant is nourished from the breast. 2. the process of milk secretion by the mammary glands.

lacteal ('lakti·əl) 1. consisting of milk. 2. a lymphatic duct in the small intestine which absorbs chyle.

lactic ('laktik) pertaining to milk. *L. acid* an acid formed by the fermentation of lactose or milk sugar. It is produced naturally in the body as a result of glucose metabolism. An excess of the acid accumulating in the muscles may cause cramp.

lactiferous (lak'tifə·rəs) conveying or secreting milk.

lactifuge ('laktifyooj) a drug or agent which retards the secretion of milk.

Lactobacillus (,laktohbə'siləs) a genus of Gram-positive, rod-shaped bacteria, many of which produce fermentation.

lactoferrin (,laktoh'ferin) an iron-binding protein found in neutrophils and bodily secretions (milk, tears, saliva, bile, etc.), having bactericidal activity and acting as an inhibitor of colony formation by granulocytes and macrophages.

lactogenic (ˌlaktə'jenik) stimulating the production of milk. *See* LUTEOTROPHIN.

lactometer (lak'tomitə) an instrument for measuring the specific gravity of milk.

lactose ('laktohz, -tohs) milk sugar consisting of glucose and galactose.

lactosuria (ˌlaktə'syooə·ri·ə) lactose in the urine.

lactovegetarian (ˌlaktoh,veji'tair-·ri·ən) 1. a person who subsists on a diet of milk or milk products and vegetables. 2. pertaining to such a diet.

lactulose ('laktyuhlohz) a synthetic disaccharide which is used as a laxative.

lacuna (lə'kyoonə) a small cavity or depression in any part of the body.

Laënnec's disease (ˌla·e'nek) *R.T.H. Laënnec, French physician, 1781–1826.* The commonest type of cirrhosis of the liver, frequently attributable to high alcohol consumption.

Laetrile ('laytriel) American trade name for a substance derived from apricot stones, alleged to have antineoplastic activity.

laevulose ('levyuh,lohz) fruit sugar; fructose.

laked (laykt) descriptive of blood when haemoglobin has separated from the red blood cells.

laking ('layking) haemolysis of the red blood cells. The cells swell

and burst and the haemoglobin is released.

lallation (la'layshən) a babbling, infantile form of speech.

Lamaze method (la'mayz) *F. Lamaze, French obstetrician, 1890–1957.* A method of preparations for NATURAL CHILDBIRTH developed by the French obstetrician Fernand Lamaze, and based on the technique of training the mind and body for the purpose of modifying perception of pain during labour and delivery.

lambda ('lamdə) the posterior fontanelle of the skull, so called from its resemblance to the Greek letter lambda (λ).

lambdoid ('lamdoyd) shaped like the Greek letter lambda Λ or λ. *L. suture* the junction of the occipital bone with the parietals.

lambliasis (lam'blieəsis) giardiasis.

lamella (lə'melə) 1. a thin layer, membrane or plate, as of bone. 2. a thin medicated disc of gelatin used in applying drugs to the eye. The gelatin dissolves and the drugs are absorbed.

lamina ('laminə) a bony plate or layer.

laminectomy (ˌlami'nektəmee) excision of the posterior arch of a vertebra, sometimes performed to relieve pressure on the spinal cord or nerves.

lanatoside (la'natohsied) a cardiac glycoside drug similar to digitalis and used in the treatment of heart failure.

Lancefield's groups ('lansfeeldz) *R.C. Lancefield, American bacteriologist, 1895–1981.* Divisions of β-haemolytic streptococci, which are classified on the basis of serological action into groups A–R. Most human infections are due to group A.

Landry's paralysis (lan'dreez) *J.B.G. Landry, French physician, 1826–1865.* Guillain–Barré syndrome; acute ascending polyneuritis.

Landsteiner's classification ('landstienəz) *K. Landsteiner, Austrian biologist, 1868–1943.* A system of blood groups; the ABO system, consisting of groups A, B, AB and O.

Lange colloidal gold test ('langə) *C.F.A. Lange, German physician, b.1883.* A test made on cerebrospinal fluid to detect syphilis, disseminated sclerosis, meningitis and other neurological conditions.

Langerhans, islet of ('langə,hanz) *P. Langerhans, German pathologist, 1847–1888.* One of a group of cells in the pancreas which produce insulin.

Langhans' cell ('langhanz) *T. Langhans, Swiss pathologist, 1834–1915.* A deep cell of a chorionic villus.

lanolin ('lanəlin) a fat obtained from sheep's wool, and used as a basis for ointments, salves, creams and cosmetics.

lanugo (lə'nyoogoh, -noo-) the fine hair that covers the body of the fetus and newly born infants, especially those who are premature. Called also *down*.

laparoscopy (,lapə'roskəpee) viewing of the abdominal cavity by passing an endoscope through the abdominal wall.

laparotomy (,lapə'rotəmee) incision of the abdominal wall for exploratory purposes.

laryngeal (lə'rinji·əl, ,larin'jeeəl) pertaining to the larynx.

laryngectomy (,larin'jektəmee) excision of the larynx.

laryngismus (,larin'jizməs) a spasmodic contraction of the larynx. *L. stridulus* a crowing sound on inspiration following a period of apnoea due to spasmodic closure of the glottis. It occurs in children, particularly those suffering from rickets. Croup.

laryngitis (,larin'jietis) inflammation of the larynx causing hoarseness or loss of voice due to acute infection or irritation by gases.

laryngologist (,laring'goləjist) a specialist in diseases of the larynx.

laryngopharynx (lə,ring'goh'faringks) the lower part of the pharynx.

laryngoscope (lə'ring·goh,skohp) an endoscopic instrument for examining the larynx or for aiding the insertion of endotracheal tubes or the bronchoscope.

laryngospasm (lə'ring·goh,spazəm) a reflex prolonged contraction of the laryngeal muscles that is liable to occur on insertion or withdrawal of an intratracheal tube.

laryngostenosis (lə,ring·gohstə-'nohsis) contraction or stricture of the larynx.

laryngostomy (,laring'gostəmee) the making of an opening into the larynx to provide an artificial air passage.

laryngotomy (,laring'gotəmee) an

incision into the larynx to make a temporary opening in an emergency when the larynx is obstructed. Tracheostomy.

laryngotracheal (lə,ring·goh'traki-·əl) referring to both the larynx and trachea.

laryngotracheitis (lə,ring·goh,tra-ki'ietis) inflammation of both the larynx and trachea.

laryngotracheobronchitis (lə ,ring·goh,trakiohbrong'kietis) an acute viral infection of the respiratory tract which occurs particularly in young children.

larynx ('laringks) [Gr.] the muscular and cartilaginous structure, lined with mucous membrane, situated at the top of the trachea and below the root of the tongue and the hyoid bone. The larynx contains the vocal cords, and is the source of the sound heard in speech; it is called also the voice box.

laser ('layzə) *l*ight *a*mplification by *s*timulated *e*mission of *r*adiation. An apparatus producing an extremely concentrated beam of light that can be used to cut metals. Used in the treatment of neoplasms, of detached retina, diabetic retinopathy and macular degeneration, and of some skin conditions.

Lassa fever ('lasə) a West African viral haemorrhagic fever with insidious onset and an incubation period of 6–21 days. It is a zoonosis, the reservoir of infection of which is the multimammate rat. Devastating outbreaks of person-to-person transmission have occurred in hospital in West Africa by accidental inoculation of blood and tissue fluid from infected patients. In the UK prevention is dependent on the early detection of cases and their isolation, and strict precautions to protect health care staff caring for febrile patients from Africa from inoculation or other accidents.

Lassar's paste ('lasəz) *G. Lassar, German dermatologist, 1849–1907.* A soothing paste used in skin diseases, containing salicylic acid, zinc oxide, starch and soft paraffin.

lassitude ('lasi,tyood) a feeling of extreme weakness and apathy.

latent ('laytənt) temporarily concealed; not manifest. *L. heat* the heat absorbed by a substance during a change in state, e.g. from water into steam. When condensation occurs this heat is released. *L. period* 1. the incubation period of an infectious disease. 2. the time between the application of a nerve stimulus and the reaction.

lateral ('latə·rəl) situated at the side; therefore, away from the centre.

lateroversion (,latə·roh'vərshən, -zhən) a turning to one side, such as may occur of the uterus.

laudanum ('lawd'nəm) tincture of opium; a preparation formerly used as a narcotic.

laughing gas ('lahfing) nitrous oxide.

lavage ('lavij, la'vahzh) the washing out of a cavity. *Colonic l.* the washing out of the colon. *Gastric l.* the washing out of the stomach.

laxative ('laksətiv) a medicine that loosens the bowel contents and

281

encourages evacuation. A laxative with a mild or gentle effect on the bowels is also known as an asperient; one with a strong effect is referred to as a cathartic or a purgative.

LE lupus erythematosus. *LE cell* a mature neutrophilic polymorphonuclear leukocyte, which has phagocytized a large, spherical inclusion derived from another neutrophil; a characteristic of lupus erythematosus, but also found in analogous connective tissue disorders.

lead (led) *symbol* Pb. A metallic element, many of the compounds of which are highly poisonous. *L. lotion* lead subacetate solution used externally on bruises. *L. poisoning* a condition which usually occurs in children as the result of excessive lead in the atmosphere, or from chewing objects covered with paint containing lead. The symptoms and signs include malaise, diarrhoea and vomiting, and sometimes encephalitis. There is often pallor and a blue line around the gums.

Leber's disease (laybərz) *T.B. Leber, German ophthalmologist, 1840–1917.* Hereditary optic atrophy.

lecithin ('lesithin) one of a group of phospholipids that are found in the cell tissues and are concerned in the metabolism of fat.

leech ('leech) *Hirudo medicinalis,* an aquatic worm which sucks blood and secretes hirudin (an anticoagulant) in its saliva. On rare occasions used to withdraw blood from patients.

leg (leg) the lower limb, from knee to ankle. *Barbados l.* elephantiasis. *Bow l.* genu varum. *Scissor l.* condition in which the patient is cross-legged, such as occurs in cerebral diplegia. *White l.* phlegmasia alba dolens.

Legionella pneumophila (,leejə-'nelə nyoo'mofilə) a species of Gram-negative, non-acid-fast, rod-shaped bacteria which require both cysteine and iron for growth; it is the causative agent of LEGIONNAIRES' DISEASE and PONTIAC FEVER.

legionellosis (,leejəne'lohsis) disease caused by infection with *Legionella* species, such as *L. pneumophila.* A notifiable disease in Scotland.

legionnaires' disease (leegən'airz) a pulmonary form of legionellosis, resulting from infection with *Legionella pneumophila.* It is contagious and symptoms include fever, pain in the muscles and across the chest, a dry cough and a partial loss of kidney function. The prevalence of legionnaires' disease is not certain but it is estimated that between 5 and 10 per cent of the annual cases of pneumonia in the UK are caused by *L. pneumophila.*

leiomyoma (,lieohmie'ohmə) a benign smooth muscle tumour (fibroid) most commonly found in the uterus.

leiomyosarcoma (,lieoh,mieohsah-'kohmə) a malignant muscle tumour.

Leishman–Donovan bodies (,leeshman'donəvən) *Sir W.B. Leishman, British pathologist, 1865–1926; C. Donovan, Irish* *physician, 1863–1951*. The intracellular forms of *Leishmania donovani*, the parasite producing kala-azar. These bodies occur in the spleen and liver.

Leishmania (leesh'mayni·ə) a genus of parasitic protozoa having flagella which infect the blood of man and are the cause of leishmaniasis.

leishmaniasis (ˌleeshmə'nieəsis) a group of diseases caused by one of the protozoan *Leishmania* parasites. *See* KALA-AZAR.

Lembert's suture (lanh'bairz) *A. Lembert, French surgeon, 1802–1851*. A series of stitches used for wounds of the intestine. So arranged that the edges are turned inwards and the peritoneal surfaces are in contact.

lens (lenz) 1. a piece of glass or other material shaped to transmit light rays in a particular direction. 2. the transparent crystalline body situated behind the pupil of the eye. It serves as a refractive medium for rays of light. *Contact l.* a thin sheet of glass or plastic moulded to fit directly over the cornea. Worn instead of spectacles.

lentigo (len'tiegoh) a brownish or yellowish spot on the skin. A freckle. *L. maligna* Hutchinson's melanotic freckle. *See* FRECKLE.

leontiasis (ˌlien'tieəsis) an osseous deformity of the face which produces a lion-like appearance. It occurs sometimes in leprosy and rarely in osteitis deformans.

lepidosis (ˌlepi'dohsis) any scaly eruption of the skin.

leprosy ('leprəsee) Hansen's disease. An incurable, chronic infection of the skin, mucous membrane and nerves with *Mycobacterium leprae*. It is predominantly a tropical disease which is transmitted by direct contact. There is an insidious onset of symptoms, mainly involving the skin and nerves, after an incubation period of between one and thirty years. The disease can be classified into three types: (1) *Lepromatous*, which is a steadily progressive form, often resulting in paralysis, disfigurement and deformity. This form is often complicated by tuberculosis. (2) *Tuberculoid*, which is often self-limiting and generally runs a more benign course. (3) *Indeterminate*, in which there are skin symptoms representative of both lepromatous and tuberculoid forms. Leprosy can be controlled by the use of sulphone drugs.

leptomeningitis (ˌleptoh,menin-'jietis) inflammation of the pia mater and arachnoid membranes of the brain and spinal cord.

Leptospira (ˌleptoh'spierə) a genus of spirochaetes. *L. icterohaemorrhagiae* the cause of spirochaetal jaundice (Weil's disease).

leptospirosis (ˌleptohspie'rohsis) any of a group of notifiable infectious diseases due to serotypes of *Leptospira*. The best known is Weil's disease, or leptospiral jaundice; others are mud fever, autumn fever and swineherd's disease. The aetiological agent is a spiral organism that is common in water. Initially the symptoms include fever, rigors, vomiting, headache and often jaundice.

Diagnosis may be difficult because the symptoms resemble those of several other diseases. Jaundice is a key symptom. Sanitation measures can reduce the spread of the disease in both man and animals.

Leriche's syndrome (lə'reeshiz) *R. Leriche, French surgeon, 1879–1955.* A condition in which atherosclerosis of peripheral arteries is accompanied by obstruction of the lower end of the aorta.

lesbianism ('lezbi·ənizəm) sexual attraction of one woman to another; female homosexuality.

Lesch–Nyhan syndrome (,lesh-'niehan) *M. Lesch, American physician, b. 1939; W.L. Nyhan Jr., American physician, b. 1926.* A hereditary disorder of purine metabolism transmitted as an X-linked recessive trait with physical and mental handicap, compulsive self-mutilation of fingers and lips by biting, choreoathetosis, spastic cerebral palsy, and impaired renal function.

lesion ('leezhən) any pathological or traumatic discontinuity of tissue or loss of function of a part. Lesion is a broad term, including wounds, sores, ulcers, tumours, cataracts and any other tissue damage. Lesions range from the skin sores associated with eczema to the changes in lung tissue that occur in tuberculosis.

lethargy ('lethəjee) a condition of drowsiness or stupor which cannot be overcome by the will.

Letterer–Siwe disease (,letə·rə-'seevə) *E. Letterer, German physician, b. 1895; S.A. Siwe, German*

physician, b. 1897. Reticuloendotheliosis of early childhood, marked by a haemorrhagic tendency, eczematoid skin eruption, hepatosplenomegaly with lymph node involvement, and progressive anaemia.

leucine ('looseen) a naturally occurring essential amino acid, vital for growth in infants and for nitrogen equilibrium in adults.

leukaemia (loo'keemi·ə) a progressive, malignant disease of the blood-forming organs, marked by abnormal proliferation and development of leukocytes and their precursors in the blood and bone marrow. It is accompanied by a reduced number of erythrocytes and blood platelets, resulting in anaemia and increased susceptibility to infection and haemorrhage. Other typical symptoms include fever, pain in the joints and bones and swelling of the lymph nodes, spleen and liver. Leukaemia is classified clinically on the basis of (1) the duration and character of the disease (acute or chronic); (2) the cell line involved, i.e. myeloid (myelocytic, myeloblastic, granulocytic) or lymphoid (lymphatic, lymphoblastic, lymphocytic). A widely used classification of acute leukaemia based on cell type is the French American British (FAB) classification. The incidence of the disease is growing and the increase is only partially explained by increased efficiency of detection.

leukocyte ('lookə,siet) a white blood corpuscle. There are three types: (1) granular (polymorpho-

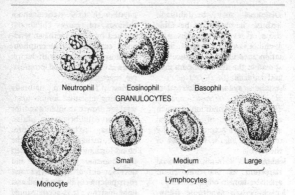

Neutrophil   Eosinophil   Basophil
GRANULOCYTES

Monocyte   Small   Medium   Large
Lymphocytes

AGRANULOCYTES

TYPES OF LEUKOCYTES

nuclear cells) formed in bone marrow, consisting of neutrophils, eosinophils and basophils; (2) lymphocytes (formed in the lymph glands); and (3) monocytes. Normal leukocyte count is as follows:

Type of leukocyte	No of cells per litre
Neutrophils	$2.5–7.4 \times 10^9$
Eosinophils	$4–44 \times 10^9$
Basophils	$0–1 \times 10^9$
Lymphocytes	$1.5–3.5 \times 10^9$
Monocytes	$2–8 \times 10^9$

leukocytolysis (,lookohsie'tolisis) destruction of white blood cells.

leukocytopoiesis (,lookoh,sietohpoy'eesis) leukopoiesis.

leukocytosis (,lookohsie'tohsis) an increase in the number of leukocytes in the blood. Often a response to infection.

leukoderma (,lookoh'dərmə) an absence of pigment in patches or bands, producing abnormal whiteness of the skin. Vitiligo.

leukodystrophy (,lookoh'distrəfee) a degenerative disorder of the brain which starts during the first few months of life and leads to mental, visual and motor deterioration.

leukoma (loo'kohmə) a white spot on the cornea, usually following an injury to the eye.

leukonychia (,lookoh'niki·ə) white patches on the nails due to air underneath.

leukopenia (,lookoh'peeni·ə) a decreased number of white cells, usually granulocytes, in the blood.

leukophoresis (ˌlookohfəˈreesis) withdrawal of blood for the selective removal of leukocytes. The remaining blood is re-transfused.

leukoplakia (ˌlookohˈplaykiˈə) a chronic inflammation, characterized by white thickened patches on the mucous membranes, particularly of the tongue, gums and inside of the cheeks. *L. vulvae* thickening of the mucous membrane of the labia with the appearance of scattered white patches.

leukopoiesis (ˌlookohpoyˈeesis) the formation of white blood cells. Leukocytopoiesis.

leukorrhoea (ˌlookəˈreeə) a viscid, whitish discharge from the vagina.

leukotomy (looˈkotəmee) a psychosurgical operation in which the white nerve fibres within the brain are severed. Prefrontal leukotomy has been largely replaced by a variety of stereotatic surgical techniques, where carefully controlled and very small lesions are made in one or more of the pathways of the limbic system. Now rarely used.

levator (ləˈvaytə) a muscle which raises a structure or organ of the body.

levels of care (ˈlevˈlz) the six division of the HEALTH CARE SYSTEM: preventive care, primary care, secondary or acute care, tertiary care, restorative care and continuing care.

levodopa (ˌleevohˈdohpə) L-dopa; a synthetic drug used in the treatment of parkinsonism.

levonorgestrel (ˌleevohnorˈjestrel) a potent progestin used in combination with an oestrogen as an oral contraceptive.

levorphanol (leˈvorfənol) an analgesic somewhat resembling morphine in its action and addiction potentialities. It is used to relieve severe pain.

Li symbol for *lithium*.

libido (liˈbeedoh) 1. the vital force or impulse which brings about purposeful action. 2. sexual drive in freudian psychoanalysis, the motive force of all human beings.

lichen (ˈliekən, ˈlichən) a group of inflammatory affections of the skin in which the lesions consist of papular eruptions. *L. planus* raised flat patches of dull, reddish-purple colour, with smooth or scaly surface.

lichenification (lieˌkenifiˈkayshən) the stage of an eruption when it resembles lichen.

lid (lid) eyelid. *Granular l.* trachoma. *L. lag* jerky movement of the upper lid when it is being lowered. A sign of exophthalmic goitre (thyrotoxicosis).

lie (lie) a position or direction. *L. of fetus* the position of the fetus in the uterus. The normal lie is longitudinal.

Lieberkühn's glands (ˈleebəˌkoonz) *J.N. Lieberkühn, German anatomist, 1711–1756.* Tubular glands of the small intestine.

lien (ˈlieˈen) the spleen.

lienculus (lieˈengkyuhləs) an accessory spleen.

lienitis (lieəˈnietis) inflammation of the spleen; splenitis.

lienorenal (ˌlieənohˈreenˈl) relating to the spleen and kidneys; splenorenal; splenonephric.

lientery (ˈlieəntəˌree) diarrhoea

consisting mainly of undigested food.

life event ('lief) a sociological term used to describe major events in a person's life, e.g. leaving home for the first time, getting married, moving house, changing a job.

life expectancy the average length of life based upon prevailing mortality trends.

ligament ('ligəmənt) 1. a band of fibrous tissue connecting bones forming a joint. 2. a layer or layers of peritoneum connecting one abdominal organ to another or to the abdominal wall. *Annular l.* the ring-like band which fixes the head of the radius to the ulna. *Cruciate l.* crossed ligaments within the knee joint. *Inguinal l.* that between the pubic bone and anterior iliac crest. *Round l.* for example, one of the two anterior ligaments of the uterus, passing through the inguinal canal and ending in the labia majora. There are also round ligaments of the femur and of the liver.

ligation (lie'gayshən) the application of a ligature.

ligature ('ligəchə) a thread of silk, catgut or other material used for tying round a blood vessel to stop it bleeding.

light (liet) electromagnetic waves which stimulate the retina of the eye. *L. adaptation* the changes that take place in the eye when the intensity of the light increases or decreases. *L. coagulation* a method of treating retinal detachment by directing a beam of strong light from a carbon arc through the pupil to the affected area.

lightening ('lietəning) the relief experienced in pregnancy, 2 to 3 weeks before labour, when the uterus sinks into the pelvis and ceases to press on the diaphragm.

lignocaine ('lignoh,kayn) a local anaesthetic administered by injection and by surface application. Also used intravenously in cases of cardiac arrhythmia, especially myocardial infarction.

limbus ('limbəs) an edge or border. *Corneal l.* the border where the cornea joins the sclera.

lime (liem) 1. a citrus fruit resembling a small lemon. 2. calcium oxide, the salts of which help to form bone. Quicklime. *Chlorinated l.* bleaching powder. *Slaked l.* calcium hydroxide. *L. water* calcium hydroxide solution. Given to counteract acidity.

liminal ('limin'l) pertaining to the threshold of perception.

lincomycin (,linkoh'miesin) an antibiotic derived from the *Streptomyces* genus. Used in the treatment of streptococcal bone and joint infections, including osteomyelitis.

linctus ('lingktəs) a thick syrup given to soothe and allay coughing.

linea ('lini·ə) [L] *a line. L. alba* the tendinous area in the centre of the abdominal wall into which the transversalis and part of the oblique muscles are inserted. *L. albicantes* white streaks that appear on the abdomen when it is distended by pregnancy or a tumour. *L. aspera* the rough ridge on the back of the femur into which muscles are inserted.

L. nigra the pigmented line which often appears in pregnancy on the abdomen between the umbilicus and the pubis.

linear ('lini·ə) pertaining to line. *L. accelerator* a mega-voltage machine for accelerating electrons so that powerful X-rays are given off for use in the treatment of deep-seated tumours.

lingual ('ling·gwəl) pertaining to the tongue.

lingula ('ling·gyuhlə) a tongue-like structure such as the projection of lung tissue from the left upper lobe.

liniment ('linimənt) a liquid to be applied externally by rubbing on to the skin.

lip (lip) 1. the upper or lower fleshy margin of the mouth. 2. any liplike part; labium. *Cleft l.* congenital fissure of the upper lip.

lip reading (lip 'reeding) understanding of speech through observation of the speaker's lip movements; called also speech reading.

lipaemia (li'peemi·ə) the presence of excess fat in the blood. Sometimes a feature of diabetes. *L. retinalis* condition in which the retinal blood vessels appear to be filled with milk due to the presence of an excess of fat in the blood.

lipase ('lipayz, -pays) fat-splitting enzyme; any enzyme that catalyses the splitting of fats into glycerol and fatty acids. Measurement of the serum lipase level is an important diagnostic test for acute and chronic pancreatitis.

lipid ('lipid) one of a group of fatty substances that are insoluble in water but soluble in alcohol or chloroform. They form an important part of the diet and are normally present in the body tissues.

lipochondrodystrophy (,lipoh-,kondroh'distrəfee) a congenital condition affecting the metabolism of fat and producing bone deformities, dwarfism, facial abnormalities and learning difficulties. Hurler's syndrome.

lipodystrophy (,lipoh'distrəfee) a disorder of fat metabolism. *Progressive l.* a rare condition occurring mainly in females in which there is progressive loss of fat over the upper half of the body.

lipoidosis (,lipoy'dohsis) a group of diseases in which there is an error in lipoid metabolism producing reticuloendothelial hyperplasia. Xanthomas are common.

lipolysis (li'polisis) the breakdown of fats by the action of bile salts and enzymes to a fine emulsion and fatty acids.

lipoma (li'pohmə) a benign tumour composed of fatty tissue, arising in any part of the body, and developing in connective tissue. *Diffuse l.* a tumour of fat in an irregular mass, without a capsule, occurring above the pelvis.

lipoprotein (,lipoh'prohteen) one of a group of fatty proteins that are present in blood plasma.

liposarcoma (,liposah'kohmə) a malignant tumour of the fat cells.

lipuria (li'pyooə'ri·ə) the presence of fat in urine.

liquefaction (,likwi'fakshən) reduction to liquid form.

liquid ('likwid) 1. a substance that flows readily in its natural state. 2. flowing readily, neither solid nor gaseous. *L. diet* a diet limited to the intake of liquids or foods that can be changed to a liquid state. A liquid diet may be restricted to clear liquids or it may be a full liquid diet.

liquor ('likə, 'liekwor) a watery fluid; a solution. *L. amnii* the fluid in which the fetus floats; amniotic fluid.

Listeria (listiə·ri·ə) *Baron J. Lister, British surgeon, 1827–1912.* A genus of Gram-negative bacteria which produce upper respiratory disease, septicaemia and encephalitic disease in humans. They can be transmitted by the consumption of infected, unpasteurized dairy produce, or by direct contact with infected animals or contaminated soil. Newborn infants, pregnant women, the elderly and the immunosuppressed are more susceptible to infection.

listeroisis (lis,tiə·ri'ohsis) infection with organisms of the genus *Listeria*

lithagogue ('lithə,gog) a drug which helps to expel calculi.

lithiasis (li'thieəsis) the formation of calculi. *Conjunctival l.* the formation of small white chalky areas on the inner surface of the eyelids.

lithium ('lithi·əm) *symbol* Li. An alkaline metallic element. *L. carbonate* a drug used in the treatment of manic-depressive illness.

litholapaxy (li'tholə,paksee) the removal of fragments of a calculus from the bladder after litho-tripsy.

lithonephrotomy (,lithohnə'frotəmee) incision into the kidney to remove a stone; nephrolithotomy.

lithopedion (,lithoh'peedi·ən) a dead fetus that has been retained and has become calcified.

lithosis (li'thohsis) pneumoconiosis resulting from inhalation of particles of silica, etc., into the lungs.

lithotomy (li'thotəmee) incision into the bladder for the removal of calculi.

lithotripsy ('lithoh,tripsee) the crushing of calculi in the bladder; lithotrity.

lithotrite ('lithoh,triet) an instrument used for lithotripsy.

lithuresis (,lithyuh'reesis) passage of small calculi or gravel in the urine.

litmus ('litməs) a blue pigment obtained from lichen and used for testing the reaction of fluids. *Blue l.* is turned red by an acid. *Red l.* is turned blue by an alkali.

litre ('leetə) *symbol* l. The SI unit of capacity. One cubic decimetre.

Little's disease ('lit'lz) *W.J. Little, British surgeon, 1810–1894.* Spastic diplegia. A congenital muscle rigidity of the lower limbs, causing 'scissor leg' deformity.

liver ('livə) the large gland situated in the right upper area of the abdominal cavity. Its chief functions are: (1) the secretion of bile, (2) the maintenance of the composition of the blood, and (3) the regulation of metabolic processes. *Cirrhotic l.* fibrotic changes which occur in the liver as the result of degeneration of the liver cells, often as a result of alcoholism. *L. transplant* the transplantation of a liver from a suitable donor who has recently died.

livid ('livid) descriptive of the bluish-grey discoloration of the skin produced by congestion of blood.

LOA left occipito-anterior. Refers to a possible position of the fetus in the uterus.

lobar (lohbə) relating to a lobe.

lobe (lohb) a section of an organ, separated from neighbouring parts by fissures. The liver, lungs and brain are divided into lobes.

lobectomy (loh'bektəmee) removal of a lobe, e.g. of the lung.

lobular ('lobyuhlə) relating to a lobule.

lobule ('lobyool) a small lobe, particularly one making up a larger lobe.

local supervising authority ('lohk'l) the authority (since 1974, the regional health authority) designated to undertake the statutory supervision of midwifery, according to the rules of the United Kingdom Central Council (UKCC). It is usually delegated to district level.

localize ('lohkə,liez) 1. to limit the spread, e.g. of disease or infection, to a certain area. 2. to determine the site of a lesion.

lochia ('lohki·ə) the discharge of blood and tissue debris from the uterus following childbirth and lasting for 2–3 weeks. Initially lochia is bright red and gradually becomes paler.

lochiometra (,lohkioh'meetrə) the

retention of lochia in the uterus, causing its distension.

lockjaw ('lok,jor) tetanus.

locomotor (,lohkə'mohtə) pertaining to movement from one place to another. *L. ataxia* tabes dorsalis. *See* ATAXIA.

loculated ('lokyuh,laytid) divided into small locules or cavities.

loculus ('lokyuhləs) a small cystic cavity, one of a number.

log roll ('log ,roll) a nursing technique used to turn a reclining patient from one side to the other. The patient lies on his back with arms folded across the chest, and legs extended. The nurses manipulate the underlying drawsheet so that the patient is rolled on to one side or the other.

logorrhoea (,logə'reeə) excessive and often unintelligible volubility.

loiasis (loh'ieəsis) infestation of the conjunctiva and eyelids with a parasite worm, *Loa loa*. A tropical condition.

loin (loyn) the area of the back between the thorax and the pelvis.

Lomotil ('lomətil) trade name for preparations of diphenoxylate, an antidiarrhoeal.

long sight (long siet) hypermetropia.

loosening ('loosəning) in psychiatry, a disorder of thinking in which associations of ideas become so shortened, fragmented and disturbed as to lack logical relationship.

LOP left occipitoposterior. Refers to a possible position of the fetus in the uterus.

lorazepam (lo'razipam, -ayzipam)

a minor tranquillizer used to treat anxiety and insomnia.

lordosis (lor'dohsis) a form of spinal curvature in which there is an abnormal forward curve of the lumbar spine.

lotion ('lohshən) a medicinal solution for external application to the body. Lotions usually have a soothing or antiseptic effect. *Calamine l.* a soothing mixture containing calamine and zinc oxide. *Evaporating l.* a dilute alcoholic solution applied to bruises. *Lead l.* a weak solution of lead acetate used for sprains and bruises where the skin is unbroken.

loupe (loop) a magnifying lens which may be used in eye examination.

louse (lows) a general term covering a number of small insects which are parasitic to man and to other mammals and birds. Three varieties are parasitic to man: (1) *Pediculus capitis*, the head louse; (2) *Pediculus corporis*, the body louse; and (3) *Phthirus pubis* which infects the coarse hair on the body and also the eyebrows. Diseases known to be transmitted by lice are typhus fever, relapsing fever and trench fever.

lozenge ('lozinj) a medicated tablet with sugar basis, used to treat mouth and throat conditions.

LSD *see* LYSERGIDE.

lubb-dupp (lub'dup) representation of the sounds heard through the stethoscope when listening to the normal heart: *lubb* when the atrioventricular valves shut, and *dupp* when the semilunar valves meet each other.

lucid ('loosid) clear, particularly of the mind. *L. interval* period of clear thinking that may occur in cerebral injury between two periods of unconsciousness or as a sane interval in a mental disorder.

Ludwig's angina ('luhdvigz) *W.F. von Ludwig, German surgeon, 1790–1865. See* ANGINA.

lues ('looeez) syphilis.

Lugol's solution ('loogolz) *J.G.A. Lugol, French physician, 1786–1851.* A preparation of iodine and potassium iodide. It is best given in milk and is frequently used in the treatment of toxic goitre.

lumbago (lum'baygoh) pain in the lower part of the back. It may be caused by muscular strain or by a prolapsed intervertebral disc ('slipped disc').

lumbar ('lumbə) pertaining to the loins. *L. puncture* insertion of a trocar and cannula into the spinal canal in the lower back and withdrawal of cerebrospinal fluid for diagnostic purposes.

lumbosacral (,lumboh'saykrəl) relating to both the lumbar vertebrae and the sacrum. *L. support* a corset aimed at both supporting and restricting movement in that region. *L. vertebra* one of the five vertebrae in the lower back lying between the thoracic vertebrae and the sacrum.

Lumbricus ('lumbrikəs) 1. a genus of annelids, including the earthworm. 2. *Ascaris lumbricoides*, a species of nematode which is parasitic in the intestine of man.

lumen ('loomin) the space inside a tube.

lumpectomy (,lump'ektəmee) the surgical excision of only the local lesion (benign or malignant) of the breast.

lunacy ('loonəsee) an obsolete term formerly applied to insanity.

Lund and Browder chart (luhnd ənd 'browdə) a chart that has been adopted by many burn centres in the UK for calculation of the surface area of a burn in a child. At birth the size and area of the head is large compared with the adult, and the legs and thighs constitute a much smaller proportion of the total body surface. On admission to a Burns Unit or ward the area of the body burned is mapped on to the Lund and Browder chart and the area of the burn affecting each portion of the body surface is calculated.

lung (lung) one of a pair of conical organs of the respiratory system, consisting of an arrangement of air tubes terminating in air vesicles (alveoli) and filling almost the whole of the thorax. The right lung has three lobes and the left lung two. They are connected with the air by means of the bronchi and trachea.

lunula ('loonyuhlə) the white semicircle near the root of each nail.

lupus ('loopəs) a chronic skin disease having many manifestations. *L. erythematosus* an inflammatory disease, affecting both the internal organs and the skin, which finally produces a round plaque-like area of hyperkeratosis. It is thought to be due to an autoimmune reaction to sunlight, infec- tion or other unknown cause. *L. vulgaris* a tuberculous disease of the skin producing brownish nodules, frequently on the nose or cheek, and severe scarring.

luteinizing hormone ('lootee·i-,niezing) abbreviated LH. One of three hormones produced by the anterior pituitary gland which control the activity of the gonads.

luteotrophin (,lootioh'trohfin) an anterior pituitary hormone which stimulates the formation of the corpus luteum and the production of milk. Prolactin.

luxation (luk'sayshən) the dislocation of a joint. *L. of the lens* displacement of the lens of the eye into the anterior chamber or posteriorly into the vitreous humour.

Lyme disease (liem) a zoonosis transmitted by ticks and characterized by rash (erythema chronicum migrans), arthritis and aseptic meningitis, caused by the spirochaete *Borrelia burgdorferi*.

lymph (limf) the fluid from the blood which has transuded through capillary walls to supply nutriment to tissue cells. It is collected by lymph vessels which ultimately return it to the blood. *L. nodes* or *glands* structures placed along the course of lymph vessels, through which the lymph passes and is filtered of foreign substances, e.g. bacteria. These nodes also make lymphocytes. *Plastic l.* an inflammatory exudate which tends to cause adhesion between structures and so limit the spread of infection. *Vaccine l.* a lymph preparation obtained from calves or other

Name _____ Age _____ Number _____

Burn record Ages Birth – 7½ Date of observation _____

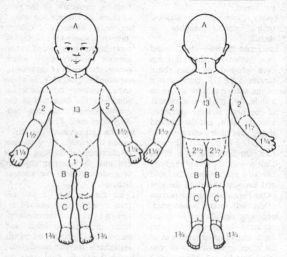

RELATIVE PERCENTAGES OF AREAS AFFECTED BY GROWTH

Area	Age	0	1	5
A = ½ of head		9½	8½	6½
B = ½ of one thigh		2¾	3¼	4
C = ½ of one leg		2½	2½	2¾

% BURN BY AREAS

Lund and Browder chart: estimation of extent of burn (birth–7½ yrs)

animals and used for vaccination.

lymphadenectomy (ˌlimfadə-ˈnektəmee) excision of a lymph gland or nodes.

lymphadenitis (ˌlimfadəˈnietis) inflammation of a lymph gland.

lymphadenoma (ˌlimfadəˈnohmə) lymphoma. *Multiple l.* Hodgkin's disease.

lymphadenopathy (ˌlimfadə-ˈnopəthee) any disease condition of the lymph nodes.

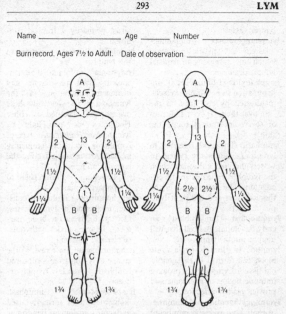

Name _____ Age _____ Number _____

Burn record. Ages 7½ to Adult. Date of observation _____

RELATIVE PERCENTAGES OF AREAS AFFECTED BY GROWTH

Area	Age 10	15	Adult
A = ½ of head	5½	4½	3½
B = ½ of one thigh	4¼	4½	4¾
C = ½ of one leg	3	3¼	3½

% BURN BY AREAS

Lund and Browder chart: estimation of extent of burn (7½ yrs–adult)

lymphangiectasis (ˌlimfənji-ˈektasis) dilatation of the lymph vessels due to some obstruction of the lymph flow. It may be congenital.

lymphangiography (ˌlimfanji-ˈogrəfee) radiographic examination of lymph vessels following the insertion of a radio-opaque contrast medium.

lymphangioma (ˌlimfanji'ohma) a swelling composed of dilated lymph vessels.

lymphangioplasty (lim'fanjioh-,plastee) any plastic operation which aims at making an artificial lymph drainage.

lymphangitis (,limfan'jietis) inflammation of lymph vessels, manifested by red lines on the skin over them. It occurs in cases of severe infection through the skin.

lymphatic (lim'fatik) referring to lymph. *L. system* the system of vessels and glands through which the lymph is returned to the circulation. The vessels end in the thoracic duct and the right lymphatic duct.

lymphoblast ('limfoh,blast) an early developmental cell that will mature into a lymphocyte.

lymphocyte ('limfoh,siet) a white blood cell formed in the lymphoid tissue. Lymphocytes produce immune bodies to overcome and protect against infection.

lymphocythaemia (,limfohsie-'theemi·ə) an excessive number of lymphocytes in the blood. Lymphocytosis.

lymphocytopenia (,limfoh'sietoh-'peeni·ə) absence or scarcity of lymphocytes in the blood. Lymphopenia.

lymphocytosis (,limfohsie'tohsis) lymphocythaemia.

lymphoedema (,limfi'deemə) a condition in which the intercellular spaces contain an abnormal amount of lymph due to obstruction of the lymph drainage.

lymphogranuloma (,limfoh-'granyuh'lohmə) Hodgkin's disease. *L. venereum* a sexually transmitted disease due to a virus, primarily a tropical condition.

lymphoid ('limfoyd) relating to the lymph.

lymphoma (lim'fohmə) lymphadenoma. Used to denote any malignant condition of the lymphoid tissue. Generally these diseases are classified as either Hodgkin's or non-Hodgkin's lymphomas. *Burkitt's l.* a type of lymphoma found predominantly in East Africa and affecting the jaws of children.

lymphopenia (,limfoh'peeni·ə) lymphocytopenia.

lymphopoiesis (,limfohpoy'eesis) the production of lymphocytes. Occurs chiefly in the bone marrow, lymph nodes, thymus, spleen and gut wall.

lymphorrhagia (,limfə'rayji·ə) the escape of lymph from a ruptured lymphatic vessel. Lymphorrhoea.

lymphosarcoma (,limfohsah'kohmə) a term formerly used to denote a malignant lymphoma (with the exception of Hodgkin's disease).

lynoestrenol (li'neestrə,nol) a synthetic drug similar in action to progesterone, used chiefly in oral contraceptives.

lyophilization (lie,ofilie'zayshən) a method of preserving biological substances in a stable state by freeze-drying. It may be used for plasma, sera, bacteria, viruses and tissues.

lysergide (lie'sərjied) lysergic acid diethylamide (LSD). A hallucinogenic drug that can cause visual hallucinations and increased auditory acuity but may prove very disrupting to the personality and affect mental ability.

lysin ('liesin) a specific antibody present in the blood that can destroy cells. *See* BACTERIOLYSIN.

lysine ('lieseen) an essential amino acid formed by the digestion of dietary protein. It is vital for normal health.

lysis ('liesis) 1. the gradual decline of a disease, especially of a fever. The temperature falls gradually, as in typhoid. *See* CRISIS. 2. the destruction of cells.

lysosome ('liesə,sohm) a particle found in the cytoplasm of cells which causes the breakdown of metabolic substances and foreign particles (e.g. bacteria) within the cell.

lysozyme ('liesə,ziem) an enzyme present in tears, nasal mucus and saliva that can kill most bacteria coming into contact with it.

lytic cocktail ('litik) a combination of chlorpromazine, promethazine and pethidine used in the treatment of severe pre-eclampsia and eclampsia. It induces deep sleep, aids muscular relaxation and lowers the blood pressure. Used also during the induction and maintenance of hypothermia.

M

M symbol for *molar*.

m symbol for *metre* and *misce* (mix).

McArdle's disease (mə'kahd'lz) *B. McArdle, British biochemist.* Myopathy resulting from the congenital absence in voluntary muscle of the enzyme phosphorylase.

McBurney's point (mək'bərniz) *C. McBurney, American surgeon, 1845–1913.* The spot midway between the anterior iliac spine and the umbilicus where pain is felt on pressure if the appendix is inflamed.

McNaghten's Rules on Insanity at Law (mək'nawtənz) the rules which define the factors on which a defence to a charge of murder on grounds of insanity may be established. These were evolved after Sir Robert Peel's Secretary was killed by McNaghten in 1843. He was suffering from delusions and the judge ordered that he be found not guilty. The Homicide Act 1957 provided for a defence based on 'diminished responsibility', i.e. the accused was suffering from such abnormality of mind as to impair his mental responsibility for his actions.

maceration (,masə'rayshən) softening of a solid by soaking it in liquid. *Neonatal m.* the natural softening of a dead fetus in the uterus.

Mackenrodt's ligaments ('maken-,rohts) *A.K. Mackenrodt, German gynaecologist, 1859–1925.* The transverse or cardinal ligaments that support the uterus in the pelvic cavity.

Macmillan nurses (mak'milən) qualified nurses who have also received special training in the management of pain relief and in the provision of emotional support to cancer patients and their families. This nursing service is provided either in the patient's home through the Macmillan home visiting service or in a hospice.

macrocheilia (,makroh'kieli-ə) a congenital condition in which there is excessive development of the lips.

macrocyte ('makroh,siet) an abnormally large red corpuscle found in the blood in some forms of anaemia.

macrocythaemia (,makrohsie-'theemi-ə) the presence of abnormally large red cells in the blood. Macrocytosis.

macrodactylism (,makroh'dak-tilizəm) abnormal enlargement of one or more of the fingers or toes.

macromastia (,makroh'masti·ə) abnormal increase in the size of the breast.

macromelia (ˌmakroh'meeli·ə) abnormal enlargement of one or more of the hands or legs.

macronutrient (ˌmakroh'nyootri-·ənt) an essential nutrient that has a large minimal daily requirement (greater than 100 mg); calcium, phosphorus, magnesium, potassium, sodium and chloride are macronutrients.

macrophage ('makroh,fayj) a large reticuloendothelial cell which has the power to ingest cell debris and bacteria. It is present in connective tissue, especially when there is inflammation.

macrophthalmia (ˌmakrof'thalmi·ə) a congenital condition of abnormally large eyes.

macroscopic (ˌmakroh'skopik) discernible with the naked eye. The opposite of microscopic.

macrostomia (ˌmakroh'stohmi·ə) an abnormal development of the mouth in which the mandibular and maxillary processes do not fuse and the mouth is excessively wide.

macula ('makyuhlə) a spot or discoloured area of the skin, not raised above the surface; a macule. *M. corneae* a small area of opacity in the cornea, seen through an ophthalmoscope as a deeper red. *M. lutea* the yellow central area of the retina, where vision is clearest.

maculopapular (ˌmakyuhloh-'papyuhlə) displaying both maculae and papules. *M. eruption* a rash comprised of both, as in measles.

Maddox rod test ('madəks) *E.E.*

Maddox, British ophthalmologist, 1860–1933. A test for muscle balance of the eyes using a tube comprised of red glass cylinders. *M. wing test* a method of measuring the amount of heterophoria.

Madura foot (mə'dyooə·rə) mycetoma of the foot.

Madurella (ˌmadyuh'relə) a genus of fungi causing mycetoma.

maduromycosis (mə,dyooə·rohmie'kohsis) a chronic disease caused by *Madurella mycetoma*. The commonest form is Madura foot.

Magendie's foramen (ˌmazhon-'deez) *F. Magendie, French physiologist, 1783–1855.* Aperture in the roof of the fourth ventricle of the brain through which cerebrospinal fluid passes into the subarachnoid space.

magnesium (mag'neezi·əm) *symbol Mg.* A bluish white metallic element. It occurs widely in mineral sources and is present in some of the body tissues. *M. carbonate* and *M. hydroxide* neutralizing antacids used in hyperacidity. *M. sulphate* a saline purgative. Epsom salts. *M. trisilicate* an antacid powder taken after food for dyspepsia and peptic ulceration.

magnet ('magnit) in ophthalmology, an instrument used for removing metallic foreign bodies that have penetrated the eye.

magnetic resonance imaging (mag'netik) abbreviated MRI. An imaging technique based on the NUCLEAR MAGNETIC RESONANCE properties of the hydrogen nucleus. Cross-sectional images in any plane of the body for examination may be obtained. MRI is without hazard to the patient.

Makaton (ˌmak'əton) one of the sign languages.

mal (mal) [Fr.] *disease. M. de mer* sea-sickness. *Grand m., petit m.* forms of epilepsy.

malabsorption (ˌmaləb-'sawpshən, -zaw-) inability of the small intestine to absorb certain substances. It may be the cause of a deficiency disease due to the lack of an essential factor.

malacia (mə'layshi·ə) softening of tissues. *Kerato-m.* softening of the cornea. *Osteo-m.* softening of bone tissue.

maladjustment (ˌmalə'justmənt) in psychiatry, a failure to adjust to the environment.

malaise (ma'layz) a feeling of general discomfort and illness.

malalignment (ˌmalə'lienmənt) displacement, especially of the teeth from their normal relation to the line of the dental arch.

malar ('maylə) relating to the cheek or cheek-bone.

malaria (mə'lair·ri·ə) a serious, notifiable infectious illness characterized by periodic chills, fever, sweating and splenomegaly. Serious and often fatal complications may arise in falciparum malaria. It is endemic in parts of Africa, Asia and Central and South America, and is estimated to occur at the rate of 100 million cases each year throughout the world. Some 2000 imported cases per year are reported in the UK, with up to ten deaths. Epidemics usually occur in areas where mosquitoes persist in large numbers.

The disease is caused by a parasite of the genus *Plasmodium* introduced into the blood by mosquitoes of the genus *Anopheles*. The attacks are periodic every 48 to 72 h according to the type of plasmodium. For *P. vivax* it lasts 48 h. *P. malariae* 72 h, and *P. falciparum* 36–48 h. *Airport m.* a term sometimes used to describe malaria occurring at or near an airport, in a country normally free of the disease, and spread by infected mosquitoes brought in on an aeroplane from an endemic area. Control measures include disinsectization of aircraft where appropriate.

malformation (ˌmalfaw'mayshən) deformity; a structural defect.

malignant (mə'lignənt) tending to become progressively worse and to result in death; having the properties of anaplasia, invasiveness and metastasis; said of tumours.

malingering (mə'ling·gə·ring) wilful, deliberate and fraudulent feigning or exaggeration of the symptoms of illness or injury to attain a consciously desired end.

malleolus (mə'leeələs) one of the two protuberances on either side of the ankle joint. *Lateral m.* that on the outer surface at the lower end of the fibula. *Medial m.* that on the inner surface at the lower end of the tibia.

malleus ('mali·əs) the hammer-shaped bone in the middle ear.

malnutrition (ˌmalnyoo'trishən) the condition in which nutrition is defective in quantity or quality.

malocclusion (ˌmalə'kloozhən) an abnormality of dental development which causes overlapping of the bite.

malpighian body (mal'pigi·ən) *M. Malpighi, Italian anatomist, physician and physiologist, 1628–1694.* The glomerulus and Bowman's capsule of the kidney.

malposition (ˌmalpə'zishən) an abnormal position of any part of the body.

malpractice (mal'praktis) failure to maintain accepted ethical standards. Professional misconduct.

malpresentation (ˌmalprezən-'tayshən) any abnormal position of the fetus at birth which renders delivery difficult or impossible.

Malta fever ('mawltə) brucellosis; undulant fever.

maltase ('mawltayz) a sugar-splitting enzyme which converts maltose to glucose. Present in pancreatic and intestinal juice.

maltose ('mawltohz, -tohs) the sugar formed by the action of digestive enzymes on starch.

malunion (mal'yooni·ən) faulty repair of a fracture.

mamilla (mə'milə) a nipple.

mamma ('mamə) a breast; a milk-secreting gland.

mammary ('mamə·ree) relating to the breasts.

mammography (mə'mogrəfee) radiographic or infra-red examination of the breast to detect abnormalities.

mammoplasty ('mamoh,plastee) a plastic operation to reduce the size of abnormally large, pendulous breasts or augment the size of very small breasts.

mammothermography (ˌmamoh-thər'mogrəfee) an examination of the breast that depends on the more active cells producing heat that can be shown on a thermograph, and may indicate abnormalities of the breast tissue.

mandible ('mandib'l) the lower jaw-bone.

manganese (man'gan·eez) *symbol* Mn. A grey-white metallic element from the salts of which the permanganates are formed.

mania ('mayni·ə) a disordered mental state of extreme excitement; specially, the manic type of manic-depressive psychosis. Also used as a word termination to denote obsessive preoccupation with something, as in tomomania.

maniac ('mayni,ak) colloquial term for one suffering from a violent or extreme form of insanity

manic ('manik) pertaining to mania. *M.-depressive psychosis* a mental illness characterized by mania or endogenous depression. The attacks may alternate between mania and depression or the patient may just have recurrent attacks of mania or depression.

manipulation (mə,nipyuh'layshən) use of the hands to produce a desired movement, such as in reducing a fracture or a hernia or changing the position of a fetus. A skilfully applied forced movement upon a joint in order to relocate the joint or increase its range of movements by tearing adhesions round it.

mannitol ('mani,tol) a sugar alcohol occurring widely in nature; an osmotic diuretic used for forced diuresis in drug overdose and in cerebral oedema.

manometer (mə'nomitə) an instrument for measuring the pressure of liquids or gases.

Mantoux test (man'too) *C. Mantoux, French physician, 1877–1947*. A tuberculin skin test in which a solution of PPD-tuberculin is injected intradermally into either the anterior or posterior surface of the forearm. The test is read 48–72 h after injection. It is considered positive when the induration at the site of injection is more than 10 mm in diameter.

manubrium (mə'nyoobri-əm) the upper part of the sternum to which the clavicle is attached.

MAOI *see* MONOAMINE OXIDASE.

maple syrup urine disease ('mayp'l 'sirəp 'yooə-rin) an inborn error of metabolism in which there is an excess in the urine of certain amino acids. The urine smells like maple syrup and there are learning difficulties, spasticity and convulsions.

marasmus (mə'razməs) severe and chronic malnutrition producing a gradual wasting of the tissues, owing to insufficient or unassimilated food, occurring especially in infants. It is not always possible to discover the cause.

marble bone disease (mahb'l 'bohn) a condition in which there is increased density of bone, which is visible on radiographic examination. Albers–Schönberg's disease. Osteopetrosis.

Marburg virus disease ('mahbərg) a Central African viral haemorrhagic fever with acute onset and characteristic morbilliform rash. The incubation period is 3–7 days. It was first reported in Europe in 1967 associated with the importation of green monkeys from Uganda. Since then several isolated incidents have occurred in Africa. The reservoir of infection is not known. Person-to-person transmission by inoculation of blood and tissue fluid and by sexual intercourse has been reported.

Marfan's syndrome (mah'fanhz) *B.J.A. Marfan, French paediatrician, 1858–1942*. A hereditary disorder in which there is excessive height with very long digits, a high arched palate, hypertonus, dislocation of the lens of the eyes and cardiac lesions, the most common of which is atrial septal defect.

marihuana ('mariyuh'ahnə, -hwahnə) *Cannabis indica*; Indian hemp or hashish. *See* CANNABIS.

marrow ('maroh) the substance contained in the middle of long bones and in the cancellous tissue of all bones. *M. puncture* investigatory procedure in which marrow cells are aspirated from the sternum or iliac crest. *Red m.* that found in all cancellous tissue at birth. Blood cells are made in it. *Yellow m.* the fatty substance contained in the centre of long bones in later life.

masculinization (,maskyuhlinie-'zayshən) the development in a woman of male secondary sexual characteristics.

Maslow's hierachy of need ('mazlohz, hieə-rahkee əv ,need) *A.H. Maslow, American psychol-*

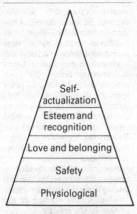

**MASLOW'S HIERARCHY
OF NEEDS**

Self-
actualization

Esteem and
recognition

Love and belonging

Safety

Physiological

ogist, *1908–1970*. A hierarchical ranking, in ascending order of importance, concerning human needs and the aim of realizing one's full potential. Physiological needs for oxygen, nutrition, shelter, sleep, etc., are the most basic and need to be met first before one is able to deal in successive order with the need for safety, security, love and belonging, self-esteem and ultimately the need for self-actualization.

masochism ('masə,kizəm) a sexual perversion in which pleasure is derived from suffering mental or physical pain.

massage ('masahzh, -sahj) a method of rubbing, kneading and manipulating the body to stimulate circulation, improve metab-

olism and break down adhesions. *External cardiac m.* the application of rhythmic pressure to the lower sternum to cause expulsion of blood from the ventricles and restart circulation in cases of cardiac arrest.

masseter (ma'seetə) the muscle of the cheek chiefly concerned in mastication.

mast cell (mahst) a large connective tissue cell found in many body tissues including the heart, liver and lungs. Most cells contain granules which release heparin, serotonin and histamine in response to inflammation or allergy.

mastalgia (ma'stalji·ə) pain in the breast.

mastatrophia (,mastə'trohfia) atrophy of the breast.

mastectomy (ma'stektəmee) amputation of the breast. *Radical m.* removal of the breast, axillary lymph glands and the pectoral muscle.

mastication (,masti'kayshən) the act of chewing food.

mastitis (ma'stietis) inflammation of the breast, usually due to bacterial infection.

mastodynia (,mastoh'dini·ə) pain in the breasts, which frequently occurs during the premenstrual phase.

mastoid ('mastoyd) breast or nipple-shaped. *M. antrum* the cavity in the mastoid process which communicates with the middle ear, and contains air. *M. cells* hollow spaces in the mastoid bone. *M. operation* drainage of mastoid cells when infection spreads from the middle ear. *M.*

process the breast-shaped prominence on the temporal bone which projects downwards behind the ear and into which the sternocleidomastoid muscle is inserted.

mastoidectomy (,mastoy'dektə-mee) removal of diseased bone and drainage of the mastoid antrum in severe purulent mastoiditis.

mastoiditis (,mastoy'dietis) inflammation of the mastoid antrum and cells.

masturbation (,mastə'bayshən) the production of sexual excitement by friction of the genitals.

materia medica (mə'tie·ri·ə 'medikə) the science of the source and preparation of drugs used in medicine.

maternal (mə'tərn'l) pertaining to the mother. *M. mortality rate* the number of deaths in childbirth per 1000 births.

matrix ('maytriks) that tissue in which cells are embedded.

matter ('matə) substance. *Grey m.* a collection of nerve cells or non-medullated nerve fibres. *White m.* medullated nerve fibres massed together, as in the brain.

maturation (,matyuh'rayshən, ,machuh-) ripening or developing.

maxilla (mak'silə) one of the pair of bones forming the upper jaw and carrying the upper teeth.

maxillary (mak'silə·ree) pertaining to the upper jaw bones.

maxillofacial (,maksiloh'fayshəl) pertaining to the maxilla and the face.

MCHC mean corpuscular haemoglobin concentration.

MCV mean corpuscular volume.

measles ('meezəlz) morbilli; rubeola. An acute, infectious statutorily notifiable disease of childhood caused by a virus spread by droplets. Endemic and worldwide in distribution. Onset is catarrhal before the rash appears at the 4th day. Koplik's spots are diagnostic earlier. Secondary infection may give rise to the serious complication of otitis media or bronchopneumonia. Vaccination provides a high degree of immunity. *German m.* See RUBELLA.

meatus (mi'aytəs) an opening or passage. *Auditory m.* the opening leading into the auditory canal. *Urethral m.* the opening of the urethra to the exterior.

mecamylamine (,mekə'milə,me-en) a ganglion-blocking drug which, given by mouth, causes a marked fall in blood pressure. Used in treating arterial hypertension.

mechanism of labour ('mekə-,nizəm) the sequence of movements whereby the fetus adapts itself to pass through the maternal passages during the process of birth.

Meckel's diverticulum ('mekəlz) *J.F. Meckel, German anatomist and surgeon, 1781–1833.* The remains of a passage which, in the embryo, connected the yolk sac and intestine, evident as an enclosed sac or tube in the region of the ileum.

meclozine ('meklohzeen, -in) an antinauseant and antihistamine.

meconium (mi'kohni·əm) the first intestinal discharges of a newly born child. Dark green in colour and consisting of epithelial cells, mucus and bile. *M. ileus* intestinal obstruction due to blockage of the bowel by a plug of meconium in a neonate with cystic fibrosis.

median ('meedi·ən) 1. placed in the centre. 2. in a series of values, the value middle in position.

mediastinum (ˌmeedi·ə'stienəm) the space in the middle of the thorax, between the two pleurae.

medical ('medik'l) pertaining to medicine. *M. audit* an evaluative process applied to the quality of clinical practice, often by peer review of routine or specially collected records of individual cases. Judgements are frequently made on the appropriateness of the processes carried out during the management of the case, in the light of the outcome. Deaths are frequently the subject of medical audit, two established examples being the Confidential Enquiry into Maternal Deaths (carried out at National level), and local reviews of perinatal deaths. *M. certificate* now replaced (since 1976) by a *m. statement*, to advise how long a patient should refrain from work. When claiming sickness benefit, the statement must be sent to the local social security office. *M. jurisprudence* medical science as applied to aid the law, e.g. in the case of death by poisoning, violence, etc. *M. Laboratory Scientific Officer* abbreviated MLSO. An allied health professional skilled in the theory and practice of clinical laboratory procedures. *M. social worker* a professionally qualified worker

who looks after the patients' socioeconomic and welfare needs. *M. statistics* that branch of statistics concerned with data relating to health and health services. Traditionally these include the use of routine data relating to death, illness and use of hospitals, clinics, etc. The term is also often used to encompass statistics derived from aspects of medical research such as the conduct of trials of new drugs or procedures.

medicament (mə'dikəmənt) any medicinal substance used in treatment.

medicated ('mediˌkaytid) impregnated with a medicinal substance.

medication (ˌmedi'kayshən) 1. a substance administered to a patient for therapeutic purposes. 2. the treatment of a patient by means of drugs.

medicinal (mə'disin'l) 1. having therapeutic qualities. 2. pertaining to a medicine.

medicine ('medisin, 'medsin) 1. any drug or remedy. 2. the art and science of the diagnosis and treatment of disease and the maintenance of health. 3. the non-surgical treatment of disease. *Community m.* that speciality which deals with all aspects of medical care in the community, including notification and control of infectious diseases, pre-school and school health care, and factors affecting the health of the population as a whole. *Emergency m.* that speciality which deals with the acutely ill or injured who require immediate medical treatment. *Family m.* family practice; the medical speciality concerned with the provision of comprehensive primary health care. *Forensic m.* the application of medical knowledge to questions of law; medical jurisprudence. Called also legal medicine. *Group m.* the practice of medicine by a group of doctors, usually representing various specialities, who are associated together for the cooperative diagnosis, treatment and prevention of disease. *Legal m.* forensic medicine. *Nuclear m.* that branch of medicine concerned with the use of radionuclides in the diagnosis and treatment of disease. *Physical m.* that branch of medicine using physical agents in the diagnosis and treatment of disease. It includes the use of heat, cold, light, water, electricity, manipulation, massage, exercise and mechanical devices. *Preventive m.* science aimed at preventing disease. *Proprietary m.* any chemical, drug, or similar preparation used in the treatment of diseases, if such article is protected against free competition as to name, product, composition, or process of manufacture by secrecy, patent, trademark or copyright, or by other means. *Psychosomatic m.* the study of the interrelations between bodily processes and emotional life. *Space m.* that branch of aviation medicine concerned with conditions to be encountered in space. *Sports m.* the field of medicine concerned with injuries sustained in athletic endeavours, including their prevention, diagnosis and treatment. **medicosocial** (,medikoh'sohshəl) applying to both medicine and the social factors involved.

medium ('meedi·əm) in bacteriology, a preparation for the culture of microorganisms. *Contrast m.* a substance used in radiography to make visible structures which could not otherwise be seen.

medroxyprogesterone (med,roksiproh'jestə,rohn) a synthetic female sex hormone used to treat menstrual disorders, endometrial carcinoma and endometriosis, and as a short-term contraceptive.

medulla (mə'dulə) 1. bone marrow. 2. the innermost part of an organ, particularly the kidneys, lymph glands and suprarenal glands. *M. oblongata* that portion of the spinal cord which is contained inside the cranium. In it are the nerve centres which govern respiration, the action of the heart, etc.

medullary (mə'dulə·ree) pertaining to the marrow or a medulla. *M. cavity* the hollow in the centre of long bones.

medullated ('medə,laytid) having a myelin covering. *M. nerve fibre* one enclosed in a myelin sheath.

medulloblastoma (mə,dulohbla-'stohmə) a rapidly growing tumour of neuroepithelial origin occurring in childhood and appearing near the fourth ventricle of the brain. The tumour is highly radiosensitive.

mefenamic acid (,mefə'namik) an analgesic and antipyretic drug used in the treatment of mild to moderate pain.

megacolon (,megə'kohlon) extreme dilatation and hypertrophy of the large intestine. When the condition is congenital it is known as Hirschsprung's disease.

megaduodenum (,megə,dyooə-'deenəm) a gross enlargement of the duodenum.

megakaryocyte (,megə'karioh-,siet) a large cell of the bone marrow, responsible for blood platelet formation.

megaloblast ('megəloh,blast) an abnormally large nucleated cell from which mature red blood cells are derived.

megalocephaly (,megəloh'kefə-lee, -'sef-) 1. abnormal largeness of the head. 2. leontiasis ossea.

megalomania (,megəloh'mayni·ə) delusions of grandeur or self-importance characteristic of general paralysis of the insane.

megaureter (megəyuh'reetə) dilatation of the ureter.

meibomian glands (mie'bohmi·ən) H. Meibom, German anatomist, 1638–1700. Small sebaceous glands situated beneath the conjunctiva of the eyelid; tarsal glands. M. cyst a small swelling of the gland caused by obstruction of its duct. If untreated, it may become infected. A chalazion.

meibomianitis (mie,bohmi·ə'nietis) a bilateral chronic inflammation of the meibomian glands.

Meigs' syndrome ('megziz) J.V. Meigs, American surgeon, 1892–1963. A fibroma or benign solid tumour of the ovary causing ascites and pleural effusion.

meiosis (mie'ohsis) 1. a stage of reduction cell division when the

chromosomes of a GAMETE are halved in number ready for union at fertilization. 2. contraction of the pupil of the eye; miosis.

melaena (mə'leenə) darkening of the faeces by blood pigments.

melancholia (,melən'kohli·ə) a state of extreme depression. See DEPRESSION.

melanin ('melənin) a dark pigment found in the hair, the choroid of the eye, the skin and in melanotic tumours.

melanism ('melə,nizəm) a condition marked by an abnormal deposit of dark pigment in the skin or other tissue. Melanosis.

melanocyte ('melənoh,siet) a cell of the skin pigment melanin. M.-stimulating hormone abbreviated MSH. Hormone produced in the pituitary gland which stimulates the formation of melanin.

melanoderma (,melənoh'dərmə) a patchy pigmentation of the skin.

melanoma (,melə'nohmə) a malignant tumour arising in any pigment-containing tissues, especially the skin and the eye. Amelanotic m. an unpigmented malignant melanoma. Juvenile m. a benign lesion which usually occurs on the face before puberty. May be mistaken for a malignant melanoma.

melanosis (,melə'nohsis) see MELANISM.

melanotic (,melə'notik) pertaining to melanosis. M. sarcoma see SARCOMA.

melanuria (,melə'nyooə·ri·ə) the presence of black pigment in the urine. Occurs in melanotic sarcoma and porphyria.

melasma (me'lazma) dark discoloration of the skin; chloasma.

melphalan ('melfəlan) a cytotoxic drug which is particularly useful in the treatment of multiple myeloma.

membrane ('membrayn) a thin elastic tissue covering the surface of certain organs and lining the cavities of the body. *Basement m.* the interface between epithelial cells and the underlying connective tissue. *Mucous m.* a membrane that secretes mucus and lines all cavities connnected directly or indirectly with the skin. *Serous m.* membrane lining the abdominal cavity and thorax and covering most of the organs within.

memory ('memə-ree) the mental faculty that enables one to retain and recall previously experienced sensations, impressions, information and ideas. The ability of the brain to retain and to use knowledge gained from past experience is essential to the process of learning. The exact way in which the brain remembers is not completely understood; it is believed that a portion of the temporal lobe of the brain acts as a memory centre, drawing on memories stored in other parts of the brain.

menarche (menar'ke) the first appearance of menstruation.

Mendel's theory ('mend'lz) *G.J. Mendel, Abbot of Brünn, 1822–1884.* The theory that the characters of sexually reproducing organisms are handed on to the offspring in fixed ratios and without blending.

Mendelson's syndrome ('mend'l-,sənz) *C.L. Mendelson, American obstetrician b. 1913.* A condition in which there is severe oedema and spasm of the bronchioles due to the inhalation of acid gastric contents.

Menière's disease or syndrome ('meni,airz) *P. Menière, French physician, 1799–1862.* A disease of the inner ear causing attacks of vertigo and tinnitus with progressive deafness.

meninges (mə'ninjeez, 'menin-) the membranes covering the brain and spinal cord. There are three: the dura mater (outer), arachnoid mater (middle) and pia mater (inner).

meningioma (mə,ninji'ohmə) a slow-growing, usually benign tumour developing from the arachnoid and pia mater.

meningism ('menin,jizəm) a condition in which there are signs of cerebral irritation similar to meningitis but where no causative organism can be isolated.

meningitis (,menin'jietis) inflammation of the meninges due to organisms, such as bacteria, viruses and fungi; chemical toxins such as lead and arsenic; contrast media used in myelography; and metastatic malignant cells. Meningitis, and its causal organism if known, is a notifiable disease. *Meningococcal m.* cerebrospinal fever. An epidemic form with a rapid onset caused by infection by *Neisseria meningitidis. Tuberculous m.* inflammation of tuberculous origin.

meningocele (mə'ning-goh,seel) a protrusion of the meninges through the skull or spinal column, appearing as a cyst filled with cerebrospinal fluid. *See* SPINA BIFIDA.

meningococcus (mə,ning·goh·'kokəs) *Neisseria meningitidis*. A diplococcus, the microorganism of cerebrospinal meningitis.

meningoencephalitis (mə,ning·goh·en,kefə'lietis, -,sef-) inflammation of the brain and meninges.

meningomyelocele (mə,ning·goh'mieəloh,seel) a protrusion of the spinal cord and meninges through a defect in the vertebral column. Myelomeningocele. *See* SPINA BIFIDA.

meniscectomy (,meni'sektəmee) surgical removal of a cartilage in a semilunar knee-joint.

meniscus (mə'niskəs) 1. the convex or concave surface of a liquid as observed in its container. 2. a lens having one convex and one concave surface. 3. a semilunar cartilage of the knee-joint.

menopause ('menə,pawz) the span of time during which the menstrual cycle wanes and gradually stops; called also change of life and climacteric. It is the period when ovaries stop functioning and therefore menstruation and childbearing cease. Usually occurs between the 45th and 50th years of life. There may be an associated hormonal imbalance which causes symptoms such as night sweats, hot flushes, diminished libido and extreme lethargy. *Artificial m.* an induced cessation of menstruation by surgery or by irradiation.

menorrhagia (,menə'rayji·ə) an excessive flow of the menses;

menorrhoea.

menses ('menseez) the discharge from the uterus during menstruation.

menstrual ('menstrooəl) relating to the menses. *M. cycle* the monthly cycle commencing with the first day of menstruation, when the endometrium is shed, through a process of repair and hypertrophy till the next period. It is governed by the anterior pituitary gland and the ovarian hormones, oestrogens and progesterone.

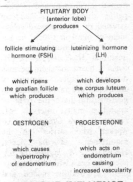

HORMONE INFLUENCE ON MENSTRUATION

menstruation (,menstroo'ayshən) the monthly discharge of blood and endometrium from the uterus, starting at the age of puberty and lasting until the menopause. *Anovular m., anovulatory m.* periodic uterine bleeding without preceding ovulation. *Vicarious m.* discharge of blood at the time of menstruation from some organ other than the uterus, e.g. epistaxis, which is not uncommon.

mental ('ment'l) 1. pertaining to the mind. *M. age* the measurement of the intelligence level of an individual in terms of the average chronological age of children showing the same mental standard, as measured by a scale of mental tests. *M. disorder* a term defined by the Mental Health Act 1983 to cover all forms of mental illness and disability, including mental impairment and psychopathic disorder. *M. handicap* arrested or incomplete development of mind in which the patient does not require compulsory detention. *M. Health Review Tribunal* a board to whom persons detained under compulsory admission orders or taken into guardianship have the right of appeal at stated intervals. *M. Health Welfare Officer* a social worker who carries out the requirements of the Mental Health Act. *M. hygiene* the science that deals with the development of healthy mental and emotional reactions. *M. illness* a term used to describe a number of disorders of the mind which affect the emotions, perceptions, reasoning or memory of the individual, e.g. psychoses and neuroses. *M. impairment* arrested or incomplete development of mind associated with abnormally aggressive or socially irresponsible conduct. If the patient is considered treatable, he may be compulsorily admitted to hospi-

tal. *M. mechanism* an unconscious and indirect manner of gratifying a repressed desire. *M. subnormality* a condition of arrested or incomplete development of the mind. The term has been superseded by mental handicap and mental impairment. 2. pertaining to the chin.

menthol ('menthol) a crystalline substance derived from oil of peppermint and used in neuralgia and rhinitis, as a local anodyne and antiseptic.

mepacrine ('mepə,krin) a synthetic drug used as an antimalarial agent and in the treatment of giardiasis.

mephenesin (mə'feni,sin) a muscle relaxant used in the treatment of parkinsonism, chorea and athetosis.

meprobamate (mə'prohbə,mayt) a tranquillizer used in the treatment of nervous anxiety.

meptazinol (mep'tazinol) a newer narcotic analgesic claimed to cause less respiratory depression than other narcotic analgesics. It has a relatively quick onset of action but a short duration of action of 2–4 h. Nausea and vomiting are quite common and the drug does not appear to have any great advantage over more established agents.

mercaptopurine (mə,kaptoh-'pyooə·reen) a drug which prevents nucleic acid synthesis and may be used in the treatment of some types of leukaemia.

mercurialism (mər'kyooə·ri·ə-,lizəm) chronic poisoning due to absorption of mercury.

mercury ('mərkyə·ree) *symbol* Hg.

Quicksilver; a heavy liquid metallic element, the salts of which are used occasionally as antiseptics and disinfectants.

mesarteritis (,mesahtə'rietis) inflammation of the middle coat of an artery.

mescaline ('meskə,leen) an alkaloid drug which produces intoxication and hallucinations. It is a drug of addiction.

mesencephalon (,mesen'kefə,lon, -'sef-) the middle brain.

mesenchyme ('meseng,kiem) in the embryo, the connective tissue developed from the mesoderm.

mesentery ('mesəntə-ree, 'mez-) a fold of the peritoneum which connects the intestine to the posterior abdominal wall.

mesmerism ('mezmə,rizəm) *F.A. Mesmer, Austrian physician, 1734–1815.* Hypnotism.

mesoderm ('mesoh,dərm) the middle of the three primary layers of cells in the embryo from which the connective tissues develop.

mesometrium (mesoh'meetri·əm) the broad ligament connecting the uterus with the abdominal wall.

mesomorph ('mesoh,mawf) a stocky individual of medium height with well developed muscles.

mesothelioma (,mesoh,theeli-'ohmə) a rapidly growing tumour of the pleura, peritoneum or pericardium which may be seen in patients with asbestosis. However, this tumour may also occur in people who have no history of exposure to asbestos.

messenger RNA (,mesinjə ,ah'en-,ay) abbreviated mRNA. The ribonucleic acid which acts as a template for the linking of amino acids during the formation of protein in the cells.

mestranol ('mestrə,nol) a synthetic oestrogen commonly used in combination with a progesterone in contraceptive pills.

metabolic (,metə'bolik) referring to metabolism.

metabolism (mə'tabə,lizəm) the sum of the physical and chemical processes by which living organized substance is built up and maintained (anabolism), and by which large molecules are broken down into smaller molecules to make energy available to the organism (catabolism). Essentially these processes are concerned with the disposition of the nutrients absorbed into the blood following digestion. *Basal m.* the minimal energy expended for the maintenance of respiration, circulation, peristalsis muscle tonus, body temperature, glandular activity and the other vegetative functions of the body. *Inborn error of m.* a genetically determined biochemical disorder in which a specific enzyme defect produces a metabolic block that may have pathological consequences at birth, as in phenylketonuria, or in later life.

metabolite (mə'tabə,liet) any product or substance taking part in metabolism. *Essential m.* a substance that is necessary for normal metabolism, e.g. a vitamin.

metacarpal (,metə'kahp'l) one of the five bones of the hand which join the fingers to the wrist.

metacarpophalangeal (,metə-,kahpohfə'lanji·əl) relating to the metacarpal bones and the phalanges.

metacarpus (,metə'kahpəs) the fives bones of the hand uniting the carpus with the phalanges of the fingers.

metamorphosis (,metə'mawfəsis) a structural change or transformation.

Metamucil (,metə'myoosil) tradename for preparations of ispaghula, a bulk laxative.

metaphase ('metə,fayz) the second stage of mitosis or cell division.

metaphysis (mə'tafisis) the junction of the epiphysis with the diaphysis in a long bone.

metaplasia (,metə'playzi·ə) abnormal change in the structure of a tissue. May be indicative of malignant change.

metastasis (mə'tastəsis) the transfer of a disease from one part of the body to another, through the blood vessels, via the lymph channels or across the body cavities. (1) Secondary deposits may occur from a primary malignant growth. (2) Septic infection may arise in other organs from some original focus.

metatarsal (,metə'tahs'l) one of the five bones of the foot which join the tarsus to the toes.

metatarsalgia (,metətah'salji·ə) pain in the metatarsal bones.

metatarsus (,metə'tahsəs) the fives bones of the foot uniting the tarsus with the phalanges of the toes.

Metazoa (,metə'zoh·ə) the division of the animal kingdom that includes the multicellular animals, i.e. all animals except the PROTOZOA.

metformin (met'fawmin) a biguanide hypoglycaemic used in the treatment of diabetes mellitus.

methadone ('methə,dohn) a powerful analgesic with no sedative action. Similar in action to morphine, it is used to relieve pain in terminal illness and also in withdrawal programmes for heroin addicts. Amidone.

methaemalbumin (,met·heem-'albyoomin) a compound of haem with plasma albumin found in the blood in some types of anaemia.

methaemoglobin (,met·heemə-'glohbin) an altered form of haemoglobin found in the blood and usually produced by the action of a drug on the red blood corpuscles. Commonly caused by phenacetin and other aniline derivatives.

methaemoglobinaemia (,met·heemə,glohbi'neemi·ə) cyanosis and inability of the red blood cells to transport oxygen due to the presence of methaemoglobin.

methandienone (,methan'dieə,nohn) an anabolic steroid used to build up body tissues in wasting diseases.

methane ('meethayn) marsh gas; an inflammable, explosive gas produced by decomposition of organic matter.

methicillin (,methi'silin) a form of penicillin that is resistant to staphylococcal penicillinase.

methimazole (mə'thiemə,zohl) a powerful drug used in the treatment of thyrotoxicosis.

methionine (me'thieoh,neen) 1.

a sulphur-containing essential amino acid occurring in proteins, which is a vital component of the diet. 2. a drug used orally in the treatment of paracetamol poisoning.

Methixene (,meth'ekseen) an atropine-like drug which relieves the tremor of parkinsonism.

methohexitone (,methoh'heksitohn) a barbiturate anaesthetic agent; given intravenously it has a quick recovery time.

methotrexate (,methoh'treksayt) a cytotoxic drug that antagonizes folic acid and prevents cell formation. It is used to treat various types of malignant disease.

methotrimeprazine (,methohtrie-'meprəzeen) a phenothiazine with sedative and analgesic properties. Useful in schizophrenia and terminal illness.

methoxamine (me'thoksə,meen) a sympathomimetic amine used for its vasopressor effects in restoring blood pressure during anaesthesia.

methyl salicylate (,methil sə'lisə,layt, ,meethiel) a compound used externally for rheumatic pains, lumbago, etc. Oil of wintergreen.

methylated spirit (,methi,laytid 'spirit) a mixture of 95 per cent ethyl alcohol and 5 per cent methyl alcohol. An industrial spirit which, taken as a drink, is poisonous.

methylcellulose (,methil'selyuhlohs, -lohz) a bulk-forming drug used as a laxative and to control diarrhoea.

methyldopa (,methil'dohpə) a hypotensive drug whose action is increased if used with thiazide diuretics.

methylene blue ('methi,leen) a synthetic organic compound, in dark green crystals or lustrous crystalline powder, used in treatment of methaemoglobinaemia, as an antidote in cyanide poisoning, as a stain in pathology and bacteriology, and as an antiseptic.

methylphenidate (,methil'feni-,dayt) a central nervous system stimulant used in the treatment of attention deficit disorder (childhood hyperactivity) and narcolepsy. Only available through hospitals.

methylphenobarbitone (,methil,fenoh'bahbitohn) a white crystalline powder used as an anticonvulsant with a slight hypnotic action. Especially useful for senile tremor.

methylprednisolone (,methilpred'nisə,lohn) a corticosteroid of the glucogenic type, having an anti-inflammatory action similar to that of prednisolone.

methyltestosterone (,methilte-'stostə-rohn) an orally effective, synthetic form of testosterone.

methyprylone (me'thiprilohn) a non-barbiturate used as a sedative and hypnotic.

methysergide (,methi'sərjied) a potent serotonin antagonist used in the prophylaxis of migraine.

metoclopramide (,metoh'klohprəmied) a drug which speeds up gastric action and is used to treat nausea, heartburn and vomiting.

metoprolol (me'tohprə,lol) a cardioselective BETA-BLOCKER having a greater effect on β_1-adrenergic receptors of the heart than on the β_2-adrenergic receptors of the bronchi and blood vessels; used for treatment of hypertension.

metra ('meetrə) the uterus.

metre ('meetə) *symbol* m. The fundamental SI unit of length.

metritis (mi'trietis) inflammation of the uterus.

metrocolpocele (,meetroh'kolpoh,seel) the protrusion of the uterus into the vagina, the wall of the latter also being pushed forward.

metronidazole (,metroh'nida-,zohl) a drug that is effective in overcoming *Trichomonas* infection of the genital tract of both sexes. Also used in the treatment of giardiasis, of acute amoebic dysentery and of infection by anaerobic bacteria.

metropathia (meetro'pathi·ə) any disorder affecting the uterus; metropathy. *M. haemorrhagica* excessive loss of blood from the uterus due to disease; uterine haemorrhage.

metroptosis (,meetrop'tohsis) prolapse of the uterus.

metrorrhagia (,meetrə'rayji·ə) irregular uterine bleeding not associated with menstruation.

metrostaxis (,meetroh'staksis) persistent slight haemorrhage from the uterus.

mexiletine (mek'siliteen) an antiarrhythmic agent used to treat ventricular arrhythmias.

mezlocillin (,mezloh'silin) an extended-spectrum penicillin used parenterally for treatment of serious infections due to susceptible organisms.

Michel's suture clips (mi'shelz) *G. Michel, French surgeon, 1875–1937.* Small metal clips used for suturing wounds.

miconazole (mie'konə,zohl) an antifungal agent used topically for dermatophytic infections such as athlete's foot or vulvovaginal candidiasis, orally for candidiasis of the mouth and gastrointestinal tract, and systemically by intravenous infusion for systemic fungal infections.

microbe ('miekrohb) a minute living organism, especially one causing disease. A microorganism.

microbiology (,miekrohbie'oləjee) the study of microorganisms and their effect on living cells.

microcephalic (,miekrohkə'falik, -sə-) having an abnormally small head.

Micrococcus (,miekroh'kokəs) a genus of bacteria, each of which has a spherical shape. The bacteria occur in pairs or in groups and are Gram-positive. Found in soil and water.

microcornea (,miekroh'kawni·ə) a condition in which the cornea is smaller than normal, producing hypermetropia and sometimes causing glaucoma.

microcythaemia (,miekrohsie-'theemi·ə) the presence of abnormally small red cells in the blood; microcytosis.

micrognathia (,miekroh'nathi·ə) failure of development of the lower jaw, causing a receding chin.

microgram ('miekroh,gram) *symbol* μg. One millionth of a gram.

micromastia (,miekroh'masti·ə)

the condition of exceptional smallness of the breasts.

micrometre ('miekroh,meetə) *symbol* μm. One millionth of a metre. Formerly called micron.

micron ('miekron) *see* MICROMETRE.

micronutrient (,miekroh'nyootri·ənt) a dietary element essential only in small quantities.

microorganism (,miekroh'awgə,nizəm) a minute animal or vegetable, particularly a virus, a bacterium, a fungus, a rickettsia or a protozoon.

microphage (,miekroh,fayj) a minute phagocyte.

microphthalmos (,miekrof'thalməs) a condition in which one or both eyes are smaller than normal. Their function may or may not be impaired.

microscope ('miekrə,skohp) an instrument which produces a greatly enlarged image of objects that are normally invisible to the human eye. *Electron m.* a microscope in which a beam of electrons is used instead of a light beam, allowing magnification of as much as 500 000 diameters.

microscopic (,miekrə'skopik) visible only by means of the microscope.

Microsporum (,miekroh'spor·rəm) a genus of fungi. The cause of some skin diseases, especially ringworm.

microsurgery (,miekroh'sərjə·ree) the carrying out of surgical procedures using a microscope and miniature instruments.

micturition (,miktyuh'rishən) the act of passing urine.

midbrain ('mid,brayn) that portion of the brain which connects the cerebrum with the pons and cerebellum. The mesencephalon.

midwife (mid,wief) the title and legal description of one who is so certified under the Midwives Act (1979)

midwifery (mid'wifə·ree, 'mid,wifə·ree) dealing with childbirth. *See* OBSTETRICS. *M. process* the application of the nursing process to midwifery. It is the systematic, cyclical method of organizing midwifery care, and is carried out by the assessment of actual and potential problems, and the planning, implementation and evaluation of care.

migraine ('meegrayn, 'mie-) paroxysmal attacks of severe headache, often with nausea, vomiting and visual disturbance.

Migravess ('miegrəves) trade name for combination preparations containing aspirin and metoclopramide, used in migraine.

Migril ('miegril) trade name for a combination preparation containing ergotamine, cyclizine and caffeine, used in migraine attacks.

milestone ('miel,stohn) one of the 'norms' against which the motor, social and psychological development of a child is measured.

miliaria (,mili'air·ri·ə) prickly heat, an acute itching eruption common among white people in tropical and subtropical areas.

miliary ('milyə·ree) resembling millet seed. *M. tuberculosis. see* TUBERCULOSIS.

milium ('mili·əm) [L.] a whitish nodule in the skin, especially of the face, usually 1–4 mm in diameter. Milia are spheroidal, epithelial cysts of lamellated keratin lying just under the epidermis, often associated with vellus hair follicles. Popularly called whitehead.

milk (milk) 1. a nutrient fluid produced by the mammary gland of many animals for nourishment of young mammals. 2. a liquid (emulsion or suspension) resembling the secretion of the mammary gland. Composition of milk (per cent):

	Cows' milk	Human milk
Protein	3.5	2.0
Fats	3.5	3.5
Carbohydrates	4.0	6.0
Mineral salts	0.7	0.2
Water	88.0	88.0

M. sugar lactose, a disaccharide present in the milk of all mammals. *M. teeth* the first set of teeth. *Witch's m.* milk secreted from the breasts of a newborn child.

Miller–Abbott tube (ˌmiləˈabət ˌtyoob) *T.G. Miller, American physician, 1886–1981; W.O. Abbott, American physician, 1902–1943.* A double-channel intestinal tube for treating obstruction, especially that due to paralytic ileus of the small intestine. It has an inflatable balloon at its distal end.

milliequivalent (ˌmili·iˈkwivələnt) *symbol* mEq. The amount of a substance that balances or is equivalent in combining power to 1 mg of hydrogen. A method of assessing the body's acid–base

balance or needs during electrolyte upset.

milligram (ˈmiliˌgram) *symbol* mg. One thousandth of a gram.

millilitre (ˈmiliˌleetə) *symbol* ml. One thousandth of a litre (one cubic centimetre).

millimetre (ˈmiliˌmeetə) *symbol* mm. One thousandth of a metre.

Millipore filter (ˈmiliˌpor) trade name for a device used to filter nutrient solutions as they are administered intravenously.

Milroy's disease (ˈmilroyz) *W.F. Milroy, American physician, 1855–1942.* A disease in which there is a congenital obstruction of the lymph channels in the legs.

Milton (ˈmiltən) trade name for an antiseptic consisting of a standardized 1 per cent solution of electrolytic sodium hypochlorite. It is used especially for the sterilization of babies' feeding bottles.

Milwaukee brace (milˈwawkee) a brace consisting of a leather girdle and neck ring connected by metal struts; used to brace the spine in the treatment of SCOLIOSIS.

mineralocorticoid (ˌminə·rəlohˈkawtiˌkoyd) a hormone produced by the adrenal cortex. Its function is to maintain the salt and water balance in the body.

Minilyn (ˈminilin) trade name for a contraceptive pill of oestrogen and progesterone combined.

Minims (minimz) trade name for eye drops packaged in single use containers.

minocycline (ˌminohˈsiekleen) a semisynthetic broad-spectrum antibiotic of the tetracycline group.

miosis (mie'ohsis) contraction of the pupil of the eye, as in reaction to a bright light; meiosis.

miotic (mie'otik) a drug which causes contraction of the pupil.

miscarriage ('miskarij) abortion; the expulsion of the fetus before the 28th week of pregnancy, ie. before it is legally viable.

Misuse of Drugs Act (1971) came into effect in 1973 to control the possession, prescribing, and sale of certain habit-forming drugs, including narcotic drugs such as papaveretum (Omnopon), cocaine, morphine, diamorphine, cannabis indica and amphetamines. These are called controlled drugs and are available for treatment only on medical prescription. Heavy penalties may follow the illegal sale or supply of these drugs.

mite (miet) a minute animal, frequently parasitic on man and animals, and causing various forms of dermatitis.

mithramycin (,mithrə'miesin) an antitumour antibiotic which is particularly helpful in the treatment of hypercalcaemia.

mitochondrion (mietoh'kondri-·ən) a body which occurs in the cytoplasm of cells and is concerned with energy production and the oxidation of food.

mitomycin (,mietoh'miesin) a group of highly toxic antineoplastics (mitomycin A, B and C), produced by *Streptomyces caespitosus*; indicated for palliative treatment of certain neoplasms that do not respond to surgery, radiation and other drugs.

mitosis (mie'tohsis) a method of multiplication of cells by a specific process of division.

mitral ('mietrəl) shaped like a mitre. *M. incompetence* the result of a defective mitral valve, when there is a back flow, or regurgitation following closure of the valve. *M.* stenosis the formation of fibrous tissue, causing a narrowing of the valve; usually due to rheumatic heart disease and endocarditis. *M. valve* the bicuspid valve between the left atrium and left ventricle of the heart. *M. valvotomy* an operation for overcoming stenosis by dividing the fibrous tissue to free the cusps.

mittelschmerz ('mit'l,shmərts) pain occurring between the menses, accompanying ovulation.

Mn symbol for *manganese.*

mobilization (,mobilie'zayshən) the bringing back into mobility of a limb by carefully applied pressure on a joint.

molar ('mohlə) a back tooth used for grinding. There are three on either side of each jaw, making twelve in all (only eight in children).

mole (mohl) 1. the molecular weight of a substance expressed in grams. 2. a pigmented naevus or dark-coloured growth on the skin. Moles are of various sizes, and are sometimes covered with hair. 3. a uterine tumour. *Carneous m.* an organized blood clot surrounding a shrivelled fetus in the uterus. *Hydatidiform m. (vesicular m.)* a condition in pregnancy in which the chorionic villi of the placenta degenerate into clusters of cysts like hydatids.

Malignant growth is very likely to follow if any remnants are left in the uterus. *See* CHORION EPITHELIOMA.

molecular (mə'lekyuhlə) pertaining to or composed of molecules. *M. weight* the weight of a molecule of a substance compared with that of an atom of carbon.

molecule ('moli,kyool) the chemical combination of two or more atoms which form a specific chemical substance, e.g. H_2O (water). The smallest amount of a substance that can exist independently.

molluscum (mo'luskəm) a skin disease characterized by the development of soft, round tumours. *M. contagiosum* a benign tumour arising in the epidermis caused by a virus, transmitted by direct contact or fomites.

monarticular (,monah'tikyuhlə) referring to one joint only.

Mönckeberg's sclerosis ('mərnkə-,bərgz) *J.G. Mönckeberg, German pathologist, 1877–1925.* Extensive degeneration of the arteries, with atrophy and calcareous deposits in the middle muscle coats. Mainly affects small and middle sized arteries.

mongolism ('mong·gə,lizəm) Down's syndrome; a type of congenital mental subnormality resulting in learning difficulties. Associated with an extra chromosome. There is retarded mental and physical growth with a characteristic facial appearance.

Monilia (mo'nili·ə) former name for the genus of fungi now known as *Candida*.

Monitor ('monitor) an adaptation for the UK of the USA Rush Medicus system of assessing quality of nursing care. It consists of 'checklists' for quality leading to a scoring system. The closer the score to 100 per cent the better the care being given. The master list has over 200 criteria which are divided into four categories based on patient dependency levels.

monitor ('monitə) 1. to check constantly on a given condition or phenomenon, e.g. blood pressure, or heart or respiration rate. 2. an apparatus by which such conditions or phenomena can be constantly observed and recorded. *Patient m.* the use of electrodes or transducers attached to the patient so that information such as temperature, pulse, respiration and blood pressure can be seen on a screen or automatically recorded.

monoamine oxidase (,monoh,a-meen 'oksidayz) an enzyme that breaks down noradrenaline and serotonin in the body. *M. o. inhibitor* abbreviated MAOI. A drug that prevents the breakdown of serotonin and leads to an increase in mental and physical activity.

monochromatism (,monoh'kro-mə,tizəm) colour-blindness. The patient sees all colours black, grey or white.

monoclonal (,monoh'klohn'l) derived from a single cell. *M. antibodies* antibodies derived from a single clone of cells. All the antibody molecules are identical and will react with the same antigenic site.

monocular (mo'nokyuhlə) pertaining to, or affecting, one eye only.

monocyte ('monoh,siet) a white blood cell having one nucleus, derived from the reticular cells, and having a phagocytic action.

mononucleosis (,monoh,nyookli-'ohsis) an excessive number of monocytes in the blood; monocytosis. *Infectious m.* an infectious disease due to the Epstein–Barr virus; glandular fever.

monoplegia (,monoh'pleeji·ə) paralysis of one limb or of a single muscle or a group of muscles.

monosaccharide (,monoh'sakə-,ried) a simple sugar. The end result of carbohydrate digestion. Examples are glucose, fructose and galactose.

monosodium glutamate (,mon-oh,sohdi·əm 'glootə,mayt) a chemical food flavour enhancer commonly added to Chinese dishes. May result in nausea, faintness with facial flushing and headache. (Sometimes called the Chinese restaurant syndrome.)

monosomy (,monoh'sohmee) a congenital defect in the number of human chromosomes. There is one less than the normal 46.

mons (monz) a prominence or mound. *M. pubis* or *m. veneris* the eminence, consisting of a pad of fat, which lies over the pubic symphysis in the female.

Montgomery's glands or tubercles (mənt'gumə·riz) *W.F. Montgomery, Irish obstetrician, 1797–1859.* Sebaceous glands around the nipple, which grow larger during pregnancy.

mood (mood) emotional reaction. Variations in mood are natural, but in certain psychiatric conditions there is severe depression in some cases and wild excitement in others, or alternations between both.

moon face ('moon ,fays) one of the features occurring in Cushing's syndrome and as a result of prolonged treatment with steroid drugs.

Mooren's ulcer ('mor-rənz) *A. Mooren, German ophthalmologist, 1829–1899.* A rare basal cell carcinoma of the cornea. The cause is unknown.

morbid ('mawbid) diseased, or relating to an abnormal or disordered condition.

morbidity (maw'biditee) the state of being diseased. *M. rate* a figure that shows the susceptibility of a population to a certain disease. Usually shown statistically as the number of cases which occur annually per thousand or other unit of population.

morbilli (mor'bilie) measles.

morbilliform (mor'bili,fawm) resembling measles.

moribund ('mo·ri,bund) in a dying condition.

morning sickness ('morning) nausea and vomiting which occurs in early pregnancy.

Moro reflex ('mo·roh) *E. Moro, German paediatrician, 1874–1951.* The reaction to loud noise or sudden movement which should be present in the newborn. Startle reflex.

morphine ('mawfeen) the principal alkaloid obtained from opium and given mainly to relieve severe pain. It is a drug of addiction. Morphia.

mortality (maw'talitee) the state of being liable to die. *M. rate* the number of deaths per 1000 occurring annually from a certain disease or condition.

mortification (,mawtifi'kayshən) gangrene or death of tissue; necrosis.

morula ('mo·ryuhlə) an early stage of development of the ovum when it is a solid mass of cells.

mosaic (moh'zayik) an individual who has cells of varying genetic composition.

motile ('mohtiel) capable of movement.

motion ('mohshən) 1. the process of moving. 2. evacuation of the bowels; defecation. *M. sickness* sickness occurring as the result of travel by land, sea or air. Appears to be caused by excessive stimulation of the vestibular apparatus within the inner ear.

motivation (,mohti'vayshən) the reason or reasons, conscious or unconscious, behind a particular attitude or behaviour.

motive ('mohtiv) the incentive that determines a course of action or its direction.

motor ('mohtə) something that causes movement. *M. end-plate* the nuclei and cytoplasm of muscle fibres at the termination of motor nerves. *M. nerve* one of the nerves which convey an impulse from a nerve centre to a muscle or gland to promote activity. *M. neurone disease* a disease in which there is progressive degeneration of the anterior cells in the spinal cord, the motor nuclei of cranial nerves and the corticospinal tracts. The cause is unknown.

mould (mohld) 1. a species of fungus. 2. the plastic shell used to immobilize a part of the body, usually the head, during radiotherapy.

moulding ('mohlding) the alteration in shape of the infant's head as it is forced through the maternal passages during labour.

mountain sickness ('mowntin) dyspnoea, headache, rapid pulse and vomiting, which occur on sudden change to the rarefied air of high altitudes.

mouth (mowth) an opening, particularly the external opening in the face, of the alimentary canal. *M.-wash* a solution for rinsing the mouth.

movement ('moovmənt) 1. an act of moving; motion. 2. an act of defecation. *Active m.* movement produced by the person's own muscles. *Associated m.* movement of parts that act together, as the eyes. *Passive m.* a movement of the body or of the extremities of a patient performed by another person without voluntary motion on the part of the patient. *Vermicular m's* the worm-like movements of the intestines in peristalsis.

mucin ('myoosin) the chief constituent of mucus.

mucinase ('myoosi,nayz) an enzyme that acts upon mucin. Contained in some aerosols and useful in the treatment of cystic fibrosis.

mucocele ('myookoh,seel) a mucous tumour. *M. of the gall-*

bladder occurs if a stone obstructs the cystic duct. *Lacrimal m.* a distension of the lacrimal sac caused by a blockage of the nasolacrimal duct.

mucocutaneous (ˌmyookohkyoo-'tayni·əs) pertaining to mucous membrane and skin.

mucoid ('myookoyd) resembling mucus.

mucolytic (ˌmyookoh'litik) a drug that has a mucous softening effect and so reduces the viscosity of the bronchial secretion in chest disorders.

mucopurulent (ˌmyookoh'pyooə-·rələnt) containing mucus and pus.

mucosa (myoo'kohsə) mucous membrane.

mucous ('myookəs) pertaining to or secreting mucus. *M. membrane* a membrane that secretes mucus and lines many of the body cavities, particularly those of the respiratory and alimentary tracts.

mucoviscidosis (ˌmyookoh,visi-'dohsis) fibrocystic disease of the pancreas. *See* FIBROCYSTIC.

mucus ('myookəs) the viscous secretion of mucous membrane.

multicellular (ˌmulti'selyuhlə) consisting of many cells.

multigravida (ˌmulti'gravida) a pregnant woman who has had two or more pregnancies.

multilocular (ˌmulti'lokyuhlə) having many locules. *M. cyst* a cyst, usually in the ovary, containing many compartments.

multinuclear (ˌmulti'nyookli·ə) possessing many nuclei.

multipara (mul'tipə·rə) a woman who has had two or more children.

multiple ('multip'l) manifold, occurring in many parts of the body at once. *M.myeloma* malignant disease of the plasma cells which invade the bone marrow and suppress its functioning. *M. sclerosis See* SCLEROSIS.

multivitamin (ˌmulti'vitamin) brown, sugar-coated tablet containing vitamin A 2500 units, thiamine hydrochloride 500 μg, ascorbic acid 12.5 mg and vitamin D 250 units.

mumps (mumps) a communicable paramyxovirus disease, which is statutorily notifiable, that attacks one or both of the parotid glands, the largest of the three pairs of salivary glands; called also epidemic parotitis or epidemic parotiditis. Most common amongst children; characterized by inflammation and swelling of the parotid glands. The symptoms are fever, and a painful swelling in front of the ears, making mastication difficult.

Munchausen's syndrome ('muhn-chowzənz) *Baron von Munchausen, 16th century German traveller noted for his lying tales.* Habitual seeking of hospital treatment for apparent acute illness, the patient giving a plausible and dramatic history, all of which is false. *M.s. by proxy* an uncommon situation in which a parent (usually the mother) or both parents fabricate symptoms or signs in a child which is then presented for hospital treatment; overlaps with other forms of child abuse, and fatal outcomes have been reported.

murmur ('mərmə) a sound, heard on auscultation, usually originating in the cardiovascular system. *Aortic m.* one indicating disease of the aortic valve. *Diastolic m.* one heard after the second heart sound. *Friction m.* one present when two inflamed surfaces of serous membrane rub on each other. *Mitral m.* a sign of incompetence of the mitral valve. *Systolic m.* one heard during systole.

Murphy's sign ('mɜrfeez) *J.B. Murphy, American surgeon, 1857–1916.* A sign denoting inflammation of the gallbladder. Continuous pressure over the organ will cause the patient to 'catch' his breath at the zenith of inspiration.

Musca ('muskə) a genus of flies. *M. domestica* the common house fly.

muscae volitantes ('muskə ‚volitanteez) black spots floating before the eyes. They do not obscure the sight.

muscarine ('muskə‧reen) a poisonous alkaloid found in certain fungi, and causing muscle paralysis.

muscle ('mus'l) strong tissue composed of fibres which have the power of contraction, and thus produce movements of the body. *Cardiac m.* muscle composed of partially striped interlocking cells. Not under the control of the will. *M. relaxant* one of a group of drugs used to reduce muscular spasm and also to relax the muscles during surgery. *Striped* or *striated m.* voluntary muscle. Transverse bands across the fibres give the characteristic appearance. It is under the control of the will. *Smooth* or *non-striated m.* involuntary muscle of

spindle-shaped cells, e.g. that of the intestinal wall. Contracts independently of the will.

muscular ('muskyuhlə) 1. pertaining to muscle. 2. well provided with strong muscles. *M. dystrophy* one of a number of inherited diseases in which there is progressive muscle wasting. *See* DUCHENNE DYSTROPHY.

musculocutaneous (‚muskyuhlohkyoo'tayni‧əs) referring to the muscles and the skin. *M. nerve* one of the nerves which supply the muscles and the skin of the arms and legs.

musculoskeletal (‚muskyuhloh-'skelit'l) referring to both the osseus and muscular systems.

mustine hydrochloride (‚musteen) nitrogen mustard. A cyotoxic drug which may be given intravenously for malignant disease of lymph glands and reticuloendothelial cells, such as Hodgkin's disease.

mutant ('myootənt) 1. in genetics, a variation that breeds true, owing to genetic changes. 2. produced by mutation.

mutation (myoo'tayshən) a chemical change in the genes of a cell causing it to show a new characteristic. Some produce evolutional changes, others disease.

mute (myoot) without the power of speech; dumb. *Deaf m.* one who cannot speak because he cannot hear.

mutilation (‚myooti'layshən) deliberate infliction of bodily injury.

mutism ('myootizəm) inability or refusal to speak. In almost all cases, mutes are unable to speak because deafness has prevented them from hearing the spoken word. Speech is learned by imitating the speech of others. May also result from disease, the most common being a stroke. *Elective m.* psychological disorder of childhood.

myalgia (mie'alji·ə) pain in the muscles.

myasthenia (,mieəs'theeni·ə) muscle weakness. *M. gravis* an extreme form of muscle weakness which is progressive. There is a rapid onset of fatigue, thought to be due to the too rapid destruction of acetylcholine at the neuromuscular junction. Commonly affected muscles are those of vision, speaking, chewing and swallowing.

mycetoma (,miesi'tohmə) a chronic fungus infection of the tissues both external and internal, but most commonly affecting the hands and feet. There is swelling and the formation of sinuses. Madura foot.

Mycobacterium (,miekohbak-'tiə·ri·əm) a genus of slender, rod-shaped, acid-fast, Gram-positive bacteria. *M. leprae* the causative organism of leprosy. *M. tuberculosis* the cause of tuberculosis.

mycology (mie'koləjee) the study of fungi.

mycosis (mie'kohsis) any disease which is caused by a fungus. *M. fungoides* a rare malignant lymphoreticular neoplasm of the skin which later progresses to the lymph nodes and viscera.

mydriasis (mi'drieəsis, mie-) abnormal dilatation of the pupil of the eye. Usually caused by injury to the pupil sphincter or by the use of mydriatic drugs.

mydriatic (,midri'atik) any drug which causes mydriasis. Used in examination of the eye and in the treatment of inflammatory conditions.

myelin ('mieəlin) the fatty covering of medullated nerve fibres.

myelitis (,mieə'lietis) 1. inflammation of the spinal cord, causing pain in the back and sometimes numbness and paralysis of the legs and the lower part of the trunk. 2. inflammation of the bone marrow; osteomyelitis.

myeloblast ('mieəloh,blast) a primitive cell in the bone marrow from which develop the granular leukocytes.

myelocyte ('mieəloh,siet) a cell of the bone marrow, derived from a myeloblast.

myelography (,mieə'logrəfee) radiographic examination of the spinal cord following the insertion of a radio-opaque substance into the subarachnoid space by means of lumbar puncture.

myeloid ('mieə,loyd) 1. pertaining to, derived from, or resembling bone marrow. 2. pertaining to the spinal cord. 3. having the appearance of myelocytes, but not necessarily derived from bone marrow. *M. leukaemia* a malignant disease in which there is excessive production of leukocytes in the bone marrow. *M. tissue* red bone marrow.

myeloma (,mieə'lohmə) a tumour composed of plasma cells. *Multiple m.* a primary malignant tumour of plasma cells usually arising in bone marrow, and usually associated with anaemia and with a paraprotein in the blood or Bence Jones protein in the urine.

myelomatosis (,mieəlohmə-'tohsis) a malignant disease of the bone marrow in which multiple myelomas are present.

myelomeningocele (,mieəlohmə-'ning·goh,seel) meningomyelocele.

myelopathy (,mieə'lopəthee) a disease affecting the spinal cord.

myocardial (,mieoh'kahdi·əl) pertaining to the myocardium. *M. infarction* necrosis of a part of the myocardium usually following a coronary thrombosis. Ventricular fibrillation may occur, followed by death.

myocarditis (,mieohkah'dietis) inflammation of the myocardium.

myocardium (,mieoh'kahdi·əm) the muscle tissue of the heart.

myocele ('mieoh,seel) protrusion of muscle through a rupture of its sheath.

myoclonus (,mieoh'klohnəs) spasmodic contraction of the muscles.

myoelectric (,mieoh·i'lektrik) pertaining to the electric properties of muscle.

myofibrosis (,mieohfie'brohsis) a degenerative condition in which there is some replacement of muscle tissue by fibrous tissue.

myogenic (,mieoh'jenik) originating in muscle tissue.

myoglobin (,mieoh'glohbin) myohaemoglobin.

myohaemoglobin (,mieoh,heemə,glohbin) a substance resembling haemoglobin, which is present in muscle cells. It is a pigment and is responsible for the colour of muscle. It acts as an oxygen store. Myoglobin.

myohaemoglobinuria (,mieoh,heemə,glohbi'nyooə·ri·ə) the presence of myohaemoglobin in the urine.

myokymia (,mieoh'kimi·ə) a benign condition in which there is persistent quivering of the muscles.

myoma (mie'ohmə) a benign tumour of muscle tissue. *See* FIBROMYOMA.

myomectomy (,mieə'mektəmee) removal of a myoma; usually referring to a uterine fibroma.

myometrium (,mieoh'meetri·əm) the muscular tissue of the uterus.

myoneural (,mieoh'nyooə·rəl) relating to both muscle and nerve. *M. junction* the point at which nerve endings terminate in a muscle; neuromuscular junction.

myopathy (mie'opəthee) any disease of the muscles. Muscular dystrophy is one of a group of inherited myopathies in which there is wasting and weakness of the muscles.

myopia (mie'ohpi·ə) shortsightedness. The light rays focus in front of the retina and a biconcave lens is needed to focus them correctly.

myoplasty ('mieoh,plastee) any operation in which muscle is detached and utilized, as may be done to correct deformities.

myosarcoma (,mieohsah'kohmə) a sarcomatous tumour of muscle.

myosin ('mieəsin) muscle protein.

myositis (,mieoh'sietis) inflammation of a muscle. *M. ossificans* a condition in which bone cells deposited in muscle continue to grow and cause hard lumps. It may occur after fractures.

myotomy (mie'otəmee) the division or dissection of a muscle.

myotonia (ˌmieə'tohni·ə) lack of muscle tone. *M. congenita* an hereditary disease in which the muscle action has a prolonged contraction phase and slow relaxation.

myringa (mi'ring·gə) the ear drum or tympanic membrane.

myringitis (ˌmirin'jietis) inflammation of the tympanic membrane.

myringoplasty (mi'ring·goh,plastee) a plastic operation to repair the tympanic membrane; tympanoplasty.

myringotome (mi'ring·gə,tohm) an instrument for puncturing the tympanic membrane in myringotomy.

myringotomy (ˌmiring'gotəmee) incision of the tympanic membrane to drain fluid from an infected middle ear.

myxoedema (ˌmiksi'deemə) a condition caused by hypothyroidism which is marked by mucoid infiltration of the skin. There is oedematous swelling of the face, limbs and hands, dry and rough skin, loss of hair, slow pulse, subnormal temperature, slowed metabolism and mental dullness. *Congenital m.* cretinism.

myxoma (mik'sohmə) a benign mucous tumour of connective tissue.

myxosarcoma (ˌmiksohsah'kohmə) a sarcoma containing mucoid tissue.

myxovirus (ˌmiksoh'vierəs) the group name of a number of related viruses, including the causal viruses of influenza, parainfluenza, mumps and Newcastle disease (of fowl).

N

N symbol for *nitrogen* and *newton*.

Na symbol for *sodium*.

Naboth's follicle or cyst ('nayboths) *M. Naboth, German anatomist, 1675–1721.* Cystic swelling of a cervical gland, the duct of which has become blocked by regenerating squamous epithelium.

naevus ('neevəs) a birthmark; a circumscribed area of pigmentation of the skin due to dilated blood vessels. A haemangioma. *N. flammeus* a flat bluish-red area, usually on the neck or face; popularly known as 'port-wine stain'. *N. pilosus* a hairy naevus. *Spider n.* a small red area surrounded by dilated capillaries. *Strawberry n.* a raised tumour-like structure of connective tissue containing spaces filled with blood.

Naffziger's operation ('nafzigəz) *H.C. Naffziger, American surgeon, 1884–1961.* Incision of the orbit transfrontally to reduce orbital pressure in exophthalmos.

naftidrofuryl (naf,tidroh'fyooəril) an agent used in the treatment of peripheral and cerebral vascular disorders.

Nägele's rule ('naygələz) rule for calculating the estimated date of labour; subtract 3 months from the first day of the last menstrual period and add 7 days.

NA non-accidental injury.

nail (nayl) the keratinized portion of epidermis covering the dorsal extremity of the fingers and toes. *N. bed* the skin underlying a nail. *Hang-n.* a strip of epidermis hanging at one side or at the root of a nail. *Ingrowing n.* a condition in which the flesh overhangs the edge of the nail, a sharp corner of which may pierce the skin, causing a wound which may become septic. *Spoon n.* a nail with a depression in the centre and raised edges. Koilonychia.

nalidixic acid (,nali'diksik) an antibacterial agent used in the treatment of urinary infections.

nalorphine ('nalawfeen) an antidote for morphine, pethidine and methadone overdosage.

naloxone (na'loksohn) a narcotic antagonist used as an antidote to narcotic overdosage and as an antagonist for pentazocine overdosage.

nandrolone ('nandrə,lohn) an anabolic steriod that promotes protein metabolism and skeletal growth.

nape (nayp) the back of the neck.

napkin rash ('napkin) an erythematous rash which may occur in infants in the napkin area. The many causes include the passage of frequent loose stools, thrush, ammoniacal dermatitis and allergy to washing powders and detergents.

narcissism ('nahsi,sizəm) the stage of infant development when the child is mainly interested in himself and his own bodily needs. In adults it may be a symptom of mental disorder. The term is derived from the Greek legend of Narcissus.

narcoanalysis (,nahkoh·ə'nalisis) a form of psychotherapy in which an injection of a narcotic drug produces a drowsy, relaxed state during which a patient will talk more freely, and in this way much repressed material may be brought to consciousness.

narcolepsy ('nahkoh,lepsee) a condition in which there is an uncontrollable desire for sleep.

narcosis (nah'kohsis) a state of unconsciousness produced by a narcotic drug. *Basal n.* a state of unconsciousness produced prior to surgical anaesthesia.

narcosynthesis (,nahkoh'sinthə-sis) the inducement of a hypnotic state by means of drugs. An aid to psychotherapy.

narcotic (nah'kotik) a drug that produces narcosis or unnatural sleep.

nares ('nair·reez) the nostrils. *Posterior n.* the opening of the nares into the nasopharynx.

nasal ('nayz'l) pertaining to the nose.

nascent ('nas'nt, 'nay-) 1. at the time of birth. 2. incipient.

Naseptin (nay'septin) trade name for a combination preparation containing chlorhexidine and neomycin, a nasal cream for the treatment of staphyloccal infections.

nasogastric (,nayzoh'gastrik) referring to the nose and stomach. *N. tube* one passed into the stomach via the nose.

nasojejunal feeding (,nayzohji-'joon'l ,feeding) a method in which a silicone-coated catheter is passed through the nose into the jejunum, to provide sufficient nutrition to a sick baby on a ventilator or receiving continuous inflating pressure (CIP) by mask or nasal tube. It is used to prevent the dangers of aspiration with a nasogastric tube feed.

nasolacrimal (,nayzoh'lakriməl) concerning both the nose and lacrimal apparatus. *N. duct* the duct draining the tears from the inner aspect of the eye to the inferior meatus of the nose.

nasopharynx (,nayzoh'faringks) the upper part of the pharynx; that above the soft palate.

nasosinusitis (,nayzoh,sienə-'sietis) inflammation of the nose and adjacent sinuses.

natural childbirth (nachər'l) a term used to describe an approach to LABOUR and delivery in which the parents are prepared for the event so that the mother is awake and cooperative and the father is able to assume an active and supportive role during the birth of their child. The underlying concept for all methods of natural childbirth is avoidance of medical interference and analgesia in labour, and education of the parents so that they can actively participate in and share the experience of childbirth.

naturopathy (,naychə'ropəthee) a drugless system of healing by a combination of diet, fasting, exercise, hydrotherapy and positive thinking.

nausea ('nawzi·ə) a sensation of sickness with an inclination to vomit.

navel ('nayv'l) the umbilicus.

navicular (nə'vikyuhlə) boat-shaped. *N. bone* one of the tarsal bones of the foot.

nebula ('nebyuhlə) a slight opacity or cloudiness of the cornea, caused by injury or by corneal ulceration.

nebulizer ('nebyuh,liezə) an apparatus for reducing a liquid to a fine spray. An atomizer.

neck (nek) 1. the narrow part of an organ or bone. 2. the part of the body which connects the head and the trunk. *Derbyshire n.* simple goitre. *Wry n.* torticollis.

necrobiosis (,nekrohbie'ohsis) localized death of a part as a result of degeneration.

necropsy ('nekropsee) autopsy; a postmortem examination of a body.

necrosis (nə'krohsis) death of a portion of tissue.

necrotizing enterocolitis ('nekrə,tiezing) abbreviated NEC. A condition of neonates in which there is severe diarrhoea and blood in the stools. It occurs in preterm or low birth weight neonates. Exact cause not known but often associated with infection.

necrotomy (nə'krotəmee) an operation to remove a dead piece of bone.

needle-stick injury (need'lstik ,injə·ree) an accidental injury with a needle that is contaminated with blood or body fluids.

The term is also used sometimes to include other sharps injuries. These injuries have been reported as a means of infecting the nurse or health care professional with hepatitis or HIV infection.

needling ('needling) discission; the operation for cataract of lacerating and splitting up the lens so that it may be absorbed.

negative ('negətiv) the opposite of positive. The absence of some quality or substance.

negativism ('negəti,vizəm) a symptom of mental illness in which the patient does the opposite of what is required of him and so presents an uncooperative attitude. Common in schizophrenia.

negligence ('neglijəns) in law, the failure to do something that a reasonable person of ordinary prudence would do in a certain situation or the doing of something that such a person would not do. Negligence may provide the basis for a lawsuit when there is a legal duty, as the duty of a doctor or nurse to provide reasonable care to patients, and when the negligence results in damage to the patient.

Neisseria (nie'siə·ri·ə) *A.L.S. Neisser, German bacteriologist, 1855–1916.* A genus of paired, spherical, Gram-negative bacteria. *N. gonorrhoeae* the causative organism of gonorrhoea. *N. meningitidis* the cause of meningococcal meningitis.

Nelson's syndrome ('nelsənz) *D.H. Nelson, American physician, b.1925.* The development of an

ACTH-producing pituitary tumour after bilateral adrenalectomy in Cushing's syndrome; it is characterized by aggressive growth of the tumour and hyperpigmentation of the skin.

Nematoda (ˌneməˈtohdə) a phylum of worms, including the *Ascaris* or roundworm and the *Enterobius* or threadworm.

neocerebellum (ˌneeohˌseriˈbeləm) the middle lobe of the cerebellum.

neocortex (ˌneeohˈkawteks) the cerebral cortex excluding the hippocampal formation and piriform area.

neoglycogenesis (ˌneeohˌgliekəˈjenəsis) the formation of liver glycogen from non-carbohydrate sources. Glyconeogenesis.

neologism (neeˈoləˌjizəm) the formation of new words, either completely new ones or ones formed by contraction of two separate words. This is done particularly by schizophrenic patients.

neomycin (ˌneeohˈmiesin) an antibiotic drug used against a wide range of bacteria, frequently those affecting the skin or the eyes. Also given orally to sterilize the bowel before surgery.

neonatal (ˌneeəˈnaytˈl) referring to the first month of life. *N. mortality rate* the number of deaths of infants up to 4 weeks old per 1000 live births in any 1 year.

neonate (ˈneeəˌnayt) newborn; specifically pertaining to a baby under 1 month old.

neonatology (ˌneeənayˈtoləjee) the branch of medicine dealing with disorders of the newborn infant.

neoplasm (ˈneeohˌplazəm) a morbid new growth; a tumour. It may be benign or malignant.

neostigmine (ˌneeohˈstigmeen) a synthetic preparation akin to physostigmine used in the treatment of myasthenia gravis and as an antidote to some musclerelaxant drugs, and as eye drops in the treatment of glaucoma.

Nepenthe (nəˈpenthee) trade name for a preparation containing opium alkaloids, used as an analgesic.

nephralgic (nəˈfraljik) relating to pain arising from the kidney. *N. crises* spasms of pain in the lumbar region in tabes dorsalis.

nephrectomy (nəˈfrektəmee) excision of a kidney.

nephritis (nəˈfrietis) inflammation of the kidney; a focal or diffuse proliferative or destructive disease that may involve the glomerulus, tubule or interstitial renal tissue. Called also *Bright's disease*. The most usual form is glomerulonephritis.

nephroblastoma (ˌnefrohblaˈstohmə) a rapidly developing malignant mixed tumour of the kidneys, made up of embryonic cells, and occurring chiefly in children before the fifth year; Wilms' tumour.

nephrocalcinosis (ˌnefrohˌkalsiˈnohsis) a condition in which there is deposition of calcium in the renal tubules resulting in calculi formation and renal insufficiency.

nephrocapsulectomy (ˌnefrohˌkapsyuhˈlektəmee) operation for removal of the capsule of the kidney.

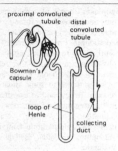

proximal convoluted tubule

distal convoluted tubule

Bowman's capsule

loop of Henle

collecting duct

NEPHRON OF KIDNEY

nephrocele ('nefroh,seel) hernia of the kidney.

nephrogram ('nefroh,gram) a radiograph of the kidney with contrast medium in the renal tubules. Usually the immediate film in an excretion urogram.

nephrolith ('nefroh,lith) stone in the kidney; renal calculus.

nephrolithiasis (,nefrohli'thieəsis) the presence of a calculus or of gravel in the kidney.

nephrolithotomy (,nefrohli'thotəmee) removal of a renal calculus by incising the kidney or by extracorporeal shock wave lithotripsy.

nephroma (ne'frohmə) tumour of the kidney.

nephron ('nefron) the functional unit of the kidney, comprising Bowman's capsule, the proximal and distal tubules, the loop of Henle and the collecting duct, which conveys urine to the renal pelvis.

nephropexy ('nefroh,peksee) the

fixation of a floating (mobile) kidney, usually by sutures to neighbouring muscle.

nephroptosis (,nefrop'tohsis) downward displacement, or undue mobility, of a kidney.

nephropyeloplasty (,nefroh'pieəloh,plastee) a plastic operation on the pelvis of the kidney performed in cases of hydronephrosis.

nephropyosis (,nefrohpie'ohsis) suppuration in the kidney.

nephrosclerosis (,nefrohsklə'rohsis) constriction of the arterioles of the kidney. Seen in benign and malignant hypertension and in arteriosclerosis in old age.

nephrosis (ne'frohsis) any disease of the kidney, especially that which is characterized by oedema, albuminuria and a low plasma albumin. Caused by noninflammatory degenerative lesions of the tubules.

nephrostomy (nə'frostəmee) creation of a permanent opening into the renal pelvis.

nephrotic (nə'frotik) referring to or caused by nephrosis. *N. syndrome* a clinical syndrome in which there are albuminuria, low plasma protein and gross oedema. Due to increased capillary permeability in the glomeruli. It may occur as a result of acute glomerulonephritis, in subacute nephritis, diabetes mellitus, amyloid disease, systemic lupus erythematosus and renal vein thrombosis.

nephrotomogram (,nefroh'tohmə,gram) a tomogram of the kidney obtained by nephrotomography.

nephrotomography (,nefrohtə'mogrəfee) radiological visualization of the kidney by tomography after introduction of a contrast medium.

nephrotomy (nə'frotəmee) incision of the kidney.

nephrotoxic (,nehfroh'toksik) poisonous or destructive to the cells of the kidney.

nephroureterectomy (,nefroh·,reetə'rektəmee) surgical removal of the kidney and the ureter.

nerve (nərv) a bundle of conducting fibres enclosed in a sheath called the epineurium. Its function is to transmit impulses between any part of the body and a nerve centre. *N. block* a method of producing regional anaesthesia by injecting a local anaesthetic into the nerves supplying the area to be operated on. *N. fibre* the prolongation of the nerve cell, which conveys impulses. Each fibre has a sheath. Medullated nerve fibres have an insulating myelin sheath. *N. gas* a gas that interferes with the functioning of the nerves and muscles. Such gases may cause death from respiratory paralysis and some of them act through the skin and cannot be avoided by the use of gas masks. *Motor (efferent) n.* one that conveys impulses causing activity from a nerve centre to a muscle or gland. *Sensory (afferent) n.* one that conveys sensation from an area to a nerve centre.

nervous ('nərvəs) 1. pertaining to, or composed of, nerves. 2. apprehensive. *N. breakdown* a popular and misleading term for any type of mental illness that interferes with a person's normal activities.

A so-called 'nervous breakdown' can include any of the mental disorders, including NEUROSIS, PSYCHOSIS or DEPRESSION, but is usually used to describe neurosis.

nervousness ('nərvəsnəs) excitability of the nervous system, characterized by a state of mental and physical unrest.

nettle rash ('net'l ,rash) an allergic skin condition; urticaria.

neural ('nyooə·rəl) pertaining to the nerves. *N. arch* the bony arch on each vertebra which encloses the spinal cord. *N. tube defect* any of a group of congenital malformations involving the neural tube, including anencephaly, hypocephalus and spina bifida.

neuralgia (nyuh'raljə, -ji·ə) a sharp stabbing pain, usually along the course of a nerve, owing to neuritis or functional disturbance.

neurapraxia (,nyooə·rə'praksi·ə) an injury to a nerve resulting in temporary loss of function and paralysis. It is usually caused by compression of the nerve, and there is no lasting damage.

neurasthenia (,nyoohə·rəs'theeni·ə) a neurosis in which there is much mental and physical fatigue, inability to concentrate, loss of appetite, and a failure of memory.

neurectomy (nyuh'rektəmee) excision of part of a nerve.

neurilemma (,nyooə·ri'lemə) the membranous sheath surrounding a nerve fibre.

neurinoma (,nyooə·ri'nohmə) a benign tumour arising in the neurilemma of a nerve fibre.

neuritis (nyuh'rietis) inflammation of a nerve, with pain, tenderness and loss of function. *Multiple n.* that involving several nerves; polyneuritis. *Nutritional (alcoholic) n.* that which may be caused by alcoholism or lack of vitamin B complex. *Optic n.* that affecting the optic disc or nerve. *Peripheral n.* that involving the terminations of nerves. *Sciatic n.* sciatica. *Tabetic n.* a type occurring in tabes dorsalis. *Traumatic n.* that which results from an injury to a nerve.

neuroblast ('nyooə-roh,blast) an embryonic nerve cell.

neuroblastoma (,nyooə-rohbla-'stohmə) a malignant tumour of immature nerve cells, most often arising in the very young.

neurodermatitis (,nyooə-roh-,dərma'tietis) a localized prurigo of somatic and psychogenic origin. It irritates, and rubbing causes thickening and pigmentation of the skin.

neuroepithelioma (,nyooə-roh,epi,theeli'ohmə) a malignant tumour of the retina of the eye, which may spread into the brain.

neurofibroma (,nyooə-rohfie-'brohmə) a benign tumour of nerve and fibrous tissue.

neurofibromatosis (,nyooə-roh-,fiebrohmə'tohsis) von Recklinghausen's disease. A generalized hereditary disease in which there are numerous fibromas of the skin and nervous system.

neurogenic (,nyooə-rə'jenik) derived from or caused by nerve stimulation. *N. bladder* a disorder of the urinary bladder caused by a lesion of the nervous system. *N. shock* shock originating in the nervous system.

neuroglia (nyuh·rogli·ə) the special form of connective tissue supporting nerve tissues.

neurohypophysis (,nyooə-roh-·hie'pofisis) the posterior lobe of the pituitary gland.

neuroleptic (,nyooə-roh'leptik) a drug which acts on the nervous system.

neurological assessment (,nyooə-·roh'lojik'l) evaluation of the health status of a patient with a nervous system disorder or dysfunction. Purposes of the assessment include establishing nursing goals to guide the nurse in planning and implementing nursing measures to help the patient cope effectively with daily living activities. Nursing assessment of a patient's neurological status is concerned with identifying functional disabilities that interfere with the person's ability to care for himself and lead an active life. A functionally oriented nursing assessment includes: (1) consciousness, (2) mental functions, (3) motor function, and (4) sensory function. Evaluation of these functions gives the nurse information about the patient's ability to perform everyday activities such as thinking, remembering, seeing, eating, speaking, moving, smelling, feeling and hearing. A patient with an acute and life-threatening alteration in neurological function is evaluated and monitored in four general areas: (1) level of consciousness, (2) sensory and motor function, (3) pupillary changes, and (4) vital signs and pattern of respiration.

neurologist (nyuh'roləjist) a medical practitioner specializing in neurology.

neurology (nyuh'roləjee) 1. the scientific study of the nervous system. 2. the branch of medicine concerned with diseases of the nervous system.

neuroma (nyuh'rohmə) a tumour consisting of nervous tissue.

neuromuscular (,nyooə-roh-'muskyuhlə) appertaining to nerves and muscles. *N. junction* the small gap between the end of the motor nerve and the motor end-plate of the muscle fibre supplied. This gap is bridged by the release of acetylcholine whenever a nerve impulse arrives.

neuromyelitis (,nyooə-roh,mieə-'lietis) neuritis associated with myelitis. It is a condition akin to multiple sclerosis. *N. optica* a disease in which there is bilateral optic neuritis and paraplegia.

neurone (neuron) ('nyooə-rohn, 'nyooə-ron) a nerve cell. *Lower motor n.* the anterior horn cell and its neurone which conveys impulses to the appropriate muscles. *Upper motor n.* that in which the cell is in the cerebral cortex and the fibres conduct impulses to associated cells in the spinal cord.

neuroparalysis (,nyooə-rohpə-'ralisis) paralysis due to disease of a nerve or nerves.

neuropathy (nyuh'ropəthee) a disease process of nerve degeneration and loss of function. *Alcoholic n.* neuropathy due to thiamine deficiency in chronic alcoholism. *Diabetic n.* that associated with diabetes. *Entrap-*

ment n. any of a group of neuropathies, e.g. carpal tunnel syndrome, due to mechanical pressure on a peripheral nerve. *Ischaemic n.* that caused by a lack of blood supply.

neuroplasty ('nyooə-roh,plastee) the surgical repair of a damaged nerve.

neurorrhaphy (nyuh'ro-rəfee) the operation of suturing a divided nerve.

neurosis (nyuh'rohsis) a mental disorder, which does not affect the whole personality, characterized by exaggerated anxiety and tension. *Anxiety n.* persistent anxiety and the accompanying symptoms of fear, rapid pulse, sweating, trembling, loss of appetite and insomnia. *Obsessive–compulsive n.* one characterized by compulsions and obsessional rumination.

neurosurgery (,nyoə-roh'sərjə-ree) that branch of surgery dealing with the brain, spinal cord and nerves.

neurosyphilis (,nyooə-roh'sifilis) a manifestation of third stage syphilis in which the nervous system is involved. The three commonest forms are: (1) meningovascular syphilis, affecting the blood vessels to the meninges, (2) tabes dorsalis (*see* ATAXIA), and (3) general paralysis of the insane.

neurotic (nyuh'rotik) a loosely applied adjective denoting association with neurosis.

neurotmesis (,nyooə-rot'meesis) degeneration of a nerve due to severance.

neurotomy (nyuh'rotəmee) the surgical division of a nerve.

neurotoxic (,nyooə·roh'toksik) poisonous or destructive to nervous tissue.

neurotransmitter (,nyooə·roh-tranz'mitə, -trahnz-) a substance (e.g. noradrenaline, acetylcholine, dopamine) that is released from the axon terminal to produce activity in other nerves.

neurotripsy ('nyooə·roh,tripsee) the surgical bruising or crushing of a nerve.

neurotropic (,nyooə·roh'tropik) having an affinity for nerve tissue. *N. viruses* those that particularly attack the nervous system.

neutropenia (,nyootrə'peeni·ə) a decrease in the number of neutrophils in the blood.

neutrophil ('nyootrə,fil) a polymorphonuclear leukocyte which has a neutral reaction to acid and alkaline dyes.

niacin ('nieəsin) nicotinic acid.

niclosamide (ni'klohsəmied) an anthelmintic used as a single dose in tapeworm infestations.

nicotine ('nikə,teen) a poisonous alkaloid in tobacco.

nicotinic acid (,nikə'tinik) niacin. A water-soluble vitamin in the B complex. A deficiency of this vitamin causes pellagra.

nictitation (,nikti'tayshən) the act of winking.

nidation (nie'dayshən) implantation of the fertilized ovum in the uterus.

nidus ('niedəs) 1. a nest. 2. a place in which an organism finds conditions suitable for its growth and development. 3. the focus of an infection.

Niemann–Pick disease (,neemən-'pik) *A. Niemann, German paedi-*atrician, 1880–1921; F. Pick, German physician, 1868–1935. A rare inherited disease occurring primarily in Jewish children and resulting in mental handicap. There is lipoid storage abnormality and widespread deposition of lecithin in the tissues.

nifedipine (nie'fedi,peen) a calcium channel blocker used as a coronary vasodilator in the treatment of angina pectoris, and in the treatment of hypertension.

night blindness (niet) nyctalopia; difficulty in seeing in the dark. This may be a congenital defect or be caused by a vitamin A deficiency. Also occurs as a result of retinal degeneration.

night sweat ('niet ,swet) profuse perspiration during sleep, especially typical of tuberculosis.

night terror ('niet ,terə) an unpleasant experience in which the subject, usually a young child, screams in his sleep and seems terrified. On waking he is unable to remember the cause of his fear.

nihilism ('nieə,lizəm) in psychiatry, a term used to describe feelings of not existing and hopelessness, that all is lost or destroyed.

nikethamide (ni'kethə,mied) a cardiac and respiratory stimulant given intravenously in cases of respiratory failure.

nipple ('nip'l) the small conical projection at the tip of the breast, through which, in the female, milk can be withdrawn. *Accessory n.* a rudimentary nipple anywhere in a line from the breast to the groin. *Depressed n.* one that does not protrude. *Retracted n.* one that is drawn inwards. It may be a sign of cancer of the breast. *N. shield* a shield fitted with a rubber teat which covers the areola of a nursing mother when her nipple is sore or not sufficiently protractile for the baby to suck.

Nissl granules ('nis'l) *F. Nissl, German neuropathologist, 1860–1919.* RNA-containing units found in the cytoplasm of cells. Probably associated with protein synthesis.

nit (nit) the egg of the head louse, attached to the hair near the scalp.

nitrazepam (nie'trazi,pam) a hypnotic and sedative drug used to treat insomnia with early morning wakening.

nitrofurantoin (,nietrohfyooə-'rantoh·in) a urinary antiseptic which is bactericidal and is effective against a wide range of organisms.

nitrofurazone (,nietroh'fyooə-rə-,zohn) an antibacterial agent used chiefly as ear drops in the treatment of otitis externa.

nitrogen ('nietrəjən) *symbol N.* A gaseous element. Air is largely composed of nitrogen, and it is one of the essential constituents of all protein foods. *N. balance* the state of the body in regard to the rate of protein intake and protein utilization. A negative nitrogen balance occurs when more protein is utilized by the body than is taken in. A positive nitrogen balance implies a net gain of protein in the body. Negative nitrogen balance can be caused by such factors as malnutrition, debilitating diseases, blood loss and glucocorticoids. A positive balance can be caused by exercise, growth hormone and testosterone. *N. mustards* a group of toxic, blistering alkylating agents, including nitrogen mustard itself (mechlorethamine hydrochloride) and related compounds; some have been used as antineoplastics in certain forms of cancer.

nitroglycerin (,nietroh'glisərin) glyceryl trinitrate. A drug which causes dilatation of the coronary arteries. In angina pectoris a tablet should be dissolved sublingually before exertion.

nitrous oxide ('nietrəs) N_2O; laughing-gas. An inhalation anaesthetic ensuring a brief spell of unconsciousness.

nociassociation (,nohsi-ə,sohsi-'ayshən) the discharge of nervous energy which occurs unconsciously in trauma, as in surgical shock. *See* ANOCIASSOCIATION.

noctambulation (,noktambyuh-'layshən) sleep-walking; somnambulism.

nocturia (nok'tyooə-ri-ə) the production of large quantities of urine at night.

nocturnal (nok'tərn'l) referring to the night. *N. enuresis* bed wetting; incontinence of urine during sleep.

node (nohd) a swelling or protuberance. *Atrioventricular n.* the specialized tissue between the right atrium and the ventricle, at the point where the coronary vein enters the atrium, from which is initiated the impulse of contraction down the atrioventricular bundle. *N. of Ranvier* a constriction occurring at intervals in a nerve fibre to enable the neurilemma with its blood supply to reach and nourish the axon of the nerve. *Sinoatrial n.* the pacemaker of the heart. The specialized neuromuscular tissue at the junction of the superior vena cava and the right atrium, which, stimulated by the right vagus nerve, controls the rhythm of contraction in the heart.

nodule ('nodyool) a small swelling or protuberance.

noma ('nohmə) a gangrenous condition of the mouth; cancrum oris.

nomogram ('nomə,gram,'noh-) a graph with several scales arranged so that a ruler laid on the graph intersects the scales at related values of the variables; the values of any two variables can be used to find the values of the others. Increasingly used in the determination of drug therapy dosage, e.g. in paediatrics.

non compos mentis (non 'kompəs 'mentis) [L.] *not of sound mind.* Applied to a person whose mental state is such that he is unable to manage his own affairs.

non-accidental injury (,nonaksi-'dent'l) injuries inflicted upon children or infants by those looking after them, usually the parents. The injuries are usually physical (beating, burnings, biting) but the term includes the giving of poisons and dangerous drugs, sexual abuse, starvation and any other form of physical assault.

non-compliance (,nonkəm'plie-ans) describes the decision made by a patient not to comply with a drug regimen, even though fully understanding the rationale for such therapy.

non-specific (,nonspə'sifik) 1. not due to any single known cause. 2. not directed against a particular agent, but rather having a general effect. *N. urethritis* a common, sexually transmitted disease which may be due to a variety of agents, e.g. *Chlamydia trachomatis* which causes 40 per cent of cases. Also called non-gonococcal urethritis.

non-steroidal anti-inflammatory drugs (non,stiə'royd'l, -,ster-) abbreviated NSAIDs. A group of drugs having analgesic, antipyretic and anti-inflammatory activity due to their ability to inhibit the synthesis of prostaglandins. It includes aspirin, phenylbutazone, indomethacin, tolmetin, ibuprofen and related drugs.

non-union (non'yooni·ən) in a fracture, failure of the two pieces of bone to unite.

noradrenaline (,nor·rə'drenəlin) a hormone present in extracts of the suprarenal medulla and at synapses in the peripheral sympathetic nervous sytem. It causes vasoconstriction and raises both the systolic and the diastolic blood pressure.

norethandrolone (,nor·rə'thandrə,lohn) an anabolic steroid that aids in the utilization of protein. May be used to treat severe wasting and in osteoporosis.

norethisterone (,nor·re'thistə-

,rohn) an anabolic steroid similar in action to progesterone. Used in the treatment of amenorrhoea. Also used in the combined contraceptive pill.

normal ('nawm'l) conforming to a standard; regular or usual. *N. flora* bacteria which normally live on body tissues and have a beneficial effect. *N. saline* isotonic solution of sodium chloride. Physiological solution.

normoblast ('nawmoh,blast) a nucleated precursor red blood cell in bone marrow. *See* ERYTHROCYTE.

normochromic (,nawmoh'krohmik) normal in colour. Applied to the blood when the haemoglobin level is within normal limits.

normocyte ('nawmoh,siet) a red blood cell that is normal in size, shape and colour.

normoglycaemia (,nawmohglie-'seemi·ə) normal blood sugar level.

normotension (,nawmoh'tenshən) normal tone, tension or pressure. Usually used in relation to blood pressure.

Norton score ('nortən) a pressure sore risk assessment scale devised by Norton, McLaren and Exton Smith and used primarily in the care of elderly patients. It comprises five health state components, each with a four-point descending scale. Maximum points are 20 and the minimum five; a 'score' of 14 and below indicates that the patient is at risk of developing pressure sores and needs 1–2 hourly changes of posture and the use of pressure-relieving aids. The system

requires weekly application and whenever a change occurs in the patient's condition and/or circumstances of care.

nortriptyline (naw'tripti,leen) a tricyclic antidepressant drug used for the relief of all types of depression.

nose (nohz) the organ of smell and the airway for respiration.

nostalgia (no'staljə) home sickness.

nostril ('nostrəl) one of the anterior orifices of the nose.

notifiable ('nohti,fieəb'l) applied to such diseases as must by law be reported to the health authorities. These include measles, scarlet fever, typhus and typhoid fever, cholera, diphtheria, tuberculosis, dysentery and food poisoning.

NSU non-specific urethritis.

nucha ('nyookə) the nape of the neck.

nuclear ('nyookli·ə) pertaining to a nucleus. *N. medicine* that branch of medicine concerned with the use of radionuclides in the diagnosis and treatment of disease.

nuclear magnetic resonance a phenomenon exhibited by atomic nuclei having a magnetic moment, i.e. those nuclei that behave as if they are tiny bar magnets. In the absence of a magnetic field these magnets are arranged randomly but when a strong magnetic field is applied they align with the field. These signals can be analysed and used for chemical analysis (NMR spectroscopy) or for imaging (magnetic resonance imaging).

nuclease ('nyookli,ayz) an enzyme

which breaks down nucleic acids.

nucleic acids (nyoo'klee·ik, -'klay-) deoxyribonucleic acid (abbreviated DNA) and ribonucleic acid (abbreviated RNA,) both of which are found in cell nuclei, and RNA in the cytoplasm also. They are composed of series of nucleotides.

nucleolus (,nyookli'ohləs, nyoo-'kleeələs) a small dense body in the cell nucleus which contains ribonucleic acid. It disappears during mitosis.

nucleoprotein (,nyooklioh'proh teen) a compound of nucleic acid and protein.

nucleotide ('nyooklioh,tied) a compound formed from pentose sugar, phosphoric acid and a nitrogen-containing base (a purine or a pyrimidine).

nucleotoxin (,nyooklioh'toksin) a toxin from cell nuclei, or one that affects cell nuclei.

nucleus ('nyookli·əs) 1. the essential part of a cell, governing nutrition and reproduction, its division being essential for the formation of new cells. 2. the positively charged centre portion of an atom. 3. a group of nerve cells in the central nervous system. *Caudate n.* and *lenticular n.* part of the basal ganglia. *N. pulposus* the jelly-like centre of an intervertebral disc.

nullipara (nu'lipə·rə) a woman who has never given birth to a child.

nurse (nərs) 1. a person who is qualified in the art and science of nursing and meets certain prescribed standards of education and clinical competence (*see also*

NURSING PRACTICE). 2. to provide services that are essential to or helpful in the promotion, maintenance, and restoration of health and well-being. 3. to nourish at the breast (*see also* BREAST FEED-ING). *Enrolled n.* a nurse who has undertaken a 2-year apprenticeship in nurse training (in Scotland 18 months) meant to provide a practical nurse who works under the supervision of the registered nurse. An enrolled nurse may undertake further training to become a registered nurse. *N. practitioner* a qualified nurse who works with general practitioners in the clinic, surgery or health centre in the community. The patients have a choice of either seeing the doctor or the nurse when they attend. *Registered n.* in the UK, a nurse whose name is on the Register held by the United Kingdom Central Council for Nurses, Midwives and Health Visitors (UKCC). *Wet n.* a woman who breast feeds the infant of another.

nursing ('nərsing) the profession of performing the functions of a NURSE. *N. audit* a systematic procedure for assessing the quality of nursing care rendered to a specific patient population. *N. care plan* devised by a nurse and based upon a nursing assessment and nursing diagnosis for an individual patient. The plan has four essential components: (1) identification of the nursing care problems; (2) an outline of the means/methods of solving these; (3) a statement of the anticipated benefit to the patient; and (4) an account of the specific actions used to achieve the goals specified. *N. diagnosis* a statement of a health problem or of a potential health problem in the patient's/client's health status that a nurse is professionally competent to treat. *N. history* a written record providing data for assessing the nursing care needs of a patient. *N. models* a conceptual framework of nursing practice based on knowledge, ideas and beliefs. A model of nursing clarifies the meaning of nursing, provides criteria for policy, gives direction to team nursing thereby obviating conflicts in approach and giving the framework for continuity of care. It identifies the nurse's role, highlights areas of practice where research is needed and can be a basis for the nursing curriculum. *N. practice* the performance or compensation of any act in the observation, care and counsel of the ill, injured or infirm, or in the maintenance of health or prevention of illness of others, or in the supervision and teaching of other personnel, or in the administration of medications and treatments as prescribed by a doctor or dentist, requiring substantial specialized judgement and skill and based on knowledge and application of the principles of biological, physical and social sciences. *N. process* a systematic approach to nursing care derived from many occupational groups. The system itself is not specific to nursing. It has been used as a framework for nursing care by American nurses and sub-

sequently its principles have been adapted to the UK's culture and health care system by British nurses. It is the vehicle for a NURSING MODEL. It is an organized approach to the identification of a patient's nursing care problems and the utilization of nursing actions that effectively alleviate, minimize or prevent the problems being presented or from developing. *Theories of n.* proposed explanations of the way in which nursing achieves its aims. They require a definition of the nurse's perception of the patient and his needs, the nurse's own role and the context in which nursing care is being performed. The understanding of the relationship of these variables enables nursing care to be planned in such a way that the outcome may be predicted and set goals achieved.

nutation (nyoo'tayshən) uncontrollable nodding of the head.

nutrient ('nyootri·ənt) food; any substance that nourishes.

nutrition (nyoo'trishən) 1. the sum of the processes involved in taking in nutriments and assimilating and utilizing them. 2. nutriment. *N. disease* one that is due to the continued absence of a necessary food factor. *Enteral n.* the provision of nutrients in fluid form to the alimentary tract by mouth, nasogastric tube, or via an opening into the tract such as through a gastrostomy. *Parenteral n.* a technique for meeting a patient's nutritional needs by means of intravenous feedings; sometimes called hyperalimentation.

nux (nuks) a nut. *N. vomica* the seed of an East Indian tree, from which strychnine is derived.

nyctalgia (nik'talji·ə) pain occurring during the night.

nyctalopia (,niktə'lohpi·ə) night blindness.

nympha ('nimfə) one of the two labia minora. *See* LABIUM.

nymphomania (,nimfə'mayni·ə) excessive sexual desire in a woman.

nystagmus (ni'stagməs) an involuntary rapid movement of the eyeball. It may be hereditary or result from disease of the semicircular canals or of the central nervous system. It can occur from visual defect or be associated with other muscle spasms.

nystatin (nie'statin, ni'-) an antibiotic drug effective against fungi. Used in the treatment of candidiasis and of fungal infections of the ear.

O

O symbol for *oxygen*.

obese (oh'bees) very fat; corpulent.

obesity (oh'beesətee) corpulence; excessive development of fat throughout the body.

objective (əb'jektiv) 1. in microscopy, the lens nearest the object being looked at. 2. a purpose; a desired end result. 3. concerning matters outside oneself. *O. signs* signs which the observer notes, as distinct from symptoms of which the patient complains (subjective).

oblique (ə'bleek) slanting. *O. muscles* 1. a pair of muscles, the inferior and the superior, which turn the eye upwards and downwards and inwards and outwards. 2. muscles found in the wall of the abdomen.

observation register (,obzə'vayshən ,rejistə) a register of children whose development may be adversely affected by problems occurring during the fetal or neonatal period. They should be carefully followed up by the health visitor, general practitioner and special paediatric department.

obsession (əb'seshən) an idea which persistently recurs to an individual although he resists it and regards it as being senseless. A compulsive thought. *See* COM-PULSION.

obstetrician (,obstə'trishən) one who is trained and specializes in obstetrics.

obstetrics (ob'stetriks) the branch of medicine and surgery dealing with pregnancy, labour and the puerperium.

obstipation (obsti,payshən) intractable constipation.

obstruction (əb'strukshən) the act of blocking or clogging; state of being clogged. *Intestinal o.* any hindrance to the passage of faeces.

obturator (,obtyuh,raytə) that which closes an opening. *O. foramen* the large hole in the hipbone closed by fascia and muscle.

obtusion (ob'tyoozhən) weakening or blunting of normal sensations, a condition produced by certain diseases.

occipital (ok'sipit'l) relating to the occiput. *O. bone* the bone forming the back and part of the base of the skull.

occipitoanterior (ok,sipitoh·an·'tie·ri·ə) referring to the position of the child's head when it is to the front of the pelvis when it comes through the birth canal. *Occipitoposterior* is the reverse position.

occiput ('oksi,puht) the back of the head.

occlusion (ə,kloozhən) closure,

applied particularly to alignment of the teeth in the jaws. *Coronary o.* obstruction of the lumen of a coronary artery. *O. of the eye* covering a good eye to improve the visual acuity of the other, lazy eye. *O. of the pupil* occlusio pupillae; obstruction of the pupil, which may be congenital or occur in iridocyclitis or after injury.

occult ('okult) hidden, concealed. *O. blood* blood excreted in the stools in such a small quantity as to require chemical tests to detect it.

occupational (okyuh'payshən'l) relating to work and working conditions. *O. disease* one likely to occur among workers in certain trades. An industrial disease. *O. therapy see* THERAPY.

ocular ('okyuhlə) relating to the eye. *O. myopathy* a gradual bilateral loss of mobility of the eyes. *O. myositis* inflammation of the orbital muscles.

oculentum (,okyuh'lentəm) an eye ointment.

oculogyric (,okyuhloh'jierik) causing movements of the eyeballs. *O. crisis* involuntary, violent movements of the eye, usually upwards.

oculomotor (,okyuhloh'mohtə) relating to movements of the eye. *O. nerves* the third pair of cranial nerves, which control the eye muscles.

Oddi, sphincter of ('odee ,sfingktə əv) *R. Oddi, Italian physician, 1864–1913.* The muscular sphincter situated at the junction of the common bile duct and the pancreatic duct.

odontalgia (,ohdon'talji·ə) toothache.

odontoid (oh'dontoyd) resembling a tooth. *O. process* a toothlike projection from the axis vertebra upon which the head rotates.

odontolith (oh'dontoh,lith) tartar, the calcareous matter deposited upon teeth.

odontology (,ohdon'toləjee) the science of treating teeth; dentistry.

odontoma (,odon'tohmə) a tumour of tooth structures.

oedema (i'deemə) an excessive amount of fluid in the body tissues. If the finger is pressed upon an affected part, the surface pits and regains slowly its original contour. *Angioneurotic o.* temporary oedema suddenly appearing in areas of skin or mucous membrane and occasionally in the viscera. *Brain o.* an excessive accumulation of fluid in the brain substance (wet brain). *Cardiac o.* a manifestation of congestive heart failure, due to increased venous and capillary pressures and often associated with renal sodium retention. *Dependent o.* oedema affecting most severely the lowermost parts of the body. *Famine o.* that due to protein deficiency. *Lymph o.* that due to blockage of the lymph vessels. *O. neonatorum* a disease of preterm and feeble infants resembling sclerema, marked by spreading oedema with cold, livid skin. *Pitting o.* oedema in which pressure leaves a persistent depression in the tissues. *Pulmonary o.* diffuse extravascular accumulation of fluid in the tissues and air spaces of the LUNG due to changes in hydrostatic forces in the capillaries or to increased capillary permeability.

Oedipus complex ('eedipəs) the suppressed sexual desire of a son for his mother, with hostility towards his father. It is a normal stage in the early development of the child, but may become fixed if the child cannot solve the conflict during his early years or during adolescence. Named after a mythical Greek hero.

oesophageal (i,sofə'jeeəl) pertaining to the oesophagus. *O. atresia* a congenital abnormality in which the oesophagus is not continuous between the pharynx and the stomach. May be associated with a fistula into the trachea. *O. varices* varicose veins of the lower oesophagus secondary to portal hypertension.

oesophagectasis (i,sofə'jektəsis) dilatation of the oesophagus.

oesophagitis (i,sofə'jietis) inflammation of the oesophagus. *Reflux o.* that caused by regurgitation of acid stomach contents through the cardiac sphincter.

oesophagocele (i,sofəgoh,seel) a protrusion of the mucous lining through a tear in the muscular wall of the oesophagus.

oesophagojejunostomy (i,sofəgoh,jejuh'nostəmee) the operation to create an anastomosis of the jejunum with the oesophagus following a total gastrectomy.

oesophagoscope (i'sofəgoh,skohp) an endoscope for viewing the inside of the oesophagus.

oesophagostomy (i,sofə'gostəmee) the making of an artificial opening into the oesophagus.

oesophagotomy (i,sofə'gotəmee) surgical incision of the oesophagus.

oesophagus (i'sofəgəs) the canal which extends from the pharynx to the stomach. It is about 23 cm long. The gullet.

oestradiol (,eestrə'dieol) the chief naturally occurring female sex hormone produced by the ovary. Prepared synthetically, it is now used to treat menopausal conditions and amenorrhoea.

oestrogen ('eestrəjən, -trə,jen) one of several steroid hormones, including oestradiol, all of which have similar functions. Although they are largely produced in the ovary, they can also be extracted from the placenta, the adrenal cortex, and the testis. They control female sexual development.

ointment ('oyntmənt) an external application with a greasy base in which the remedy is incorporated.

olecranon (oh'lekrə,non, ,ohli-'kraynən) the curved process of the ulna which forms the point of the elbow.

oleum ('ohli-əm) an oil.

olfactory (ol'faktə-ree) relating to the sense of smell. *O. nerves* the first pair of cranial nerves; those of smell.

oligaemia (,oli'geemi-ə) a deficiency in the volume of blood.

oligocythaemia (,oligohsie'theemi-ə) a cell deficiency in the blood.

oligodendroglioma (,oligoh,dendroglie'ohmə) a central nervous system tumour of the glial tissue.

oligohydramnios (,oligoh-hie-'dramnios) a deficiency in the amount of amniotic fluid.

oligomenorrhoea (,oligoh,menə-'reeə) 1. a diminished flow at the menstrual period. 2. infrequent occurrence of menstruation.

oligospermia (,oligoh'spərmi·ə) a diminished output of spermatozoa.

oliguria (,oli'gyooə·ri·ə) a deficient secretion of urine.

olivary ('olivə·ree) like an olive in shape. *O. body* a mass of grey matter situated behind the anterior pyramid of the medulla oblongata.

ombudsman ('ombuhdzmən) a person appointed to receive complaints about unfair administration. The officer in the National Health Service, appointed as 'ombudsman' or Health Service Commissioner, investigates complaints about failures in the health services. He is not able to pass judgment on clinical matters.

omentectomy (,ohmen'tektəmee) the surgical removal of all or part of the omentum.

omentopexy (oh'mentə,peksee) the surgical fixation of the omentum to some other tissue, usually the abdominal wall. *Cardio-o.* attachment of the omentum to the heart to establish a collateral circulation when there is coronary occlusion.

omentum (oh'mentəm) a fold of peritoneum joining the stomach to other abdominal organs. *Greater o.* the fold reflected from the greater curvature of the stomach and lying in front of the intestines. *Lesser o.* the fold reflected from the lesser curvature and attaching the stomach to the under surface of the liver.

omphalitis (,omfə'lietis) inflammation of the umbilicus.

omphalocele ('omfəloh,seel) an umbilical hernia.

omphalus ('omfələs) the umbilicus.

Onchocerca (,ongkoh'sərkə) a genus of filarial worms, found in tropical parts of Africa and America, which may give rise to skin and subcutaneous lesions and attack the eye.

onchocerciasis (,ongkohsər-'kieəsis) a tropical skin disease caused by infestation with *Onchocerca*.

oncogenesis (,ongkoh'jenəsis) the causation and formation of tumours.

oncogenic (,ongkoh'jenik) giving rise to tumour formation.

oncology (ong'koləjee) the scientific study of tumours.

onychia (o'niki·ə) inflammation of the matrix of a nail, with suppuration, which may cause the nail to fall off.

onychogryphosis (,onikohgri-'fohsis) enlargement of the nails, with excessive ridging and curvature, most commonly affecting the elderly.

onycholysis (,oni'kolisis) loosening or separation of a nail from its bed.

onychomycosis (,onikohmie-'kohsis) infection of the nails by a fungus.

onychosis (,oni'kohsis) a disease or deformity of the nails or of a nail.

oöcyte (,oh·ə,siet) the immature egg cell or ovum in the ovary.

oögenesis (,oh·ə'jenəsis) the development and production of the ovum.

oöphoralgia (,oh·əfə'ralji·ə) pain in an ovary.

oöphorectomy (,oh·əfə'rektəmee) excision of an ovary; ovariectomy.

oöphoritis (,oh·əfə'rietis) inflammation of an ovary.

oöphorocystectomy (oh,ofə·rohsi'stektəmee) surgical removal of an ovarian cyst.

oöphorocystosis (oh,ofə·rohsi'stohsis) the development of one or more ovarian cysts.

oöphoron (oh'ofə·ron) an ovary.

oöphoropexy (oh'ofə·roh,peksee) the surgical fixation of a displaced ovary to the pelvic wall.

oöphorosalpingectomy (oh,ofə·roh,salpin'jektəmee) removal of an ovary and its associated uterine tube.

opacity (oh'pasitee) cloudiness, lack of transparency. Opacities occur in the lens of an eye when a cataract is forming. They also occur in the vitreous humour and appear as floating objects.

operant conditioning (,opə·rənt) a form of behaviour therapy in which a reward is given when the subject performs the action required of him. The reward serves to encourage repetition of the action.

operation (,opə'rayshən) a surgical procedure in which instruments or hands are used by the operator.

ophthalmia (of'thalmi·ə) severe inflammation of the eye or of the conjunctiva or deeper structures of the eye. *O. neonatorum* any hyperacute purulent conjunctivitis which may be due to the gonococcus, *Escherichia coli*, staphylococci or *Chlamydia trachomatis*, occurring within the first 21 days of life, usually contracted during birth from infected vaginal discharge of the mother. This condition is notifiable except in Scotland. *Sympathetic o.* granulomatous inflammation of the uveal tract of the uninjured eye following a wound involving the uveal tract of the other eye, resulting in bilateral granulomatous inflammation of the entire uveal tract. Called also sympathetic uveitis.

ophthalmitis (,ofthal'mietis) inflammation of the eyeball.

ophthalmologist (,ofthal'moləjist) a specialist in diseases of the eye.

ophthalmology (,ofthal'moləjee) the study of the eye and its diseases.

ophthalmoplegia (of'thalmoh'pleeji·ə) paralysis of the muscles of the eye.

ophthalmoscope (of'thalmə,skohp) an instrument fitted with a light and lenses by which the interior of the eye can be illuminated and examined.

ophthalmotomy (,ofthal'motəmee) incision of the eyeball.

opiate (,ohp·ət, -,ayt) any medicine containing opium.

opisthotonos (,ohpis'thotənəs) a muscle spasm causing the back to be arched and the head retracted, with great rigidity of the muscles of the neck and back. This condition may be present in acute cases of meningitis, tetanus, and strychnine poisoning.

opium ('ohpi·əm) a drug derived from dried poppy juice and used as a narcotic. It produces deep sleep, slows the pulse and respiration, contracts the pupils and checks all secretions of the body except sweat. It is a highly addictive drug. Opium derivatives include apomorphine, codeine, morphine and papaverine.

opponens (o'pohnənz) opposing. A term applied to certain muscles controlling the movements of the fingers. *O. pollicis* a muscle that adducts the thumb so that it and the little finger can be brought together.

opportunistic (,opətyoo'nistik) 1. denoting a microorganism which does not ordinarily cause disease but becomes pathogenic under certain circumstances. 2. denoting a disease or infection caused by such an organism.

opsonic index (op,sonik 'indeks) a measurement of the bactericidal power of the phagocytes in the blood of an individual.

opsonin (,opsənin) an antibody present in the blood which renders bacteria more easily destroyed by the phagocytes. Each kind of bacteria has its specific opsonin.

optic ('optik) relating to vision. *O. atrophy* degeneration of the optic nerve. *O. chiasma* the crossing of the fibres of the optic nerves at the base of the brain. *O. disc* the point where the optic nerve enters the eyeball. *O. foramen* the opening in the posterior part of the orbit through which pass the optic nerve and the ophthalmic artery. *O. nerve* a bundle of nerve fibres running from the optic chiasma in the

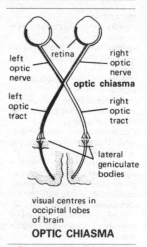

visual centres in
occipital lobes
of brain

OPTIC CHIASMA

brain to the optic disc on the eyeball.

optical ('optik'l) pertaining to sight. *O. density* the refractive power of the transparent tissues through which light rays pass, changing the direction of the ray.

optician (op'tishən) a professional trained in the detection of refractive errors and the dispensing of appropriate spectacles or contact lenses.

optimum ('optiməm) the best and most favourable.

optometry (op'tomətree) the measuring of visual acuity and the fitting of glasses to correct visual defects.

ora ('ohra) [L.] *a margin. O. serrata* the jagged edge of the retina.

oral ('or·rəl) 1. pertaining to the mouth; taken through or applied in the mouth, as an oral medication or an oral thermometer. 2. denoting that aspect of the teeth which faces the oral cavity or tongue.

orbit (,awbit) 1. the bony cavity containing the eyeball. 2. the path of an object moving around another object.

orchidalgia (,awki'dalji·ə) pain in a testicle.

orchidectomy (,awki'dektəmee) excision of a testicle. *Bilateral o.* the operation of castration.

orchidopexy (,awkidoh,peksee) an operation to free an undescended testicle and place it in the scrotum.

orchiepididymitis (,awki,epididi-'mietis) inflammation of a testicle and its epididymis.

orchis ('awkis) a testicle.

orchitis (aw'kietis) inflammation of a testicle.

orf (awf) a virus infection transmitted from sheep to man. It may give rise to a boil-like lesion on the hands of meat handlers.

organ ('awgən) a part of the body designed to perform a particular function.

organelle (,awgə'nel) a structure within a cell which has specialized functions, e.g. nucleus, endoplasmic reticulum, mitochondrion, etc.

organic (aw'ganik) 1. pertaining to the organs. *O. disease* disease of an organ, accompanied by structural changes. 2. pertaining to chemicals containing carbon.

organism ('awgə,nizəm) an individual living being, animal or vegetable.

orgasm (,awgazəm) the climax of sexual excitement.

orientation (,or·rien'tayshən) a sense of direction. 1. The ability of a person to estimate his position in regard to time, place and persons. 2. The imparting of relevant information at the onset of a course or conference so that its content and objects may be understood.

orifice ('o·rifis) any opening in the body.

origin ('o·rijin) in anatomy: 1. the point of attachment of a muscle; 2. the point at which a nerve or a blood vessel branches from the main stem.

ornithosis (,awni'thohsis) a virus disease of birds, usually pigeons, which may be transmitted to man in a form resembling bronchopneumonia.

orogenital (or·roh'jenit'l) pertaining to the mouth and external genitalia.

oropharynx (,or·rohfaringks) the lower portion of the pharynx behind the mouth and above the oesophagus and larynx.

orphenadrine (aw'fenə,drin) a drug used to treat parkinsonism, especially when accompanied by depression.

orthodontics (,awthoh'dontiks) dentistry which deals with the prevention and correction of malocclusion and irregularities of the teeth.

orthopaedics (,awthə'peediks) the science dealing with deformities, injuries and diseases of the bones and joints.

orthopnoea (,awthop'neeə) difficulty in breathing unless in an upright position, e.g. sitting up in bed.

orthoptics (aw'thoptiks) the practice of treating by non-surgical methods (usually eye exercises) abnormalities of vision such as strabismus (squint).

orthostatic (,awthoh'statik) pertaining to or caused by standing erect. *O. albuminuria see* ALBUMINURIA. *O. hypotension* low blood pressure, occurring when someone stands up.

orthotic (aw'thotik) serving to protect or to restore or improve function; pertaining to the use or application of an orthosis (an appliance which can be applied to or around the body in the care/ treatment of physical impairment or disability).

orthotist ('awthə,tist) a person skilled in orthotics and practising its application in individual cases.

Ortolani's sign (,awtoh'lahniz) *M. Ortolani, 20th century Italian orthopaedic surgeon.* A test performed soon after birth to detect possible congenital dislocation of the hip. A 'click' is felt on reversing the movements of abduction and rotation of the hip while the child is lying with knees flexed.

os¹ (ohs) pl. **ora** [L.] 1. any body orifice. 2. the mouth. *See also* CERVICAL OS.

os² (os) pl. **ossa** [L.] *a bone.*

oscillation (,osi'layshən) 1. a backwards and forwards motion. 2. vibration.

oscilloscope (ə'silə,skohp) an apparatus using a cathode-ray tube to depict visibly data fed

into it electronically, e.g. the way in which the heart is performing.

Osgood–Schlatter disease (,oz-guhd'shlatə) *R.B. Osgood, American orthopaedic surgeon, 1873–1956; C. Schlatter, Swiss surgeon, 1864–1934.* Osteochondritis of the tibial tuberosity.

Osler's nodes ('ohsləz) *Sir W. Osler, Canadian physician, 1849–1919.* Small painful swellings which occur in or beneath the skin, especially of the extremities in subacute bacterial endocarditis, caused by minute emboli. They usually disappear in 1–3 days.

osmoreceptor (,ozmohri'septə) one of a group of specialized nerve cells which monitor the osmotic pressure of the blood and the extracellular fluid. Impulses from these receptors are relayed to the hypothalamus.

osmosis (oz'mohsis, os-) the passage of fluid from a low concentration solution to one of a higher concentration through a semipermeable membrane.

osmotic (oz'motik) pertaining to osmosis. *O. pressure* the pressure exerted by large molecules in the blood, e.g. albumin and globulin proteins, which draws fluid into the bloodstream from the surrounding tissues.

osseous ('osi-əs) bony.

ossicle ('osik'l) a small bone. *Auditory o.* one of the three bones in the middle ear: the malleus, incus and stapes.

ossification (,osifi'kayshən) the process by which bone is developed; osteogenesis.

ostalgia (,osti'alji·ə) pain in a

bone.

osteitis (ˌosti'ietis) inflammation of bone. *O. deformans see* PAGET'S DISEASE. *O. fibrosa cystica* or *parathyroid o.* defects of ossification, with fibrous tissue production, leading to weakening and deformity. It affects children chiefly, and is associated with parathyroid tumour, removal of which checks it. *See* VON RECKLINGHAUSEN'S DISEASE.

osteoarthritis (ˌostioh·ah'thrietis) *see* ARTHRITIS.

osteoarthrotomy (ˌostioh·ah-'throtəmee) surgical excision of the jointed end of a bone.

osteoblast ('ostioh,blast) a cell which develops into an osteocyte and turns into bone.

osteochondritis (ˌostiohkon'drietis) inflammation of bone and cartilage, particularly a degenerative disease of an epiphysis, causing pain and deformity. *O. of the hip* Perthes' disease. *O. of the tarsal scaphoid bone* Köhler's disease. *O. of the tibial tuberosity* Osgood–Schlatter disease.

osteochondroma (ˌostiohkon-'drohmə) a tumour consisting of both bone and cartilage.

osteoclasis (ˌosti'oklɔsis) 1. the surgical fracture of bones to correct a deformity such as bow leg. 2. the restructuring of bone by osteoclasts during growth or the repair of damaged bone.

osteoclast ('ostioh,klast) 1. a large cell that breaks down and absorbs bone and callus. 2. an instrument designed for surgical fracture of bone.

osteocyte ('ostioh,siet) a bone cell.

osteodystrophy (ˌostioh'distrəfee) a metabolic disease of bone.

osteogenesis (ˌostioh'jenəsis) the formation of bone. *O. imperfecta* a congenital disorder of the bones, which are very brittle and fracture easily. Fragilitas osseum.

osteoma (ˌosti'ohmə) a benign tumour arising from bone.

osteomalacia (ˌostiohmə'layshi·ə) a disease characterized by painful softening of bones. Due to vitamin D deficiency.

osteomyelitis (ˌostioh,mieə'lietis) inflammation of bone, localized or generalized, due to a pyogenic infection. It may result in bone destruction, stiffening of joints, and, in extreme cases occurring before the end of the growth period, in the shortening of a limb if the growth centre is destroyed. Acute osteomyelitis is caused by bacteria that enter the body through a wound, spread from an infection near the bone, or come from a skin or throat infection. The infection usually affects the long bones of the arms and legs and causes acute pain and fever. It most often occurs in children and adolescents, particularly boys.

osteopath (ˌostioh,path) one who practises osteopathy.

osteopathy (ˌosti'opəthee) 1. any bone disease. 2. a system of treatment of disease by bone manipulation.

osteoperiostitis (ˌostioh,perio-'stietis) inflammation of bone and periosteum.

osteopetrosis (ˌostiohpe'trohsis) a rare congenital disease in which the bones become abnormally dense. Albers–Schönberg disease.

osteophyte ('ostioh,fiet) a small outgrowth of bone.

osteoplasty ('ostioh,plastee) a plastic operation on bone.

osteoporosis (,ostiohpor'rohsis) abnormal rarefaction of bone which may be idiopathic or secondary to other conditions. The disorder leads to thinning of the skeleton and decreased precipitation of lime salts. There also may be inadequate calcium absorption into the bone and excessive bone resorption. The principal causes are lack of physical activity, lack of oestrogens or androgens, and nutritional deficiency. There is almost always some degree of osteoporosis that occurs with ageing. Symptoms include pathological fractures and collapse of the vertebrae without compression of the spinal cord.

osteosarcoma (,ostiohsah'kohmə) an osteogenic sarcoma; a malignant bone tumour.

osteosclerosis (,ostiohsklə'rohsis) an increase in density and a hardening of bone. *O. congenita* achondroplasia. *O. fragilis* osteopetrosis.

osteotome ('ostioh,tohm) a surgical chisel for cutting bone.

osteotomy (,osti'otəmee) the cutting into or through a bone, sometimes performed to correct deformity. *O. of the hip* a method of treating osteoarthritis by cutting the bone and altering the line of weight bearing.

ostium ('osti·əm) a mouth. *Abdominal o.* the opening at the end of the uterine tube into the peritoneal cavity.

otalgia (oh'talji·ə) earache.

otic ('ohtik) relating to the ear.

otitis (oh'tietis) inflammation of the ear. *Aviation o.* a symptom complex resulting from fluctuations between atmospheric pressure and air pressure in the middle ear; called also barotitis media. *O. externa* inflammation of the external ear. *Furuncular o.* the formation of furuncles in the external ear. *O. interna, o. labyrinthica* labyrinthitis. *O. mastoidea* inflammation of the mastoid spaces. *O. media* inflammation of the middle ear, occurring most often in infants and young children, and classified as serous, secretory and suppurative.

otolaryngology (,ohtoh,laring-'goləjee) the scientific study of the ear and the larynx and the diseases affecting them.

otolith ('otoh,lith) 1. a calculus in the middle ear. 2. one of a number of small calcareous concretions of the inner ear, at the base of semicircular canals.

otology (oh'toləjee) the scientific study of the ear and its diseases.

otomycosis (,ohtohmie'kohsis) a fungal infection of the auditory canal.

otoplasty ('ohtoh,plastee) plastic surgery of the outer ear.

otorhinolaryngology (,ohtoh,rienoh,laring'goləjee) the scientific study of diseases of the ear, nose and throat.

otorrhoea (,ohtə'reeə) discharge from the ear, especially of pus.

otosclerosis (,ohthsklə'rohsis) the formation of spongy bone in the

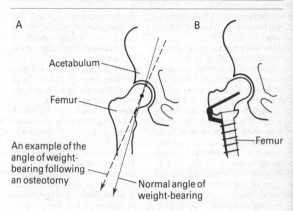

Osteotomy of Hip A showing weightbearing angle, and B showing an example of an osteotomy with fixator.

OSTEOTOMY OF HIP

labyrinth of the ear, causing the auditory ossicles to become fixed and less able to pass on vibrations when sound enters the ear. The cause of otosclerosis is still unknown. It may be hereditary, or perhaps related to vitamin deficiency or otitis media. An early symptom is ringing in the ears, but the most noticeable symptom is progressive loss of hearing.

otoscope ('ohtoh,skohp) an auriscope; an instrument for examining the ear.

otoscopy (oh'toskəpee) an examination of the tympanic membrane and auditory canal by means of an otoscope.

Otosporin (ohtə'sporin) trade name for a combination preparation of eardrops containing hydrocortisone, neomycin and polymyxin.

ototoxic (,ohtoh'toksik) anything which has a deleterious effect on the eighth cranial nerve or on the organs of hearing.

ouabain (wah'bah·in, 'wahbayn) a cardiac glycoside; its effect is similar to that of digitalis, but digitalization is achieved more rapidly.

ovarian (oh'vair·ri·ən) relating to an ovary. *O. cyst* a tumour of the ovary containing fluid.

ovariectomy (,ohvə·ri'ektəmee) oöphorectomy; excision of an ovary.

ovariotomy (oh,vair·ri'otəmee) 1. surgical removal of an ovary. 2. excision of an ovarian tumour.

ovaritis (,ohvə'rietis) oöphoritis; inflammation of an ovary.

ovary ('ohvə·ree) one of a pair of glandular organs in the female pelvis. They produce ova, which pass through the uterine tubes into the uterus, and steroid hormones which control the menstrual cycle.

overbite ('ohvə,biet) an overlapping of the lower teeth by the upper teeth.

overcompensation (,ohva,kompən'sayshən) a mental mechanism by which a person tries to assert himself by aggressive behaviour or by talking or acting 'big' to compensate for a feeling of inadequacy.

oviduct ('ohvi,dukt, 'ovi-) a uterine tube.

ovotestis (,ohvoh'testis) a gonad containing both ovarian and testicular tissue.

ovulation (,ovyuh'layshən, ,oh-) the process of rupture of the mature graafian follicle when the ovum is shed from the ovary.

ovum ('ohvəm) [L.] *an egg.* The reproductive cell of the female.

oxidization (,oksidie'zayshən) oxidation. The process by which combustion occurs and breaking up of matter takes place; e.g. oxidation of carbohydrates gives carbon dioxide and water:
$$C_6H_{12}O_6 + 6O_2 = 6CO_2 + 6H_2O$$

oximeter (ok'simitə) a photoelectric cell used to determine the oxygen saturation of blood. *Ear o.* one attached to the ear by which the oxygen content of blood flowing through the ear can be measured.

oxprenolol (oks'prenoh,lol) a beta-blocking drug used in the treatment of angina, hypertension and cardiac arrhythmias.

oxygen ('oksijən) *symbol* O. A colourless, odourless gas constituting one-fifth of the atmosphere. It is stored in cylinders at high pressure or as liquid oxygen. It is used medicinally to enrich the air when either respiration or circulation is impaired. *O. saturation* the amount of oxygen bound to haemoglobin in the blood. *O. tent* a large plastic canopy that encloses the patient in a controlled environment; used for oxygen therapy, humidity therapy or aerosol therapy. *O. therapy* supplementary oxygen administered for the purpose of relieving hypoxaemia and preventing damage to the tissue cells as a result of oxygen lack.

oxygenation (,oksijə'nayshən) saturation with oxygen; a process which occurs in the lungs to the haemoglobin of blood, which is saturated with oxygen to form oxyhaemoglobin.

oxygenator ('oksijə,naytə) a machine through which the blood is passed to oxygenate it during open heart surgery. *Pump o.* a machine which pumps oxygenated blood through the body during heart surgery.

oxyhaemoglobin (,oksi,heemə'glohbin) haemoglobin which has been oxygenated, as in arterial blood.

oxyntic (ok'sintik) acid forming. *O. cell* a parietal cell of the gastric glands which secretes hydrochloric acid.

oxypertine (ˌoksi'pərteen) an antipsychotic tranquillizing drug used in the treatment of schizophrenia and related psychoses, and of mania and hyperactivity.

oxytetracycline (ˌoksiˌtetrə'siekleen) a broad-spectrum antibiotic, chiefly used against infections caused by *Chlamydia*, *Rickettsia* and *Brucella*.

oxytocic (ˌoksi'tohsik) any drug which stimulates uterine contractions and may be used to hasten delivery.

oxytocin (ˌoksi'tohsin) a pituitary hormone which stimulates uterine contractions and the ejection

of milk. Synthetically prepared, it is used to induce labour and to control postpartum haemorrhage.

oxyuriasis (ˌoksiyuh'rieəsis) infestation by threadworms of the genus *Enterobius*.

ozaena (oh'zeenə) atrophic rhinitis. A condition of the nose in which there is loss and shrinkage of the ciliated mucous membrane and of the turbinate bones. There may be an offensive nasal discharge.

ozone ('ohzohn) an intensified form of oxygen containing three O atoms to the molecule (i.e. O_3), and often discharged by electrical machines such as X-ray apparatus. In medicine it is employed as an antiseptic and oxidizing agent.

P

P symbol for *phosphorus*.

pacemaker ('pays,maykə) an object or substance that controls the rate at which a certain phenomenon occurs. The natural pacemaker of the heart is the sinoatrial NODE. *Electronic cardiac p.* an electrically operated mechanical device which stimulates the myocardium to contract. It consists of an energy source, usually batteries, and electrical circuitry connected to an electrode which is in direct contact with the myocardium. Pacemakers may be temporary or permanent. Temporary ones usually have an external energy source whereas permanent ones have a subcutaneously implanted one. The rate the pacemaker delivers pulses may be either fixed or on demand. *Fixed* pacing means that pulses are delivered to the heart at a predetermined rate irrespective of any cardiac activity. A *demand* pacemaker is programmed to deliver pulses only in the absence of spontaneous cardiac activity. The need for replacement batteries is usually indicated when the rate of the pulse slows by five beats or more.

pachydactyly (,paki'daktilee) abnormal thickening of the fingers or toes.

pachydermia (,paki'dərmi·ə) an abnormal thickening of the skin. *P. laryngis* chronic hypertrophy of the vocal cords.

pachyonychia (,pakio'niki·ə) abnormal thickening of the nails.

pachysomia (,paki'sohmi·ə) abnormal thickening of parts of the body, as in acromegaly.

Pacini's corpuscles (pa'cheeniz) *F. Pacini, Italian anatomist, 1812–1883.* Specialized end-organs, situated in the subcutaneous tissue of the extremities and near joints, which react to firm pressure.

paediatrician (,peedi·ə'trishən) a specialist in the diseases of children.

paediatrics (,peedi'atriks) the branch of medicine dealing with the care and development of children and with the treatment of diseases that affect them.

paedophilia (,peedə'fili·ə) a sexual attraction towards young children.

Paget's disease ('pajits) *Sir J. Paget, British surgeon, 1814–1899.* 1. a chronic disease of bone in which overactivity of the osteoblasts and osteoclasts leads to dense bone formation with areas of rarefaction. Osteitis deformans. 2. an inflammation of the nipple caused by cancer of the milk ducts of the breast.

pain (payn) a feeling of distress,

suffering, or agony, caused by stimulation of specialized nerve endings. Its purpose is chiefly protective; it acts as a warning that tissues are being damaged and induces the sufferer to remove or withdraw from the source. Pain is a subjective experience and one person's pain cannot be compared to another's experience. *Bearing-down p.* pain accompanying uterine contractions during the second stage of LABOUR. *False p's* ineffective pains during pregnancy that resemble labour pains, not accompanied by cervical dilatation; called also false labour. *See also* BRAXTON HICKS CONTRACTIONS. *Gas p's* pains caused by distension of the stomach or intestine by accumulations of air or other gases, *Hunger p.* pain coming on at the time for feeling hunger for a meal; a symptom of gastric disorder. *Intermenstrual p.* pain accompanying ovulation, occurring during the period between the menses, usually about midway. Also called mittelschmerz. *Labour p's* the rhythmic pains of increasing severity and frequency due to contraction of the uterus at childbirth. See also LABOUR. *Lancinating p.* sharp, darting pain. *Phantom p.* pain felt as if it were arising in an absent (amputated) limb. *See also* AMPUTATION. *Referred p.* pain in a part other than that in which the cause that produced it is situated. Referred pain usually originates in one of the visceral organs but is felt in the skin or sometimes in another area deep inside the body. Referred pain probably occurs because pain signals from the viscera travel along the same neural pathways used by pain signals from the skin. The person perceives the pain but interprets it as having originated in the skin rather than in a deep-seated visceral organ. *Rest p.* a continuous burning pain due to ischaemia of the lower leg, which begins or is aggravated after reclining and is relieved by sitting or standing.

palate ('palət) the roof of the mouth. *Artificial p.* a plate made to close a cleft palate. *Cleft p.* a congenital deformity where there is lack of fusion of the two bones forming the palate. *Hard p.* the bony part at the front. *Soft p.* a fold of mucous membrane that continues from the hard palate to the uvula.

palatine bone ('palə,tien) one of a pair of bones which form a part of the nasal cavity and the hard palate.

palatoplegia (,palətoh'pleeji·ə) paralysis of the soft palate.

palliative ('pali·ətiv) treatment which relieves, but does not cure, disease.

pallidectomy (,pali'dektəmee) an operation performed to decrease the activity of the globus pallidus, the medial part of the lentiform nucleus in the base of the cerebrum. It has brought about a marked improvement in severely agitated cases of parkinsonism.

pallor ('palə) abnormal paleness of the skin.

palmar ('palmə) relating to the palm of the hand. *Deep and super-*

ficial p. arches the chief arterial blood supply to the hand formed by the junction of the ulnar and radial arteries. *P. fascia* the arrangement of tendons in the palm of the hand.

palpation (pal'payshən) the examination of the organs by touch or pressure of the hand over the part.

palpebral ('palpibrəl) referring to the eyelids. *P. ligaments* a band of ligaments which stretches from the junction of the upper and lower lid to the orbital bones, both medially and laterally.

palpitation (,palpi'tayshən) rapid and forceful contraction of the heart of which the patient is conscious.

palsy ('pawlzee) paralysis. *Bell's p.* paralysis of the facial muscles on one side, supplied by the seventh cranial nerve. *Crutch p.* paralysis due to pressure of a crutch on the radial nerve and a cause of 'dropped wrist'. *Erb's p.* paralysis of one arm due to a birth injury to the brachial plexus. *Shaking p.* parkinsonism; paralysis agitans.

panacea (,panə'seeə) a remedy for all diseases.

panarthritis (,panah'thrietis) inflammation of all the joints or of all the structures of a joint.

pancarditis (,pankahdi'ietis) inflammation of all the structures of the heart.

Pancoast's tumour ('pankohsts) *H.K. Pancoast, American radiologist, 1875–1939.* Pain, wasting and weakness of the arm which occur as secondary features of carcinoma of the bronchus due

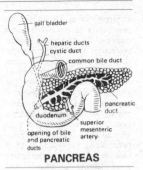

PANCREAS

to neurological involvement. The tumour is at the apex of the lung.

pancreas ('pangkri·əs) an elongated, racemose gland about 15 cm long, lying behind the stomach, with its head in the curve of the duodenum, and its tail in contact with the spleen. It secretes a digestive fluid (pancreatic juice) containing ferments which act on all classes of foods. The fluid enters the duodenum by the pancreatic duct which joins the common bile duct. The pancreas also secretes the hormones insulin and glucagon.

pancreatectomy (,pangkri·ə'tektəmee) surgical excision of the whole or a part of the pancreas.

pancreatin ('pangkri·ətin, pan-'kreeə-) an extract from the pancreas containing the digestive enzymes. Used to treat deficiency, as in cystic fibrosis, and after pancreatectomy.

pancreatitis (,pangkri·ə'tietis) inflammation of the pancreas.

Acute p. a severe condition in which the patient experiences sudden pain in the upper abdomen and back. The patient often becomes severely shocked. *Chronic p.* chronic inflammation occurring after acute attacks. Pancreatic failure may lead to diabetes mellitus.

pancreatolith (,pangkri'atoh,lith) a stone (calculus) in the pancreas.

pancreozymin (,pangkrioh'zie-min) a hormone of the duodenal mucosa that stimulates the external secretory activity of the pancreas, especially its production of amylase.

pancuronium (,pangkyuh'rohni-·əm) a neuromuscular blocking agent of the nerve depolarizing type used as a muscle relaxant during surgery. It has a relatively long duration of action, a single intravenous dose lasting 45–60 min. It is often used in poor risk patients.

pancytopenia (,pansietoh'peeni-ə) a reduction in number of all types of blood cell due to failure of bone marrow formation.

pandemic (pan'demik) an epidemic spreading over a wide area, sometimes all over the world.

panhypopituitarism (pan,hie-pohpi'tyooitə,rizəm) Simmond's disease. A deficiency of all the hormones produced by the anterior pituitary gland.

panhysterectomy (,panhistə'rektəmee) surgical removal of the whole of the uterus.

panic ('panik) an unreasoning and overwhelming fear or terror. It may occur in anxiety states and acute schizophrenia.

panleukopenia (,panlookoh'peeni-ə) a deficiency of all the white blood cells.

panmyelopathy (,panmieə'lopəthee) a disease affecting all the cells formed in the bone marrow.

panniculitis (pe,nikyuh'lietis) inflammation of the subcutaneous fat causing tender nodules on the abdomen and thorax and on the thighs.

panniculus (pə'nikyuhləs) a sheet of membrane. *P. adiposus* the fatty layer beneath the skin.

pannus ('panəs) increased vascularity of the cornea leading to granulation tissue formation and impaired vision. It occurs after inflammation of the cornea.

panophthalmia (,panof'thalmi·ə) panophthalmitis; inflammation of all the tissues of the eyeball.

panosteitis (,panosti'ietis) inflammation of all the structures of a bone.

panotitis (,panoh'tietis) inflammation of all parts of the ear.

pansystolic murmur (,pansi,stolik 'mərmə) a heart murmur heard throughout the time when the heart is in systole. *See* MURMUR.

pantothenic acid (,pantə'thenik) one of the vitamins in the B complex.

Papanicolaou test (Pap test) (,papə,nikə'layoo) *G.N. Papanicolaou, Greek physician, anatomist and cytologist, 1883–1962.* A smear test to detect diseases of the uterine cervix and endometrium.

papaveretum (pə'pahvə'reetəm) a preparation of the alkaloids of opium with an action similar to morphine. It is used to counteract severe pain.

papilla (pə'pilə) a small nipple-shaped protuberance. *Circumvallate p.* one surrounded by a ridge. A number are found at the back of the tongue arranged in a V-shape, and containing taste buds. *Filiform p.* one of the fine, slender filaments on the main part of the tongue which give it its velvety appearance. *Fungiform p.* a mushroom-shaped papilla of the tongue. *Optic p.* the optic disc, where the optic nerve leaves the eyeball. *Tactile p.* a projection on the true skin which contains nerve endings responsible for relaying sensations of pressure to the brain. A touch corpuscle.

papillitis (,papi'lietis) 1. inflammation of the optic disc. 2. inflammation of a papilla.

papilloedema (,papili'deemə) oedema and hyperaemia of the optic disc, usually associated with increased intracranial pressure; called also choked disc.

papilloma (,papi'lohmə) a benign growth of epithelial tissue, e.g. a wart.

papillomatosis (,papi,lohmə'tohsis) the occurrence of multiple papillomas.

papovavirus (pə'pohvə,vierəs) a family of DNA-producing viruses which cause tumours, usually benign, such as warts.

papule ('papyool) a pimple, or small solid elevation of the skin.

papulopustular (,papyuhloh'pustyuhla) descriptive of skin eruptions of both papules and pustules.

papulosquamous (,papyuhloh-'skwayməs) descriptive of skin eruptions which are both papular and scaly. They include such conditions as lichen planus, pityriasis and psoriasis.

para-aminobenzoic acid (,parə,-aminohben'zoh·ik) a member of the B group of vitamins. It is used in creams and lotions to prevent sunburn.

para-aminosalicylic acid (,parə,-aminoh,sali'silik) abbreviated PAS. An acid, the salts of which are used together with other drugs, usually isoniazid (INH) or streptomycin, in the treatment of tuberculosis.

paracentesis (,parəsen'teesis) puncture of the wall of a cavity with a hollow needle in order to draw off excess fluid or to obtain diagnostic material.

paracetamol (,parə'seetə,mol, -'setə-) a mild analgesic drug used to treat headaches, toothache and rheumatic pains, and also to treat pyrexia.

paracusis (,parə'kyoosis) a perverted sense of hearing. *P. of Willis* an improvement in hearing when surrounded by noise.

paradoxical sleep (,parə'doksik'l) rapid eye movement sleep (REM). *See* SLEEP.

paraesthesia (,paris'theezi·ə) an abnormal tingling sensation. 'Pins and needles'.

paraffin ('parəfin) any saturated hydrocarbon obtained from petroleum. *P. wax* a hard paraffin that can be used for wax treatment for chronic inflammation of joints. *Liquid p.* a mineral oil which is used as a laxative. *Soft p.* petroleum jelly. Used as a barrier agent to protect the skin.

paraformaldehyde (,parəfaw-'maldi,hied) paraform; a preparation of formaldehyde used as an antiseptic and also for fumigating rooms.

Paragonimus (,parə'goniməs) a genus of trematode parasites. The flukes infest the lungs and are found mainly in tropical countries.

paraldehyde (pə'raldi,hied) a sedative and hypnotic and anticonvulsant that has an unpleasant taste and imparts an unpleasant odour on the breath. It is now little used, except in the treatment of status epilepticus.

paralysis (pə'ralisis) loss or impairment of motor function in a part due to a lesion of the neural or muscular mechanism; also, by analogy, impairment of sensory function (sensory paralysis). Paralysis is a symptom of a wide variety of physical and emotional disorders rather than a disease in itself. Palsy. *P. agitans* parkinsonism. *Bulbar p.* (*labioglossopharyngeal p.*) paralysis due to changes in the motor centre of the medulla oblongata. It affects the muscles of the mouth, tongue and pharynx. *Facial p.* (*Bell's palsy*) paralysis that affects the muscles of the face and is due to injury to or inflammation of the facial nerve. *Flaccid p.* loss of tone and absence of reflexes in the paralysed muscles. *General p. of the insane* abbreviated GPI. Paralytic dementia occurring in the late stages of syphilis. *Infantile p.* the major form of poliomyelitis (*see* POLIOMYELITIS). *Spastic p.* paralysis characterized by

rigidity of affected muscles.

paralytic (,parə'litik) affected by or relating to paralysis. *P. ileus* obstruction of the ileum due to absence of peristalsis in a portion of the intestine.

paramedian (,parə'meedi·ən) situated on the side of the median line.

paramedical (,parə'medik'l) associated with the medical profession and the delivery of health care. The paramedical services include occupational and speech therapy, physiotherapy, radiography and social work.

parametritis (,parəmi'trietis) inflammation of the parametrium; pelvic cellulitis.

parametrium (,parə'meetri·əm) the connective tissue surrounding the uterus.

paramnesia (,param'neezi·ə) a defect of memory in which there is a false recollection. The patient may fill in the forgotten period with imaginary events which he describes in great detail.

paramyotonia congenita (,parə-'mieə'tohni·ə kən'jenita) a rare congenital condition in which a prolonged muscle contraction develops when the patient is exposed to cold.

paranoia (,parə'noyə) a mental disorder characterized by delusions of grandeur or persecution which may be fully systematized in logical form, with the personality remaining fairly well preserved.

paranoid ('parə,noyd) resembling paranoia. Refers to a condition that can occur in many forms of mental disease. Delusions of persecution are a marked feature. *P. schizophrenia see* SCHIZO-PHRENIA.

paraparesis (ˌparəpə'reesis) an incomplete paralysis affecting the lower limbs.

paraphasia (ˌparə'fayzi·ə) a speech disorder involving the substitution of a similar sound or word for that intended, thereby producing a nonsensical utterance.

paraphimosis (ˌparəfie'mohsis) retraction of the prepuce behind the glans penis, with inability to replace it, resulting in a painful constriction.

paraphrenia (ˌparə'freeniə) schizophrenia occurring for the first time in later life and not accompanied by deterioration of the personality.

paraplegia (ˌparə'pleeji·ə) paralysis of the lower extremities and lower trunk. All parts below the point of lesion in the spinal cord are affected. It may be of sudden onset from injury to the cord or may develop slowly as the result of disease.

paraprofessional (ˌparəprə'feshən'l) 1. a person who is specially trained in a particular field or occupation to assist a professional. 2. allied health professional. 3. pertaining to a paraprofessional.

parapsychology (ˌparəsie'koləjee) the branch of psychology dealing with psychical effects and experiences that appear to fall outside the scope of physical law, e.g. telepathy and clairvoyance.

paraquat ('parə,kwat) a poisonous compound used as a contact

herbicide. Contact with concentrated solutions causes irritation of the skin, cracking and shedding of the nails, and delayed healing of cuts and wounds. After ingestion renal and hepatic failure may develop, followed by pulmonary insufficiency and death.

parasite ('parə,siet) any animal or vegetable organism living upon or within another, from which it derives its nourishment.

parasiticide (ˌparə'siti,sied) a drug which kills parasites.

parasympathetic system (ˌparə-ˌsimpə,thetik) the craniosacral part of the autonomic nervous system.

parasympatholytic (ˌparə,simpə-thoh'litik) anticholinergic; an agent that opposes the effects of the parasympathetic nervous system.

parathormone (ˌparə'thawmohn) the endocrine secretion of the parathyroid glands.

parathyroid gland (ˌparə'thieroyd) one of four small endocrine glands, two of which are associated with each lobe of the thyroid gland, and sometimes embedded in it. The secretion from these has some control over calcium metabolism, and lack of it is a cause of tetany.

parathyroidectomy (ˌparə,thieroy'dektəmee) the surgical removal of parathyroid glands.

paratyphoid (ˌparə'tiefoyd) a notifiable infection caused by *Salmonella* of all groups except *S. typhosa*. The disease is usually milder and has a shorter incubation period, more abrupt onset, and a lower mortality rate than does typhoid. Clinically and pathologically, the two diseases cannot be distinguished. Called also paratyphoid fever.

parenchyma (pə'rengkima) the essential active cells of an organ as distinguished from vascular and connective tissue.

parenteral (pə'rentə·rel) apart from the alimentary canal. Applied to the introduction into the body of drugs or fluids by routes other than the mouth or rectum, for instance intravenously or subcutaneously.

paresis (pə'reesis, 'parəsis) partial paralysis.

paries ('pair·eez) the wall of a cavity.

parietal (pə'rieət'l) relating to the walls of any cavity. *P. bones* the two bones forming part of the roof and sides of the skull. *P. cells* the oxyntic cells in the gastric mucosa that secrete hydrochloric acid. *P. pleura* the pleura attached to the chest wall.

Parinaud's oculogranular syndrome ('pari,nohz) *H. Parinaud, French ophthalmologist, 1844–1905.* A chronic granulomatous conjunctivitis with regional lymphadenitis and pyrexia.

parity ('parətee) the classification of a woman with regard to the number of children which have been born live to her.

Parkinson's disease ('pahkinsənz) *J. Parkinson, British physician, 1755–1824.* Parkinsonism; paralysis agitans. A slowly progressive disease usually occurring in later life, characterized pathologically by degeneration within the nuclear masses of the extrapyramidal system, and clinically by masklike facies (PARKINSON'S FACIES), a characteristic tremor of resting muscles, a slowing of voluntary movements, a festinating gait, peculiar posture, and muscular weakness. When this symptom complex occurs secondarily to another disorder, the condition is called PARKINSONISM.

paronychia (,paro'nikiə) an abscess near the finger-nail; a whitlow or felon. *P. tendinosa* a pyogenic infection that involves the tendon sheath.

parosmia (pa'rozmi·ə) a disordered sense of smell.

parotid (pə'rotid) situated near the ear. *P. glands* two salivary glands, one in front of each ear.

parotitis (,parə'tietis) inflammation of a parotid gland. Caused usually by ascending infection via its duct, when hygiene of the mouth is neglected or when the natural secretions are lessened, especially in severe illness or following operation. *Epidemic p.* mumps.

parous ('parəs) having borne one or more children.

paroxysm ('parok,sizəm) 1. a sudden attack or recurrence of a symptom of a disease. 2. a convulsion.

paroxysmal (,parok'sizməl) occurring in paroxysms. *P. cardiac dyspnoea* cardiac asthma. Recurrent attacks of dyspnoea associated with pulmonary oedema and left-sided heart failure. *P. tachycardia* recurrent attacks of rapid heart beats that may occur without heart disease.

parrot disease ('parət) *see* PSITTA-COSIS.

parthenogenesis (,pahthənoh-'jenəsis) asexual reproduction by means of an egg which has not been fertilized.

particle (,pahtik'l) a minute piece of substance.

parturient (pah'tyooə·ri·ənt) giving birth; relating to childbirth.

parturition (,pahtyuh'rishən) the act of giving birth to a child.

PAS para-aminosalicylic acid.

pascal (pa'skal, 'pask'l) *symbol* Pa. The SI unit of pressure.

passive ('pasiv) not active. *P. immunity see* IMMUNITY. *P. movements* in massage, manipulation by a physiotherapist without the help of the patient.

passivity (pa'sivitee) in psychiatry, a delusional feeling that a person is under some outside control and must therefore be inactive.

Pasteurella (,pahstə'relə) L. *Pasteur, French chemist and bacteriologist, 1833–1895.* A genus of short Gram-negative bacilli. *P. pestis* the causative organism of plague transmitted by rat fleas to man.

pasteurization (,pastə·rie'zayshən, ,pahstyə-) the process of checking fermentation in milk and other fluids by heating them to a temperature of 72°C for 15–20 min or 63°C for 30 min and then rapidly cooling. This kills most pathogenic bacteria.

patch test (pach) a test of skin sensitivity in which a number of possible allergens are applied to the skin under a plaster. The causal agent of the allergy will produce an inflammation.

patella (pə'telə) the small, circular, sesamoid bone forming the kneecap.

patellar (pə'telə) belonging to the patella. *P. reflex* . a knee jerk obtained by tapping the tendon below the patella.

patellectomy (,pate'lektəmee) excision of the patella.

patent ('paytənt) open. *P. ductus arteriosus* failure of the ductus arteriosus to close, causing a shunt of blood from the aorta into the pulmonary artery and producing a continuous heart murmur.

pathogen ('pathə,jen) any disease-producing agent or microorganism.

pathogenicity (,pathəjə'nisitee) the ability of a microorganism to cause disease.

pathognomonic (,pathəgnə'monik) specifically characteristic of a disease. A sign or symptom by which a pathological condition can positively be identified.

pathological (,pathə'lojik'l) 1. pertaining to pathology. 2. causing or arising from disease. *P. fracture* a fracture occurring in diseased bone where there has been little or no external trauma.

pathology (pə'tholəjee) the branch of medicine which deals with the essential nature of disease, especially of the structural and functional changes in tissues and organs of the body which cause or are caused by disease.

pathophobia (,pathə'fohbi·ə) an exaggerated dread of disease.

patient ('payshənt) a person who is ill or is undergoing treatment

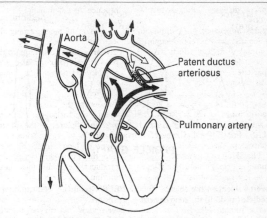

Aorta

Patent ductus arteriosus

Pulmonary artery

PATENT DUCTUS ARTERIOSUS

for disease.

patient's rights ('payshəns riets) patients have three basic rights, namely, the right to know, the right to privacy and the right to treatment. The first two are moral rights while the third is, in the UK, both a moral and legal right.

Paul–Bunnell test (,pawlbə'nel) *J.R. Paul, American physician 1893–1971; W.W. Bunnell, American physician, b. 1902).* An agglutination test which, if positive, confirms the diagnosis of glandular fever.

Pavlov's method ('pavlovz ,methəd) *I.P. Pavlov, Russian physiologist, 1849–1936.* A method for the study of the conditioned reflexes. Pavlov noticed that his experimental dogs salivated in anticipation of food when they heard a bell ring.

peau d'orange (,poh do'ronhzh) a dimpled appearance of the overlying skin. Blockage of the skin lymphatics causes dimpling of the hair follicle openings which resembles orange skin. Particularly associated with breast cancer.

pecten ('pekten) 1. the middle third of the anal canal. 2. a ridge on the pubic crest to which the inguinal ligament is attached.

pectoral ('pektə-rəl) relating to the chest. *P. muscles* two pairs of muscles, pectoralis major and pectoralis minor, which control the movements of the shoulder and upper arm.

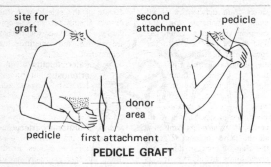

PEDICLE GRAFT

pectus ('pektəs) the chest.

pedicle ('pedik'l) the stem or neck of a tumour. *P. graft* a tissue graft that is partially detached and inserted in its new position while temporarily still obtaining its blood supply from the original source.

pediculosis (pə,dikyuh'lohsis) the condition of being infested with lice.

Pediculus (pə'dikyuhləs) genus of lice. *P. humanus* a species that feeds on human blood and is an important vector of relapsing fever, typhus, and trench fever; two subspecies are recognized; *P. humanus* var. *capitis* (head louse) found on the scalp hair, and *P. humanus* var. *corporis* (body or clothes louse) found elsewhere on the body.

peduncle (pə'dungk'l) a narrow part of a structure acting as a support. *Cerebellar p.* one of the collections of nerve fibres connecting the cerebellum with the medulla oblongata.

PEEP positive end-expiratory pressure.

peer review (piə ri'vyoo) a basic component of a QUALITY ASSURANCE programme in which the results of health and/or nursing care given to a specific patient population are evaluated according to defined criteria established by the peers of the professionals delivering the care. Peer review is focused on the patient and on the results of care given by a group of professionals rather than on individual professional practitioners.

Pel–Ebstein syndrome (pel'ebstein) *P.K. Pel, Dutch physician, 1852–1919; W. Ebstein, German physician, 1836–1912.* A recurrent pyrexia having a cycle of 15–21 days which occurs in cases of lymphadenoma.

pellagra (pə'lagrə, -lay-) a syndrome caused by a diet seriously deficient in niacin (or by failure to convert tryptophan to niacin). Most persons with pellagra also suffer from deficiencies of vitamin B_2 (riboflavin) and other essential vitamins and minerals. The disease also occurs in persons suffering from alcoholism and drug addiction. Characterized by debility, digestive disorders, peripheral neuritis, ataxia, mental disturbance and erythema with exfoliation of the skin.

pelvic ('pelvik) pertaining to the pelvis. *P. exenteration* removal of all the pelvic organs. *P. girdle* the ring of bone to which the lower limbs are jointed. It consists of the two hip bones and the sacrum and coccyx.

pelvimetry (pel'vimətree) measurement of the pelvis.

pelvirectal (,pelvi'rekt'l) pertaining to the flexure where the pelvic colon joins the rectum at an acute angle.

pelvis ('pelvis) a basin-shaped cavity. *Bony p.* the pelvic girdle formed of the hip bones and the sacrum and coccyx. *Contracted p.* narrowing of the diameter of the pelvis. *See* CONJUGATE. It may be of the true conjugate or the diagonal. Effective antenatal care will recognize this condition, and caesarean section may be necessary. *False p.* the part formed by the concavity of the iliac bones above the ileopectineal line. *Renal p.* the dilatation of the ureter which, by enclosing the hilus, surrounds the pyramids of the kidney substance. *True p.* the basin-like cavity below the false pelvis, its upper limit being the pelvic brim.

pemphigoid ('pemfi,goyd) 1. resembling pemphigus. 2. a bullous disease of the elderly with the blisters arising beneath the epidermis. The skin and the mucosa are affected, and sometimes the conjunctiva.

pemphigus ('pemfigəs) a distinctive group of rare but serious diseases characterized by successive crops of large bullae ('water blisters'); the name is derived from the Greek word for blister: *pemphix*. Clusters of blisters usually appear first near the nose and mouth (sometimes inside them) and then gradually spread over the skin of the rest of the body. When the blisters burst, they leave round patches of raw and tender skin. Pemphigus is considered to be an autoimmune disorder.

pendulous ('pendyuhləs) hanging down. *P. abdomen* the hanging down of the abdomen over the pelvis, due to weakness and laxity of the abdominal muscles.

penicillamine (,peni'silə,meen) a chelating agent that is used in heavy metal poisoning to aid excretion of the metal and in the treatment of hepatolenticular degeneration (Wilson's disease). Also used in the treatment of severe rheumatoid arthritis.

penicillin (,peni'silin) an antibiotic cultured from certain moulds of the genus *Penicillium*. The drug is used in various forms to treat a wide variety of bacterial infections. Discovered by Fleming in 1929, it was first used therapeutically in 1941. Varieties of the drug include: benethamine penicillin, benzylpenicillin, benzathine penicillin, procaine penicillin, cloxacillin, ampicillin and amoxycillin.

penicillinase (,peni'sili,nayz) an enzyme that inactivates penicillin. Many bacteria, particularly staphylococci, produce this enzyme.

Penicillium (,peni'sili·əm) a genus of mould-like fungi from some of which the penicillins are derived. Some species are pathogenic to man.

penis ('peenis) the male organ of copulation and of urination.

pentagastrin (,pentə'gastrin) a synthetic hormone with a similar structure to gastrin. It has largely replaced histamine in gastric secretion tests as it has no apparent side-effects.

pentamidine (pen'tamideen) an antiprotozoal drug used mainly in the treatment of *Pneumocystis carinii* infections.

pentazocine (pen'tazoh,seen) an analgesic similar to morphine and used in the treatment of moderate to severe pain.

pentose ('pentohz) a monosaccharide containing five carbon atoms in a molecule.

pentosuria (,pentoh'syooə·ri·ə) a benign inborn error of metabolism due to a defect in the activity of the enzyme L-xylulose dehydrogenase resulting in pentose in the urine.

pepsin ('pepsin) an enzyme found in gastric juice. It partially digests proteins in an acid solution.

pepsinogen (pep'sinəjən) the precursor of pepsin, activated by hydrochloric acid.

peptic ('peptik) relating to pepsin

or the action of the gastric juices in promoting digestion. *P. ulcer* an ulcer, usually in the stomach or the duodenum, caused by an excess of acid in the gastric juices.

peptide ('peptied) any of a class of compounds of low molecular weight which yield two or more amino acids on hydrolysis. Peptides form the constituent parts of proteins.

peptone ('peptohn) a substance produced by the action of pepsin on protein.

peptonuria (,peptə'nyooə·ri·ə) presence of peptones in urine.

per os (pər os) [L.] *by the mouth.*

percept; perception ('pərsept; pə-'sepshən) an awareness and understanding of an impression that has been presented to the senses. The mental process by which we perceive.

percussion (pə'kushən) a method of diagnosis by tapping with the fingers or with a light hammer upon any part of the body. Information can thus be gained as to the condition of underlying organs.

percutaneous (,pərkyoo'tayni·əs) through the skin, particularly in relation to ointments that are applied to unbroken skin.

perforation (,pərfə'rayshən) a hole or break in the containing walls or membranes of an organ or structure of the body. Perforation occurs when erosion, infection or other factors create a weak spot in the organ and internal pressure causes a rupture. It also may result from a deep penetrating wound.

performance indicators 'package' of routine statistics derived nationally by the Department of Health and visually presented in ways which highlight the relative efficiency of health services in each Health Authority compared with other Authorities. Performance indicators are intended to identify aspects which merit further scrutiny locally with a view to changes in organization or practice.

perfusion (pə'fyoozhən) the passage of liquid through a tissue or an organ, particularly the passage of blood through the lung tissue.

perianal (,peri'ayn'l) surrounding or located around the anus. *P. abscess* a small subcutaneous pocket of pus near the anal margin.

periarteritis (,peri,ahtə'rietis) inflammation of the outer coat and surrounding tissues of an artery.

periarthritis (,periah'thrietis) inflammation of the tissues surrounding a joint.

pericardiectomy (,peri,kahdi'ektəmee) surgical removal of the pericardium; pericardectomy. Used in the treatment of chronic constrictive pericarditis.

pericardiocentesis (,peri,kahdiohsen'teesis) drainage of fluid from the pericardium.

pericarditis (,perikah'dietis) inflammation of the pericardium. *Adhesive p.* the presence of adhesions between the two layers of pericardium owing to a thick fibrinous exudate. *Bacterial p.* inflammation of the pericardium due to bacterial infection. *Chronic constrictive p.* thickening and sometimes calcification of the pericardium, which inhibits the action of the heart. *Rheumatic p.* pericarditis due to rheumatic fever.

pericardium (,peri'kahdi·əm) the smooth membranous sac enveloping the heart, consisting of an outer fibrous and an inner serous coat. The sac contains a small amount of serous fluid.

perichondrium (,peri'kondri·əm) the membrane covering cartilaginous surfaces.

pericolpitis (,perikol'pietis) inflammation of the tissues around the vagina.

pericranium (,peri'krayni·əm) the periosteum of the cranial bones.

pericyazine (,peri'sieə,zeen) a phenothiazine stronger than chlorpromazine; used in behavioural disturbances, schizophrenia and related psychoses.

perilymph ('peri,limf) the fluid which separates the bony and the membranous labyrinths of the ear.

perimeter (pə'rimitə) 1. the line marking the boundary of any area or geometrical figure; the circumference. 2. an instrument for measuring the field of vision.

perimetrium (,peri'meetri·əm) the peritoneal covering of the uterus.

perinatal (,peri'nayt'l) relating to the period shortly before and 7 days after birth. *P. mortality rate* the number of stillbirths plus deaths of babies under 7 days old per 1000 total births in any one year.

perinatologist (,perinay'toləjist) a specialist in perinatology.

perinatology (,perinay'toləjee) the

branch of medicine (obstetrics and paediatrics) dealing with the fetus and infant during the perinatal period.

perineal (,peri'neeəl) relating to the perineum.

perineorrhaphy (,perini'o·rəfee) suture of the perineum to repair a laceration caused during childbirth.

perinephrium (,peri'nefri·əm) the tissue surrounding the kidney.

perineum (,peri'neeəm) the tissues between the anus and external genitals. *Lacerated p.* a torn perineum, which may result from childbirth, but is often forestalled by performing an episiotomy. Treatment is by perineorrhaphy.

periodic (,pie·ri'odik) recurring at regular or irregular intervals. *P. apnoea of the newborn* occurring in the normal full-term infant, periodic episodes of rapid breathing followed by a brief period of apnoea which is associated with rapid eye movements. *P. syndrome* recurrent head, limb or abdominal pains in children for which no organic cause can be found. It often leads to migraine in adult life.

periodontitis (,peri·ədon'tietis) inflammation of the periodontium

periodontium (,peri·ə'donshi·əm) the connective tissue between the teeth and their bony sockets.

perioperative (,peri'opə·rətiv) pertaining or relating to the period immediately before or after an operation, as perioperative care.

periosteal (,peri'ostiəl) pertaining to or composed of periosteum.

P. elevator an instrument for separating the periosteum from the bone.

periosteum (,peri'osti·əm) the fibrous membrane covering the surface of bone. It consists of two layers, the inner or osteogenetic, which is closely adherent, and which forms new cells (by which the bone grows in girth), and in close contact with it the fibrous layer richly supplied with blood vessels.

periostitis (,perio'stietis) inflammation of the periosteum.

peripheral (pə'rifə·rəl) relating to the periphery. *P. iridectomy* excision of a small piece of iris from its peripheral edge. *P. nervous system* those parts of the nervous system lying outside the central nervous system. *P. neuritis* inflammation of terminal nerves. *P. resistance* the resistance in the walls of the arterioles, which is a major factor in the control of blood pressure.

periphery (pə'rifə·ree) the outer surface or circumference.

peristalsis (,peri'stalsis) a wave-like contraction, preceded by a wave of dilatation, which travels along the walls of a tubular organ, tending to press its contents onwards. It occurs in the muscle coat of the alimentary canal. *Reversed p.* a wave of contraction in the alimentary canal which passes *towards* the mouth. *Visible p.* a wave of contraction in the alimentary canal that is visible on the surface of the abdomen.

peritomy (pe'ritəmee) excision of a portion of the conjunctiva at the edge of the cornea, for the cure of pannus.

peritoneal (ˌperitəˈneeəl) referring to the peritoneum. *P. cavity* the cavity between the parietal and the visceral peritoneum. *P. dialysis* a method of removing waste products from the blood by passing a cannula into the peritoneal cavity, running in a dialysing fluid, and after an interval, draining it off.

peritoneoscopy (ˌperitəniˈoskəpee) visual examination of the peritoneum by means of a peritoneoscope.

peritoneum (ˌperitəˈneeəm) the serous membrane lining the abdominal cavity and forming a covering for the abdominal organs. *Parietal p.* that which lines the abdominal cavity. *Visceral p.* the inner layer which closely covers the abdominal organs, and includes the mesenteries.

peritonitis (ˌperitəˈnietis) inflammation of the peritoneum. *Acute p.* this may be produced by inflammation of abdominal organs, by irritating substances from a perforated gallbladder or gastric ulcer, by rupture of a cyst, or by irritation from blood, as in cases of internal bleeding. *Chronic p.* this is comparatively rare, and is often associated with tuberculosis. Less frequently it may result from long-standing irritation caused by the presence in the abdomen of a foreign body such as gunshot, or by chronic peritoneal dialysis.

peritonsillar (ˌperiˈtonsilə) around the tonsil. *P. abscess* quinsy.

perlèche (pərˈlesh) inflammation with fissuring at the angles of the mouth; often due to vitamin B deficiency, poorly fitting dentures or thrush infection.

permeability (ˌpərmi-əˈbilitee) the degree to which a fluid can pass from one structure through a wall or membrane to another.

pernicious (pəˈnishəs) highly destructive; fatal. *P. anaemia* an anaemia due to lack of absorption of vitamin B_{12} for the formation of red blood cells.

perniosis (ˌpərniˈohsis) a condition resulting from persistent exposure to cold which produces vascular spasm in the superficial arterioles of the hands and feet, causing thrombosis and necrosis. Perniosis includes chilblains and Raynaud's disease.

peromelia (ˌpeerohˈmeeli-ə) a congenital malformation of a limb which resembles an amputation, although bud-like remnants of the peripheral segments may exist.

peroral (pərˈror-rəl) by the mouth.

perphenazine (pərˈfenəˌzeen) an antiemetic and tranquillizing drug similar to chlorpromazine. Used in the treatment of nausea and vomiting, and of schizophrenia and other psychoses.

perseveration (pərˌsevəˈrayshən) the constant recurrence of an idea or the tendency to keep repeating the same words or actions.

personality (ˌpərsəˈnalitee) the sum total of heredity and inborn tendencies, with influences from environment and education, which goes to form the mental make-up of a person and influence his attitude to life. *Antisocial p.* a personality disorder in which repetitive antisocial behaviour is associated with ego eccentricity, lack of guilt or anxiety, and imperviousness to punishment. Called also sociopathic (psychopathic) personality. *Cyclothymic p.* a personality marked by alternate moods of elation and dejection. *Double p., dual p.* multiple personality. *Multiple p.* a dissociative reaction in which an individual adopts two or more personalities alternatively, in none of which is he aware of the experiences of the other(s). *Psychopathic p.* antisocial personality, sociopathic personality. *Schizoid p.* a personality disorder marked by timidity, self-consciousness, introversion, feelings of isolation and loneliness, and failure to form close interpersonal relationships; the individual is frequently ambitious, meticulous, and a perfectionist.

perspiration (ˌpərspi'rayshən) sweat or the act of sweating. *Insensible p.* water evaporation from the moist surfaces of the body, such as the respiratory tract and skin, that is not due to the activity of the sweat glands. It occurs at a constant rate of about 500 ml/day. When treating dehydration this loss must be taken into account. *Sensible p.* sweat which is visible as droplets on the skin. Part of the mechanism for regulation of body temperature.

Perthes' disease ('pərtayz) *G.C. Perthes, German surgeon, 1869–*

1927. Osteochondritis of the head of the femur. Pseudocoxalgia (Legg–Calvé–Perthes disease).

pertussis (pə'tusis) whooping cough.

perversion (pə'vərshən) morbid diversion from a normal course. *Sexual p.* abnormal sexual desires and behaviour. A deviation.

pes (payz, peez) the foot, or any foot-like structure. *P. cavus* a foot with an abnormally high arch. Claw-foot. *P. malleus valgus* hammer toe. *P. planus* flat foot.

pessary ('pesə-ree) 1. a plastic or metal ring-shaped device which is inserted in the vagina to support a prolapsed uterus. 2. a medicated suppository inserted into the vagina for antiseptic or contraceptive purposes.

pesticide ('pesti,sied) a chemical agent that destroys pests.

petechia (pə'teeki-ə) a small spot due to an effusion of blood under the skin, as in purpura.

pethidine ('pethi,deen, -in) a synthetic narcotic analgesic, less potent than morphine with quicker onset but shorter duration of action, used in obstetrics and pre- and postoperative medication. Particularly useful, as it relaxes smooth muscle, in patients with ureteric and biliary colic and as an analgesic in patients with asthma.

petit mal (ˌpeti 'mal) a mild form of epilepsy common in children and characterized by a sudden and brief loss of consciousness.

pétrissage (paytri'sahzh) a kneading action used in massage.

petrositis (ˌpetroh'sietis) inflammation of the petrous portion of the temporal bone usually spread from a middle-ear infection.

petrous ('petrəs) resembling a stone. *P. bone* that part of the two temporal bones that forms the base of the skull and contains the middle and inner ear.

Peyer's glands or patches ('pieəz) *J.C. Peyer, Swiss anatomist, 1653–1712.* Small lymph nodules situated in the mucous membrane of the lower part of the small intestine.

Peyronie's disease ('payrəneez) induration of the corpora cavernosa of the penis, producing a fibrous chordee leading to painful erection.

pH a measure of the hydrogen ion concentration, and so the acidity or alkalinity of a solution. Expressed numerically 1 to 14; 7 is neutral, below this is acid and above alkaline. *See* HYDROGEN ION CONCENTRATION.

phacoanaphylactic uveitis (,fakoh,anəfi,laktik ,yoovi'ietis) inflammation of the uveal tract occurring as a result of an allergy to lens protein following rupture of the lens capsule or after an extracapsular extraction.

phacoemulsification (,fakohi,mulsifi'kayshən) a technique of CATARACT extraction, utilizing high-frequency ultrasonic vibrations to fragment the lens nucleus, combined with controlled irrigation to maintain normal pressure in the anterior chamber and suction to remove lens fragments and irrigating fluid.

phacoma (fə'kohmə) a congenital tumour of the lens of the eye.

phaeochromocytoma (,feeoh-,krohmohsie'tohmə) a tumour of the adrenal medulla which gives rise to paroxysmal hypertension.

phage (fayj, fahzh) bacteriophage. A virus which lives on bacteria but is confined to a particular strain. *P.-typing* the identification of certain bacterial strains by determining the presence of strain-specific phages. Used in detecting the causative organisms of epidemics, especially food poisoning.

phagocyte ('fagə'siet) a blood cell that has the power of ingesting bacteria, protozoa and foreign bodies in the blood.

phagocytosis (,fagəsie'tohsis) the engulfing and destruction of microorganisms and foreign bodies by phagocytes in the blood.

phalanges (fa'lanjeez) the bones of the fingers or toes.

phalloplasty ('fahloh,plastee) a plastic operation on the penis to repair deformity or after injury.

phallus ('faləs) the penis.

phantasy ('fantəsee) *see* FANTASY.

phantom ('fantəm) 1. an image or impression not evoked by actual stimuli. 2. a model of the body or of a specific part thereof. 3. a device for simulating the in vivo interaction of radiation with tissues. *P. pain* pain felt as if it were arising in an absent (amputated) limb. *P. pregnancy* see PSEUDOCYESIS. *P. tumour* a tumour-like swelling of the abdomen caused by contraction of the muscles or by localized gas.

pharmacogenetics (,fahməkohjə'netiks) the study of genetically determined variations in drug metabolism and the response of the individual.

pharmacology (,fahmə'koləjee) the science of the nature and preparation of drugs and particularly of their effects on the body.

pharmacopoeia (,fahmәkә'pee·ə) an authoritative publication which gives the standard formulae and preparations of drugs used in a given country. *British P.* that authorized for use in the United Kingdom.

pharmacy ('fahmәsee) 1. the art of preparing, compounding and dispensing medicines. 2. the place where drugs are stored and dispensed.

pharyngeal (,farin'jeeәl, fә'rinji·әl) relating to the pharynx. *P. pouch* dilatation of the lower part of the pharynx.

pharyngectomy (,farin'jektәmee) excision of a section of the pharynx.

pharyngitis (,farin'jietis) inflammation of the pharynx.

pharyngolaryngeal (,fә,ring-goh-,larin'jeeәl) referring to both the pharynx and larynx.

pharyngotympanic tube (fә,ring-gohtim'panik) the tube which joins the middle ear to the pharynx; the eustachian tube.

pharynx ('faringks) the muscular tube lined with mucous membrane situated at the back of the mouth. It leads into the oesophagus, and also communicates with the nose through the posterior nares, with the ears through the pharyngotympanic (eustachian) tubes, and with the larynx. *See* LARYNGOPHARYNX, NASOPHARYNX and OROPHARYNX.

phenazocine (fe'nazoh,seen) an analgesic drug used to relieve severe pain. It is a drug of addiction.

phenelzine (fe'nelzeen) a monoamine oxidase inhibitor used in the treatment of depressive illness.

phenformin (fen'fawmin) an oral hypoglycaemic drug. A biguanide that aids the entry of glucose into the cells. Used in the treatment of diabetes mellitus.

phenindione (,fenin'dieohn) an anticoagulant drug used in the treatment of deep vein thrombosis.

phenobarbitone (,feenoh'bahbi-,tohn) a long-lasting barbiturate drug used to treat severe insomnia and also as an anticonvulsant drug in the treatment of epilepsy.

phenol ('feenol) carbolic acid. A disinfectant derived from coaltar.

phenolphthalein (,feenol'thalee·in, -,leen, -'thay-) a cathartic. Its use should be avoided as it may cause rashes, albuminuria and haemoglobinuria. Its laxative effects may continue for several days.

phenomenon (fi'nominәn) an objective sign or symptom. A noteworthy occurrence.

phenoperidine (,feenoh'perideen) synthetic narcotic analgesic used intraoperatively to supplement general anaesthesia. Also used in the intensive care unit to facilitate patients accepting mechanical ventilation.

phenothiazine (,feenoh'thieәzeen) one of a group of drugs used in the treatment of severe psychiatric disorders. The first to be used was chlorpromazine.

phenotype ('feenoh,tiep) the characteristics of an individual that are due both to his environment and to his genetic make-up.

phenoxybenzamine (fee,noksi-'benzəmeen) a vasodilator drug used in the treatment of peripheral conditions such as Raynaud's disease.

phenoxymethylpenicillin (fe-,noksi,methil,peni'silin) a penicillinase-sensitive antibiotic similar in action to benzylpenicillin. Used mainly against streptococcal infections in children, it is taken orally. Penicillin V.

phentermine ('fentə,meen) an appetite-suppressant drug used in the treatment of obesity.

phentolamine (fen'tolə,meen) a vasodilator, used to reduce blood pressure in treating phaeochromocytoma.

phenylalanine (,feenil'aləneen) an essential amino acid that cannot be properly metabolized in persons suffering from phenylketonuria.

phenylbutazone (,feenil'byootəzohn) an analgesic antipyretic drug used in the treatment of gout and rheumatic disorders.

phenylketonuria (,feenil,keetə-'nyooə·ri·ə) abbreviated PKU. A congenital disease due to a defect in the metabolism of the amino acid phenylalanine. The condition is hereditary. It results from lack of an enzyme, phenylalanine hydroxylase, necessary for the conversion of the amino acid phenylalanine into tyrosine. Thus there is accumulation of phenylalanine in the blood with eventual excretion of phenylpyruvic acid in the urine. If untreated, the condition results in mental handicap and other abnormalities. The condition can be detected soon after birth and screening of newborns for PKU entails a simple blood test. A sample of blood is taken from infants' heels at approximately 2 weeks and phenylalanine levels are assessed (Guthrie test). Treatment is with a diet low in phenylalanine.

phenylpyruvic acid (,feenilpie-'roovik) an abnormal constituent of the urine present in phenylketonuria.

phenytoin (,feni'toh·in) an anticonvulsant drug used in the treatment of major epileptic fits.

phimosis (fie'mohsis) constriction of the prepuce so that it cannot be drawn back over the glans penis. The usual treatment is circumcision.

phlebectomy (fli'bektəmee) excision of a vein or a portion of a vein.

phlebitis (fli'bietis) inflammation of a vein, usually in the leg, which tends to lead to the formation of a thrombus. The symptoms are: pain and swelling, and redness along the course of the vein, which is felt later as a hard, tender cord.

phlebography (fli'bogrəfee) 1. Radiographic examination of a vein containing a contrast medium. 2. the graphic representation of the venous pulse.

phlebolith ('fleboh,lith) a stone formed in a vein by calcification of a blood clot.

phlebothrombosis (ˌfleboh-throm'bohsis) obstruction of a vein by a blood clot, without local inflammation. It is usually in the deep veins of the calf of the leg, causing tenderness and swelling. The clot may break away and cause an embolism.

Phlebotomus (flə'botəməs) a genus of sandflies, the various species of which transmit leishmaniasis in its many forms, and also sandfly fever.

phlebotomy (fli'botəmee) the puncture of a vein for the withdrawal of blood. Venesection.

phlegm (flem) mucus secreted by the lining of the air passages.

phlegmasia (fleg'mayzi·ə) an inflammation. *P. alba dolens* acute oedema in a leg due to lymphatic blockage. 'White leg'. Rarely occurs now but was seen most frequently in women after childbirth.

phlegmatic (fleg'matik) dull and apathetic.

phlycten ('fliktən) 1. a small blister caused by a burn. 2. a small vesicle containing lymph occurring in the conjunctiva or cornea of the eye. Often associated with tuberculosis.

phlyctenule ('fliktən,yool) a small vesicle on the conjunctiva or cornea.

phobia (fohbi·ə) an irrational fear produced by a specific situation which the patient attempts to avoid.

phocomelia (ˌfohkə'meeli·ə) a congenital deformity in which the long bones of the limbs are minimal or absent and the individual has hands or feet resembling the flippers of seals, or stump-like limbs of various lengths. The drug thalidomide, taken by the mother early in pregnancy, has produced this deformity.

pholcodine ('folkoh,deen) a linctus for the suppression of a dry or painful cough.

phonation (foh'nayshən) the art of uttering meaningful vocal sounds.

phonocardiogram (ˌfohnoh'kah-dioh,gram) a record of the heart sounds made by a phonocardiograph.

phonocardiograph (ˌfohnoh'kah-dioh,grahf, -graf) an instrument that records graphically heart sounds and murmurs.

phonology (fə'noləjee) the study of speech sounds, their production and the relationship between sounds as elements of language.

phosphatase ('fosfə,tayz) one of a group of enzymes involved in the metabolism of phosphate. *Alkaline p.* one formed by osteoblasts in the bone and by liver cells and excreted in the bile.

phosphate ('fosfayt) a salt or ester of phosphoric acid.

phosphaturia (ˌfosfə'tyooə·ri·ə) excess of phosphates in the urine.

phospholipid (ˌfosfə'lipid) a lipid of glycerol fats found in cells, especially those of the nervous system.

phosphonecrosis (ˌfosfənə'krohsis) necrosis, usually of the jawbone, due to an excessive intake of phosphorus. An industrial disease, occurring in workers engaged in the chemical industry.

phosphorus ('fosfə·rəs) *symbol* P. Phosphorus is an essential element in the diet. It is a major component of bone and is involved in almost all metabolic processes and also plays an important role in cell metabolism. It is obtained by the body from milk products, cereals, meat and fish. Its use by the body is controlled by vitamin D and calcium. Phosphorus is very inflammable and exceedingly poisonous. Inhalation of its vapour by workers in chemical industries may cause necrosis of the mandible (phosphonecrosis or phossy jaw). Free phosphorus causes fatty degeneration of the liver and other viscera.

phosphorylase (fos'fo·ri,layz) an enzyme found in the liver and kidneys, which catalyses the breakdown of glycogen into glucose 1-phosphate.

photalgia (foh'talji·ə) pain in the eyes from exposure to too much light.

photocoagulation (,fohtohkoh-,agyuh'layshən) the use of a powerful light source to induce inflammation of the retina and choroid to treat retinal detachment.

photophobia (,fohtoh'fohbi·ə) intolerance of light. It can occur in many eye conditions including conjunctivitis, corneal ulceration, iritis and keratitis.

photophthalmia (,fohtof'thalmi·ə) inflammation of the eye due to overexposure to bright light, especially to ultraviolet light.

photopic (foh'topik, -'toh-) pertaining to bright light. *P. vision* vision in bright light when the cones of the retina provide the visual appreciation of colour and shape.

photopsia (foh'topsi·ə) a sensation of flashes of light sometimes occurring in the early stages of retinal detachment.

photosensitivity (,fohtoh,sensi-'tivitee) an abnormal degree of sensitivity of the skin to sunlight.

phototherapy (,fohtoh'therəpee) treatment using fluorescent light, containing a high output of blue light, to reduce the amount of unconjugated bilirubin in the skin of a mildly jaundiced neonate. Phototherapy also may be used prophylactically in preterm infants with bruising, and in babies affected by rhesus incompatibility.

phrenemphraxis (,frenem'fraksis) an operation in which a phrenic nerve is crushed to paralyse one half of the diaphragm.

phrenic ('frenik) 1. relating to the mind. 2. pertaining to the diaphragm. *P. avulsion* the surgical extraction of a part of the phrenic nerve. *P. nerve* one of a pair of nerves controlling the muscles of the diaphragm.

phrenicectomy (,freni'sektəmee) the excision of a part of the phrenic nerve.

phrenicotomy (,freni'kotəmee) division of a phrenic nerve.

phthalylsulpathiazole (,thalilsul-'fonə,zohl) an insoluble sulphonamide, poorly absorbed in the intestine and so used to kill intestinal bacteria prior to surgery.

Phthirus pubis ('thirəs 'pyoobis) the crab louse.

phthisis (thie'sis) pulmonary tuberculosis. *P. bulbi* a shrinking of the eyeball following inflammation or injury.

physical ('fisik'l) in medicine, relating to the body as opposed to the mental processes. *P. examination* examination of the bodily state of a patient by ordinary physical means, as inspection, palpation, percussion and auscultation. *P. handicap* a term used when a physical disadvantage is due to impairment of physiological or anatomical structure or function. *P. medicine* the treatment and rehabilitation of patients with physical disabilities. It includes physiotherapy and manipulation. *P. signs* those observed by inspection, percussion, etc.

physician (fi'zishən) one who practises medicine as opposed to surgery. *Community p.* a doctor who practises community MEDICINE. *Consultant p.* senior doctor in overall charge of patients within a specialist medical field, and responsible for directing junior medical staff working for the same firm. *House p.* a junior doctor, resident in hospital whilst on duty acting under the orders of a consultant physician.

physiological (,fizi·ə'lojik'l) relating to physiology. Normal, as opposed to pathological. *P. jaundice see* JAUNDICE. *P. solutions* those of the same salt composition and same osmotic pressure as blood plasma.

physiology (,fizi'oləjee) the science of the functioning of living organisms.

physiotherapy (,fizioh'therəpee) treatment and rehabilitation by natural forces, e.g. heat, light, electricity, massage, manipulation and remedial exercises.

physique (fi'zeek) the structure of the body.

physostigmine (,fiesoh'stigmeen) eserine, an alkaloid from the calabar bean. It is an antidote to curare; it constricts the pupils and is used with pilocarpine in the treatment of glaucoma.

phytomenadione (,fietoh,menə-'dieohn) an intravenous preparation of vitamin K, effective in treating haemorrhage occurring during anticoagulant therapy.

pia mater (,piea 'maytə) [L.] the innermost membrane enveloping the brain and spinal cord consisting of a network of small blood vessels connected by areolar tissue. This dips down into all the folds of the nerve substance.

pica ('piekə) an unnatural craving for strange foods and for things not fit to be eaten. It may occur in pregnancy, and sometimes in mentally handicapped children.

Pick's disease (piks) *A. Pick, Czechoslovakian physician, 1851–1924.* A form of presenile brain failure (dementia) with an age of onset between 50 and 60. There is shrinkage of the brain and loss of cortical cells.

pickwickian syndrome (pik'wiki·ən) (named after the fat boy 'Joe' in *Pickwick Papers*). A condition in which extreme obesity is associated with severe congestive cardiac failure. The victims are cyanosed and have polycythaemia and marked oedema.

picornavirus (pie'kawnə,vierəs) a family of small RNA-containing viruses including echoviruses and rhinoviruses.

PID prolapse of an intervertebral disc.

pigeon breast ('pijən) a deformity in which the sternum is unduly prominent.

pigment ('pigmənt) colouring matter. *Bile p's* bilirubin and biliverdin. *Blood p.* haemoglobin. *Melanotic p.* melanin.

pigmentation (,pigmen'tayshən) the deposition in the tissues of an abnormal amount of pigment.

pile (piel) a haemorrhoid.

pill (pil) a rounded mass of one or more drugs sometimes coated with sugar. Taken orally.

pilocarpine (,pieloh'kahpeen) an alkaloid prepared from jaborandi leaves. It is used to constrict the pupils in the treatment of glaucoma.

pilomotor (,pieloh'mohtə) capable of moving the hair. *P. nerves* sympathetic nerves which control muscles in the skin connected with hair follicles. Stimulation causes the hair to be erected, and also the condition of 'gooseflesh' of the skin.

pilonidal (,pieloh'nied'l) having a growth of hair. *P. cyst* a congenital infolding of hair-bearing skin over the coccyx. It may become infected and lead to sinus formation.

pilosebaceous (,pielohsi'bayshəs) applied to sebaceous glands that open into the hair follicles.

pilosis (pie'lohsis) an abnormal growth of hair.

pimple ('pimp'l) a small papule or pustule.

pineal ('pini·əl, 'pie-) shaped like a pine cone. *P. body* a small cone-shaped structure attached by a stalk to the posterior wall of the third ventricle of the brain and composed of glandular substance.

pinguecula (ping'gwekyuhlə) [L.] a small, benign, yellowish spot on the bulbar conjunctiva, seen usually in the elderly. Caused by degeneration of elastic tissue of conjunctiva.

pink disease (pink) acrodynia.

pinkeye ('pingk,ie) acute contagious conjunctivitis.

pinna ('pinə) the projecting part of the external ear; the auricle.

pinocytosis (,pienohsie'tohsis) a process similar to phagocytosis by which molecules of protein enter or are absorbed by cells.

pinta ('pintə) a non-venereal skin infection caused by *Treponema carateum* which is similar to the causative agent of syphilis. It is prevalent in the West Indies and Central America.

pinworm ('pin,wərm) a threadworm; *Enterobius vermicularis*.

piperacillin (pie,perə'silin, pi-) a broad-spectrum semi-synthetic penicillin active against a wide variety of Gram-negative, Gram-positive and anaerobic bacteria.

piperazine (pie'perə,zeen, pi-) an anthelmintic drug used in the treatment of threadworms and roundworms.

pirenzepine (pi'renzə,peen) a drug which inhibits gastric acid secretion and promotes ulcer healing in the stomach.

piriform ('piri,fawm) pear-shaped.

P. fossa one of a pair of depressions lying on either side of the opening into the larynx.

Piriton ('piriton) trade name for chlorpheniramine maleate; a preparation used for the relief of allergy and the emergency treatment of anaphylactic reactions.

piroxicam (pi'roksikam) a nonsteroidal anti-inflammatory drug used in the treatment of rheumatic diseases.

pituitary (pi'tyooitə‧ree) an endocrine gland suspended from the base of the brain and protected by the sella turcica in the sphenoid bone. It consists of two lobes: (1) the anterior, which secretes a number of different hormones including adrenocorticotrophic hormone (ACTH), gonadotrophin, thyroid stimulating hormone (TSH) and prolactin; (2) the posterior, which secretes oxytocin and vasopressin.

pityriasis (,piti'rieəsis) a skin disease characterized by fine scaly desquamation. *P. alba* a condition common in children, when white scaly patches appear on the face. *P. capitis* dandruff. *P. rosea* an inflammatory form, in which the affected areas are macular and ring-shaped.

place of safety order a court order whereby a child is arbitrarily removed from the care of its parents in the interests of the child's safety.

placebo (plə'seeboh) [L.] a substance given to a patient as medicine or a procedure performed on a patient that has no intrinsic therapeutic value and relieves symptoms or helps the patient in some way only because the patient believes or expects that it will. A placebo may be prescribed to satisfy a patient's psychological need for drug therapy and may also be given during controlled experiments.

placenta (plə'sentə) the afterbirth. A vascular structure inside the pregnant uterus supplying the fetus with nourishment through the connecting umbilical cord. The placenta develops about the third month of pregnancy, and is expelled after the birth of the child. *Battledore p.* one in which the cord is attached to the margin and not the centre. *P. praevia* one attached to the lower part of the uterine wall. It may cause severe antepartum haemorrhage.

Placido's disc ('plasidohz) *A. Placido, Portuguese ophthalmologist, 1882–1916.* A disc marked with black and white circles used in the diagnosis of corneal distortion.

plagiocephaly (,playjioh'kefəlee, -'sef-) asymmetry of the head resulting from the irregular closing of the sutures.

plague (playg) an acute febrile, infectious, highly fatal disease caused by the bacillus *Yersinia pestis*. It is a notifiable disease. Transmitted to man by the bites of fleas that have derived the infection from diseased rats. *Bubonic p.* type in which the lymph glands are infected and buboes form in the groins and armpits. Known in mediaeval times as 'The Black Death'. *Pneumonic p.* type in which the infection attacks chiefly the lung tissues. A fatal form. *Septicaemic p.* a very severe and fatal form when the infection enters the bloodstream.

plantar ('plantə) relating to the sole of the foot. *P. arch* the arch made by anastomosis of the plantar arteries. *P. flexion* bending of the toes downward and so arching the foot. *P. reflex* contraction of the toes on stroking the sole of the foot. *P. wart* a common WART located on the sole of the foot. Plantar warts are epidermal tumours caused by a virus which may be picked up by going barefoot. Called also verruca plantaris.

plaque (plak, plahk) 1. a flat patch on the skin. 2. a deposit of food and bacteria on the enamel of teeth which may produce tartar and caries.

plasma ('plazmə) the fluid portion of the blood in which corpuscles are suspended. Plasma is to be distinguished from serum, which is plasma from which the fibrinogen has been separated in the process of clotting. *Reconstituted p.* dried plasma when again made liquid by addition of distilled water. *P. proteins* those present in the blood plasma; albumin, globulin and fibrinogen. *P. volume expander* a solution transfused instead of blood to increase the volume of fluid circulating in the blood vessels. Called also artificial plasma extender.

plasmacytoma (,plazməsie'tohmə) a malignant tumour of plasma cells akin to multiple myeloma.

plasmapheresis (,plazməfə'reesis)

a method of removing a portion of the plasma from circulation. Venesection is performed, the blood is allowed to settle, the plasma is removed, and the red blood cells are returned to the circulation. Used in the treatment of those diseases caused by antibodies circulating in the patient's plasma.

plasmin ('plazmin) a fibrinolysin found in blood plasma which can dissolve fibrin clots.

plasminogen (plaz'minəjən) the inactive precursor of plasmin.

Plasmodium (plaz'mohdi·əm) a genus of protozoan parasites in the red blood cells of animals and man. Four species, *P. falciparum, P. malariae, P. ovale* and *P. vivax,* cause the four specific types of human malaria.

plaster ('plahstə, 'plastə) 1. a mixture of materials that hardens; used for immobilizing or making impressions of body parts. 2. an adhesive substance spread on fabric or other suitable backing material, for application to the skin. *Bohler's p.* plaster for Pott's fracture. A leg splint of plaster of Paris, in which is embedded an iron stirrup extending below the foot, which enables the patient to walk without putting weight on the joint. *Corn p.* one impregnated with salicylic acid. *Frog p.* a plaster of Paris splint used to maintain the position after correction of the deformity due to congenital dislocation of the hip. *P. of Paris* calcium sulphate or gypsum which sets hard when water is added to it and is used to form a plaster cast to immobilize a part and in dentistry for taking dental impressions.

plastic ('plastik) 1. constructive; tissue-forming. 2. capable of being moulded; pliable. *P. lymph* the exudate which in wounds and inflamed serous tissues is organized into fibrous tissue and promotes healing. *P. surgery* the branch of surgery which deals with the repair and reconstruction of deformed or injured parts of the body, including their replacement, by tissue grafting or other means.

platelet ('playtlət) a disc-shaped structure present in the blood and concerned in the process of clotting. A thrombocyte.

platyhelminth (,plati'helminth) a flat-bodied worm. The flatworms include tapeworms and flukes.

play group (play) a session of care and activities for preschool children. It can be organized by any interested person at home or in other premises, but it must be registered by the social services department.

play specialist a person who is qualified to use play constructively to help children come to terms with illness and hospitalization.

play therapist one trained in the skills of play therapy.

play therapy a technique used in child psychotherapy in which play is used to reveal unconscious material. Play is the natural way in which children express and work through unconscious conflicts; thus play therapy is analogous to the technique of free association used in adult psycho-

therapy.

pleomorphism (,pleeoh'mawfizem) occurring in more than one form. The existence of several distinct types of the same species.

pleoptics (pli'optiks) an orthoptic method of improving the sight in cases of strabismus by stimulating the use of the macular part of the retina.

plethora ('plethə·rə) a general term denoting a red, florid complexion, or specifically, an exccessive amount of blood.

plethysmography (,plethiz'mogrəfee) the measurement of changes in the volume of a limb due to alterations in blood pressure, using an oncometer.

pleura ('plooə·rə) the serous membrane lining the thorax and enveloping each lung. *Parietal p.* the layer which lines the chest wall. *Visceral p.* the inner layer which is in close contact with the lung.

pleurisy, pleuritis ('plooə·riseey; plooə'rietis) inflammation of the pleura; it may be caused by infection, injury, or tumour. It may be a complication of lung diseases, particularly of pneumonia, or sometimes of tuberculosis, lung abscess, or influenza. The symptoms are cough, fever, chills, sharp, sticking pain that is worse on inspiration, and rapid shallow breathing. *Dry (fibrinous) p.* pleurisy in which the membrane is inflamed and roughened, but no fluid is formed. *P. with effusion (wet p.)* type that is characterized by inflammation and exudation of serous fluid into the pleural cavity. *Purulent p.* or *empyema* the formation of pus in the pleural cavity. An operation for drainage is usually necessary.

pleurocele ('plooə·roh,seel) hernia of the lung or pleura.

pleurodynia (,plooə·roh'dini·ə) pain in the intercostal muscles, probably rheumatic in origin.

plexus ('pleksəs) a network of veins or nerves. *Auerbach's p.* the nerve ganglion situated between the longitudinal and circular muscle fibres of the intestine. They are motor nerves. *Brachial p.* the network of nerves of the neck and axilla. *Choroid p.* a capillary network situated in the ventricles of the brain which forms the cerebrospinal fluid. *Meissner's p.* the sensory nerve ganglion situated in the submucous layer of the intestinal wall. *Rectal p.* the network of veins which surrounds the rectum and forms a direct communication between the systemic and portal circulations. *Solar* or *coeliac p.* the network of nerves and ganglia at the back of the stomach, which supply the abdominal viscera.

plication (plie'kayshən) the taking of tucks in a structure to shorten it; a folding to decrease the size of a structure or organ during a surgical procedure.

plumbism ('plumbizəm) lead poisoning.

Plummer–Vinson syndrome (,pluma'vinsən) *H.S. Plummer, American physician, 1874–1936; P.P. Vinson, American physician, 1890–1959.* Difficulty in swallowing associated with glossitis and iron deficiency anaemia.

pneumatocele (nyoo'matoh,seel) 1. a swelling containing a collec-

tion of gas. 2. hernia of the lung.

pneumaturia (,nyoomə'tyooə·ri·ə) the passing of flatus with the urine owing to a vesico-intestinal fistula and air from the bowel entering the bladder.

pneumocephalus (,nyoomoh-'kefələs, -'sef-) the presence of air in the ventricles of the brain caused usually by an anterior fracture of the base of the skull.

pneumococcus (,nyoomoh'kokəs) the causative agent of lobar and bronchopneumonia and of other bronchial diseases. A Gram-positive, ovoid diplococcus, *Streptococcus pneumoniae*.

pneumoconiosis (,nyoomoh,kohni'ohsis) an industrial disease of the lung due to inhalation of dust particles over a period of time. *See* ANTHRACOSIS, ASBESTOSIS and SILICOSIS.

Pneumocystis (,nyoomooh'sistis) a genus of microorganisms of uncertain status, but usually considered to be protozoans. *P. carinii* the causative organism of interstitial plasma cell pneumonia, particularly in immunosuppressed patients, people with HIV infection or small children.

pneumodynamics (,nyoomohdie-'namiks) the mechanics of respiration.

pneumoencephalography (,nyoomoh·en,kefə'lografee, ,sef-) *see* ENCEPHALOGRAPHY.

pneumogastric (,nyoomoh'gastrik) pertaining to lungs and stomach. *P. nerve* the tenth cranial nerve to the lungs, stomach, etc. The vagus nerve.

pneumolysis (nyoo'molisis) the operation of detaching the pleura from the chest wall in order to collapse the lung when the two pleural layers are adherent. Pleurolysis.

pneumomycosis (ˌnyoomohmie-ˈkohsis) infection of the lung by microfungi. *See* BRONCHOMYCOSIS.

pneumonectomy (ˌnyooməˈnektəmee) partial or total removal of a lung.

pneumonia (nyooˈmohni·ə) inflammation of the lung with consolidation and exudation. *Aspiration p.* an acute condition caused by the aspiration of infected material into the lungs. *Broncho-p.* a descending infection starting around the bronchi and bronchioles. *Hypostatic p.* a form which occurs in weak, bedridden patients. *Lobar p.* an acute infectious disease caused by a pneumococcus and affecting whole lobes of either or both lungs. *Virus p.* inflammation of the lung occurring during some virus disease and secondary to it.

pneumonitis (ˌnyooməˈnietis) an imprecise term denoting any inflammatory condition of the lung.

pneumoperitoneum (ˌnyoomohˌperitəˈneeəm) the presence of air or gas in the peritoneal cavity, occurring pathologically or introduced intentionally for diagnostic or therapeutic purposes.

pneumoradiography (ˌnyoomoh-ˌraydiˈografee) radiographic examination of a cavity or part after air or a gas has been injected into it.

pneumotaxic (ˌnyoomohˈtaksik) regulating the rate of repiration.

P. centre the centre in the pons that influences inspiratory effort during respiration.

pneumothorax (ˌnyoomohˈthor-·raks) accumulation of air or gas in the pleural cavity, resulting in collapse of the lung on the affected side. The condition may occur spontaneously, as in the course of a pulmonary disease, or it may follow trauma to, and perforation of, the chest wall. *Artificial p.* is a surgical procedure sometimes used in the tratment of tuberculosis or following pneumonectomy. *Spontaneous p.* sometimes occurs when there is an opening on the surface of the lung allowing leakage of air from the bronchi into the pleural cavity. *Tension p.* is a particularly dangerous form of pneumothorax that occurs when air escapes into the pleural cavity from a bronchus but cannot regain entry into the bronchus. As a result, continuously increasing air pressure in the pleural cavity causes progressive collapse of the lung tissue.

podagra (pəˈdagrə) gout, particularly of the big toe.

podalic (pəˈdalik) relating to the feet. *P. version* a method of changing the lie of a fetus so that its feet will present.

podarthritis (ˌpodahˈthrietis) inflammation of any of the joints of the foot.

poikilocyte (ˈpoykilohˌsiet) an irregularly shaped red blood cell.

poikilocytosis (ˌpoykilosieˈtohsis) the presence of poikilocytes in the blood; poikilocythaemia.

pointillage (ˌpwanhtiˈahzh) [Fr.] a method of massage using the tips of the fingers.

poison ('poyzən) any substance which, applied to the body externally or taken internally, can cause injury to any part or cause death.

poisoning ('poyzəning) the morbid condition produced by a poison. The poison may be swallowed, inhaled (as in CARBON MONOXIDE POISONING), injected by a stinging insect as in a BEE STING, or spilled or otherwise brought into contact with the skin.

polioencephalitis (,pohlioh·en-,kefə'lietis, -,sef-) acute inflammation of the cortex of the brain.

poliomyelitis (,pohlioh,miеə-'lietis) an acute, notifiable, infectious viral disease that attacks the central nervous system, injuring or destroying the nerve cells that control the muscles and sometimes causing paralysis; called also polio, infantile paralysis and HEINE–MEDIN DISEASE. Paralysis most often affects the limbs but can involve any muscles, including those that control breathing and swallowing. Since the development and the use of vaccines against poliomyelitis, the disease has been virtually eliminated in Western countries, where vaccination rates are high, but is still common in many other parts of the world.

poliovirus (,pohlioh'vierəs) a small RNA-containing virus which causes poliomyelitis.

Politzer's bag ('politsez) *A. Politzer, Australian otologist, 1835–1920.* A rubber bag attached to a eustachian catheter, for forcing air into the pharyngotympanic tube to clear it.

politzerization (,politsə·rie'zay-shən) insufflation of the middle ear and the pharyngotympanic tube by a Politzer bag.

pollinosis (,poli'nohsis) hay fever; an allergy caused by various kinds of pollen. Pollenosis.

pollution (pə'looshən) the act of destroying the purity of or contaminating something.

polyarteritis (,poli,ahtə'rietis) inflammatory changes in the walls of the small arteries.

polyarthralgia (,poliah'thralji·ə) pain in several joints.

polyarthritis (,poliah'thrietis) inflammation of several joints at the same time, as seen in rheumatoid arthritis.

polycoria (,poli'kor·ri·ə) a congenital abnormality in which there are one or more holes in the iris in addition to the pupil.

polycystic (,poli'sistik) containing many cysts. *P. ovary disease* Stein–Leventhal syndrome. *P. renal disease* a hereditary disease in which there is massive enlargement of the kidney with the formation of many cysts. Severe bleeding into cysts can occur. End-stage renal disease can affect many members of one family.

polycythaemia (,polisie'theemi·ə) an abnormal increase in the number of red cells in the blood. Erythrocythaemia. *P. vera* a rare disease in which there is a greatly increased production of red blood cells and also of leukocytes and platelets. The skin becomes flushed, with cyanosis, thrombosis and splenomegaly.

polydactylism (ˌpoli'dakti,lizəm) the condition of having more than the normal number of fingers or toes.

polydipsia (ˌpoli'dipsi·ə) abnormal thirst. It may be a symptom of diabetes.

polymastia (ˌpoli'masti·ə) the presence in a human being of more than two mammary glands. Pleomastia.

polymorphonuclear (ˌpoli,maw-foh'nyookli·ə) 1. having nuclei of many different shapes. 2. a polymorphonuclear leukocyte.

polymorphous (ˌpoli'mawfəs) occurring in several or many different forms.

polymyalgia rheumatica (ˌpoli-mie,alji·ə roo'matika) persistent aching pain in the muscles often involving the shoulder or the pelvic girdle.

polymyositis (ˌpoli,mieoh'sietis) a generalized inflammation of the muscles with weakness and joint stiffness, particularly around the hips and shoulders.

polymyxin (ˌpoli'miksin) an antibiotic drug, used in the treatment of Gram-negative bacteria, particularly *Pseudomonas*.

polyneuritis (ˌpolinyuh'rietis) inflammation of many nerves at the same time.

polyneuropathy (ˌpolinyuh'rop-əthee) a number of disease conditions of the nervous system.

polyopia (ˌpoli'ohpi·ə) the perception of two or more images of the same object. Multiple vision.

polyp ('polip) a pedunculated tumour of mucous membrane. A polypus.

polypharmacy (ˌpoli'fahməsee) 1.

the administration of many drugs together. This increases the likelihood of side-effects from drug interactions and of non-compliance by the patient. 2. the administration of excessive medication.

polyposis (ˌpoli'pohsis) the presence of many polyps in an organ. *Familial p.* an hereditary condition in which large numbers of polyps develop in the colon, which may become malignant.

polyuria (ˌpoli'yooə·ri·ə) an abnormally large output of urine due to either an excessive intake of liquid or to disease, often diabetes.

pompholyx ('pomfəliks) an intensely pruritic skin condition in which vesicles appear on the hands and feet, particularly on the palms and soles. Typically occurring in repeated, self-limiting attacks.

pons (ponz) a bridge of tissue connecting two parts of an organ. *P. varolii* the part of the brain which connects the cerebrum, cerebellum and medulla oblongata.

Pontiac fever ('ponti,ak) an influenza-like illness with little or no pulmonary involvement, caused by *Legionella pneumophila*. It is not life threatening as is the pulmonary form known as legionnaires' disease. The name Pontiac fever comes from an outbreak of the disease in Pontiac, Michigan.

popliteal (ˌpopli'teeəl, pop'liti·əl) relating to the posterior part of the knee joint.

popliteus (ˌpopli'teeəs, pop'liti·əs)

the flat triangular muscle at the back of the knee joint.

pore (por) a minute circular opening on a surface. *Sweat p.* an opening of a sweat gland on the skin surface.

porphyria (paw'firi·ə) an inborn error in the metabolism of porphyrins, resulting in porphyrinuria. Two general types of porphyria are known: erythropoietic porphyrias, which are concerned with the formation of erythrocytes in the bone marrow; and hepatic porphyrias, which are responsible for liver dysfunction. The manifestations of porphyria include gastrointestinal, neurological and psychological symptoms, cutaneous photosensitivity, pigmentation of the face (and later of the bones), and anaemia with enlargement of the spleen.

porphyrin ('pawfirin) one of a number of pigments used in the production of the haem portion of haemoglobin.

porphyrinuria (,pawfiri'nyooə·ri·ə) the presence of an excess of porphyrin in the urine.

porta (pawtə) an opening in an organ through which pass the main vessels.

Portacath (pawtə,kath) a catheter to provide a central venous line; attached to it is an injectable depot which is placed under the skin.

portacaval (,pawtə'kayv'l) pertaining to the portal vein and the inferior vena cava. *P. anastomosis* the joining of the portal vein to the inferior vena cava so that much of the blood bypasses the liver. It is used in the treatment of portal hypertension.

Portage system ('pawtij ,sistəm) a method of behaviour modification taught to family members to enable them to assist their handicapped child in developing and acquiring skills for everyday living.

position (pə'zizhən) attitude or posture. *Dorsal p.* lying flat on the back. *Genupectoral* or *knee–chest p.* resting on the knees and chest with arms crossed above the head. *Lithotomy p.* lying on the back with thighs raised and knees supported and held widely apart. *Prone p.* face down. *Sims' p.* or *semi-prone p.* lying on the left side with the right knee well flexed and the left arm drawn back over the edge of the bed. *Trendelenburg p.* lying down on a tilted plane (usually an operating table at an angle of 45° to the floor), with the head lowermost and the legs hanging over the raised end of the table.

positive ('pozətiv) having a value greater than zero; indicating existence or presence, as chromatin-positive or Wassermann-positive; characterized by affirmation or cooperation.

positive end-expiratory pressure abbreviated PEEP. In mechanical ventilation, a positive airway pressure maintained until the end of expiration. A PEEP higher than the critical closing pressure holds alveoli open until the end of expiration and can markedly improve the arterial Po_2 in patients with a lowered functional residual capacity (FRC), as in acute respiratory failure.

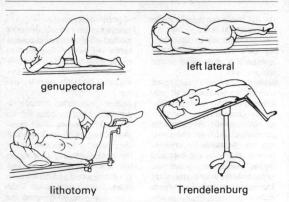

genupectoral

left lateral

lithotomy

Trendelenburg

GYNAECOLOGICAL POSITIONS

posseting (positing) regurgitation of a small amount of milk by an infant immediately after a feed.

Possum ('posəm) Patient-Operated Selector Mechanism; a machine that can be operated with a very slight degree of pressure, or suction, using the mouth, if no other muscle movement is possible. It may transmit messages from a lighted panel or be adapted for typing, telephoning, or working certain machinery.

postconcussional syndrome (,pohstkən'kushən'l) constant headaches with mental fatigue, difficulty in concentration and insomnia that may persist after head injury.

posterior (po'stiə·ri·ə) behind a part. Dorsal. *P. chamber* that part of the aqueous chamber that lies behind the iris, but in front of the lens.

posteroanterior (,postə·roh·an-'tie.ri·ə) from the back to the front.

postganglionic (,pohstgang·gli-'onik) situated posterior or distal to a ganglion. *P. fibre* a nerve fibre posterior to a ganglion of the autonomic nervous system.

postgastrectomy syndrome (,pohstga'strektəmee) *see* DUMI·ING.

posthitis (pos'thietis) inflammation of the prepuce.

posthumous ('postyuhməs) occurring after death. *P. birth* one occurring after the death of the father, or by caesarean section after the death of the mother.

postmature (postmə'tyooə) a state in which the pregnancy is prolonged after the expected date of delivery. Owing to the many variables it is difficult to estimate, but may exist when a pregnancy has lasted 41–42 weeks from the last menstrual period. There is a danger of hypoxia to the fetus.

postmortem (pohst'mawtəm) after death. *P.-m. examination* autopsy.

postnatal (pohst'nayt'l) after childbirth. *P. care* includes the care of the mother for at least 6 weeks after delivery. *P. clinic* an examination centre where the patient can be examined (postnatally), preferably 6 weeks following childbirth: (1) regarding her general health; (2) specifically, to find out the state of the uterus, pelvic floor and vagina. *P. depression* a low mood experienced by some mothers for a few days after the birth of their baby. Sometimes called 'baby blues'. *P. period* defined in law as a period of not less than 10 days and not more than 28 days after the end of labour, during which the continued attendance of a midwife on the mother and baby is requisite.

postpartum (pohst'pahtəm) occurring after labour.

postprandial (pohst'prandi·əl) occurring after a meal.

postural ('postyuhrəl) relating to a position or posture. *P. drainage* drainage of secretions from specific lobes or segments of the lung, aided by careful positioning of the patient.

potassium (pə'tasi·əm) *symbol* K. A metallic alkaline element which is a constituent of all plants and animals. Its salts are widely used in medicine. *P. chloride* a compound used orally or intravenously as an electrolyte replenisher. *P.*

citrate a diuretic, expectorant, and systemic alkalizer. *P. gluconate* an electrolyte replenisher used in the prophylaxis and treatment of hypokalaemia. *P. iodide* an expectorant and antithyroid agent. *P. permanganate* a topical antiinfective, oxidizing agent, and antidote for many poisons. *P. sodium tartrate* a compound used as a saline cathartic and also in combination with sodium bicarbonate and tartaric acid.

Pott's disease (pots) *P. Pott, British surgeon, 1714–1788.* Tuberculosis of the spine.

Pott's fracture a fracture-dislocation of the ankle, involving fracture of the lower end of the tibia, displacement of the talus and sometimes fracture of the medial malleolus.

pouch (powch) a pocket-like space or cavity. *P of Douglas,* the lowest fold of the peritoneum between the uterus and rectum. *Morison's p.* a fold of peritoneum below the liver.

poultice ('pohltis) a soft, moist, mass about the consistency of cooked cereal, spread between layers of muslin, linen, gauze or towels and applied hot to a given area in order to create moist local heat or counterirritation.

Poupart's ligament ('poopahts) *F. Poupart, French anatomist, 1616–1708.* The inguinal ligament. The tendinous lower border of the external oblique muscle of the abdominal wall, which passes from the anterior spine of the ilium to the os pubis.

povidone–iodine (,pohvidohn'ieə,deen) a complex of iodine with the polymer povidone; used as a topical anti-infective and in pre-operative skin preparation.

practice ('praktis) the exercise of a profession. *Family p.* the medical speciality concerned with the planning and provision of comprehensive primary health care, regardless of age or sex, on a continuing basis.

practitioner (prak'tishənə) a person who practises a profession. *See* NURSE PRACTITIONER.

PPR price precipitation reaction.

PPS pelvic pain syndrome.

practolol ('praktoh,lol) a drug used in the treatment of tachycardia and irregular heart rhythms. It is a beta-blocker and can only be given by injection.

precancerous (pree'kansə-rəs) applied to conditions or histological changes that may precede cancer.

precipitate (pri'sipi,tayt) a deposit of solid matter which was previously in solution.

precipitate labour unusually rapid labour with extremely quick delivery. There is danger to the mother of severe perineal lacerations, and to the child of intracranial trauma as a result of the rapid passage through the birth canal.

precipitin (pri'sipitin) an antibody, present in the blood, which when mixed in solution with its antigen forms a precipitate.

precocious (pri'kohshəs) developed in advance of the norm either mentally or physically or both.

precognition (,preekog'nishən) a direct perception of a future

event which is beyond the reach of inference.

precordium (pree'kawdi·əm) the area lying over the heart.

prediabetes (pree,die·ə'beetis, -teez) a state which precedes diabetes mellitus, in which the disease is not yet clinically manifested. In pregnancy the diabetes may become evident, or the patient may remain well but give birth to an unusually large child. Screening by urine testing can detect the condition.

predigestion (,preedie'jeschən, -di-) partial digestion of food by artificial means before it is taken into the body.

predisposition (,preedispə,zishən) susceptibility to a specific disease.

prednisolone (pred'nisəlohn) a synthetic corticosteroid used in the treatment of inflammatory and rheumatic conditions and of asthma and allergic skin diseases.

prednisone ('preni,sohn) a synthetic drug with an action and usage similar to prednisolone.

pre-eclampsia (,pree·i'klampsi·ə) a condition occurring in late pregnancy. The symptoms include proteinuria, hypertension and oedema.

pregnancy ('pregnənsee) being with child; the condition from conception to the expulsion of the fetus. The normal period is 280 days or 40 weeks. *Ectopic* or *extrauterine p.* pregnancy occurring outside the uterus, as in the uterine tube (*tubal p.*) or very rarely in the abdominal cavity. *P. tests* tests used to demonstrate whether conception has occurred. These detect the human chorionic gonadotrophin (HCG) produced by the embryo 8 days after the first missed period. Immunological laboratory tests are more accurate and less likely to give a false–positive result than an over-the-counter kit.

premature (,premə'tyooə) occurring before the anticipated time. *P. contraction* a form of cardiac irregularity in which the ventricle contracts before its anticipated time. *See* SYSTOLE. *P. ejaculation* emission of semen before or at the beginning of sexual intercourse. *P. infant* a child weighing 2500 g or less at birth. *See also* PRETERM INFANT.

premedication (,preemedi'kayshən) drugs given preoperatively in order to reduce fear and anxiety and to facilitate the induction and maintenance of, and recovery from, anaesthesia.

premenstrual (pree'menstrooəl) preceding menstruation. *P. endometrium* the hypertrophied and vascular mucous lining of the uterus immediately before the menstrual flow starts. *P. tension* feelings of nervousness, depression and irritability experienced by some women in the days before their menstrual periods. Emotional and physical symptoms usually disappear with the onset of menstruation.

premolar (pree'mohlə) a bicuspid tooth in front of the molars on each side of the upper and lower jaws.

prenatal (pree'nayt'l) preceding birth; antenatal. *P. care* care of the pregnant woman before delivery of the infant.

prepuce ('preepyoos) foreskin; the loose fold of skin covering the glans penis.

presbycusis (,presbi'koosis) progressive bilateral deafness in old age.

presbyopia (,presbi'ohpi·ə) diminution of accommodation of the lens of the eye, due to a loss of elasticity, occurring normally with ageing, and usually resulting in hyperopia, or farsightedness.

prescription (pri'skripshən) a formula written by a physician, directing the pharmacist to supply the medication.

presenile (pree'seeniel) prematurely aged in mind and body. *See* DEMENTIA.

presentation (,prezən'tayshən) in obstetrics, that portion of the fetus which appears in the centre of the neck of the uterus.

pressor ('presə) a substance that can cause a rise in the blood pressure.

pressure ('preshə) stress or strain. The force exerted by one object upon another. *P. areas* areas of the body where the tissues may be compressed between the bed and the underlying bone, especially the sacrum, greater trochanters and heels; the tissues become ischaemic. *P. point* the point at which an artery can be compressed against a bone in order to stop bleeding. *P. sore* a decubitus ulcer; a bedsore. Ulceration of the skin due to pressure, which causes interference with the blood supply to the area.

presystole (pree'sistəlee) the per-

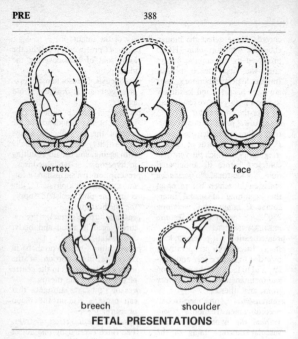

vertex   brow   face

breech   shoulder

FETAL PRESENTATIONS

iod in the cardiac cycle just before systole.

preterm infant ('preetərm) one with a gestational age of less than 37 weeks.

priapism ('prieə,pizəm) persistent erection of the penis, usually without sexual desire. It may be caused by local or spinal cord injury.

Price precipitation reaction (pries) *I.N.O. Price, British physician*, abbreviated PPR; a serological test for syphilis.

prickle cell ('prik'l) a cell from the inner layer of the epidermis possessing delicate rod-shaped processes, by which it is connected to other cells. *P.c. layer* the layer of the epidermis immediately above the basal-cell layer.

prickly heat ('priklee) miliaria; heat rash. A skin eruption characterized by minute red spots with central vesicles.

primaquine ('primə,kween) a drug used in the treatment of benign tertian malaria after initial treatment with other antimalarial drugs.

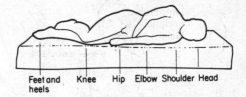

(a)

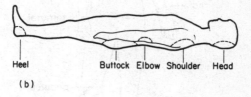

(b)

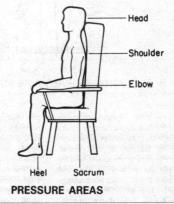

(c)

PRESSURE AREAS

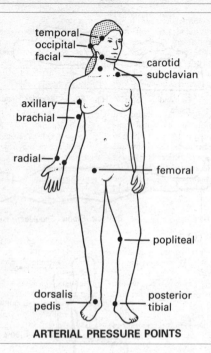

temporal
occipital
facial
carotid
subclavian
axillary
brachial
radial
femoral
popliteal
dorsalis pedis
posterior tibial

ARTERIAL PRESSURE POINTS

primary care ('priemǝree) the level of care in the HEALTH CARE SYSTEM that consists of initial care outside institutions. *P. health care* the care given to individuals in the community at the first point of contact with the primary health care team. First contact may be the general practitioner, a health visitor or a district nurse. *P. health care team* usually made up of a general practitioner, dis-

trict nurses, health visitors and possibly paramedical staff, such as a physiotherapist. They may serve a geographical area and be based in a health centre or a general practice area.

primary nurse a named nurse who is responsible for the planning, implementation and evaluation of nursing care for one or more patients/clients for the duration of their stay in hospital. The primary nurse delegates to an associate nurse when off duty but the primary nurse remains responsible and accountable for the patient's nursing care. *See* Appendix 1.

primary nursing Manthey (1980) described a system for delivering nursing care that consists of four design elements: (1) allocation and acceptance of individual responsibility for decision making to one individual; (2) individual assignment of daily care; (3) direct communication channels; and (4) one person responsible for the quality of care administered to patients on a unit 24 h a day, 7 days a week. *See* Appendix 1.

primidone ('primi,dohn) an anticonvulsant drug used in the treatment of major epilepsy.

primigravida (,priemi'gravidə) a woman who is pregnant for the first time.

primipara (prie,mipə·rə) a woman who has given birth to her first child.

probenecid (proh'benisid) a drug which increases the excretion of uric acid and is used between attacks of gout to prevent their occurrence.

problem-oriented record ('probləmorientid) a multiprofessional approach to patient care record keeping that focuses on the patient's specific health problems requiring immediate attention, and the structuring of a health care plan designed to cope with the identified problems.

procainamide (proh'kaynə,mied) a cardiac depressant drug used in the treatment of abnormal heart rhythms.

procaine ('prohkayn) a local anaesthetic used by infiltration. *P. penicillin* a long-acting antibiotic drug, chiefly used in the treatment of venereal diseases.

procarbazine (proh'kahbə,zeen) a monoamine oxidase inhibitor used in the treatment of some malignant conditions such as lymphadenoma.

process ('prohses) in anatomy, a prominence or outgrowth of any part. *P. of nursing see* NURSING PROCESS and Appendix 2.

prochlorperazine (,prohklor'perə,zeen) a tranquillizing drug used in the treatment of schizophrenia and other psychoses and also of vertigo, nausea and vomiting.

procidentia (,prohsi'denshi·ə) complete prolapse of an organ, particularly the uterus so that the cervix extrudes through the vagina.

proctalgia (prok'talji·ə) pain in the rectum and anus; proctodynia.

proctectomy (prok'tektəmee) surgical removal of the rectum.

proctitis (prok'tietis) inflammation of the rectum.

proctocele ('proktoh,seel) prolapse of a part of the rectum into the vagina; rectocele.

proctocolectomy (,proktohkə'lektəmee) surgical removal of the rectum and colon.

proctodynia (,proktoh'dini·ə) pain in the rectum and anus; proctalgia.

proctorrhaphy (prok'to·rəfee) suture of a wound in the rectum or anus.

proctoscope ('proktə,skohp) an

instrument for examination of the rectum. *Tuttle's p.* a speculum illuminated by an electric bulb, combined with an arrangement by which the rectum can be dilated with air.

proctosigmoiditis (‚proktoh‚sigmoy'dietis) inflammation of the rectum and sigmoid colon.

proctotomy (prok'totəmee) incision of the rectum or anus to relieve stricture.

procyclidine (proh'siekli‚deen) a drug used in the treatment of parkinsonism as it reduces muscle tremor and rigidity.

prodrome ('prohdrohm) a symptom which appears before the true diagnostic signs of a disease.

prodrug ('proh‚drug) a compound that, on administration, must undergo chemical conversion by metabolic processes before becoming an active pharmacological agent, thus avoiding gastrointestinal side-effects.

professional (prə'feshən'l) 1. pertaining to one's profession or occupation. 2. one who is a specialist in a particular field or occupation. *Allied health p.* a person with special training and licensed when necessary, who works under the supervision of a health professional with responsibilities bearing on patient care.

progeria (proh'jeeri·ə) premature senility, the signs of which appear in childhood.

progesterone (proh'jestə‚rohn) a hormone of the corpus luteum, which plays an important part in the regulation of the menstrual cycle and in pregnancy.

progestogen (proh'jestəjən) one of a group of steroid hormones having an action similar to that of progesterone.

proglottis (proh'glotis) a mature segment of a tapeworm.

prognathism ('prognə‚thizəm) enlargement and protrusion of one or both jaws.

prognosis (prog'nohsis) a forecast of the probable course and outcome of an attack of disease and the prospects of recovery as indicated by the nature of the disease and the symptoms of the case. *Nursing p.* the application of information obtained during a nursing assessment in order to determine the prospect for altering, through nursing intervention; a client's/patient's response to illness or injury. The prognosis provides a rationale for setting priorities for meeting a particular client's/patient's nursing care needs and enhances continuity of nursing care by clearly indicating the agreed-upon priorities.

proguanil (proh'gwahnil) a widely used drug which is taken daily to prevent malarial infection.

Project 2000 ('projekt too'thowzənd) Project 2000 (1986) is the title of the proposal of the United Kingdom Central Council (UKCC) altering radically the process of nursing education. *See* Appendix 11.

projection (prə'jekshən) in psychology, an unconscious process by which painful thoughts or impulses are made acceptable by transferring them on to another person or object in the environment.

prolactin (proh'laktin) a milk-producing hormone of the anterior lobe of the pituitary body, which stimulates the mammary gland. Now termed luteotrophin as it also stimulates the continued secretion of the corpus luteum.

prolapse ('prohlaps) the downward displacement of an organ or part of one. *P. of the cord* expulsion of the umbilical cord before the fetus presents. *P. of an intervertebral disc* abbreviated PID. Displacement of part of an intervertebral disc; 'slipped disc'. *P. of the iris* protrusion of a part of the iris through a wound in the cornea. *P. of the rectum* protrusion of the mucous membrane, through the anal canal to the exterior. *P. of the uterus* descent of the cervix or of the whole uterus into the vagina owing to a weakening of its supporting ligaments.

proliferation (prə,lifə'rayshən) rapid multiplication of cells, as may occur in a malignant growth and during wound healing.

promazine ('prohmə,zeen) a tranquillizing drug used to treat confusion and anxiety in elderly patients.

promethazine (proh'methə,zeen) a powerful long-acting antihistamine drug used in conditions of hypersensitivity, e.g. hay fever, contact dermatitis, drug rashes, etc.

prominence ('prominəns) in anatomy, a projection, usually on a bone.

pronation (proh'nayshən) turning the palm of the hand downward.

prone (prohn) lying face downward.

propantheline (proh'panthə,leen) an antispasmodic drug that blocks the impulses from the vagus nerve to the stomach and is used in the treatment of peptic ulcer and spastic colon.

prophylactic (,profi'laktik) 1. relating to prophylaxis. 2. a drug used to prevent a disease developing.

prophylaxis (,profi'laksis) measures taken to prevent a disease.

propranolol (proh'pranə,lol) a beta-blocking drug used in the treatment of cardiac arrhythmias, angina, thyrotoxicosis and also of anxiety states.

proprietary name (prə'prieətə-·ree) the name assigned to a drug by the firm which first made it. A drug may have several different proprietary names.

proprioceptor (,prohprioh'septə) one of the sensory end-organs that provide information about movements and position of the body. They occur chiefly in the muscles, tendons, joint capsules and labyrinth.

proptosis (prop'tohsis) forward displacement of the eyeball; exophthalmus.

propylthiouracil (,prohpil,thieoh-'yooə-rəsil) a thyroid inhibitor used in the treatment of thyrotoxicosis.

prostacyclin (,prostə'sieklin) an intermediate in the metabolic pathway of arachidonic acid, formed from prostaglandin endoperoxides in the walls of arteries and veins; it is a potent vasodilator and a potent inhibitor of platelet aggregation.

prostaglandin (ˌprostəˈglandin) one of several hormone substances produced in many body tissues including the brain, lungs, uterus and semen. They are active in many ways, having cardiac, gastric and respiratory effects and causing uterine contractions. They are sometimes used for the induction of abortion. Chemically they are fatty acids.

prostate ('prostayt) the gland surrounding the male urethra at its junction with the bladder; during ejaculation it produces a fluid which forms part of the semen. It often becomes enlarged after middle age and may require removal if it causes obstruction to the outflow of urine.

prostatectomy (ˌprostəˈtektəmee) surgical removal of the whole or a part of the prostate gland. *Retropubic p.* removal of the gland by incising the capsule of the prostate after making a suprapubic abdominal incision. *Transurethral p.* resection of the gland through the urethra using a resectoscope. *Transvesical p.* removal of the gland by incising the bladder following a low abdominal incision.

prostatitis (ˌprostəˈtietis) inflammation of the prostate gland.

prostatorrhoea (ˌprostətəˈreeə) a thin urethral discharge from the prostate gland, occurring in prostatitis.

prosthesis ('pros·theesis) [Gr.] 1. the replacement of an absent part by an artificial substitute. 2. an artificial substitute for a missing part.

prostration (proˈstrayshən) a condition of extreme exhaustion.

protamine ('prohtəˌmeen) one of a number of proteins occurring only in fish sperm. *P. sulphate* a drug used to neutralize circulating heparin should haemorrhage arise during anticoagulant therapy.

protanopia (ˌprohtəˈnohpi-ə) partial colour blindness for red hues.

protease ('prohtiˌayz) a proteolytic enzyme in the digestive juices that causes the breakdown of protein.

protective isolation (prətektiv ˌiesəˈlayshən) a type of ISOLATION designed to prevent contact between potentially pathogenic microorganisms and uninfected persons who have seriously impaired resistance. Called also reverse isolation.

protein ('prohteen) one of a group of complex organic nitrogenous compounds formed from amino acids and occurring in every living cell of animal and vegetable tissue. *Bence Jones p.* an abnormal protein found in the urine of patients suffering from multiple myeloma. *First class p.* one that provides the essential amino acids. Sources are meat, poultry, fish, cheese, eggs and milk. *Second class p.* one that comes from a vegetable source (e.g. peas, beans and whole cereal), which cannot supply all the body's needs. *P.-bound iodine* the iodine in the plasma which is combined with protein. Measurement of this is made when assessing thyroid function. *P.-losing enteropathy* a condition in which protein is lost from the lumen of the intestine. This causes hypo-proteinaemia and oedema.

proteinuria (,prohti'nyooə·ri·ə) an excess of serum proteins in the urine.

proteolysis (,prohti'olisis) the processes by which proteins are reduced to an absorbable form by digestive enzymes in the stomach and intestines.

proteolytic (,prohtioh'litik) 1. pertaining to, characterized by, or promoting proteolysis. 2. a proteolytic enzyme.

proteose ('prohti,ohz) one of the first products in the breakdown of proteins.

Proteus ('prohti·əs) a genus of Gram-negative bacteria common in the intestines of man and animals and in decaying matter. They are frequently to be found in secondary infections of wounds and in the urinary tract.

prothrombin (proh'thrombin) a constituent of blood plasma, the precursor of thrombin, which is formed in the presence of calcium salts and thrombokinase when blood is shed. *P. time* a test to measure the activity of clotting factors. Deficiency of any of these factors leads to a prolongation of clotting time. This test is widely used for the establishment and maintenance of anticoagulant therapy.

protoplasm ('prohtə,plazəm) the essential chemical compound of which living cells are made.

prototype ('prohtə,tiep) the original form from which all other forms are derived.

Protozoa (,prohtə'zoh·ə) a phylum comprising the unicellular

eukaryotic organisms; most are free-living but some lead commensalistic, mutualistic or parasitic existences. Pathogenic protozoa include *Entamoeba histolytica* (cause of amoebic dysentery) and *Plasmodium vivax* (cause of malaria). *See* METAZOA.

protriptylene (proh'triptə,leen) an antidepressant drug used in the treatment of extreme apathy and withdrawal.

protuberance (prə'tyoobə·rəns) in anatomy, a rounded projecting part.

provitamin (proh'vitamin) a precursor of a vitamin. *P. 'A'* carotene. *P. 'D'* ergosterol.

proximal ('proksiməl) in anatomy, nearest that point which is considered the centre of a system; the opposite to distal.

prurigo (prooə'riegoh) a chronic skin disease with an irritating papular eruption.

pruritus (prooə'rietis) great irritation of the skin. It may affect the whole surface of the body, as in certain skin diseases and nervous disorders, or it may be limited in area, especially involving the anus and vulva.

prussic acid ('prusik) hydrocyanic acid.

pseudarthrosis (,syoodah'throhsis) a false joint formed when the two parts of a fractured bone have failed to unite together.

pseudoangina (,syoodoh·an'jienə) false angina. Precordial pain occurring in anxious individuals without evidence of organic heart disease.

pseudocoxalgia (,syoodohkok-'salji·ə) osteochondritis of the head of the femur. Perthes' disease.

pseudocrisis (,syoodoh'kriesis) a false crisis which is sometimes accompanied by the symptoms of true crisis, but in which the temperature rises again almost at once, and there is continuation of the disease.

pseudocyesis (,syoodohsie'eesis) false pregnancy; development of all the signs of pregnancy without the presence of an embryo.

pseudogynaecomastia (,syoodoh-,gienəkoh'masti·ə) the deposition of adipose tissue in the male breast that may give the appearance of enlarged mammary glands.

pseudohermaphroditism (,syoodoh·hər'mafrədi,tizəm) a congenital abnormality in which the external genitalia are characteristic of the opposite sex and confusion may arise as to the true sex of the individual.

pseudoisochromatic chart (,syoodoh,iesohkrə'matik) a chart of coloured dots for testing colour-blindness. Ishihara colour chart.

Pseudomonas (,syoodoh'mohnəs) a genus of Gram-negative motile bacilli commonly found in decaying organic matter. *P. pyocyanea* (*P. aeruginosa*) one found in pus from wounds ('blue pus') and also in urinary tract infections.

pseudomyopia (,syoodohmie'ohpi·ə) spasm of the ciliary muscle causing the same focusing defect as in myopia.

pseudoparalysis (,syoodohpə'ralisis) apparent loss of muscular power without real paralysis. *Arthritic general p.* a condition resembling dementia paralytica,

dependent on intracranial atheroma in arthritic patients. Called also Klippel's disease. *Parrot's p.*, *syphilitic p.* pseudoparalysis of one or more extremities in infants, due to syphilitic osteochrondritis of an epiphysis.

pseudoplegia (,syoodoh'pleeji·ə) hysterical paralysis.

pseudopodium (,syoodoh'pohdi·əm) a temporary protrusion of a part of an amoeba which enables it to move and to ingest food.

psittacosis (,sitə'kohsis) a disease of parrots and budgerigars due to *Chlamydia psittaci*. Communicable to man, the symptoms resemble paratyphoid fever with bronchopneumonia.

psoas ('soh·əs) a long muscle originating from the lumbar spine with insertion into the lesser trochanter of the femur. It flexes the hip joint. *P. abscess* one that arises in the lumbar region and is due to spinal caries as a result of tuberculous infection.

psoriasis (sə'rieəsis) a chronic, recurrent skin disease characterized by reddish marginated patches with profuse silvery scaling on extensor surfaces like the knees and elbow, but which may be more widespread. It is noninfectious and the cause is unknown. It tends to occur in families; about one-third of the cases are believed to be related to a hereditary factor.

psyche ('siekee) the mind, both conscious and unconscious.

psychedelic (,siekə'delik) mind-altering; a term applied to hallucinatory or psychotomimetic drugs capable of profound effects upon the nature of perception and conscious experience. *See also* HALLUCINOGEN.

psychiatrist (sie'kieətrist) a doctor who specializes in psychiatry.

psychiatry (sie'kieətree) the branch of medicine that deals with the study, treatment and prevention of mental illness.

psychoanalysis (,siekoh·ə'nalisis) 1. a method of investigating mental processes, developed by Sigmund Freud, which uses the techniques of free association, interpretation, and dream analysis. 2. a system of theoretical psychology formulated by Freud based on the recognition of unconscious mental processes, such as resistance, repression, and transference, and of the importance of infantile experience as a determinant of adult behaviour. 3. a method of psychotherapy based on the psychoanalytical method and psychoanalytical psychology.

psychoanalyst (,siekoh'anə,list) one who specializes in psychoanalysis.

psychodrama (,siekoh'drahmə) group PSYCHOTHERAPY in which patients dramatize their individual conflicting situations of daily life.

psychodynamics (,siekohdie'namiks) the understanding and interpretation of psychiatric symptoms or abnormal behaviour in terms of unconscious mental mechanisms.

psychogenic (,siekoh'jenik) originating in the mind. *P. illness* a disorder having a psychological origin as opposed to an organic basis.

psychogeriatrics (,siekoh,jeri-'atriks) the study and treatment of the psychological and psychiatric problems of the aged.

psychologist (sie,koləjist) one who studies normal and abnormal mental processes, development and behaviour.

psychology (sie'koləjee) the study of the mind and mental processes.

psychometrics (,siekoh'metriks) the measurement of mental characteristics by means of a series of tests.

psychomotor (,siekoh'mohtə) related to the motor effects of mental activity. The term is applied to those mental disorders which affect muscular activity.

psychoneurosis (,siekohnyuh-'rohsis) a mental disorder characterized by an abnormal mental response to a normal stimulus. The psychoneuroses include anxiety states, depression, hysteria and obsessive-compulsive neurosis.

psychopath ('siekoh,path) *see* SOCIOPATH.

psychopathic disorder (,siekoh-'pathik) a persistent disorder or disability of the mind (whether or not including significant impairment of intelligence) which results in abnormally aggressive or seriously irresponsible conduct on the part of the patient (Mental Health Act 1983).

psychopathology (,siekohpə'tholəjee) the study of the causes and processes of mental disorders.

psychopharmacology (,siekoh-,fahmə'koləjee) the study of drugs which have an action on the mind and how such action is produced.

psychoprophylaxis (ˌsiekoh.profiˈlaksis) 1. a psychological technique used to prevent emotional disturbances. 2. a technique involving breathing control and exercises used to relieve pain during childbirth.

psychosexual (ˌsiekoh'seksyooəl) relating to the mental aspects of sex. *P. development* the stages through which an individual passes from birth to full maturity, especially in regard to sexual urges, in the total development of the person.

psychosis (sie'kohsis) any major mental disorder of organic or emotional origin, marked by derangement of the personality and loss of contact with reality, often with delusions, hallucinations or illusions. Psychoses are usually classified as functional psychoses, those for which no physical cause has been discovered, and organic psychoses, which are the result of organic damage to the brain.

psychosomatic (ˌsiekohsə'matik) relating to the mind and the body. *P. disorders* those illnesses in some individuals in which emotional factors (either causative or aggravating) have a profound influence, including anorexia nervosa and asthma respectively.

psychotherapy (ˌsiekoh'therəpee) any of a number of related techniques for treating mental illness by psychological methods. These techniques are similar in that they all rely mainly on establishing communication between the therapist and the patient as a means of understanding and modifying the patient's behaviour. On occasion, drugs may be used, but only in order to make this communication easier.

psychotomimetic (sie'kotohmiˈmetik) a drug that produces symptoms similar to those of a psychosis with an abnormal mental state, mood changes, and delusions.

psychotrophic (ˌsiekoh'trohfik) pertaining to drugs that have an effect on the psyche. These include antidepressants, stimulants, sedatives and tranquillizers.

pterygium (tə'riji.əm) a winglike structure, especially an abnormal triangular fold of membrane from the conjunctiva to the cornea.

pteroylglutamic acid (ˌteroh.il.gloo'tamik) folic acid.

ptosis ('tohsis) 1. dropping of the upper eyelid due to paralysis of the third cranial nerve. It may be congenital or acquired. 2. prolapse of an organ; e.g. gastroptosis.

ptyalin ('tieəlin) an eyzyme (amylase) in saliva which metabolizes starches.

ptyalism ('tieə.lizəm) an abnormally large secretion of saliva; sialorrhoea.

ptyalolith ('tieəloh'lith) a salivary calculus; a sialith.

puberty ('pyoobətee) the period during which secondary sexual characteristics develop and the reproductive organs become functional. Generally between the 12th and 17th year.

pubes ('pyoobeez) pubic hair or the area on which it grows.

pubic ('pyoobik) pertaining to the pubis.

pubiotomy (,pyoobi'otəmee) surgical division of a pubic bone during labour to increase the pelvic diameter.

pubis ('pyoobis) the anterior part of a hip bone. The left and right pubic bones meet at the front of the pelvis at the pubic symphysis.

public health ('publik) the field of medicine that is concerned with safeguarding and improving the physical, mental and social well-being of the community as a whole. Environmental aspects are the responsibility of the district local authority, whereas communicable disease control is supervised by the Medical Officer for Environmental Health, from the District Health Authority. Central government formulates national policy and is responsible for international aspects.

pudendal block (pyoo'dend'l blok) a form of local analgesia induced by injecting a solution of 0.5 or 1 per cent lignocaine around the pudendal nerve. Used mainly for episiotomy and forceps delivery.

pudendum (pyoo'dendəm) the external genitalia, especially those of a woman.

puerperal (pyoo'ərpə·rəl) pertaining to childbirth. *P. fever* or *sepsis* infection of the genital tract following childbirth.

puerperium (,pyooə'piə·ri·əm) a period of about 6 weeks following childbirth when the reproductive organs are returning to their normal state.

Pulex ('pyooleks) a genus of fleas. *P. irritans* that parasitic on man. The type which infests rats may transmit plague to man.

pulmonary ('pulmə,nə·ree, 'puhl-) pertaining to or affecting the lungs. *P. embolism* obstruction of the pulmonary artery or one of its branches by an embolus. *P. hypertension* an increase of blood pressure in the lungs usually following disease of the lung. *P. oedema* an excess of fluid in the lungs. *P. stenosis* a narrowing of the passage between the right ventricle of the heart and the pulmonary artery. The condition is frequently congenital. *P. tuberculosis see* TUBERCULOSIS. *P. valve* the valve at the point where the pulmonary artery leaves the heart.

pulp (pulp) any soft, juicy animal or vegetable tissue. *P. cavity* the centre of a tooth containing blood tissue and nerves. *Digital p.* the soft pads at the ends of the fingers and toes. *Splenic p.* the reddish-brown tissue of the spleen.

pulsation (pul'sayshən) a beating or throbbing.

pulse (puls) the local rhythmic expansion of an artery, which can be felt with the finger, corresponding to each contraction of the left ventricle of the heart. It may be felt in any artery sufficiently near the surface of the body which passes over a bone, and the normal adult rate is about 72/min. In childhood it is more rapid, varying from 130 in infants to 80 in older children. *Alternating p.* alternate strong and weak beats; pulsus alternans. *P.*

deficit a sign of atrial fibrillation; the pulse rate is slower than the apex beat. *High-tension p.* cordy pulse The duration of the impulse in the artery is long, and the artery feels firm and like a cord between the beats. *Low-tension p.* one easily obliterated by pressure. *Paradoxical p.* pulsus paradoxus; the pulse rate slows on inspiration and quickens on expiration. It may occur in constrictive pericarditis. *Running p.* little distinction between the beats. It occurs in haemorrhage. *Thready p.* thin and almost imperceptible pressure. *Venous p.* that felt in a vein; it is usually taken in the right jugular vein.

pulseless disease ('pulsləs) progressive obliteration of the vessels arising from the aortic arch, leading to loss of the pulse in both arms and carotids and to symptoms associated with ischaemia of the brain, eyes, face and arms. Called also Takayasu's arteritis or disease.

punctate ('pungktayt) dotted. *P. erythema* a rash of very fine spots.

punctum ('pungktəm) a point or small spot. *P. lacrimalis* one of the two openings of the lacrimal ducts at the inner canthus of the eye.

puncture ('pungkchə) 1. the act of piercing with a sharp object. 2. the wound so produced. *Cisternal p.* the withdrawal of fluid from the cisterna magna. *Lumbar p.* the removal of cerebrospinal fluid by puncture between the third and fourth lumbar vertebrae. *Sternal p.* the withdrawal of bone marrow from the

manubrium of the sternum. *Ventricular p.* the withdrawal of cerebrospinal fluid from a cerebral ventricle.

pupil ('pyoop'l) the circular aperture in the centre of the iris, through which light passes into the eye. *Argyll Robertson p.* absence of response to light but not to accommodation; characteristic of syphilis of the central nervous system. *Artificial p.* one made by cutting a piece out of the iris when the centre part of the cornea or the lens is opaque. *Fixed p.* one that fails to respond to light or convergence. *Multiple p.* two or more openings of the iris. *Tonic p.* one that reacts slowly to light or to convergence or both.

pupillary (pyoo'pilə·ree) referring to the pupil.

purgative ('pərgətiv) a laxative; an aperient drug. Purgatives may be: (1) irritants like cascara, senna, rhubarb and castor oil; (2) lubricants like liquid paraffin; (3) mechanical agents that increase bulk like bran and agar preparations.

purine (,pyooə·reen) a heterocyclic compound that is the nucleus of the purine bases (or purines) such as adenine and guanine, which occur in DNA and RNA. See PYRIMIDINE.

purpura (,pərpyuhrə) a condition characterized by extravasation of blood in the skin and mucous membranes, causing purple spots and patches. There are two general types of purpura: primary or idiopathic (usually autoimmune) thrombocytopenic purpura, in which the cause is unknown, and secondary or symptomatic thrombocytopenic purpura, which may be associated with exposure to drugs or other chemical agents, systemic diseases such as systemic lupus erythematosus, diseases affecting the bone marrow, such as leukaemia, and infections such as septicaemia and viral infections. *Allergic p.*, *anaphylactic p.* Schönlein–Henoch purpura; also called Henoch–Schönlein. *Idiopathic thrombocytopenic p.* abbreviated ITP. An acquired thrombocytopenia which may be acute or chronic in its course. Acute ITP is common in young children. The disorder is usually self-limiting and rarely fatal. Chronic ITP is more insidious in onset, and is more common in young adult women. *Schönlein–Henoch p.* non-thrombocytopenic purpura of unknown cause, most often seen in children, associated with various clinical symptoms, such as urticaria and erythema, arthropathy and arthritis, gastrointestinal symptoms and renal involvement. *P. senilis* dark purplish red ecchymoses occurring on the forearms and backs of the hands in the elderly; the platelet count is normal. *Steroid p.* purpura secondary to prolonged use of steroids. The platelet count is normal, the basic defect being the loss of supporting connective tissue. *Thrombocytopenic p.* purpura associated with a decrease in the number of platelets in the blood.

purulent (,pyooə·rələnt) containing or resembling pus.

pus (pus) a thick, yellow semi-liquid substance consisting of dead leukocytes and bacteria, debris of cells, and tissue fluids. It results from inflammation caused by invading bacteria, mainly *Staphylococcus aureus* and *Streptococcus haemolyticus* which have destroyed the phagocytes and set up local suppuration. *Blue p.* that produced by infection with *Pseudomonas pyocyanea*.

pustule ('pustyool) a small pimple or elevation of the skin containing pus. *Malignant p. see* ANTHRAX.

putative ('pyootətiv) supposed, reputed. *P. father* the man believed to be the father of an illegitimate child.

putrefaction (,pyootri'fakshən) decomposition of animal or vegetable matter under the influence of microorganisms, usually accompanied by an offensive odour due to gas formation.

pyaemia (pie'eemi·ə) a condition resulting from the circulation of pyogenic microorganisms from some focus of infection. Multiple abscesses occur, the development of which causes rigor and high fever. *Portal p.* pylephlebitis.

pyarthrosis (,pieah'throhsis) suppuration in a joint.

pyelitis (,pieə'lietis) inflammation of the renal pelvis. Pyelitis is a fairly common disease, particularly among young children, affecting girls more often than boys. The most common presentation includes urgency of micturition, frequency and dysuria. Pyuria is present.

pyelography (,pieə'logrəfee) *see* UROGRAPHY.

pyelolithotomy (,pieəlohti'thot-əmee) the surgical removal of a stone from the renal pelvis.

pyelonephritis (,pielohnə'frietis) inflammation of the renal pelvis and renal substance characterized by fever, acute loin pain, and increased frequency of micturition with the presence of pus and albumin in the urine.

pyeloplasty ('pieəloh,plastee) plastic repair of the renal pelvis.

pylephlebitis (,pielifli'bietis) inflammation of the portal vein which gives rise to severe symptoms of septicaemia or pyaemia.

pylethrombosis (,pielithrom-'bohsis) thrombosis of the portal vein.

pyloric (pie'lo·rik) relating to the pylorus. *P. stenosis* stricture of the pyloric orifice. It may be: (1) Hypertrophic, when there is thickening of normal tissue. This is congenital and occurs in infants from 4–7 weeks old, usually males and first babies. (2) Cicatricial, when there is ulceration or a malignant growth near the pylorus.

pyloromyotomy (pie,lo·rohmie-'otəmee) Ramstedt's operation; an incision of the pylorus performed to relieve congenital pyloric stenosis.

pyloroplasty (pie'lo·roh,plastee) plastic operation on the pylorus to enlarge the outlet. A longitudinal incision is made and it is re-sutured transversely.

pylorospasm (pie'lo·roh,spazəm) forceful muscle contraction of the pylorus that delays emptying of the stomach and causes vomiting.

pylorus (pie'lor·əs) the opening into the duodenum at the lower end of the stomach. It is surrounded by a circular muscle, the *pyloric sphincter*, which contracts to close the opening.

pyocolpos (,pieoh'kolpos) an accumulation of pus in the vagina.

pyoderma (,pieoh'dərmə) any purulent skin disease. *P. gangrenosum* a rapidly evolving cutaneous ulcer or ulcers, with undermining of the border. Once regarded as a complication peculiar to ulcerative colitis, it is now known to occur in other wasting diseases.

pyogenic (,pieoh'jenik) producing pus.

pyometra (,pieoh'meetrə) the presence of pus in the uterus.

pyonephrosis (,pieohnə'frohsis) obstruction and infection of the pelvis of the kidney. The calyces and pelvis are dilated, and contain pus.

pyopericarditis (,pieoh,perikah-'dietis) suppurative infection of the pericardium.

pyopneumothorax (,pieoh,nyoo-moh'thor·raks) pus and gas or air in the pleural cavity, usually associated with the partial or total collapse of the lung.

pyorrhoea (pieə'reeə) a discharge of pus. *P. alveolaris* pus in the sockets of the teeth; suppurative periodontitis.

pyosalpinx (,pieoh'salpingks) the presence of pus in a uterine tube.

pyosis (pie'ohsis) suppuration; the formation of pus.

pyothorax (,pieoh'thor·raks) the presence of pus in the pleural cavity; empyema.

pyramidal (pi'ramid'l) of pyramid shape. *P. cells* cortical cells

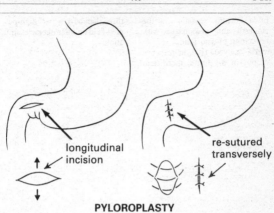

longitudinal incision

re-sutured transversely

PYLOROPLASTY

shaped like a pyramid from which originate nerve impulses to voluntary muscle. *P. tract* the nerve fibres which transmit impulses from pyramidal cells through the cerebral cortex to the spinal cord.

pyrazinamide (,pirə'zinəmied) a drug used in the treatment of tuberculosis, especially tuberculous meningitis.

pyrexia (pie'reksi·ə) fever; a rise of body temperature to any point between 37 and 40°C; above this is hyperpyrexia.

pyridostigmine (,piridoh'stigmeen) a drug that prevents destruction of acetylcholine at the neuromuscular junctions and is used in treating myasthenia gravis. It is less powerful than neostigmine but has a more prolonged action.

pyrixodine (,piri'dokseen) vitamin B₆. This vitamin is concerned with protein metabolism and blood formation. It is found in many types of food and deficiency is rare.

pyrimethamine (,pieri'methəmeen) a folic acid antagonist used as an antimalarial, especially for suppressive prophylaxis, and also used concomitantly with a sulphonamide in the treatment of toxoplasmosis.

pyrimidine (pie'rimi,deen) a nitrogen-containing organic compound. Thymine and cytosine are essential constituents of DNA, and uracil and cytosine of RNA. *See* PURINE.

pyrogen ('pieroh,jen) a substance that can produce fever.

pyromania (,pieroh'mayni·ə) an irresistible desire to set things on fire.

pyrosis (pie'rohsis) heartburn; a symptom of indigestion marked by a burning sensation in the stomach and oesophagus with eructation of acid fluid.

pyuria (pie'yoo‌·ri‌·ə) the presence of pus in the urine; more than three leukocytes per high-powered field on microscopic examination.

Q

Q fever ('kyoo ,feeva) an acute infectious disease of cattle which is transmitted to man usually by infected milk. It is caused by a rickettsia, *Coxiella burnetii*, and has symptoms resembling pneumonia.

QRS complex a group of waves depicted on an electrocardiogram; called also the QRS wave. It actually consists of three distinct waves created by the passage of the cardiac electrical impulse through the ventricles and occurs at the beginning of each contraction of the ventricles. In a normal ELECTROCARDIOGRAM the R wave is the most prominent of the three; the Q and S waves may be extremely weak and sometimes are absent.

quadrantanopia (,kwodrantə'nohpi·ə) loss of one quarter of the visual field.

quadratus (kwod'raytəs) four-sided. The term is used to describe a number of four-sided muscles.

quadriceps ('kwodri,seps) four-headed. *Q. femoris muscle* the principal extensor muscle of the thigh.

quadriplegia (,kwodri'pleeji·ə) paralysis in which all four limbs are affected; tetraplegia.

quality assurance ('kwolitee) in the health care field, a pledge to the public by those within the various health disciplines that they will work towards the goal of an optimal achievable degree of excellence in the services rendered to every patient. *See* COST EFFECTIVENESS and PERFORMANCE INDICATORS.

quarantine ('kwo·rən,teen) the period of isolation of an infectious or suspected case, to prevent the spread of disease. For contacts, this is the longest incubation period known for the specific disease.

quartan ('kwawtan) 1. recurring in 4-day cycles (every third day). 2. a variety of intermittent fever of which the paroxysms recur on every third day (*see* MALARIA).

Queckenstedt's test ('kweken-,stets) *H.H.G. Queckenstedt, German physician, 1876–1918.* A test carried out during lumbar puncture by compression of the jugular veins. When normal there is a sharp rise in pressure, followed by a fall as the compression is released. Blockage of the spinal canal or thrombosis of the jugular vein will result in an absence of rise, or only a sluggish rise and fall.

'quickening' ('kwikəning) the first perceptible fetal movement, felt by the mother usually between the fourth and fifth months of pregnancy.

quiescent (kwi'es'nt) inactive or at rest. Descriptive of a time when the symptoms of a disease are not evident.

quinalbarbitone (,kwinal'bahbi-,tohn) an intermediate-acting barbiturate drug used in the treatment of severe insomnia.

quinestrol (kwi'neestrol) a synthetic oestrogen used for the suppression of lactation after childbirth.

quinidine ('kwini,deen) an alkaloid obtained from cinchona. It is used in the treatment of cardiac arrhythmias.

quinine ('kwineen, kwi'neen) an alkaloid obtained from cinchona. Formerly used in the prevention and treatment of malaria. Still used to treat malignant tertian malaria.

quinsy ('kwinzee) a peritonsillar abscess; acute inflammation of the tonsil and surrounding cellular tissue with suppuration.

quotidian (kwo'tidi·ən) recurring every day. *Q. fever* a variety of malaria in which the fever recurs daily.

quotient ('kwohshənt) a number obtained by dividing one number by another. *Intelligence q.* abbreviated IQ. The degree of intelligence estimated by dividing the mental age reckoned from standard tests by the age in years. *Respiratory q.* the ratio between the carbon dioxide expired and the oxygen inspired during a specified time.

R

R symbol for the *roentgen* unit.

rabid ('rabid) infected with rabies.

rabies ('raybeez) hydrophobia; an acutely notifiable infectious disease of the central nervous system of animals, especially dogs, foxes, wolves and bats. The virus is found in the saliva of infected animals and is usually transmitted by a bite. Symptoms include fever, muscle spasms and intense excitement, followed by convulsions and paralysis, and death usually occurs. Vaccines are available.

racemose ('rasi,mohz) grape-like. *R. gland* a compound gland composed of a number of small sacs, e.g. the salivary gland.

radiant ('raydi·ənt) emitting rays.

radiation (,raydi'ayshən) the emanation of energy in the form of electromagnetic waves, including gamma rays, X-rays, infra-red and ultraviolet rays, and visible light rays. Radiation may cause damage to living tissues. *R. pneumonitis* inflammatory changes in the alveoli and interstitial tissue due to radiation which may lead to fibrosis later. *R. sickness* a toxic reaction of the body to radiation. Any or all of the following may be present: anorexia, nausea, vomiting and diarrhoea.

radical ('radik'l) dealing with the root or cause of a disease. *R.*

cure one which cures by complete removal of the cause.

radioactivity (,raydioh·ak'tivitee) disintegration of certain elements to ones of lower atomic weight, with the emission of alpha and beta particles and gamma rays. *Induced r.* that brought about by bombarding the nuclei of certain elements with neutrons.

radiobiology (,raydiohbie'oləjee) the branch of medical science that studies the effect of radiation on live animal and human tissues.

radiocolloid (,raydioh'koloyd) a radioactive isotope in the form of a large molecule solution which can be instilled into the body cavities to treat malignant ascites.

radiodermatitis (,raydioh,dərmə-'tietis) a late skin complication of radiotherapy in which there is atrophy, scarring, pigmentation and telangiectases of the skin.

radiograph ('raydioh,grahf, -,graf) skiagram; the picture obtained on a sensitive plate by X-rays passing through the body.

radiographer (,raydi'ogrəfə) a professional health care worker in a diagnostic X-ray department (diagnostic radiographer) or in a radiotherapy department (therapy radiographer).

radiography (,raydi'ogrəfee) the making of film records (radiographs) of internal structures of the body by exposure of film specially sensitized to X-rays or gamma rays. *Body-section r.* a special technique to show in detail images and structures lying in a predetermined plane of tissue, while blurring or eliminating detail in images in other planes; various mechanisms and methods for such radiography have been given various names, e.g. laminagraphy, tomography, etc. *Double contrast r.* a technique for revealing any abnormality of the intestinal mucosa, involving injection and evacuation of a barium enema, followed by inflation of the intestine with air under light pressure. *Neutron r.* that in which a narrow beam of neutrons from a nuclear reactor is passed through tissues; especially useful in visualizing bony tissue. *Serial r.* the making of several exposures of a particular area at arbitrary intervals.

radioisotope (,raydioh'iesə,tohp) an isotope of an element that emits radioactivity. These isotopes may occur naturally or be produced artificially by bombardment with neutrons.

radiologist (,raydi'oləjist) a doctor who specializes in the science of radiology.

radiology (,raydi'oləjee) the science of radiation. In medicine the term refers to its use in the diagnosis and treatment of disease.

radiomimetic (,raydiohmi'metik) producing effects similar to those of ionizing radiations.

radionuclide (,raydioh'nyooklied) a radioactive substance which is inherently unstable. It is used in both radiodiagnosis and in radiotherapy.

radioscopy (,raydi'oskəpee) the examination of X-ray images on a fluorescent screen.

radiosensitive (,raydioh'sensitiv) pertaining to those structures that respond readily to radiotherapy.

radiotherapist (,raydioh'therəpist) a doctor specializing in radiotherapy.

radiotherapy (,radioh'therəpee) treatment of disease by X-rays or radioactive isotopes.

radium (,raydi·əm) *symbol* Ra. A radioactive element obtained from uranium ores, which gives off emanations of great radioactive power. Used in the treatment of some malignant diseases.

râle (rahl) an abnormal rattling sound, heard on auscultation of the chest during respiration when there is fluid in the bronchi.

Ramsay Hunt syndrome (,ramzi 'hunt) *J.Ramsay Hunt, American neurologist, 1872–1937.* Facial paralysis accompanied by otalgia and a vesicular eruption involving the external canal of the ear, sometimes extending to the auricle, due to herpes zoster virus.

Ramstedt's operation ('ramshtets) *W.C. Ramstedt, German surgeon, 1867–1963.* Operation for congenital stricture of the pylorus in which the fibres of the sphincter muscle are divided leaving the mucous lining intact.

ranula (,ranyuhlə) a retention cyst usually under the tongue when blockage occurs in a submaxillary or sublingual duct, or in a mucous gland.

Ranvier's node ('ronhvi,ayz) *L.A. Ranvier, French pathologist, 1835–1922. See* NODE.

rape (rayp) sexual assault or abuse; criminal forcible sexual intercourse (i.e. penetration) without the consent of the adult or child. Many cases are not reported because of feelings of shame, guilt, embarrassment or fear. Although rape can occur between men (homosexual rape), it is usually associated with victims who are women.

raphe ('rayfee) a seam or ridge of tissue indicating the junction of two parts.

rapport (ra'por) in psychiatry, a satisfactory relationship between two persons, either the doctor and patient or nurse and patient, or the patient with any other person significant to him.

rarefaction (,rair-ri'fakshən) the process of becoming less dense.

rash (rash) a superficial eruption on the skin, frequently characteristic of some specific fever.

Rashkind catheter ('rashkint) *W.J. Rashkind, American paediatric cardiologist, b. 1922.* A balloon catheter used to increase the size of the atrial septal defect in children who have transposition of the great vessels.

rationalization (,rashənəlie'zayshən) in psychiatry, the mental process by which an individual explains his behaviour, giving reasons that are advantageous to himself or are socially acceptable. It may be a conscious or an unconscious act.

Rauwolfia (raw'wuhlfi·ə, row-) a genus of tropical trees and shrubs. The dried root of *R. serpentina* is sometimes used as an antihypertensive and sedative, e.g. reserpine.

ray (ray) a straight beam of electromagnetic radiation, which includes light and heat.

Raynaud's phenomenon (disease) ('raynohz) *M. Raynaud, French physician, 1834–1881.* Raynaud's phenomenon is characterized by episodic digital ischaemia provoked by stimuli such as emotion, cold, trauma, hormones and drugs. It includes both Raynaud's disease, where no underlying cause can be found, and Raynaud's syndrome, where there is an associated underlying disorder. These disorders include scleroderma, mixed connective tissue disease, systemic lupus erythematosus (SLE), polymyositis, rheumatoid arthritis, neurovascular entrapment syndromes and occlusive arterial disease.

RDS respiratory distress syndrome (infants).

reaction (ri'akshən) counteraction; a response to the application of a stimulus.

reactive (ri'aktiv) in psychiatry, used to describe a mental condition brought about by adverse external circumstances. *R. depression* one that arises in this way and is not endogenous.

reagent (ri'ayjənt) a substance employed to produce a chemical reaction.

recall (ri'kawl, 'reekawl) to bring back to consciousness.

receptaculum (,reesep'takyuhləm) a vessel or receptacle, *R. chyli* the pouch-like end of the thoracic duct.

receptor (ri'septə) 1. a sensory nerve ending that receives stimuli for transmission through the sensory nervous system. 2. a molecule on the surface or within a cell that recognizes and binds with specific molecules, producing some effect in the cell.

recessive (ri'sesiv) tending to recede. The opposite to dominant. *R. gene* a gene which will produce its characteristics only when present in a homozygous state; both parents need to possess the particular gene, and there is a 1 in 4 chance of a child inheriting it homozygously.

recipient (ri'sipi·ənt) one who receives, as a blood transfusion, or a tissue or organ graft. *Universal r.* a person thought to be able to receive blood of any 'type' without agglutination of the donor cells.

Recklinghausen's disease ('rekling,howzənz) *F.D. von Recklinghausen, German pathologist, 1833–1910.* Called also *von Recklinghausen's disease.* 1. neurofibromatosis. 2. OSTEITIS FIBROSA CYSTICA.

recrudescence (,reekroo'des'ns) renewed aggravation of symptoms following an interval of abatement.

rectal ('rekt'l) relating to the rectum. *R. examination* inspection by insertion of a glove-covered finger or with the aid of a proctoscope.

rectocele (,rektoh,seel) hernia or prolapse of the rectum usually caused by overstretching of the vaginal wall at childbirth. Procto-

cele.

rectoperineorrhaphy (,rektoh-,perini'o·rəfee) the operation for repair of the perineum and rectal wall.

rectopexy ('rektoh,peksee) the operation for fixation of a prolapsed rectum.

rectosigmoid (,rektoh'sigmoyd) the junction of the pelvic colon to the rectum.

rectovaginal (,rektovə'jien'l) concerning the rectum and vagina.

rectovesical (,rektoh'vesik'l) concerning the rectum and bladder.

rectum ('rektəm) the lower end of the large intestine from the sigmoid flexure to the anus.

recumbent (ri'kumbənt) lying down in the dorsal position.

recuperation (ri,koopə'rayshən) convalescence; recovery of health and strength.

recurrent (ri'kurənt) liable to recur. *R. fever* relapsing fever.

Redivac drainage tube ('redi,vak) a proprietary closed drainage system used mainly postoperatively for abdominal wounds.

reduction (ri'dukshən) 1. the correction of a fracture, dislocation or hernia. 2. the addition of hydrogen to a substance, or more generally, the gain of electrons; the opposition of oxidation. *Closed r.* the manipulative reduction of a fracture without incision. *Open r.* reduction of a fracture after incision into the fracture site.

re-education (,ree·edyuh'kayshən) the education and training of the physically or mentally handicapped person to enable him to develop his potential.

referred pain (ri,fərd 'payn) that which occurs at a distance from the place of origin due to the sensory nerves entering the cord at the same level, e.g. the phrenic nerve supplying the diaphragm enters the cord in the cervical region, as do the nerves from the shoulder, and so an abscess on the diaphragm may cause pain in the shoulder. Synalgia.

reflex ('reefleks) reflected or thrown back. *Accommodation r.* the alteration in the shape of the lens according to the distance of the image viewed. *R. action* an involuntary action following immediately upon some stimulus, e.g. the knee jerk, or the withdrawal of a limb from a pinprick. *R. arc* the sensory and motor neurones together with the connector neurone which carry out a reflex action. *Conditioned r.* that which is not natural, but is developed by association and frequent repetition until it appears natural. *Corneal r.* the automatic reaction of closing the eyelids following light pressure on the cornea. This is a test for unconsciousness which is absolute when there is no response. *Deep r.* a muscle reflex elicited by tapping the tendon or bone of attachment. *Light r.* alteration of the size of the pupil in response to exposure to light.

reflux (reefluks) a backward flow; regurgitation.

refraction (ri'frakshən) 1. the bending or deviation of rays of light, as they pass obliquely through one transparent medium and penetrate another of different

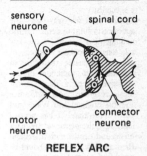

REFLEX ARC

density. 2. in ophthalmology, the testing of the eyes to ascertain the amount and variety of refractive error that may be present in each of them.

refractory (ri'fraktə-ree) not yielding to, or resistant to, treatment. *R. period* the period immediately after some activity during which a nerve or muscle is unable to react to a fresh impulse.

refrigeration (ri,frijə'rayshən) the therapeutic cooling of a part to reduce the metabolic requirements.

regeneration (ri,jenə'rayshən) renewal, as in new growth of tissue in its specific form after injury.

region ('reejən) a defined area of the body.

register ('rejistə) an epidemiological term meaning an index on file of all cases with a particular disease or condition in a defined population.

registrar (,reji'strah) 1. an official keeper of records. 2. in British hospitals, a doctor training to be a specialist.

registration (ˌrejiˈstrayshən) the act of recording; in dentistry, the making of a record of the jaw relations present or desired, in order to transfer them to an articulator to facilitate proper construction of a dental prosthesis. *R. of births and death* since 1837 in England and Wales and 1855 in Scotland it has been a legal requirement to register births and deaths with a General Register Office. Births should be registered within 6 weeks in England (21 days in Scotland). Without a death certificate which indicates that the death has been registered it is illegal to dispose of the body.

regression (riˈgreshən) 1. a return to a previous state of health. 2. in psychiatry, a tendency to return to primitive or child-like modes of behaviour. Some degree of regression frequently accompanies physical illness and hospitalization. Patients who are mentally ill may exhibit regression to an extreme degree, reverting all the way back to infantile behaviour (atavistic regression).

regurgitation backward flow, e.g. of food from the stomach into the mouth. Fluids regurgitate through the nose in paralysis affecting the soft palate. *Aortic r.* backward flow of blood into the left ventricle when the aortic valve is incompetent. *Mitral r.* mitral incompetence. *See* MITRAL.

rehabilitation (ˌreeəˌbiliˈtayshən) re-education, particularly of one who has been ill or injured, so

that he may become capable of useful activity. *R. centre* one which provides for organized employment within the capacity of the patient, and with especial regard to the psychical influence of the work.

rehabilitation evaluation of Hall and Baker (REHAB) an assessment system to identify the patient's level of normal, everyday living and work skills, and of any disturbed behaviour.

reinforcement (ˌree-inˈfawsmənt) the increasing of force or strength. In behavioural science, the process of presenting a reinforcing stimulus so as to strengthen a response. *See* CONDITIONING. A positive reinforcer is a stimulus that is added to the environment immediately after the desired response. It serves to strengthen the response, that is, to increase the likelihood of its occurring again. Examples of a positive reinforcer are food, money, a special privilege, or some other reward that is satisfying to the subject.

Reiter's protein complement fixation (ˈrietəz) *H. Reiter, German bacteriologist, 1881–1969.* Abbreviated RPCF. A serological test used to aid the diagnosis of syphilis.

Reiter's syndrome a non-specific urethritis, affecting males, in which there is also arthritis and conjunctivitis.

rejection (riˈjekshən) in immunology, the formation of antibodies by the host against transplanted tissue with eventual destruction of the transplanted tissue.

relapse (ri'laps, 'ree,laps) the return of a disease, after an interval of convalescence.

relapsing fever (ri'lapsing) one of a group of similar notifiable infectious diseases transmitted to man by the bites of ticks. Marked by alternating periods of normal temperature and periods of fever relapse. The diseases in the group are caused by several different species of spirochaetes belonging to the genus *Borrelia*. Called also recurrent fever.

relaxant (ri'laks'nt) a drug or other agent that brings about muscle relaxation or relieves tension.

relaxin (ri'laksin) a hormone that is produced by the corpus luteum of the ovary; it softens the cervix and loosens the pelvic ligaments to aid the birth of the baby.

releasing factor (ri'leesing) a substance produced in the hypothalamus which causes the anterior pituitary gland to release hormones.

REM rapid eye movement, a phase of SLEEP associated with dreaming and characterized by rapid movements of the eyes. Paradoxical sleep.

reminiscence therapy (remi'nisəns) measures to stimulate long-term elderly patients with memorabilia, films and songs meaningful to their generation. Used in conjunction with or as a prelude to reality orientation therapy.

remission (ri'mishən) subsidence of the symptoms of a disease for a long time.

remittent (ri'mitənt) decreasing at intervals *R. fever* one in which a partial fall in the temperature occurs daily.

remotivation (ree,mohti'vayshən) in psychiatry, a group therapy technique administered by the nursing staff in a psychiatric hospital or department, which is used to stimulate the communication skills and an interest in the environment of long-term, withdrawn patients.

renal ('reen'l) relating to the kidney. *R. calculus* stone in the kidney. *R. clearance tests* laboratory tests that determine the ability of the kidney to remove certain substances from the blood. *R. dialysis* the application of the principles of dialysis for treatment of renal failure (*see* below). *See also* HAEMODIALYSIS and PERITONEAL DIALYSIS. *R. failure* inability of the kidney to maintain normal function. It may be *acute* or *chronic*. Acute renal failure is a sudden, severe interruption of kidney function. It is normally the complication of another disorder and is reversible. Chronic renal failure is a progressive loss of kidney function. In its early stage, renal function can remain adequate, but the glomerular filtration ' rate (GFR) is depressed and plasma chemistry begins to show abnormalities as waste products accumulate. In the later stage, known as end-stage renal disease (ESRD), the GFR deteriorates and when URAEMIA becomes evident and the patient becomes symptomatic, dialysis is commenced or the patient transplanted. *R. threshold* the level of the blood sugar beyond which it is excreted in the urine; normally 0.18. *R. tubule* the thin tubular part of a nephron. A uriniferous tubule.

renin ('reenin) a proteolytic enzyme released into the bloodstream when the kidneys are ischaemic. It causes vasoconstriction and increases the blood pressure.

rennin ('renin) an enzyme present in gastric juice that curdles milk.

reorganization (,ri·awgənie'zayshən) healing by formation of new tissue identical to that which was injured or destroyed.

reovirus (,reeoh'vierəs) any of a group of RNA viruses isolated from healthy children, children with febrile and afebrile upper respiratory disease or children with diarrhoea.

repetitive strain injury (re'petitiv) a soft tissue disorder produced by repetitive use of muscle or tendon. Includes lateral epicondylitis of elbow (tennis elbow), medial epicondylitis (golfer's elbow), tenosynovitis of abductor pollicis longus and extensor pollicis brevis (de Quervain's syndrome), and achilles tendinitis.

replication (,repli'kayshən) 1. the turning back of a tissue on itself. 2. the process by which DNA duplicates itself when the cell divides.

replogle tube (ri'plohg'l) a double-lumen aspiration catheter attached to low pressure suction apparatus.

repression (ri'preshən) 1. the act of restraining, inhibiting or suppressing. 2. in psychiatry, a defence mechanism whereby a person unconsciously banishes unacceptable ideas, feelings or impulses from consciousness. A person using repression to obtain relief from mental conflict is unaware that he is 'forgetting' unpleasant situations as a way of avoiding them (motivated forgetting).

reproductive system (,reeprə-'duktiv) all those parts of the male and female body associated with the production of children.

resection (ri'sekshən) surgical removal of a part. *Submucous r.* removal of part of a deflected nasal septum, from beneath a flap of mucous membrane which is then replaced. *Transurethral r.* a method of removing portions of an enlarged prostate gland via the urethra.

resectoscope (ri'sektə,skohp) a telescopic instrument by which pieces of tissue can also be removed. Used for transurethral prostatectomy.

reserpine ('rezə,peen) an alkaloid from *Rauwolfia*, a drug used to reduce the blood pressure in hypertension.

reservoir ('rezə,vwah) 1. a storage place or cavity. 2. the host or environment in which an organism lives and from which it is able to infect susceptible individuals, e.g. hands, skin, nose and bowel.

residential care (,rezi'denshəl) the provision of care for frail, elderly people in a variety of settings, e.g. long stay hospital wards, local authority residential homes for the elderly or private nursing homes.

residual (ri'zidyooəl) remaining. *R. air, r. volume* the amount of air remaining in the lungs after breathing out fully. *R. urine* urine remaining in the bladder after voiding; seen with bladder outlet obstruction and disorders affecting nerves controlling bladder function.

resistance (ri,zistəns) the degree of opposition to a force. (1) In electricity, the opposition made by a non-conducting substance to the passage of a current. (2) In psychology, the opposition, stemming from the unconscious, to repressed ideas being brought to consciousness. *Drug r.* the ability of a microorganism to withstand the effects of a drug that are lethal to most members of its species. *Peripheral r.* that offered to the passage of blood through small vessels and capillaries. *R. to infection* the natural power of the body to withstand the toxins of disease.

resolution (,rezə'looshən) 1. in medicine, the process of returning to normal. 2. the disappearance of inflammation without the formation of pus.

resonance ('rezənəns) in medicine, the reverberating sound obtained on percussion over a cavity or hollow organ, such as the lung.

resorcinol (ri'zawsi,nol) resorcin; a phenol compound used in ointments and hair lotions in skin diseases.

respiration (,respi'rayshən) the gaseous interchange between the tissue cells and the atmosphere. *Artificial r.* the production of respiratory movements by external effort. *External r.* breathing, which comprises inspiration, when the external intercostal muscles and the diaphragm contract and air is drawn into the lungs, and expiration, when the air is breathed out. *Intermittent positive pressure r.* abbreviated IPPR. Respiration produced by a ventilator. *Internal* or *tissue r.* the interchange of gases which occurs between tissues and blood through the walls of capillaries. *Laboured r.* that which is difficult and distressed. *Stertorous r.* snoring; a noisy breathing. *See* CHEYNE–STOKES RESPIRATION.

respirator ('respi,raytə) an apparatus to qualify the air breathed through it, or a device for giving artificial respiration or to assist pulmonary ventilation (*see also* VENTILATOR). *R. shock* circulatory SHOCK due to interference with the flow of blood through the great vessels and chambers of the heart, causing pooling of blood in the veins and the abdominal organs and a resultant vascular collapse. The condition sometimes occurs as a result of increased intrathoracic pressure in patients who are being maintained on a mechanical VENTILATOR.

respiratory (ri'spiritə-ree, 'rəspirətree) pertaining to respiration. *Adult r. distress syndrome* abbreviated ARDS. A group of signs and symptoms resulting in acute respiratory failure; characterized clinically by tachypnoea, dyspnoea, tachycardia, cyanosis, and low Pao_2 that persists even with oxygen therapy. *R. distress syndrome of newborn* (abbreviated RDS), *idiopathic r. distress syndrome*, *infant r. distress syndrome* (abbreviated IRDS) a condition occurring in preterm infants, full-term infants of diabetic mothers, and infants delivered by caesarean section and associated with pulmonary maturity and inability to produce sufficient lung surfactant. Also called hyaline membrane disease. *R. failure* a life-threatening condition in which respiratory function is inadequate to maintain the body's need for oxygen supply and carbon dioxide removal while at rest; called also acute ventilatory failure. *R. insufficiency* a condition in which respiratory function is inadequate to meet the body's needs when increased physical activity places extra demands on it. *R. quotient* the ratio of the volume of expired carbon dioxide to the volume of oxygen absorbed by the lungs per unit of time. *R. syncytial virus* a virus isolated from children with bronchopneumonia and bronchitis, characteristically causing severe respiratory infection in very young children but less severe infections as the children grow older. *R. therapy* the technical speciality concerned with the treatment, management and care of patients with respiratory problems including administration of medical gases.

resuscitation (ri,susi'tayshən) restoration to life or consciousness of one apparently dead, or whose respirations have ceased. *See also* ARTIFICIAL RESPIRATION. *Cardiopulmonary r.* an emergency technique used in cardiac arrest to reestablish heart and lung function until more advanced life support is available.

retardation (,reetah'dayshən) delay; hindrance; delayed development. *Mental r.* subnormal general intellectual development, associated with impairment either of learning and social adjustment or of maturation, or of both.

retching ('reching) strong, involuntary effort to vomit.

retention (ri'tenshən) holding back. *R. cyst see* CYST. *R. defect* a defect of memory. Inability to retain material in the mind so that it can be recalled when required. *R. of urine* inability to pass urine from the bladder which may be due to obstruction or be of nervous origin.

reticular (rə,tikyuhlə) resembling a network. *R. formation* areas in the brain stem from which nerve fibres extend to the cerebral cortex.

reticulocyte (rə'tikyuhloh,siet) a red blood cell that is not fully mature; it retains strands of nuclear material.

reticulocytosis (rə,tikyuhlohsie-'tohsis) the presence of an increased number of immature red cells in the blood, indicating overactivity of the bone marrow.

reticuloendothelial system (rə-'tikyuhloh,endə'theeli-əl) a collection of endothelial cells in the liver, spleen, bone marrow and lymph glands that produce large mononuclear cells or macrophages. These are phagocytic; they destroy red blood cells and have the power of making some antibodies.

retina ('retinə) the innermost coat of the eyeball, formed of nerve cells and fibres, and from which the optic nerve leaves the eyeball and passes to the visual area of the cerebrum. The impression of the image is focused upon it.

retinal ('retinəl) relating to the retina. *R. detachment* partial detachment of the retina from the underlying choroid layer, resulting in loss of vision. It may result from the presence of a tumour, from trauma or from high myopia.

retinitis (,reti'nietis) inflammation of the retina. *R. pigmentosa* a group of diseases, frequently hereditary, marked by progressive loss of retinal function, especially associated with contraction of the visual field and impairment of vision. The disorder often follows a slow course over a period of many years, but there is considerable variation in the progression of the disease.

retinoblastoma (,retinohbla'stohmə) a malignant tumour arising from retinal cells. Occurs in infancy and may be hereditary. Treatment includes cryosurgery, irradiation and photocoagulation, but enucleation may be required.

retinopathy (,reti'nopəthee) any non-inflammatory disease of the retina. *Diabetic r.* a complication occurring in diabetes. Retinal haemorrhages occur, resulting in permanent visual damage and retinal detachment may follow.

Hypertensive r. retinal change occurring as a result of high blood pressure.

retinoscope ('retinə,skohp) an instrument which illuminates the retina and is used to detect and measure refractive errors. Retinoscopy.

retractile (ri'traktiəl) capable of being drawn back.

retractor (ri'traktə) a surgical instrument for drawing apart the edges of a wound to allow the deep structures to be more accessible.

retrobulbar (,retroh'bulbə) pertaining to the back of the eyeball. *R. neuritis* dimness of vision due to inflammation of the optic nerve.

retroflexion (,retroh'flekshən) a bending back, particularly of the uterus when it is bent backward at an acute angle, the cervix being in its normal position. *See* RETRO-VERSION.

retrograde ('retrə,grayd) going backwards. *R. amnesia* forgetfulness of events occurring immediately before an illness or injury. *R. urography* radiographic examination of the kidney by injecting an opaque substance into the renal pelvis through the urethra, using ureteric catheters.

retrolental fibroplasia (,retroh-'lent'l) a fibrous condition of the anterior vitreous body which develops when a premature infant is given too much oxygen. The condition now seldom occurs. Both eyes are affected and it may cause blindness.

retroperitoneal (,retroh,peritə-'neeəl) behind the peritoneum.

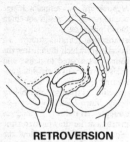

**RETROVERSION
OF UTERUS**

---

retropharyngeal (,retrohfə'rin-ji·əl, -,farin'jeeəl) behind the pharynx.

retropubic (,retroh'pyoobik) behind the pubic bone.

retrospection (,retroh'spekshən) a morbid dwelling on memories.

retrosternal (,retroh'stərnəl) behind the sternum.

retroversion (,retroh'vərshən) a lifting backwards, particularly of the uterus when the whole organ is tilted backward. *See* RETROFLEXION.

Reverdin's graft ('revərdanhz) *J.L. Reverdin, Swiss surgeon, 1842–1929.* A form of skin graft in which pieces of skin are placed as islands over the area. *See* THIERSCH'S GRAFT.

Reye's disease (riez) *R.D.K. Reye, 20th century Australian pathologist.* An acute, potentially fatal disease occurring in children in which there is fatty degeneration of the liver and the brain and raised intracranial pressure, accompanied by vomiting, con-

vulsions and coma. The cause of Reye's syndrome is unknown but administration of salicylates in children under the age of 12 is not recommended. This follows evidence that aspirin may be a contributory factor in the development of Reye's syndrome.

rhabdomyosarcoma (,rabdoh-,mieohsah'kohmə) a rare malignant growth of striated muscle. It grows rapidly and metastasizes early.

rhagades ('ragə,deez) cracks or fissures in the skin, especially those round the mouth.

rhesus factor ('reesəs) abbreviated Rh factor. The red blood cells of most humans carry a group of genetically determined antigens and are said to be rhesus positive (Rh^+). Those that do not are said to be rhesus negative (Rh^-). This is of importance as a cause of anaemia and jaundice in the newly born when the infant is Rh^+ and the mother Rh^-. The result of this incompatibility (isoimmunization) is the formation of an antibody which causes excessive haemolysis in the child's blood. *See* ANTI-RHESUS SERUM.

rheumatism ('roomə,tizəm) any of a variety of disorders marked by inflammation, degeneration, or metabolic derangement of the connective tissue structures, especially the joints and related structures, and attended by pain, stiffness, or limitation of motion. *Acute r.* or *rheumatic fever* an acute fever associated with previous streptococcal infection and occurring most commonly in children. The onset is usually sudden with pain, swelling and stiffness in one or more joints. There is fever, sweating and tachycardia, and carditis is present in most cases. Sometimes the symptoms are minor and ignored. This disease is the commonest cause of mitral stenosis as scar tissue results from the inflammation.

rheumatoid ('roomǝ,toyd) resembling rheumatism. *R. arthritis see* ARTHRITIS.

rheumatology (,roomǝ'tolǝjee) the branch of medicine dealing with disorders of the joints, muscles, tendons and ligaments.

rhinitis (rie'nietis) inflammation of the mucous membrane of the nose.

rhinopathy (rie'nopǝthee) any disease of the nose.

rhinoplasty ('rienoh,plastee) a plastic operation on the nose; repairing a part or forming an entirely new nose.

rhinorrhoea (,rienǝ'reeǝ) an abnormal discharge of mucus from the nose.

rhinoscopy (rie'noskǝpee) examination of the interior of the nose. *Anterior r.* examination through the nostrils with the aid of a speculum. *Posterior r.* examination through the nasopharynx by means of a rhinoscope.

rhinovirus (,rienoh'vierǝs) one of a genus of small RNA-containing viruses that cause respiratory diseases, including the common cold.

Rhipicephalus (,riepi'kefǝlǝs, -'sef-) a genus of ticks which can transmit the rickettsiae which

cause typhus and relapsing fever.

rhizodontropy (,riezoh'dontrǝpee) the fixing of an artificial crown on to a natural tooth root.

rhizotomy (rie'zotǝmee) division of a spinal nerve root for the relief of pain or of tic douloureux.

rhodopsin (roh'dopsin) the visual purple of the retina, the formation of which is dependent upon vitamin A in the diet.

rhomboid ('romboyd) any one of two pairs of muscles in the upper back which control the shoulder blades.

rhonchus ('rongkǝs) a wheezing sound produced in the bronchial tubes which is caused by partial obstruction and can be heard on auscultation.

rhythm ('ridhǝm) a regular recurring action. *Cardiac r.* the smooth action of the heart when systole is followed by diastole. *R. method* a contraceptive technique in which intercourse is limited to the 'safe period' (avoiding the 2–3 days immediately preceding and following ovulation).

rib (rib) any one of the twelve pairs of long, flat curved bones of the thorax, each united by cartilage to the spinal vertebrae at the back. *Cervical r.* elongation of the cervical processes towards the front of the chest. Pressure on this may cause impairment of nerve or vascular function. *See* SCALENUS SYNDROME. *False r.* the last five pairs, the upper three of which are attached by cartilage to each other. *Floating r.* the last two pairs, connected only to the vertebrae. *True r.* the seven pairs attached directly to the sternum.

riboflavin (‚rieboh'flayvin) a chemical factor in the vitamin B complex.

ribonuclease (‚rieboh'nyookli‚ayz) an enzyme from the pancreas which is responsible for the breakdown of nucleic acid.

ribonucleic acid (‚riebohnyoo-'klee·ik, -'klay-) abbreviated RNA. A complex chemical found in the cytoplasm of animal cells and concerned with protein synthesis. Certain viruses contain RNA.

ribosome ('riebə‚sohm) an RNA and protein-containing particle which is the site of protein synthesis in the cell.

rickets ('rikits) a condition of infancy and childhood caused by deficiency of vitamin D, which leads to altered calcium and phosphorus metabolism and consequent disturbance of ossification of bone, resulting in deformity such as bowing of the legs. Since the action of sunlight on the skin produces vitamin D in the human body, rickets often occurs in parts of the world where the winter is especially long, and where smoke and fog constantly intercept the sun. *Adult r.* osteomalacia; a rickets-like disease affecting adults. *Fetal r.* achondroplasia. *Late r.* OSTEOMALACIA, that occurring in older children. *Vitamin D-resistant r.* a condition almost indistinguishable from ordinary rickets clinically but resistant to unusually large doses of vitamin D; it is often familial.

Rickettsia (ri'ketsi·ə) a genus of microorganisms which are parasitic in lice and similar insects. The bite of the host is thus the means of transmitting the organisms, some of which are responsible for the typhus group of fevers.

rifampicin (ri'fampisin) an antibiotic drug used in leprosy and, with other drugs, in the treatment of tuberculosis.

rigor ('riegor) an attack of intense shivering occurring when the heat regulation is disturbed. The temperature rises rapidly and may either stay elevated or fall rapidly as profuse sweating occurs. *R. mortis* stiffening of the body which occurs soon after death.

Ringer's solution ('ringəz) *S. Ringer, British physiologist, 1835–1910.* A physiological solution of saline for topical use to which small amounts of calcium and potassium salts have been added.

ringworm ('ring‚wərm) tinea. A contagious skin disease, characterized by circular patches, pinkish in colour, with a desquamating surface, and due to a parasitic fungus.

Rinne's test ('rinəz) *H.A. Rinne, German biologist, 1819–1868.* A test for deafness in which the degree of conductivity through bone is tested by holding a vibrating tuning fork alternately in front of the ear and over the mastoid bone.

risk (risk) hazard, or chance of developing a disease or of complications following or during treatment. This may arise because of inherent problems with the treatment itself (e.g. drug side-effects) or because of the frailty of the patient. *R. factor* a factor which, when added to others, increases the likelihood of a disease or complication (e.g. smoking and obesity are risk factors for the development of coronary artery disease). *Relative r.* the likelihood of developing a disease after a given exposure; in epidemiological terms, calculated as: incidence rate of disease in an exposed group divided by incidence rate in the non-exposed group.

risus ('riesəs) laughter. *R. sardonicus* a peculiar grin caused by muscle spasm around the mouth, seen in tetanus and in strychnine poisoning.

RNA ribonucleic acid. *RNA viruses* viruses which contain ribonucleic acid as their genetic material.

Rocky Mountain spotted fever ('rokee 'mowntən, -tayn) a tick-borne infection caused by a *Rickettsia*, common in the USA, with rash, fever, muscle pain and often an enlarged liver. The disease lasts about 3 weeks.

rod (rod) a straight thin structure. *Retinal r.* one of the two types of light-sensitive end-organs of the retina, which contain rhodopsin and are responsible for night vision.

role (rohl) a pattern of behaviour developed in response to the demands or expectations of others; the pattern of responses to the persons with whom an individual interacts in a particular situation. *Sick r.* the role played by a person who has defined himself as ill. Adoption of the sick role changes the behavioural expectations of others towards the sick person. He is exempted from normal social responsibilities and is not held responsible for his condition; he is obliged to 'want to get well' and to seek competent medical help.

Romberg's sign ('rombərgz) *M.H. Romberg, German physician, 1795–1853.* Inability to stand erect without swaying if the eyes are closed. A sign of tabes dorsalis.

Rorschach test ('rorshahk) *H. Rorschach, Swiss psychiatrist, 1884–1922.* A personality trait test that consists of ten ink-blot designs, some in colours and some in black and white.

rosacea (roh'zayshi·ə) *see* ACNE ROSACEA.

roseola (roh'zeeələ) 1. a rose-coloured rash. 2. roseola infantum. *R. infantum* a common acute viral disease that usually occurs in children less than 24 months old; it attacks suddenly but disappears in a few days, leaving no permanent marks. *Syphilitic r.* an eruption of rose-coloured spots in early secondary syphilis.

Roth's spots (rohts) *M. Roth, Swiss physician, 1839–1915.* Small white spots seen in the retina early in the course of subacute bacterial endocarditis.

roughage ('rufij) coarse vegetable fibres and cellulose that give bulk to the diet and stimulate peristalsis.

rouleau ('rooloh) a rounded formation found in blood caused by red cells piling on each other.

roundworm ('rownd,wɜrm) any of various types of parasitic nematode worms, somewhat resembling the common earthworm, which sometimes invade the human intestinal tract and multiply there. Very common among them is the pinworm, or threadworm.

Rovsing's sign ('rohvsingz) *N.T. Rovsing, Danish surgeon, 1868–1927.* A test for acute appendicitis in which pressure in the left iliac fossa causes pain in the right iliac fossa.

RPCF Reiter's protein complement fixation.

rubefacient (,roobi'fayshənt) an agent causing redness of the skin.

rubella (roo'belə) German measles. An acute, notifiable virus infection of short duration, characterized by pyrexia, enlarged cervical lymph glands and a transient rash. The greatest risk from this disease is to the offspring of mothers who contract it during the early weeks of pregnancy. The child may be born with cataract or deformities, be a deaf mute or have other congenital defects.

rumination (,roomi'nayshən) recurring thoughts. *Obsessional r.* thoughts which persistently recur against the patient's will and from which he cannot rid himself.

rupture ('rupchə) 1. tearing or bursting of a part, as in rupture of an aneurysm; of the membranes during labour; or of a tubal pregnancy. 2. a term commonly applied to hernia.

Russell traction ('rus'l) *R.H. Russell, Australian surgeon.* A form of extension by use of skin traction and sling supports without the use of a splint. *See* TRACTION.

Ryle's tube ('rieəlz) *G.A. Ryle, British physician, 1889–1950.* A thin tube with a weighted end, introduced via the nose into the stomach. It may be used for the withdrawal of gastric contents or for the administration of fluids.

S

Sabin vaccine ('saybin) *A.B. Sabin, American biologist, b. 1906.* A live oral attenuated poliovirus vaccine active against poliomyelitis.

saccharide ('sakə,ried) one of a series of carbohydrates, including the sugars.

saccharin (,sakə·rin) gluside; a crystalline substance used as a substitute for sugar.

Saccharomyces (,sakə·roh'mie·seez) a genus of fungi, of which yeast is an example.

saccule ('sakyool) a small sac, particularly the smaller of the two sacs within the membranous labyrinth of the ear.

sacral ('saykrəl) relating to the sacrum.

sacroiliac (,saykroh'ili,ak) relating to the sacrum and the ilium.

sacrum ('saykrəm) a triangular bone composed of five united vertebrae, situated between the lowest lumbar vertebra and the coccyx. It forms the back of the pelvis.

sadism ('saydizem) a form of sexual perversion in which the individual takes pleasure in inflicting mental and physical pain on others.

sagittal ('sajit'l) arrow-shaped. *S. suture* the junction of the parietal bones.

salbutamol (sal'byootəmol) a sympathomimetic drug used in the treatment of bronchospasm.

salicylate (sə'lisə,layt) a salt of salicylic acid. *Methyl s.* the active ingredient in ointments and lotions for joint pains and sprains. *Sodium s.* the specific drug used for rheumatic fever. It reduces the pyrexia and relieves the pain but does not prevent cardiac complications.

salicylic acid (,sali'silik) a drug with bacteriostatic and fungicidal properties used in the treatment of skin diseases and, in concentrated form, to remove warts and corns.

saline ('saylien) a solution of sodium chloride and water. *Hypertonic s.* a stronger than normal strength. *Hypotonic s.* a weaker than normal strength. *Normal* or *physiological s.* a 0.9, solution which is isotonic with blood.

saliva (sə'lievə) the secretion of the salivary glands. When food is taken, it moistens and partially digests carbohydrates by the action of its enzyme, ptyalin (amylase).

salivary (sə'lievə·ree, 'salivə·ree) relating to saliva. *S. calculus* a stony concretion in a salivary duct. *S. fistula* an unnatural opening on the skin of the face leading into a salivary duct or gland. *S.*

glands the parotid, submaxillary and sublingual glands.

salivation (,sali'vayshən) 1. the process of salivating. 2. excessive salivation that may lead to soreness of mouth and gums. Ptyalism.

Salk vaccine (sawlk) *J.E. Salk, American virologist, b. 1914.* The first poliomyelitis vaccine of killed viruses, given by injection. *See* VACCINE.

Salmonella (,salmə'nelə) any of the genus of Gram-negative, nonsporing, rod-like bacteria that are parasites of the intestinal tract of man and animals. *S. typhi* and *S. paratyphi* are exclusively human pathogens which cause typhoid and paratyphoid fevers.

salmonellosis (,salmə ne'lohsis) infection with the genus *Salmonella*, usually caused by the ingestion of food containing salmonellae or their products. The organisms can be found in raw meats, raw poultry, eggs, and dairy products; they multiply rapidly at temperatures between 7 and 46°C. Symptoms of salmonellosis include violent diarrhoea attended by abdominal cramps, nausea and vomiting, and fever. It is rarely fatal and can be prevented by adequate cooking.

salpingectomy (,salpin'jektəmee) excision of one or both of the uterine tubes.

salpingitis (,salpin'jietis) 1. inflammation of the uterine tubes. *Acute s.* most often a bilateral ascending infection due to a streptococcus or a gonococcus. *Chronic s.* a less acute form that

may be blood borne. 2. inflammation of the pharyngotympanic (eustachian) tubes.

salpingography (,salping'gografee) radiographic examination of the uterine tubes after injection of a radio-opaque substance to determine their patency.

salpingo-oöphorectomy (sal,ping-goh,oh-əfə'rektəmee) removal of a uterine tube and its ovary.

salpingostomy (,salping'gostəmee) the making of a surgical opening in a uterine tube near the uterus to restore patency.

salpinx ('salpingks) a tube. Applied to the uterine or pharyngotympanic (eustachian) tubes.

salt (sawlt) 1. sodium chloride, common salt, used in solution as a cleansing lotion, a stimulating bath, or for infusion into the blood, etc. 2. any compound of an acid with an alkali or base. 3. a saline purgative such as Epsom salts. *S. depletion* a loss of salt from the body due to sweating or persistent diarrhoea or vomiting. Common in hot climates when it may be prevented by the taking of salt tablets. *Smelling s's* aromatic ammonium carbonate. A restorative in fainting.

salve (salv, sahv) an ointment.

sandfly ('sand,flie) a very small fly of the genus *Phlebotomus*, common in tropical climates and the vector of most types of leishmaniasis. *S. fever* a fever transmitted by the bites of sandflies, and common in Mediterranean countries. Similar to dengue and sometimes known as three-day fever.

sanguineous (sang'gwini·əs) pertaining to or containing blood.

saphena (sə'feenə) one of two superficial veins that carry blood from the foot upwards.

saphenous (sə'feenəs) relating to the saphena.

saponaceous (,sapə'nayshəs) soapy; having the nature of soap.

saponification (sə,ponifi'kayshən) the making of soap by combining a fat and an alkali.

sapphism ('safizm) female homosexuality; lesbianism.

sapraemia (sa'preemi·ə) a form of toxaemia. The toxins are produced by saprophytes and circulate in the blood.

saprophyte ('saproh,fiet) an organism bred in and living on putrefying animal or plant matter.

sarcoid (,sahkoyd) 1. tuberculoid; characterized by non-caseating epithelioid cell tubercles. 2. pertaining to or resembling sarcoidosis. 3. sarcoidosis.

sarcoidosis (,sahkoy'dohsis) a chronic, progressive, generalized disease resembling tuberculosis that may affect any part of the body but most frequently involves the lymph nodes, liver, spleen, lungs, skin, eyes and small bones of the hands and feet.

sarcoma (sah'kohmə) a malignant tumour developed from connective tissue cells, and their stroma. *Chondro-s.* one arising in cartilage. *Fibro-s.* one containing much fibrous tissue; this may arise in the fibrous sheath of a muscle. *Kaposi's s.* one principally involving the skin, although visceral lesions may be present; it usually begins on the distal parts of the extremities, most often on the toes or feet, as reddish-blue or brownish soft nodules and tumours. It is viral in origin and is frequently seen in AIDS. *Melanotic s.* a highly malignant type, pigmented with melanin. *Round-celled s.* a highly malignant growth, composed of a primitive type of cell.

sarcomatosis (,sahkohmə'tohsis) multiple sarcomatous growths in various parts of the body.

Sarcoptes (sah'kopteez) a genus of mites. *S. scabiei* the cause of scabies.

sardonic (sah'donik) pertaining to the grinning expression sometimes displayed in tetanus. *See* RISUS SARDONICUS.

sartorius (sah'tor·ri·əs) a long muscle of the thigh, which flexes both the thigh and the lower leg.

satyriasis (,sati'rieəsis) abnormally excessive sexual appetite in men.

scab (skab) the crust on a superficial wound consisting of dried blood, pus, etc.

scabies ('skaybeez) 'the itch'; a contagious skin disease caused by the itch mite (*Sarcoptes scabiei*), the female of which burrows beneath the skin and deposits eggs at intervals. It is intensely irritating, and the rash is aggravated by scratching. The sites affected are chiefly between the fingers and toes, the axillae and groins.

scald ('skawld) a burn caused by hot liquid or vapour.

scale (skayl) 1. a scheme or instrument by which something can be measured. A pair of scales is a balance for measuring weight. 2. compact layers of dead epithelial tissue shed from the skin. 3. to scrape deposits of tartar from the teeth.

scalenus (skə'leenəs) one of four muscles which move the neck to either side and raise the first and second ribs during inspiration. *S. syndrome* symptoms of pain and tenderness in the shoulder, with sensory loss and wasting of the medial aspect of the arm. It may be caused by pressure on the brachial plexus, by spasm of the scalenus anterior muscle or by a cervical rib.

scalp (skalp) the hairy skin which covers the cranium.

scalpel ('skalp'l) a small pointed surgical knife with a convex edge to the blade.

scan (skan) an image produced using a moving detector or a sweeping beam of radiation, as in scintiscanning. B-mode ultrasonography, scanography, or computed tomography.

scanning ('skaning) 1. visual examination of an area. 2. a speech disorder that may be present in cerebellar disease. The syllables are inappropriately separated from each other and are evenly stressed with rhythmically occurring pauses between them.

scaphocephaly (,skafoh'kefəlee, -'sef-) abnormal boat-shape of the head due to premature closure of the sagittal suture of the skull. Learning difficulties are usually experienced.

scaphoid (,skafoyd, 'skay-) boat-shaped. *S. bone* a boat-shaped bone of the wrist which articu-lates with the radius and with the trapezium and the trapezoid bones.

scapula ('skapyuhla) the large flat triangular bone forming the shoulder-blade.

scar (skah) the mark left after a wound has healed with the formation of connective tissue.

scarification (,skarifi'kayshən, ,skair·ri-) the making of small cuts or punctures of the skin to allow a vaccine to enter the body.

scarlet fever ('skahlət) scarlatina; an acute, notifiable, rare, infectious disease of childhood. It is caused by group A beta-haemolytic streptococcus. There is sore throat, high fever and a punctate rash. Now it is readily treated by antibiotics and the complications of nephritis and middle ear infection are less common.

Scheuermann's disease ('shoyə-,manz) *H.W. Scheuermann, Danish surgeon, 1877–1960.* Osteochondritis of the spine affecting the ring epiphyses of the vertebral bodies in adolescents.

Schick test (shik) *B. Schick, Austrian paediatrician, 1877– 1967.* A skin test of susceptibility to diphtheria. A small amount of diphtheria toxin is injected intradermally.

Schilling test ('shiling) *R.F. Schilling, American haematologist, b. 1919.* A test used to confirm the diagnosis of pernicious anaemia by estimating the absorption of ingested radioactive vitamin B_{12}.

Schirmer's test ('shiəməz) *O.W. Schirmer, German ophthalmologist, b. 1864.* A method of determining the quantity of lacrimal secretion by using standard-sized pieces of filter paper to collect the liquid produced in 5 min.

Schistosoma (,shistoh'sohmə) a genus of minute blood flukes, some of which are parasitic in man. *S. haematobium* a species which infests the urinary bladder; widely found in Africa and the Middle East, especially in Egypt. *S. japonicum* and *S. mansoni* species which infest the large intestine. They are found respectively in China, Japan and the Philippines, and in Africa, the West Indies and tropical America.

schistosomiasis (,shistəsoh'mieəsis) a parasitic infection of the intestinal or urinary tract by *Schistosoma*. The parasite enters the skin from contaminated water, and causes diarrhoea, haematuria and anaemia. The secondary hosts are freshwater snails.. Bilharziasis.

schizoid ('skitsoyd) resembling schizophrenia. *S. personality* one that is marked by introspection, self-consciousness, solitariness and a failure in affection towards others. Some schizophrenics have this personality, but only a few who are schizoid become schizophrenic.

schizophrenia (,skitsoh'freeni-ə) a general term encompassing a large group of mental disorders (the schizophrenic disorders) characterized by mental deterioration from a previous level of functioning and characteristic disturbances of multiple psychological processes, including delusions, loosening of associations, poverty of the content of speech, auditory hallucinations, inappropriate affect, disturbed sense of self, and withdrawal from the external world. *Paranoid s.* predominance of delusions of a persecutory nature. *Simple s.* a progressive deterioration of the patient's efficiency with increasing social withdrawal. *See* HEBEPHRENIA and CATATONIA.

Schlatter's disease ('shlatəz) *C. Schlatter, Swiss surgeon, 1864–1934.* Osteochondrosis of the tibial tuberosity.

Schlemm's canal (shlemz) *F. Schlemm, German anatomist, 1795–1858.* A venous channel at the junction of the cornea and sclera for the draining of aqueous humour.

Schönlein–Henoch purpura or **syndrome** (,shərnlien'henok) *J.L. Schönlein, German physician, 1793–1864; E.H. Henoch, German paediatrician, 1820–1910. See* PURPURA.

school health service the provision of medical and dental inspection and treatment in schools maintained by local education authorities. The National Health Service Reorganisation Act 1977 made this service a duty of the Department of Health and Social Security. It is now provided by the district health authority.

school nurse an RGN who has undertaken further training to specialize in the health care of school age children. Responsibilities include health promotion and education, monitoring growth and development, and screening and caring for those with special educational needs.

Schwartze's operation ('shwaw-tsəz) *H.H.R. Schwartze, German otologist, 1837–1910.* Opening of the mastoid cells, without involvement of the middle ear, in order to drain a mastoid abscess.

sciatica (sie'atikə) pain down the back of the leg in the area supplied by the sciatic nerve. It is usually caused by pressure on the nerve roots by a protrusion of an intervertebral disc.

scintigraphy (sin'tigrəfee) the recording of the distribution of radioactivity in an organ following injection of a small dose of a radioactive substance that is specifically taken up by that organ.

scirrhous (,sirəs) hard; indurated; resembling a scirrhus.

scirrhus ('sirəs) a hard carcinoma containing much connective tissue.

sclera ('skliə·rə) the fibrous coat of the eyeball, the white of the eye, which covers the posterior part and in front becomes the cornea.

scleroderma (,skliə·roh'dərmə) a disease marked by progressive hardening of the skin in patches or diffusely, with rigidity of the underlying tissues. It is often a chronic condition. *See* RAYNAUD'S PHENOMENON.

scleroma (sklə'rohmə) a patch of hardened tissue.

sclerosis (sklə'rohsis) the hardening of any part from an overgrowth of fibrous and connective tissue, often due to chronic inflammation. *Amyotrophic lateral s.* rapid degeneration of the pyr-amidal (motor nerves) tract and anterior horn cells in the spinal cord. Characterized by weakness and spasm of limb muscles with wasting of the muscle, difficulty with talking and swallowing. *Arterio-s.* the changes occurring in walls of arteries which cause hardening and loss of elasticity. *Athero-s.* the deposition of fatty plaques and hardening and fibrosis of the artery lining. *Disseminated s. see* MULTIPLE S. *Mönckeberg's s.* extensive degeneration with atrophy and calcareous deposits in the middle muscle coat of arteries, especially of the small ones. *Multiple s.* scattered (disseminated) patches of degeneration in the nerve sheaths in the brain and spinal cord. Characterized by relapses and remissions. Symptoms include disturbances of speech, vision and micturition and muscular weakness of a limb or limbs. *Systemic s. (scleroderma)* a generalized multisystem disease characterized by dense fibrosis of involved organs and a widespread vascular disorder. *See* RAYNAUD'S PHENOMENON.

sclerotherapy (,sklə·roh'therəpee) treatment of varicose veins and haemorrhoids by the injection of sclerosing solutions to produce fibrosis.

sclerotic (sklə'rotik) 1. hard; indurated; affected by sclerosis. 2. pertaining to the sclera of the eye. *S. coat* the tough membrane forming the outer covering of the eyeball, except in front of the iris, where it becomes the clear horny cornea.

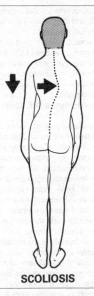

SCOLIOSIS

sclerotomy (sklə'rotəmee) incision of the sclerotic coat, usually for the removal of a foreign body or for the relief of glaucoma.

scolex ('skohleks) the head of a tapeworm. It is provided with hooks and suckers with which to hold on to the wall of the intestine.

scoliosis (,skohli'ohsis) lateral curvature of the spine. *See* LORDOSIS and KYPHOSIS.

scopolamine (skoh'polə,meen) hyoscine.

scorbutic (skaw'byootik) affected with or related to scurvy.

scotoma (skoh'tohmə) a blind area in the field of vision, due to some lesion of the retina. It is also found in glaucoma and in detachment of the retina.

screening ('skreening) 1. fluoroscopy. 2. the carrying out of a test on a large number of people to determine the proportion of them that have a particular disease.

scrotum ('skrohtəm) the pouch of skin and soft tissues containing the testicles.

scurf (skərf) dandruff.

scurvy ('skərvee) avitaminosis C. A deficiency disease due to lack of vitamin C found in raw fruits and vegetables. Clinical features include fatigue, oozing of blood from the gums and bruising. It rapidly improves with adequate diet.

scybalum ('sibələm) a mass of abnormally hard faecal matter in the intestine.

sebaceous (si'bayshəs) fatty, or pertaining to the sebum. *S. glands* are found in the skin, communicating with the hair follicles and secreting sebum. *S. cyst see* CYST.

seborrhoea (,sebə'reeə) a disease of the sebaceous glands, marked by an excessive secretion of sebum which collects on the skin in oily scales.

sebum ('seebəm) the fatty secretion of the sebaceous glands.

secondary ('sekəndree) second in order of time or importance. *S. deposits see* METASTASES.

secretin (si'kreetin) the hormone originating in the duodenum which, in the presence of bile salts, is absorbed into the bloodstream and stimulates the secretion of pancreatic juice.

secretion (si'kreeshən) a substance formed or concentrated in a gland and passed into the alimentary tract, the blood or to the exterior. The secretions of the endocrine glands include various hormones and are important in the overall regulation of body processes.

sedation (si,dayshən) the allaying of irritability or the relief of pain or mental distress, particularly by drugs.

sedative ('sedətiv) a drug or agent which lessens excitement and relieves tension. Sedative drugs are used to induce sleep.

sedentary ('sed'nt-ə-ree) pertaining to sitting; physically inactive.

sedimentation (,sedimen'tayshən) the deposit of solid particles at the bottom of a liquid. *Erythrocyte s. rate* abbreviated ESR. *See* ERYTHROCYTE.

segment ('segmənt) a small piece separated from any part by an actual or imaginary line.

segregation (,segri'gayshən) the separation during meiosis of allelic genes as the chromosomes migrate towards opposite poles of the cell.

Seldinger technique ('seldingə) the technique of percutaneous insertion of a special catheter into an artery along which it is passed.

self (self) 1. a term used to denote an animal's own antigenic constituents, in contrast to 'not-self', denoting foreign antigenic constituents. 2. the complete being of an individual, comprising both physical and psychological

characteristics, and including both conscious and unconscious components.

self-actualization (self,aktyooə-lie'zayshən) a level of psychological development in which innate potential is realized to the full, allowing transcendance of the environment.

self-examination of breast *see* BREAST.

self-examination of testes in order to ensure early detection of cancer of the testis, men should be urged to conduct a monthly self-examination of the testes. The self-examination involves the use of both hands to examine each of the testes. The index and middle fingers are placed below the testis and thumbs on top. With a gentle motion each testis is rolled between the thumbs and fingers to discover any lump (usually about the size of a pea), thickening, or change in the consistency of the tissues. It is important that the man become familiar with the feel of the epididymis so that he doesn't confuse this normal structure with an abnormal lump. Should a lump or any other abnormality be found, a doctor should be consulted immediately. An increasing awareness of testicular cancer has resulted in some educational material on testicular self-examination (TSE).

sella turcica (,selə 'tərsika) a depression in the sphenoid body which protects the pituitary gland.

semen ('seemen) the secretion of the testicles containing spermatozoa, which is ejaculated from the penis during sexual intercourse. Seminal fluid.

semicircular (‚semi'sərkyuhlə) formed in a half-circle. *S. canals* part of the labyrinth of the internal ear, consisting of three canals in the form of arches which contain fluid, and by their nerve supply are connected with the cerebellum. Impressions of change of position of the body are registered in these canals by oscillation of the fluid, and are conveyed by the nerves to the cerebellum.

semicomatose (‚semi'kohmə-tohs, -tohz) in a condition of unconsciousness from which the patient can be roused.

semilunar (‚semi'loonə) shaped like a half-moon. *S. cartilages* two crescent-shaped cartilages in the knee-joint. *S. valve see* VALVE.

seminoma (‚semi'nohmə) a malignant tumour of the testis, which is highly radiosensitive.

semipermeable (‚semi'pərmi·əb'l) of a membrane, permitting the passage of some molecules and hindering that of others.

semiprone (‚semi'prohn) partly prone. Applied to a position in which the patient is lying face down but the knees are turned to one side.

senescence (sə'nes'ns) the process of growing old.

Sengstaken–Blakemore tube (‚sengztayken 'blaykmor) *R.W. Sengstaken, American neurosurgeon, b. 1923; A.H. Blakemore, American surgeon, 1879–1970.* A compression tube used in the treatment of bleeding oeso-

SENGSTAKEN–BLAKEMORE TUBE

phageal varices.

senile ('seeniel) related to the involutional changes associated with old age. *S. dementia* deterioration of mental activity in the elderly associated with an impaired blood supply to the brain.

senna ('senə) a laxative derived from the cassia plant. Proprietary standardized preparations are available as tablets or granules.

sensation (sen'sayshən) a feeling

resulting from impulses sent to the brain by the sensory nerves.

sense (sens) the faculty by which conditions and properties of things are perceived, e.g. hunger or pain. *Special s.* any one of the faculties of sight, hearing, touch, smell, taste and muscle sense, through which the consciousness receives impressions from the environment. *S. organ* one which receives a sensory stimulus, for instance the eyes and ears.

sensible ('sensib'l) 1. capable of being perceived. *S. perspiration* that obvious on the skin as moisture. 2. sensitive.

sensitization (,sensitie'zayshən) 1. the process of rendering susceptible. 2. an increase in the body's response to a certain stimulus, as in the development of an allergy. *Protein s.* the condition occurring in an individual when a foreign protein is absorbed into the body, e.g. shellfish causing urticaria when eaten. *See* DESENSITIZATION.

sensory ('sensə·ree) relating to sensation. *S. cortex* that part of the cerebral cortex to which information is relayed by the sensory nerves. *S. nerve* an afferent nerve conveying impressions from the peripheral nerve endings to the brain or spinal cord.

sentiment ('sentimənt) an emotion directed towards some object or person. Sentiments are acquired and profoundly influence a person's actions.

sepsis ('sepsis) an infection of the body by pus-forming bacteria. *Focal s.* a local focus of infection which produces general symptoms. *Oral s.* infection of the mouth which causes general ill-health by absorption of toxins. *Puerperal s.* infection of the uterus occurring after labour.

septicaemia (,septi'seemi·ə) the presence in the blood of large numbers of bacteria and their toxins. The symptoms are: a rapid rise of temperature, which is later intermittent, rigors, sweating, and all the signs of acute fever.

septum ('septəm) a division or partition. *Atrial s., atrioventricular s., ventricular s.* the partitions dividing the various cavities of the heart. *Nasal s.* the structure made of bone and cartilage which separates the nasal cavities.

sequela (si'kweelə) a morbid condition following a disease and resulting from it.

sequestrectomy (,seekwe'strektəmee) the removal of a sequestrum.

sequestrum (si'kwestrəm) a piece of dead bone. Inflammation in bone leads to thrombosis of blood vessels resulting in necrosis of the affected part, which separates from the living structure.

serological (,siə·rə'lojik'l) relating to serum. *S. tests* those that are dependent on the formation of antibodies in the blood as a response to specific organisms or proteins.

serology (si'roləjee) the scientific study of sera.

serosa (si'rohsə) a serous membrane. It consists of two layers: the visceral, in close contact with the organ, and the parietal, lining the cavity.

serotonin (,sie·roh'tohnin, ,serə-)

an amine present in blood platelets, the intestine and the central nervous system, which acts as a vasoconstrictor. It is derived from the amino acid tryptophan and is inactivated by monoamine oxidase.

serous ('siə·rəs) related to serum. *S. effusion* an effusion of serous exudate.

serpiginous (sər'pijinəs) creeping from one place to another. Applied to skin lesions such as those of ringworm.

serum ('siə·rəm) the clear, fluid residue of blood, from which the corpuscles and fibrin have been removed. *S. hepatitis* jaundice caused by hepatitis B virus, usually following a blood transfusion or an inoculation with contaminated material. *S. sickness* an allergic reaction usually 8 to 10 days after a serum injection. It may be manifest by an irritating urticaria, pyrexia and painful joints. It readily responds to adrenaline and antihistaminic drugs. *See* ANAPHYLAXIS.

sessile ('sesiel) attached by a base. *S. tumour* a tumour without a stalk or peduncle.

sex (seks) 1. either of the two divisions of organic organisms described respectively as male and female. *S. chromosome* a chromosome that determines sex. Women have two X chromosomes and men have one X chromosome and one Y chromosome. *S. hormone* a steroid hormone produced by the ovaries or the testes and controlling sexual development. *S.-limited* pertaining to a characteristic found in only one sex. *S.-linked* pertaining to a characteristic that is transmitted by genes that are located on the sex chromosomes, e.g. haemophilia. 2. to discover the sex of an organism.

sexual ('seksyooəl) pertaining to sex. *S. development* the biological and psychosocial changes that lead to sexual maturity. *S. deviation* aberrant sexual activity; expression of the sexual instinct in practices which are socially prohibited or unacceptable, or biologically undesirable.

sexuality (,seksyoo'alitee) 1. the characteristic quality of the male and female reproductive elements. 2. the constitution of an individual in relation to sexual attitudes and behaviour.

sexually transmitted disease ('seksyooəlee) abbreviated STD. An infectious disease that is usually transmitted by means of sexual intercourse, either between heterosexual or homosexual individuals, or by intimate contact with the genitals, mouth, and rectum. Within the category of STD are the three legally defined VENEREAL DISEASES (VDs). The currently preferred term is genitourinary medicine.

SGOT serum glutamic–oxalacetic transaminase, an enzyme excreted by damaged heart muscle. A raised serum level occurs in myocardial infarction.

SGPT serum glutamic–pyruvic transaminase, an enzyme excreted by the parenchymal cells of the liver. There is a raised blood level in infectious hepatitis.

shared care (shaird kair) in

obstetrics, a term used to describe antenatal care carried out by an obstetrician and a general practitioner. The latter usually carries out the care following the booking until some time in the third trimester.

Sheehan's syndrome ('sheeənz) *H.L. Sheehan, British pathologist, b. 1900.* Hypopituitarism caused by thrombosis of the pituitary blood supply. It occurs in association with postpartum haemorrhage.

Shigella (shi'gelə) a genus of Gram-negative rod-like bacteria. Some species cause bacillary dysentery. *S. flexneri* and *S. shiga* are common in Asia, *S. dysenteriae* in the USA, and *S. sonnei* in Western Europe.

shin (shin) the bony front of the leg below the knee. The tibia.

shingles ('shing·g'lz) herpes zoster.

Shirodkar's suture (shi'rodkəz) *Shirodkar, Indian obstetrician.* A 'purse-string' suture that is placed round an incompetent cervix during pregnancy to prevent abortion. It is removed at the thirty-eighth week.

shock (shok) a condition produced by severe illness or trauma in which there is a sudden fall in blood pressure. This leads to lack of oxygen in the tissues and greater permeability of the capillary walls, so increasing the degree of shock, by greater loss of fluid. The patient has a cold moist skin, a feeble pulse, a low blood pressure and is distressed, thirsty and restless. *Allergic* or *anaphylactic s.* shock produced by the injection of a protein to which the patient is sensitive. *Cardiogenic s.* shock as a result of an acute heart condition such as myocardial infarction. *Hypovolaemic s.* shock resulting from a reduction in the volume of blood in circulation, following haemorrhage or severe burns. *Neurogenic s.* shock due to nervous or emotional factors. *Shell s.* a psychoneurotic condition caused by the stresses of warfare.

short-sightedness (,shawt'sietidnəs) myopia.

shoulder ('shohldə) the junction of the clavicle and the scapula where the arm joins the body. *S. lift see* AUSTRALIAN LIFT.

show (shoh) the blood-stained discharge which occurs at the onset of labour.

shunt (shunt) a diversion, particularly of blood, due to a congenital defect, disease or surgery.

sialogogue (sie'alə,gog, 'sieələ-) a drug increasing the flow of saliva.

sialography (,sieə'logrəfee) radiographic examination of the salivary ducts following the insertion of a radio-opaque contrast medium

sialolith ('sieəloh,lith) a salivary calculus.

sibling ('sibling) one of a family of children having the same parents. Applied in psychology to one of two or more children of the same parent or substitute parent figure. *S. rivalry* jealousy, compounded of love and hate of one child for its sibling.

sickle-cell anaemia ('sik'l) an inherited blood disease. *See* ANAEMIA.

siderosis (ˌsidəˈrohsis) 1. chronic inflammation of the lung due to inhalation of particles of iron. 2. excess iron in the blood. 3. the deposit of iron in the tissues.

sigmoid ('sigmoyd) shaped like the Greek letter Σ. *S. colon* or *flexure* that part of the colon in the left iliac fossa just above the rectum.

sigmoidoscope (sigˈmoydəˌskohp) an instrument by which the interior of the rectum and sigmoid colon can be seen.

sigmoidostomy (ˌsigmoyˈdostəmee) the making of an artificial opening between the sigmoid colon and the skin.

sign (sien) 1. any objective evidence of disease or dysfunction. 2. an observable physical phenomenon so frequently associated with a given condition as to be considered indicative of its presence. *S. language* hand and body language used by totally deaf people to communicate with others. *Vital s's* the signs of life, namely pulse, respiration and temperature.

silicosis (ˌsiliˈkohsis) fibrosis of the lung due to the inhalation of silica dust particles. It occurs in miners, stone masons and quarry workers.

Sims' position (simz) *J.M. Sims, American gynaecologist, 1813–1883.* A semi-prone position. *See* POSITION.

sinew ('sinyoo) a tendon or ligament.

sinoatrial (ˌsienohˈaytri·əl) situated between the sinus venosus and the atrium of the heart. *S. node* the pacemaker of the heart.

See NODE.

sinus ('sienəs) 1. a cavity in a bone. *Air s.* a cavity in a bone containing air. *Ethmoidal s.* air spaces in the ethmoid bone. *Frontal s.* air spaces in the frontal bone. *Sphenoidal s.* air spaces in the sphenoid bone. 2. a venous channel, especially within the cranium. *S. arrhythmia see* ARRHYTHMIA. *Cavernous s.* a venous sinus of the dura mater which lies along the body of the sphenoid bone. *Coronary s.* the vein which returns the blood from the heart muscle into the right atrium. *S. thrombosis* clotting of blood in a cranial venous channel. In the lateral sinus it is a complication of mastoiditis. 3. an unhealed passage leading from an abscess or internal lesion to the surface.

sinusitis (ˌsienəˈsietis) inflammation of the lining of a sinus, especially applied to the bony cavities of the face.

sinusoid ('sienəˌsoyd) like a sinus. Used to describe the irregular channels by which blood vessels anastomose in certain organs, such as the liver and suprarenal glands.

Sjögren's disease (shərgrenz) *H.S.C. Sjögren, Swedish ophthalmologist, b. 1899.* A deficiency in lacrimation usually found in women in middle age. Keratoconjunctivitis, rhinitis or laryngitis may occur.

skeleton ('skelitən) the bony framework of the body, supporting and protecting the organs and soft tissues.

Skene's gland (skeenz) *A.J.C.*

Skene, American gynaecologist, 1838–1900. One of a pair of glands which open into the posterior urethral orifice in the female.

skin (skin) the outer protective covering of the body. It consists of an outer layer, the epidermis or cuticle, and an inner layer, the dermis or corium, which is known as 'true skin'. *S. grafting* transplantation of pieces of healthy skin to an area where loss of surface tissue has occurred. *S. patch* a drug-impregnated adhesive patch which is applied to the skin. The drug is slowly absorbed, allowing its level in the blood to be maintained over a given period of time. *S. test* application of a substance to the skin, or intradermal injection of a substance, to permit observation of the body's reaction to it.

skull (skul) the bony framework of the head, consisting of the cranium and facial bones.

sleep (sleep) a period of rest for the body and mind, during which volition and consciousness are in partial or complete abeyance and the bodily functions partially suspended. It occurs in a 24 h biological rhythm. Sleep occurs in cycles which have two distinct phases. Each phase lasts approximately 60–90 min: orthodox or non-rapid eye movement sleep (NREM), and paradoxical or rapid eye movement sleep (REM).

sleeping sickness ('sleeping) trypanosomiasis. A tropical fever occurring in parts of Africa, caused by a protozoal parasite (*Trypanosoma*) which is conveyed by the tsetse fly.

slipped disc (slipt) a prolapsed intervertebral disc which causes pressure on the spinal nerves. It may be very painful.

slit lamp ('slit ,lamp) a special light source so arranged with a microscope that examination of the interior of the eye can be carried out at the level of each layer.

slough (sluf) dead tissue caused by injury or inflammation. It separates from the healthy tissue and is ultimately washed away by exuded serum, leaving a granulating surface.

smallpox ('smawl,poks) variola. Eradicated from the world in 1980. Smallpox vaccination is no longer required for travellers to any part of the world.

smear (smiə) a specimen for microscopic examination that has been prepared by spreading a thin film of the material across a glass slide.

smegma ('smegmə) the secretion of sebaceous glands of the clitoris and prepuce.

Smith-Petersen nail (,smith-'peetəsən) *M.N. Smith-Petersen, American surgeon, 1886–1953.* A metal nail used to fix the fragments of bone in intracapsular fracture of the head of the femur.

smoking ('smohking) the act of drawing into the mouth and puffing out the smoke of tobacco contained in a cigarette, cigar, or pipe. A close relationship between smoking and lung cancer and heart disease has definitely

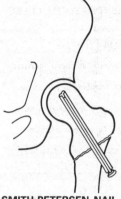

SMITH-PETERSEN NAIL

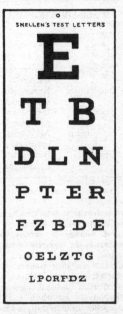

SNELLEN'S TEST LETTERS

been established.

snake (snayk) a limbless reptile; a serpent. The bites of many snakes are poisonous to man. *S. venom antitoxin* antivenin. A serum made from animals, usually horses, which have been immunized against the venom of a specific type of snake.

Snellen's test letters ('snelənz) *H. Snellen, Dutch ophthalmologist, 1834–1908*. Square-shaped letters on a chart, used for sight testing.

snow (snoh) frozen water vapour. *S. blindness* photophobia due to the glare of snow. *Carbon dioxide s.* solid CO_2 which is used as a refrigerant; 'dry ice'.

snuffles ('snuf'lz) a chronic discharge from the nose occurring in children, usually those with **congenital syphilis**, due to infec-

tion of the nasal mucous membrane.

social class ('sohshəl) a category arising from the division of society into economic or occupational groupings. Since 1911, the office of the Registrar General in the UK (since 1969 the Office of Population Censuses and Surveys) has used a five-category

SCALE SHOWING MEASUREMENT OF SOCIAL CLASS

Social class	Occupation (examples)
1. Professional	Doctors, dentists, lawyers, architects, university teachers
2. Intermediate	Nurses, pharmacists, members of parliament, school teachers
3. Skilled	Clerical workers, police, shop assistants, sales representatives
4. Semi-skilled	Agricultural workers, bartenders, telephone operators, postmen
5. Unskilled	Porters, labourers, cleaners, bus conductors, packers, messengers

measurement of social class based on occupational groupings.

social worker a professional trained in the treatment of individual and social problems of patients and their families. *See also* MEDICAL SOCIAL WORKER.

socialization (ˌsohshəlie'zayshən) the process by which society integrates the individual, and the individual learns to behave in socially acceptable ways.

sociology (ˌsohsi'oləjee) the scientific study of the development of man's social relationships and organization, i.e. interpersonal and intergroup behaviour as distinct from the behaviour of an individual.

sociopath ('sohsioh,path) a person with an antisocial personality; a psychopath.

sodium ('sohdi·əm) *symbol* Na. A metallic alkaline element widely distributed in nature, and form-ing an important constituent of animal tissue. *S. aminosalicylate* an antituberculous drug used in conjunction with streptomycin and isoniazid. *S. bicarbonate* an antacid widely used to treat digestive disorders, especially flatulence. Repeated use can cause alkalosis. *S. chloride* common salt. Its presence in the diet is necessary to health. *S. citrate* compound used to prevent clotting of blood during blood transfusions. *S. cromoglycate* a drug used as an inhalant in the treatment of asthma. *S. fluoride* a salt used in the fluoridation of water and also in toothpastes to prevent the formation of caries. *S. hydroxide* caustic soda. A powerful corrosive drug used to destroy warts. It can cause severe chemical burns. *S. hypochlorite* a compound with germicidal properties used in solution to disinfect utensils and diluted as a topical antibacterial agent. *S. phosphate* a purgative. *S. salicylate* an antipyretic drug used in the treatment of rheumatic fever. *S. sulphate* a purgative; also used in 25% solution as a wound dressing. *S. valproate* a drug used in the treatment of epilepsy.

solar plexus ('sohlǝ) coeliac plexus. A network of sympathetic nerve ganglia in the abdomen; the nerve supply to abdominal organs below the diaphragm.

solution (sǝ'looshǝn) a liquid in which one or more substances have been dissolved.

solvent ('solvǝnt) a liquid which dissolves or has power to dissolve. *S. abuse see* ABUSE.

soma ('sohmǝ) 1. the body as distinct from the mind. 2. the body tissue as distinct from the germ cells.

somatic (soh'matik) 1. relating to the body as opposed to the mind. 2. relating to the body wall as distinct from the viscera.

somnambulism (som'nambyuh,-lizǝm) walking and carrying out other complex activities during a state of sleep.

Somogyi effect (soh'mohgee) *M. Somogyi, American biochemist, 1883–1971.* A rebound phenomenon occurring in diabetes mellitus; overtreatment with insulin induces hypoglycaemia, resulting in rebound hyperglycaemia and ketosis.

Sonne dysentery (soni) *C.O. Sonne, Danish bacteriologist, 1882–1948.* Bacillary dysentery which is common in the UK. The symptoms are diarrhoea, vomiting and abdominal pain. The causative agent is *Shigella sonnei*.

sorbitol ('sawbit,tol) a sweetening agent which is converted into sugar in the body though it is slowly absorbed from the intestine. It is used in some diabetic foods and in intravenous feeding.

sordes ('sawdeez) brown crusts which form on the teeth and lips of unconscious patients, or those suffering from acute or prolonged fevers.

sore (sor) a general term for any ulcer or open skin lesion. *Cold s.* herpes simplex. *Hard s.* a syphilitic chancre. *Pressure s.* a sore caused by pressure from the bed (decubitus ulcer) or a splint. *Soft s.* a chancroid ulcer. *S. throat* inflammation of the larynx or pharynx, including tonsillitis.

souffle ('soof'l) a blowing sound heard on auscultation. *Uterine s.* is due to the blood passing through the uterine arteries of the mother, particularly over the placental site. It is synchronous with the maternal pulse.

sound (sownd) an instrument shaped like a probe for exploring cavities, detecting the presence of foreign bodies or dilating a stricture.

spasm ('spazǝm) a sudden involuntary muscle contraction. *Carpopedal s.* spasm of the hands and feet. A sign of tetany. *Clonic s.* alternate muscle rigidity and relaxation. *Habit s.* a tic. *Nictitating s.* spasmodic twitching of the eyelid. *Tetanic s.* violent muscle spasms, including opisthotonos. *Tonic s.* a sustained muscle rigidity.

spasmolytic (,spazmə'litik) a drug which reduces spasm.

spastic (,spastik) 1. caused by spasm; convulsive. *S. colon* irritable bowel syndrome. *S. paralysis* paralysis associated with lesions of the upper motor neurone as in cerebral vascular accidents and characterized by increased muscle tone and rigidity. 2. one affected by spasticity, often applied to persons suffering from congenital paralysis due to some cerebral lesion or impairment.

spasticity (spa'stisitee) marked rigidity of muscles.

spatial ('spayshəl) pertaining to space.

spatula ('spatyuhlə) 1. a flexible, blunt blade used for spreading ointment. 2. a rigid blade-shaped instrument for depressing the tongue in throat examination, etc.

species ('speesheez) a subdivision of a genus.

specific (spə'sifik) 1. relating to a species. 2. a remedy which has a distinct curative influence on a particular disease, e.g. quinine in malaria. 3. related to a unit mass of a substance. *S. gravity* the density of fluid compared with that of an equal volume of water.

specimen ('spesimən) a sample or part taken to show the nature of the whole, e.g. for chemical testing or microscopic survey.

spectacles ('spektək'lz) a frame containing lenses worn in front of the eyes to correct errors of vision or to protect from glare.

spectrometer (spek'tromitə) an instrument for measuring the strength and wavelengths of visible or invisible electromagnetic radiations.

spectroscope ('spektrə,skohp) an instrument used for analysing the spectra of light and other radiations.

speech (speech) the act of communicating by sounds by means of a linguistic code. *Clipped s.* speech in which the words are cut short. *Deaf s.* the characteristic utterance of people with severe hearing loss. *Explosive s.* loud, sudden utterances; a sign of mental disorder. *Incoherent s.* disconnected utterances made when the sequence of thought is disturbed, as in delirium. *Oesophageal s.* speech produced following laryngectomy by swallowing air and using it to vibrate within the oesophagus against the closed cricopharyngeal sphincter. *Scanning s.* speech in which the syllables are inappropriately separated from each other and are evenly stressed. Characteristic of cerebellar damage. *Staccato s.* speech in which each syllable is separately pronounced. Characteristic of multiple sclerosis. *S. therapist* a professional trained to identify, assess, and rehabilitate persons with speech or language disorders and feeding difficulties.

sperm (spərm) 1. a spermatozoon. 2. the semen.

spermatocele ('spərmətoh,seel) a cystic swelling in the epididymis, containing semen.

spermatorrhoea (,spərmətə'reeə) an involuntary discharge of semen, without orgasm.

spermatozoon (,spərmətoh'zoh-·on) a mature male germ cell consisting of a flat-shaped head, a short middle part and a long tail. There are 300–500 million sperms in a normal ejaculate.

spermicide ('spərmi,sied) any agent which will destroy spermatozoa.

sphenoid ('sfeenoyd) wedge-shaped. *S. bone* the central part of the base of the skull.

spherocytosis (,sfiə·rohsie'tohsis) the presence in the blood of erythrocytes which are more nearly spherical than biconcave. Characteristic of acholuric jaundice, it may also be hereditary.

sphincter (,sfingktə) a ring-shaped muscle, contraction of which closes a natural orifice.

sphincterectomy (,sfingktə'rektəmee) 1. the excision of a sphincter. 2. in ophthalmology, an operation to free the sphincter of the iris when it has become attached to the back of the cornea.

sphincterotomy (,sfingktə'rotəmee) the incision of a sphincter to relieve constriction.

sphygmic ('sfigmik) relating to the pulse.

sphygmocardiograph (,sfigmoh'kahdioh,grahf, -,graf) an instrument that records both the pulse waves and heartbeat.

sphygmograph ('sfigmoh,grahf, -,graf) an instrument which registers graphically the force and character of the arterial pulse.

sphygmomanometer (,sfigmohmə'nomitə) an instrument for measuring the arterial blood pressure.

spica ('spiekə) a bandage applied to a joint in a series of 'figures of eight'.

spicule ('spikyool) a splinter-like fragment of bone.

spigot ('spigət) a small plastic peg to close the opening of a tube.

spina ('spienə) spine; a slender, thorn-like projection that occurs on many bones. *S. bifida* a congenital defect of non-union of one or more vertebral arches, allowing protrusion of the meninges and possibly their contents. *See* MENINGOCELE and MENINGO-MYELOCELE.

spinal ('spien'l) relating to the spine. *S. anaesthesia see* ANAES-THESIA. *S. canal* the hollow in the spine formed by the neural arches of the vertebrae. It contains the spinal cord, meninges, and cerebrospinal fluid. *S. caries* disease of the vertebrae, usually tuberculous. *See* POTT'S DISEASE. *S. column* the backbone; the vertebral column. *S. cord see* CORD. *S. curvature* abnormal curving of the spine. If associated with caries, it is known as Pott's disease. *See* KYPHOSIS, LORDOSIS and SCOLIOSIS. *S. jacket* a support for the spine, made of plaster of Paris, or other material, and used to give rest after injury to or operation on the spine. *S. nerves* the 31 pairs of nerves which leave the spinal cord at regular intervals throughout its length. They pass out in pairs, one on either side between each of the vertebrae, and are distributed to the periphery. *S. puncture* lumbar or cisternal puncture.

spine (spien) 1. the backbone or

vertebral column, consisting of 33 vertebrae, separated by fibrocartilaginous discs, and enclosing the spinal cord. 2. a sharp process of bone.

Spinhaler ('spinhaylə) a nebulizing device which delivers a preset dose of the contained drug.

spinnbarkeit ('spinbah,kiet) [G.] a thread of mucus secreted by the cervix uteri. Used to determine ovulation as this usually coincides with the time at which the mucus can be drawn out on a glass slide to its maximum length.

Spirillum (spie'riləm) a genus of spiral-shaped bacteria. *S. minus* a species carried by rats and causing one type of rat-bite fever.

spirochaete ('spieroh,keet) one of a group of microorganisms in the form of a spiral, some of which are found in impure fresh or salt water. The group includes the species *Treponema, Borrelia* and *Leptospira*.

spirograph ('spieroh,grahf, -,graf) an instrument for registering respiratory movements.

spirometer (spie'romitə, spi'rom-) an instrument for measuring the air capacity of the lungs.

spironolactone (,spierənoh'lak-tohn) a diuretic drug used when there is excess secretion of aldosterone. It promotes the excretion of sodium and water but the retention of potassium.

Spitz–Holter valve (,spits 'holtə) *Spitz, American engineer; J.W. Holter, American engineer.* A device used in the treatment of hydrocephalus to drain the cerebrospinal fluid from the ventricles into the superior vena cava or the right atrium.

splanchnic ('splangknik) pertaining to the viscera. *S. nerves* sympathetic nerves to the viscera.

spleen (spleen) a large, vascular gland-like but ductless organ, coloured a reddish purple and situated in the left hypochondrium under the border of the stomach. It manufactures lymphocytes and breaks down red blood corpuscles.

splenectomy (spli'nektəmee) excision of the spleen.

splenitis (spli'nietis) inflammation of the spleen.

splenomegaly (,spleenoh'megəlee) enlargement of the spleen.

splenorenal (,spleenoh'reen'l) relating to the spleen and the kidney. *S. anastomosis* an operation carried out to treat portal hypertension. The spleen is excised and the splenic vein is inserted into the renal vein.

splint (splint) an appliance used to support or immobilize a part while healing takes place or to correct or prevent deformity.

spondylitis (,spondi'lietis) inflammation of the vertebrae. *Ankylosing s.* a rheumatic disease, chiefly of young males, in which there is abnormal ossification with pain and rigidity of the intervertebral, hip and sacroiliac joints.

spondylolisthesis (,spondilohlis-'theesis) a sliding forwards or displacement of one vertebra over another, usually the fifth lumbar over the sacrum, causing symptoms such as low back pain due to pressure on the nerve roots.

spondylosis (,spondi'lohsis) ankylosis of the vertebral joints usually caused by a degenerative disease of the intervertebral discs, such as osteoarthritis.

spongioblastoma (,spunjiohbla-'stohmə) a rapidly growing brain tumour that is highly malignant. A glioma.

spontaneous (spon'tayni·əs) occurring without apparent cause. Applied to certain types of fracture and to recovery from a disease without any specific treatment.

sporadic (spə'radik) pertaining to isolated cases of a disease which occurs in various and scattered places (compare endemic and epidemic).

spore (spor) 1. a reproductive stage of some of the lowest forms of vegetable life, e.g. moulds. 2. a protective state which some bacteria are able to assume in adverse conditions, such as lack of moisture, food or heat. In this form the organism can remain alive, but inert, for years.

sporotrichosis (,spor·rohtri'kohsis) a chronic fungal infection caused by *Sporothrix schenckii*.

spotted fever ('spotid) a febrile disease characterized by a skin eruption, such as Rocky Mountain spotted fever, boutonneuse fever, and other infections due to tickborne rickettsiae.

sprain (sprayn) wrenching of a joint, producing laceration of the capsule or stretching of the ligaments, with consequent swelling, which is due to effusion of fluid into the affected part.

Sprengel's deformity ('sprengəlz) *O.G.K. Sprengel, German surgeon, 1852–1915.* A congenital condition in which one shoulder blade is higher than the other, causing some limitation of abduction power.

sprue (sproo) a disease of malabsorption in the intestine, which may be tropical or non-tropical in form. There is steatorrhoea, diarrhoea, glossitis and anaemia.

sputum ('spyootəm) material expelled from the air passages through the mouth. It consists chiefly of mucus and saliva, but in diseased conditions of the air passages it may be purulent, blood-stained and frothy and contain many bacteria. It must always be regarded as highly infectious. *Rusty s.* that in which altered blood permeates the mucus. Characteristic of acute lobar pneumonia.

squamous ('skwayməs) scaly. *S. bone* the thin part of the temporal bone which articulates with the parietal and frontal bones. *S. cell carcinoma* a malignancy of the squamous cells of the bronchus. *S. epithelium* epithelium composed of flat and scale-like cells.

squint (skwint) *see* STRABISMUS.

staging ('stayjing) 1. the determination of distinct phases or periods in the course of a disease. 2. the classification of neoplasms according to the extent of the tumour. *TNM s.* staging of tumours according to three basic components: primary tumour (T), regional nodes (N), and metastasis (M). Subscripts are used to denote size and degree of involvement; for example, 0 indicates undetectable, and 1, 2, 3, and 4 a progressive increase in size or involvement.

stammering ('stamə·ring) stuttering; a speech disorder in which the utterance is broken by hesitation and repetition or prolongation of words and syllables.

stapedectomy (ˌstaypi'dektəmee) removal of the stapes and insertion of a vein graft or other device to re-establish conduction of sound waves in otosclerosis.

stapediolysis (stəˌpeedi'olisis) an operation in which the footpiece of the stapes is mobilized to aid conduction in deafness from otosclerosis.

stapes ('staypeez) the stirrup-shaped bone of the middle ear.

staphylectomy (ˌstafi'lektəmee) surgical removal of the uvula; uvulectomy.

Staphylococcus (ˌstafiloh'kokəs) a genus of Gram-positive non-mobile bacteria which, under the microscope, appear grouped together in small masses like bunches of grapes. They are normally present on the skin and mucous membranes. *S. pyogenes* (or *S. aureus*) is a common cause of boils, carbuncles and abscesses.

staphyloma (ˌstafi'lohmə) a protrusion of the cornea or the sclerotic coat of the eyeball as the result of inflammation or wound.

staphylorrhaphy (ˌstafi'lo·rəfee) an operation to suture a cleft soft palate and uvula.

starch (stahch) a carbohydrate occurring in many vegetable tissues.

stasis (ˌstaysis) the stagnation or stoppage of the flow of a fluid. *Intestinal s.* sluggish movement of faeces through the bowel, due to partial obstruction or to impairment of the action of the intestinal muscles. *Venous s.* congestion of blood in the veins.

status (ˌstaytəs) condition. *S. asthmaticus* a severe and prolonged attack of asthma. *S. epilepticus* a condition in which there is rapid succession of epileptic fits. *S. lymphaticus* a condition in which all lymphatic tissues are hypertrophied, especially the thymus gland.

STD sexually transmitted disease.

steapsin (sti'apsin) the fat-splitting enzyme (LIPASE) of the pancreatic juice.

steatoma (stie'tohma) 1. a sebaceous cyst. 2. a lipoma; a fatty tumour.

steatopygia (ˌstiətoh'piji·ə) excessive deposit of fat in the buttocks.

steatorrhoea (ˌstiətə'reeə) the presence of an excess of fat in the stools due to malabsorption of fat by the intestines.

steatosis (stiə'tohsis) fatty degeneration.

Stein–Leventhal syndrome (ˌstien-'levənthal) *I.F. Stein, American gynaecologist, b. 1887; M.L. Leventhal, American gynaecologist, 1901–1971.* Condition affecting females in which obesity, hirsutism and sterility are associated with polycystic ovaries and menstrual irregularities.

Steinmann pin ('stienmən) *F. Steinmann, Swiss surgeon, 1872–1932.* A fine metal rod, passed through bone, by which extension is applied to overcome muscle contraction in certain fractures.

See KIRSCHNER'S WIRE.

stellate ('stelayt) star-shaped. *S. fracture* a radiating fracture of the patella. *S. ganglion* the inferior cervical ganglion. A star-shaped collection of nerve cells at the base of the neck.

Stellwag's sign ('stelvahgz) *C. Stellwag von Carion, Austrian ophthalmologist, 1823–1904.* A 'widening' of the eyes with infrequent blinking, as may occur in exophthalmos.

stenocardia (,stenoh'kahdi·ə) angina pectoris.

stenosis (stə'nohsis) abnormal narrowing or contraction of a channel or opening. *Aortic s.* narrowing of the opening of the aortic valve due to scar tissue formation as the result of inflammation. *Mitral s.* narrowing of the orifice of the mitral valve, usually following rheumatic fever. *Pulmonary s.* a congenital narrowing of the opening from the right ventricle of the heart into the pulmonary artery. *Pyloric s.* narrowing of the pyloric orifice of the stomach due to scar tissue, new growth, or congenital hypertrophy.

Stensen's duct ('stensənz) *H. Stensen, Danish physician, 1638–1686.* The duct of the parotid gland, opening into the mouth opposite the second upper molar.

stercobilin (,stərkoh'bielin) a brown-orange pigment derived from bile and present in faeces.

stercoraceous (,stərkə'rayshəs) faecal, or containing faeces. *S. vomit* vomit containing faeces.

stereognosis (,steriog'nohsis, ,stiə-) the ability to visualize the shape of an object by touch alone.

stereotypy ('sterioh,tiepee, 'stiə-) repetitive actions carried out or maintained for long periods in a monotonous fashion.

Sterets (ste'rets) a proprietary brand of swabs impregnated with 70, isopropyl alcohol. These swabs are rubbed on to a skin site prior to an injection.

sterile ('steriel) 1. aseptic; free from microorganisms. 2. barren; incapable of producing young.

sterility (stə'rilətee) 1. the state of being free from microorganisms. 2. the inability of a woman to become pregnant, or of a man to produce potent spermatozoa.

sterilization (,sterilie'zayshən) 1. rendering dressings, instruments, etc. aseptic by destroying or removing all microbial life. 2. rendering incapable of reproduction by any means.

sterilizer ('steri'liezə) an apparatus in which objects can be sterilized. *See* AUTOCLAVE.

Steri-Strips ('steri ,strips) proprietary skin closure strips which are placed across a wound with a space between the edges to allow for drainage. A final strip is placed on either side parallel to the wound.

sternocleidomastoid (,stərnoh,kliedoh'mastoyd) a muscle group stretching from the mastoid process to the sternum and clavicle.

sternotomy (stər'notəmee) the operation in which the sternum is cut through to enable the heart to be reached.

sternum ('stərnəm) the breastbone; the flat narrow bone in the centre of the anterior wall of the thorax.

steroid ('steroyd, 'stiə-) one of a group of hormones chemically related to cholesterol. They include oestrogen and androgen, progesterone and the corticosteroids. They may be naturally occurring or they may be synthesized.

sterol ('sterol, 'stiə·rol) one of a group of steroid alcohols which includes cholesterol and ergosterol.

stertorous ('stərtə·rəs) snore-like; applied to a snoring sound produced in breathing during sleep or in coma.

stethoscope ('stethə,skohp) the instrument used for listening to internal body sounds, especially from the heart and lung. It consists of a hollow tube, one end of which is placed over the part to be examined and the other at the ear of the examiner.

Stevens–Johnson syndrome (,steevənz'jonsən) *A.M. Stevens, American paediatrician, 1884–1945; F.C. Johnson, American paediatrician, 1894–1934.* A severe form of erythema multiforme in which the lesions may involve the oral and anogenital mucosa, eyes and viscera, associated with such constitutional symptoms as malaise, headache, fever, arthralgia and conjunctivitis.

stibophen ('stiboh,fen) a sodium salt of antimony given intramuscularly in the treatment of schistosomiasis.

stigma (,stigmə) 1. a small spot or mark on the skin. 2. any mark characteristic of a condition or defect, or of a disease. It refers to visible signs rather than symptoms.

stilboestrol (stil'beestrol) a synthetic oestrogen preparation used in the treatment of cancer of the prostate and less commonly for postmenopausal breast cancer.

stillbirth ('stil,bərth) a baby which has issued forth from its mother after the 28th week of pregnancy and has not, at any time after being completely expelled from its mother, breathed or shown any sign of life. *S. certificate* a certificate issued to the parents by a registered medical practitioner who was present at the birth, or examined the body.

Still's disease (stilz) *Sir G.F. Still, British paediatrician, 1868–1941.* A form of rheumatoid arthritis in children sometimes associated with enlargement of the lymph glands.

stimulant ('stimyuhlənt) an agent which causes increased energy or functional activity of any organ.

stimulus ('stimyuhləs) *pl. stimuli* (L.) any agent, act, or influence that produces functional or trophic reaction in a receptor or an irritable tissue. *Conditioned s.* a neutral object or event that is psychologically related to a naturally stimulating object or event and which causes a CONDITIONED RESPONSE (*see also* CONDITIONING). *Discriminative s.* a stimulus associated with reinforcement, which exerts control over a particular form of behaviour; the subject discriminates between closely related stimuli and responds positively only in the presence of that stimulus. *Eliciting s.* any stimulus, conditioned or unconditioned, which elicits a response. *Structured s.* a well-organized and unambiguous stimulus, the perception of which is influenced to a greater extent by the characteristics of the stimulus than by those of the perceiver. *Threshold s.* a stimulus that is just strong enough to elicit a response. *Unconditioned s.* any stimulus that is capable of eliciting an unconditioned response (*see also* CONDITIONING). *Unstructured s.* an unclear or ambiguous stimulus, the perception of which is influenced to a greater extent by the characteristics of the perceiver than by those of the stimulus.

stitch (stich) 1. a sudden sharp pain usually due to spasm of the diaphragm. 2. a suture. *S. abscess* pus formation where a stitch has been inserted.

Stokes–Adams syndrome (,stohks-'adəmz) *Sir W. Stokes, Irish surgeon, 1804–1878; R. Adams, Irish physician, 1791–1875.* Attacks of syncope or fainting due to cerebral anaemia in some cases of complete heart block. The heart stops temporarily but breathing continues. It is treated by using an artificial pacemaker.

stoma ('stohmə) 1. a mouth or mouth-like opening. 2. an artificial opening in the skin surface leading into one of the tubes forming the alimentary canal. *See* COLOSTOMY and ILEOSTOMY.

stomach ('stumək) the dilated portion of the alimentary canal between the oesophagus and the duodenum, just below the diaphragm. *Bilocular* or *hour-glass s.* one divided into two parts by a constriction. *Leather bottle s.* induration and thickening of the gastric wall, usually the result of malignant disease. *S. pH electrode* apparatus used to measure gastric contents in situ. *S. pump* one that removes the contents of the stomach by suction. *S. tube* a flexible tube used for washing out the stomach, or for the administration of liquid food.

stomatitis (,stohmə'tietis) inflammation of the mouth, either simple or with ulceration caused by a vitamin deficiency or by a bacterial or fungal infection. *Angular s.* cracking at the corners of the mouth, usually due to riboflavin deficiency. *Aphthous s.* that characterized by small, white, painful ulcers on the mucous membrane. *Ulcerative s.* painful shallow ulcers on the tongue, cheeks and lips. A severe type which may produce serious constitutional effects.

stone (stohn) a calculus.

stool (stool) a motion or discharge from the bowels. *Fatty s.* that which contains undigested fat. *Hunger s.* stool passed by underfed infants: frequent, small and green. *Rice-water s.* the watery stool, containing small white flakes, seen in cholera. *Tarry s.* a black tarry stool due to the presence of blood from a peptic ulcer.

strabismus (strə'bizməs) squint; heterotropia. A deviation of the eye from its normal direction. It is called convergent when the eye turns in toward the nose, and divergent when it turns outward. *Concomitant s.* a squint in which the angle of deviation stays constant.

strabotomy (strə'botəmee) the division of ocular muscles in the treatment of strabismus.

strain (strayn) 1. overuse or stretching of a part, e.g. a muscle or tendon. 2. a group of microorganisms within a species. 3. to pass a liquid through a filter.

stramonium (strə'mohni-əm) a vegetable drug containing the alkaloid hyoscyamine, which in its action resembles belladonna.

strangulated (,strang·gyuh'laytid) compressed or constricted so that the circulation of the blood is arrested. *S. hernia see* HERNIA.

strangulation (,strang·gyuh'layshən) 1. choking caused by compression of the air passages. 2. arrested circulation to a part, which will result in gangrene.

strangury ('strang·gyuhree) a painful, frequent desire to micturate, but in which only a few drops of urine are passed with difficulty.

stratified ('strati,fied) arranged in layers. *S. tissue* a covering tissue in which the cells are arranged in layers. The germinating cells are the lowest, and as surface cells are shed there is continual replacement.

stratum ('strahtəm, 'stray-) a layer; applied to structures such as the skin and mucous membranes. *S. corneum* the outer, horny layer of the epidermis.

Streptococcus (,streptoh'kokəs) a genus of Gram-positive spherical bacteria occurring in chains or pairs. Divided into various groups. The first group includes the beta-haemolytic human and animal pathogens; the second and third include alpha-haemolytic parasitic forms occurring as normal flora in the body; and the fourth is made up of saprophytic forms. *S. mutans* implicated in dental caries. *S. pneumoniae* pneumococcus, the most common cause of lobar pneumonia; also causes serious forms of meningitis, septicaemia, empyema and peritonitis. *S. pyogenes* beta-haemolytic, toxigenic, pyogenic streptococci causing septic sore throat, scarlet fever, rheumatic fever, puerperal fever and acute glomerulonephritis.

streptodornase (,streptoh'dornayz) an enzyme produced by some haemolytic streptococci. It is capable of liquefying pus and blood clots. Used in combination with streptokinase.

streptokinase (,streptoh'kienayz) an enzyme derived from a streptococcal culture and used to liquefy clotted blood and pus.

Streptomyces (,streptoh'mieseez) a genus of soil bacteria from which a large number of antibiotics are derived.

streptomycin (,streptoh'miesin) an antibiotic drug derived from *Streptomyces griseus*; used particularly in the treatment of tuberculosis, when treatment is combined with other drugs to reduce drug resistance.

stress (stres) any factor, mental or physical, the pressure of which can adversely affect the functioning of the body. *S. disorders* those resulting from an individual's inability to withstand stress. *S. incontinence* incontinence, usually of urine, when the intra-abdominal pressure is raised such as in coughing, sneezing or laughing.

stria ('strieə) *pl.* striae. A line or stripe. *Striae gravidarum* the lines which appear on the abdomen of pregnant women. They are red in first pregnancy, but white subsequently and are due to stretching and rupture of the elastic fibres.

striated (strie'aytid) striped. *S. muscle* voluntary muscle. *See* MUSCLE.

stricture ('strikchə) a narrowing or local contraction of a canal. It may be caused by muscle spasm, new growth, or scar tissue formation following inflammation.

stridor ('striedor) a harsh, vibrating, shrill sound, produced during respiration when there is partial obstruction of the larynx or trachea.

stroke (strohk) a popular term to describe the sudden onset of symptoms, especially those of cerebral origin. *Apoplectic s.* cerebral haemorrhage. *Heat s.* a hyperpyrexia accompanied by cerebral symptoms. It may occur in someone newly arrived in a very hot climate.

stroma ('strohmə) the connective tissue forming the ground substance, framework, or matrix of an organ, as opposed to the functioning part or parenchyma.

Strongyloides (stronji'loydeez) a genus of nematode worms, one of which, *S. stercoralis*, is common

in tropical countries and causes diarrhoea and intestinal ulcers.

strontium ('stronti·əm) *symbol* Sr. A metallic element. Isotopes of strontium are used in bone scanning to detect abnormalities. *S.-90* a radioactive isotope used in radiotherapy in the treatment of skin and eye malignancies.

strychnine ('strikneen) a highly poisonous alkaloid made from the seeds of *Strychnos nux-vomica*. Formerly used in small amounts in 'tonics'.

Stryker frame ('striekə) an apparatus specially designed for care of patients with injuries of the spinal cord or paralysis. It is constructed of pipe and canvas and is designed so that one nurse can turn the patient without difficulty.

stupor ('styoopə) a state of semi-unconsciousness occurring in the course of many varieties of mental illness, where the patient does not move or speak, and makes no response to stimuli.

Sturge–Weber syndrome (,stərj-'webə) *W.A. Sturge, British physician, 1850–1919; Sir H.D. Weber, British physician, 1824–1918.* A congenital abnormality in which there is a port wine stain on the face with an angioma of the meninges on the same side. Common symptoms are epilepsy, hemiplegia, and mental handicap.

stuttering (,stutə·ring) *see* STAMMERING.

stye *see* HORDEOLUM.

stylet ('stielit) a wire or rod for keeping clear the lumen of catheters, cannulae and hollow needles.

styloid ('stieloyd) like a pen. *S. process* a long pointed spine, particularly one projecting from the temporal bone. Also processes on the ulna and radius.

styptic ('stiptik) an astringent which, applied locally, arrests haemorrhage, e.g. alum and tannic acid.

subacute (,subə'kyoot) moderately acute. Applied to a disease that progresses moderately rapidly, but does not become acute.

subarachnoid (,subə'raknoyd) below the arachnoid. *S. space* between the arachnoid and pia mater of the brain and spinal cord, and containing cerebrospinal fluid.

subclavian (sub'klayvi·ən) beneath the clavicle. *S. artery* the main vessel of supply to the neck and arms.

subclinical (sub'klinik'l) without clinical manifestations; said of the early stages or a very mild form of a disease.

subconscious (sub'konshəs) 1. not conscious yet able to be recalled to consciousness. 2. in psychoanalysis, the part of the mind that retains memories which cannot without much effort be recalled to mind.

subcutaneous (,subkyoo'tayni·əs) beneath the skin. *S. injection* one given hypodermically.

subdural (sub'dyooə·rəl) below the dura mater. *S. haematoma* a blood clot between the arachnoid and dura mater. It may be acute or arise slowly from a minor injury.

subinvolution (,subinvə,looshən) incomplete or delayed return of

the uterus to its pre-gravid size during the puerperium, usually due to retained products of conception and infection.

subjective (səb'jektiv) related to the individual. *S. symptoms* those of which the patient is aware by sensory stimulation, but which cannot easily be seen by others. *See also* OBJECTIVE.

sublimate ('subli,mayt) a substance obtained by sublimation.

sublimation (,subli'mayshən) 1. the vaporization to a solid and its condensation into a solid deposit. 2. in psychoanalysis, a redirecting of energy at an unconscious level. The transference into socially acceptable channels of tendencies that cannot be expressed. An important aspect of maturity.

subliminal (sub'limin'l) below the threshold of perception.

sublingual (sub'ling-gwəl) beneath the tongue. *S. glands* two small salivary glands in the floor of the mouth.

subluxation (,subluk'sayshən) partial dislocation of a joint.

submaxillary (,submak'silə·ree) beneath the lower jaw. *S. glands* two salivary glands situated under the lower jaw.

submucous (sub'myookəs) beneath mucous membrane. *S. resection* an operation to correct a deflected nasal septum.

subnormality (,subnaw'malitee) a state less than normal of that usually encountered, as mental subnormality, generally considered characterized by an intelligence quotient under 69.

subphrenic (sub'frenik) beneath the diaphragm. *S. abscess* one which develops below the diaphragm, usually after peritonitis or from postoperative infection.

substitution (,substi'tyooshən) the act of putting one thing in place of another. In psychology, this may be the nurse or foster mother in the place of the child's own mother. In psychotherapy, the nurse or therapist may be substituted for someone in the patient's background.

substrate (,substrayt) a substance on which an enzyme acts.

succus ('sukəs) a juice. *S. entericus* a digestive fluid secreted by intestinal glands. *S. gastricus* gastric juice.

succussion (su'kushən) a method of determining when free fluid is present in a cavity in the body. A sound of splashing is heard when the patient moves or is deliberately moved.

sucrose ('sookrohz, -ohs) a disaccharide obtained from cane or beet sugar.

suction ('sukshən) 1. the process of sucking. 2. the removal of gas or fluid from a cavity or other container by means of reduced pressure. *Post-tussive s.* a sucking noise heard in the lungs just after a cough.

sudamen (soo'daymən) a small white vesicle formed in the sweat glands after prolonged sweating.

sudden infant death syndrome (sud'n) abbreviated SIDS. The sudden and unexpected death of an apparently healthy infant, typically occurring between the ages of 3 weeks and 5 months, and not explained by careful postmortem studies. Called also

crib or cot death because the infant often is found dead in the cot.

sudor ('syoodor) sweat; perspiration.

sudorific (,syoodə'rifik) diaphoretic; an agent causing sweating.

suffocation (,sufə'kayshən) asphyxiation; a cessation of breathing caused by occlusion of the air passages, leading to unconsciousness and ultimately to death.

suffusion (sə'fyoozhən) a process of diffusion or overspreading as in flushing of the skin; blushing.

sugar ('shyhgə) a group of sweet carbohydrates classified chemically as monosaccharides or disaccharides. The following are included: *beet s.* obtained from sugar beet; *cane s.* obtained from sugar cane; *fructose* fruit sugar; *grape s.* dextrose, glucose; *milk s.* lactose. *Muscle s.* inositol; a sugarlike compound found in animal tissue, particularly in muscle, and also in many plant tissues.

suggestibility (sə,jestə'bilətee) inclination to act on suggestions of others.

suggestion (sə'jeschən) a tool of psychotherapy in which an idea is presented to a patient and accepted by him. *Posthypnotic s.* one implanted in a patient under hypnosis, which lasts after his return to normal condition.

suicide ('sooi,sied) the taking of one's own life; also any person who voluntarily and intentionally takes his own life. Legally, a death suspected of being due to violence that is self-inflicted is not termed a suicide unless there is positive evidence of the victim's intent to destroy himself, or the method of death is such that a verdict of suicide is inevitable. Some religious faiths consider it to be a sin and may refuse a consecrated burial.

sulcus ('sulkəs) a furrow or fissure; applied especially to those of the brain.

sulphacetamide (,sulfə'setə,mied) a soluble sulphonamide used as eyedrops to treat corneal and conjunctival infections.

sulphadiazine (,sulfə'dieə,zeen) a slow-acting sulphonamide drug which is relatively non-toxic. Used in the treatment of meningococcal meningitis.

sulphadimidine (,sulfə'diemi,deen) a sulphonamide of which a high blood level can be obtained with reduced incidence of side-effects. Used in the treatment of urinary tract infections.

sulphaemoglobin (,sulfheemə'glohbin) the substance produced in the blood by an excess of sulphur, which gives rise to sulphaemoglobinaemia. Sulphmethaemoglobin.

sulphaemoglobinaemia (,sulfheemə,glohbi,neemi·ə) a condition of sulphmethaemoglobin circulating in the blood.

sulphafurazole (,sulfə'fyooə·rə,zohl) a soluble, rapidly excreted sulphonamide useful in treating urinary tract infections.

sulphaguanidine (,sulfə'gwahni,deen) a mild sulphonamide used in the treatment of bacillary dysentery.

sulphamethizole (,sulfə'methi,zohl) a sulphonamide used in urinary infection as it is rapidly

excreted in an active form.

sulphasalazine (,sulfə'salə,zeen) a sulphonamide used in the treatment of ulcerative colitis.

sulphmethaemoglobin (,sulfmet,heemə'globin) see SULPHAEMO-GLOBIN.

sulphonamide (sul'fonə,mied) the generic term for all aminobenzene-sulphonamide preparations, including the bactericidal sulpha drugs.

sulphone ('sulfohn) one of a group of drugs which with prolonged use have been successful in treating leprosy. Dapsone is the most widely used.

sulphonylurea (,sulfoni'lyooə·ri·ə) one of a group of oral hypoglycaemic agents used in the treatment of diabetes mellitus.

sulphuric acid (sul'fyooə·rik) H_2SO_4; oil of vitriol. A heavy colourless liquid and corrosive poison, which burns any organic substance with which it comes into contact.

sulthiame (sul'thie,aym) an anticonvulsant drug used in the treatment of epilepsy.

sunburn ('sun,bərn) a dermatitis due to exposure to the sun's rays, causing burning and redness.

sunstroke ('sun,strohk) a profound disturbance of the body's heat-regulating mechanism caused by prolonged exposure to excessive heat from the sun. Persons over 40 and those in poor health are most susceptible to it.

supercilium (,soopə'sili·əm) the eyebrow.

superego (,soopə'reegoh, -'regoh) that part of the personality that is concerned with moral standards and ideals that are derived unconsciously from the parents, teachers and environment, and influence the person's whole mental make-up, acting as a control on impulses of the ego.

superfecundation (,soopə,fekən-'dayshən, -,fee-) the fertilization of two or more ova, produced during the same menstrual cycle, by spermatozoa from separate coital acts.

superfetation (,soopəfee'tayshən) the fertilization of a second ovum when pregnancy has already started, producing two fetuses of different maturity.

superior (soo'pie·ri·ə) above; the upper of two parts.

supine ('soopien) 1. lying on the back, with the face upward. 2. the turning of the palm of the hand upwards. *See* PRONATION.

suppository (sə'pozitə·ree) a medicated solid substance, prepared for insertion into the rectum or vagina, which will dissolve at body temperature.

suppression (sə'preshən) 1. complete cessation of a secretion. *S. of urine* no secretion of urine by the kidneys. 2. in psychology, conscious inhibition as distinct from repression, which is unconscious.

suppuration (,supyuh'rayshən) the formation of pus.

supracondylar (,sooprə'kondilə) above the condyles. *S. fracture* one above the lower end of the humerus or femur.

supraorbital (,sooprə'awbit'l) above the orbit of the eye.

suprapubic (,sooprə'pyoobik) above the pubic bones. *S. cys-*

totomy surgical incision of the urinary bladder just above the pubic bones.

suprarenal (,sooprə'reen'l) above the kidney. *S. gland* adrenal gland. One of a pair of triangular endocrine glands situated on the upper surface of the kidneys. *See* ADRENAL.

surfactant (sər'faktənt) a surface-active agent. A mixture of phospholipids secreted into the pulmonary alveoli which reduces the surface tension of pulmonary fluids and thus contributes to the elastic properties of pulmonary tissue. Surfactant can be instilled via a tracheal catheter as treatment for respiratory distress syndrome. *See also* RESPIRATORY DISTRESS SYNDROME.

surgeon ('sərjən) a medical practitioner who specializes in surgery. By custom the surgeon's title is Mr, Mrs or Miss, as opposed to physicians who are called Doctor.

surgery ('sərjə·ree) the branch of medicine that treats disease by operative measures.

surrogate ('surəgət) a real or imaginary substitute for a person or object in someone's life. *S. mother* a woman who carries a child for another (the commissioning mother) with the intention that the child be handed over after birth.

susceptibility (sə,septə'bilitee) lack of resistance to infection. The opposite to immunity.

suspensory (sə'spensə·ree) supporting a part. *S. bandage* one applied to support a part of the body, particularly the scrotum or the lower jaw. *S. ligament* a ligament that supports or suspends an organ, e.g. that of the lens of the eye.

suture ('soochə) 1. a stitch or series of stitches used to close a wound. *Atraumatic s.* a suture fused to the needle to obtain a single thickness through each puncture of the needle. *Continuous s.* a form of oversewing with one length of suture. *Everting s.* a type of mattress stitch that turns the edges outwards to give a closer approximation. *Fascial s.* a strip of fascia taken from the patient and used to form a suture. *Interrupted s.* a series of separate sutures. *Mattress s.* one in which each suture is taken twice through the wound, giving a loop one side and a knot the other. *Purse-string s.* a circular continuous suture round a small wound or appendix stump. *Subcuticular s.* a continuous suture placed just below the skin. *Tension s.* or *relaxation s.* one taking a large bite and relieving the tension on the true stitch line. 2. the jagged line of junction of the bones of the cranium. *Coronal s.* the junction between the frontal and parietal bones. *Lambdoid s.* the junction between the parietal and occipital bones. *Sagittal s.* the junction between the two occipital bones.

suxamethonium (‚suksəmee'thohni·əm) a short-acting muscle-relaxant drug that may be used to get good muscle relaxation during surgery performed under general anaesthesia and during electroconvulsive therapy.

swab (swob) 1. a small piece

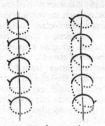

interrupted   continuous

mattress

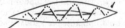

subcuticular

SUTURES

of cotton wool or gauze. 2. in pathology, a dressed stick used in taking bacteriological specimens.

swallowing ('swoloh·ing) the taking in of a substance through the mouth and pharynx and into the oesophagus. It is a combination of a voluntary set and a series of reflex actions. Once begun, the process operates automatically. Called also deglutition.

sweat (swet) perspiration; a clear watery fluid secreted by the sweat glands. *S. glands* coiled tubular glands situated in the dermis with long ducts to the skin surface.

sycosis (sie'kohsis) a pustular inflammation of the hair follicles, usually of the beard and moustache. *S. barbae* a staphylococcal infection affecting the beard. Scrupulous cleanliness is necessary to prevent reinfection. Now rare. Barber's itch.

Sydenham's chorea ('sid'n'mz) *T. Sydenham, British physician, 1624–1689.* A disorder of the central nervous system closely linked with rheumatic fever; called also Saint Vitus' dance. The condition, usually self-limited, is characterized by purposeless, irregular movements of the voluntary muscles that cannot be controlled by the patient.

symbiosis (,simbie'ohsis) in parasitology, an intimate association between two different organisms for the mutual benefit of both.

symblepharon (sim'blefə·ron) adhesion of an eyelid to the eyeball.

symbolism ('simbə,lizəm) in psychology, an abnormal mental condition in which events or objects are interpreted as symbols of the patient's own thoughts. In psychiatry, the re-entry into consciousness of repressed material in an acceptable form.

Syme's amputation (siemz) *J. Syme, British surgeon, 1799–1870.* Amputation of the foot at the ankle joint.

sympathectomy (,simpə'thektə-mee) division of autonomic nerve fibres which control specific involuntary muscles. An operation performed for many conditions, among them Raynaud's disease.

sympathetic (,simpə'thetik) 1. exhibiting sympathy. *S. ophthalmia* inflammation leading to loss of sight in the opposite eye following a perforating injury in the ciliary region. 2. relating to the autonomic nervous system. *S. nervous system* one of the two divisions of the autonomic nervous system. It supplies involuntary muscle and glands; it stimulates the ductless glands and the circulatory and respiratory systems, but inhibits the digestive system.

sympatholytic (,simpəthoh'litik) pertaining to drugs which oppose the action of the sympathetic nervous system.

sympathomimetic (,simpəthohmi-'metik) pertaining to drugs which produce effects similar to those caused by a stimulation of the sympathetic nervous system.

symphysis ('simfisis) a cartilaginous joint along the line of union of two bones. *S. pubis* the cartilaginous junction of the two pubic bones.

symptom ('simptəm) any indication of disease perceived by the patient. *Cardinal s's* 1. symptoms of greatest significance to the doctor, establishing the identity of the illness. 2. the symptoms shown in the temperature, pulse and respiration. *Dissociation s.* anaesthesia to pain and to heat and cold, without impairment of tactile sensibility. *Objective s.* one perceptible to others than the patient, as pallor, rapid pulse or respiration, restlessness, etc. *Presenting s.* the symptom or group of symptoms about which the patient complains or from which he seeks relief. *Signal s.* a sensation, aura or other subjective experience indicative of an impending epileptic or other seizure. *Subjective s.* one perceptible only to the patient, as pain, pruritus, vertigo, etc. *Withdrawal s's* symptoms which follow sudden abstinence from a drug on which a person is dependent.

symptomatology (,simptəmə'tolǝjee) 1. the study of the symptoms of a disease. 2. the symptoms of a particular disease, taken together.

synalgia (si'nalji·ǝ) pain felt in one part of the body but caused by inflammation of or injury to another part. Referred pain.

synapse ('sienaps) the termination of an axon with the dendrites of another nerve cell. Chemical transmitters pass the impulse across the space.

synchysis ('singkisis) liquefaction of the vitreous humour of the eye.

syncope ('singkǝpee) a simple faint or temporary loss of consciousness due to cerebral ischaemia, often caused by dilatation of the peripheral blood vessels and a sudden fall in blood pressure.

syndactylism (sin'dakti,lizǝm) possessing webbed fingers or toes. A condition in which two or more fingers or toes are joined together.

syndrome ('sindrohm) a group of signs or symptoms typical of a distinctive disease, which frequently occur together and form a distinctive clinical picture.

synechia (si'neeki·ǝ) adhesion of the iris to the cornea in front (*anterior s.*) or the capsule of the lens behind (*posterior s.*).

synergist (,sinǝ,jiist, si,nǝr-) 1. a muscle which works in conjunction with another muscle. 2. a drug which works in combination with another drug, the two drugs having a greater effect when taken together than when taken separately.

synovectomy (,sienoh'vektǝmee, ,si-) excision of a diseased synovial membrane to restore joint movement.

synovial fluid (sie'nohvi·ǝl, si-) the fluid which surrounds a joint and is secreted by the synovial membrane. It is a thick, colourless, lubricating substance.

synovial membrane a serous membrane lining the articular capsule of a movable joint, and terminating at the edge of the articular cartilage.

synovitis (,sienoh'vietis) inflammation of a synovial membrane, usually with an effusion of fluid within the joint.

synthesis ('sinthǝsis) the building up of a more complex structure from simple components. This may apply to drugs or to plant or animal tissues.

syphilid ('sifilid) a skin rash occurring during the secondary stage of syphilis.

syphilis ('sifilis) an infectious venereal disease leading to many structural and cutaneous lesions; called also lues. Syphilis is caused by a spiral-shaped bacterium (spirochaete), *Treponema pallidum*. It is a SEXUALLY TRANSMITTED DISEASE (STD), with the exception of congenital syphilis acquired by an infant from the mother in utero. There is an early infectious stage, followed by a latent period of many years before the non-infectious late stage when serious disorders of the nervous and vascular systems arise. *Congenital s.* that transmitted by the mother to the fetus; it is preventable if the mother receives a full course of penicillin during her pregnancy. *Non-venereal s.* a chronic treponemal infection mainly seen in children, occurring in many areas of the world, caused by an organism indistinguishable from *Treponema pallidum*, and transmitted by direct non-sexual contact. Lesions are usually oral mucous patches; subsequent lesions occur in the axillae, inguinal region and rectum. Then, after a latent period, destructive lesions of the skin and bones develop.

syringe (si'rinj) an instrument for injecting fluids or for aspirating or irrigating body cavities. It consists of a hollow tube with a tight-fitting piston. A hollow needle or a thin tube can be fitted to the end.

syringomyelia (si,ring-gohmie-'eeli-ə) the formation of cavities filled with fluid inside the spinal cord. Impairment of muscle function and sensation result at the level of and below the lesion. Painless injury may be the first symptom. It is a progressive disease.

syringomyelitis (si,ring-goh,mieə-'lietis) inflammation of the spinal cord, as the result of which cavities are formed in it.

syringomyelocele (si,ring-goh-'mieəloh,seel) a type of spina bifida in which the protruded sac of fluid communicates with the central canal of the spinal cord.

systemic (si'stemik) pertaining to or affecting the body as a whole. *S. circulation* circulation of the blood throughout the whole body, other than the pulmonary circulation. *See* SCLEROSIS.

systole ('sistəlee) the period of contraction of the heart. *See* DIASTOLE. *Atrial s.* the contraction of the heart by which the blood is pumped from the atria into the ventricles. *Extra-s.* a premature contraction of the atrium or ventricle, without alteration of the fundamental rhythm of the pacemaker. *Ventricular s.* the contraction of the heart by which the blood is pumped into the aorta and pulmonary artery.

systolic (si'stolik) relating to a systole. *S. murmur* an abnormal sound produced during systole, in heart affections. *S. pressure* the highest pressure of the blood reached during systole.

T

T symbol for *thymine*.

T cell (te sel) a lymphocyte which is derived from the thymus and is responsible for cell-mediated immunity.

TAB typhoid–paratyphoid A and B vaccine. A sterile suspension of the killed salmonellae causing these diseases. Used as a preventive it provides an active immunity.

tabes ('taybeez) a wasting away. *T. dorsalis* locomotor ataxia. A slowly progressive disease of the nervous system affecting the posterior nerve roots and spinal cord. It is a late manifestation of syphilis.

taboparesis (,taybohpə'reesis) the presence of the symptoms of both tabes dorsalis and general paralysis of the insane in a patient suffering from late syphilis.

tachycardia (,taki'kahdi·ə) abnormally rapid action of the heart and consequent increase in pulse rate. *See* BRADYCARDIA. *Paroxysmal t.* spasmodic increase in cardiac contractions of sudden onset lasting a variable time from a few seconds to hours.

tachylalia (,taki'layli·ə) extreme rapidity of speech.

tachyphasia (tachyphrasia) (,taki-'fayzi·ə; ,taki'frayzi·ə) extreme volubility of speech. It may be a sign of mental disorder.

tachyphrenia (,taki'freeni·ə) hyperactivity of the mental processes.

tachypnoea (,takip'neeə) rapid, shallow respirations; a reflex response to stimulation of the vagus nerve endings in the pulmonary vessels.

tactile ('taktiel) relating to the sense of touch.

Taenia ('teeni·ə) a genus of tapeworms. *T. saginata* the beef tapeworm. The commonest type of tapeworm found in the human intestine. *T. solium* the pork tapeworm. Can also be parasitic in man, causing cysticercosis. *See* TAPEWORM.

taeniacide ('teeni·ə,sied) an agent that is lethal to tapeworms.

taeniafuge ('teeni·ə,fyooj) a drug which expels tapeworms.

taeniasis (tee'nieəsis) an infestation with tapeworms.

TAF toxoid–antitoxin floccules. A vaccine used for diphtheria immunization. *See* TOXOID.

talipes ('talipeez) club-foot. A deformity caused by a congenital or acquired contraction of the muscles or tendons of the foot. *T. calcaneous* the heel alone touches the ground on standing. *T. equinus* the toes touch the ground but not the heel. *T. valgus* the inner edge of the foot only is in contact with the ground. *T. varus* the person

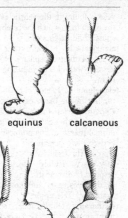

equinus   calcaneous

valgus   varus

TALIPES

walks on the outer edge of the foot.

talus ('tayləs) the astragalus or ankle bone.

tampon ('tampon) a plug of absorbent material inserted in the vagina, the nose or other orifice to restrain haemorrhage or absorb secretion.

tamponade ('tampə,nayd) the surgical use of tampons. *Cardiac t.* impairment of heart action by haemorrhage or effusion into the pericardium; may be due to a stab wound or follow surgery.

tannic acid ('tanik) a yellowish powder prepared from bark and the fruit of many plants. A

powerful astringent.

tantalum ('tantələm) *symbol* Ta. Metallic element used for prostheses and wire sutures.

tantrum ('tantrəm) an outburst of ill temper. *Temper t.* a behaviour disorder of childhood. A display of bad temper in which the child performs uncontrolled actions in a state of emotional stress.

tapeworm ('taypwərm) any of a group of cestode flatworms, including the *Taenia* genus, which are parasitic in the intestines of man and many animals. The adult consists of a round head with suckers or hooklets for attachment (scolex). From this numerous segments (proglottids) arise, each of which produces ova capable of independent existence for a considerable length of time. Treatment is by anthelmintic drugs.

tapotement (,tapoht'monh) [Fr.] a tapping movement used in massage.

tapping ('taping) *see* PARACENTESIS.

tarsal ('tahs'l) relating to a tarsus. *T. bones* the seven small bones of the ankle and instep. *T. cyst* meibomian cyst; chalazion. *T. glands* meibomian glands of the eyelids. *T. plates* small cartilages in the upper and lower eyelids.

tarsalgia (tah'salji·ə) pain in the foot, usually associated with flattening of the arch.

tarsoplasty ('tahsoh,plastee) plastic surgery of the eyelid.

tarsorrhaphy (tah'so·rəfee) stitching of the eyelids together to protect the cornea or to allow healing of an abrasion.

tartar ('tahtə) a hard incrustation deposited on the teeth and on dentures. *T. emetic* antimony potassium tartrate. A salt used in the treatment of schistosomiasis and leishmaniasis.

taste (tayst) the sense by which it is possible to identify what is eaten and drunk. Taste receptors (buds) lie on the tongue and give the sensations of sweet, sour, salt and bitter.

taxis ('taksis) manipulation by hand to restore any part to its normal position. It can be used to reduce a hernia or a dislocation.

taxonomy (tak'sonəmee) in biology, the classification of animals and plants.

Tay–Sachs disease (,tay'saks) *W. Tay, British physician, 1843–1927; B. Sachs, American neurologist, 1858–1944. See* AMAUROTIC FAMILIAL IDIOCY.

tears (tiəz) the watery, slightly alkaline and saline secretion of the lacrimal glands that moistens the conjunctiva.

teat (teet) 1. a nipple of the breast. 2. a manmade nipple used on infants' feeding bottles.

technetium (tek'neeshi·əm) *symbol* Tc. A metallic element. *Radioactive t.* isotope (^{99m}Tc) used in a number of diagnostic tracer tests. As it has a short half-life (6 h), a high dose for scanning organs may be given whilst the patient receives only a low radiation dose.

teeth (teeth) *see* DENTITION.

tegument ('tegyuhmənt) the skin.

tela ('teelə) a web-like tissue. *T. choroidea* a fold of pia mater containing a network of blood vessels found in the ventricles of the brain from which the cerebrospinal fluid originates.

telangiectasis (tə,lanji'ektəsis) a group of dilated capillary blood vessels, web-like or radiating in form.

telangioma (tə,lanji'ohmə) a tumour of the blood capillaries.

telepathy (tə'lepəthee) the transmission of thought without any normal means of communication between two persons.

telereceptor (,teliri'septə) a sensory nerve ending which can respond to distant stimuli. Those of the eyes, ears and nose are examples. Teleceptor.

teletherapy (,teli'therəpee) treatment in which the source of the therapeutic agent, e.g. radiation, is at a distance from the body.

telophase ('teloh,fayz) the last stage in the division of cells when the chromosomes have been reconstituted in the nuclei at either end of the cell and the cell cytoplasm divides to form two new cells.

temperature ('temprəchə) the degree of heat of a substance or body as measured by a thermometer. *Normal t.* of the human body is 37°C (98.6°F) with a slight decrease in the early morning, and a slight increase at night. It indicates the balance between heat production and heat loss.

template ('templayt) a mould or pattern. In radiotherapy, a map of the area of the patient requiring treatment and of those areas to be protected from radiation.

temple ('temp'l) the region on either side of the head above the zygomatic arch.

temporal ('tempə·rəl) pertaining to the side of the head. *T. arteritis* giant cell arteritis. A chronic inflammatory condition of the carotid arterial system, occurring usually in elderly people. There is persistent headache and partial or total blindness may result. *T. bone* one of a pair of bones on either side of the skull and containing the organ of hearing. *T. lobe* the part of the cerebrum below the lateral sulcus.

temporomandibular (,tempə·roh·man'dibyuhlə) relating to the temporal bone and the mandible. *T. joint* the hinge of the lower jaw. *T. j. syndrome* painful dysfunction of the temporomandibular joint, marked by a clicking or grinding sensation in the joint; commonly caused by malocclusion of the teeth.

tenacious (tə'nayshəs) thick and viscid, as applied to sputum or other body fluids.

tendinitis (,tendi'nietis) inflammation of a tendon and its attachments.

tendon ('tendən) a band of fibrous tissue, forming the termination of a muscle and attaching it to a bone. *Achilles t.* that inserted into the calcaneum. *T. grafting* an operation which repairs a defect in one tendon by a graft from another. *T. insertion* the point of attachment of a muscle to a bone which it moves. *T. reflex* the muscular contraction produced on percussing a tendon.

tenesmus (tə'nezməs) a painful ineffectual straining to empty the bowel or bladder.

tennis elbow ('tenis) a painful disorder which affects the extensor muscles of the forearm at their attachment to the external epicondyle.

Tenon's capsule (tə'nonhz) *J.R. Tenon, French surgeon, 1724–1816.* The fibrous tissue in which the eyeball is situated.

tenonitis ('tenə'nietis) inflammation of Tenon's capsule. Proptosis of the eyeball occurs, often accompanied by pain and pyrexia.

tenorrhaphy (te'no·rəfee) the suturing together of the ends of a divided tendon.

tenosynovitis (,tenoh,sienoh'vietis) inflammation of a tendon sheath.

tenotomy (tə'notəmee) the surgical division of a tendon, to correct a deformity caused by its shortening. In ophthalmology, performed to correct a squint.

tension ('tenshən) the act of stretching or the state of being stretched. *Arterial t.* the pressure of blood on the vessel wall during cardiac contraction. *Intraocular t.* the pressure of the contents of the eye on its walls, measured by a tonometer. *Intravenous t.* the pressure of blood within the veins. *Premenstrual t.* symptoms of abdominal distension, headache, emotional lability and depression occurring a few days before the onset of menstruation. *See* PREMENSTRUAL. *Surface t.* tension or resistance which acts to preserve the integrity of a surface, particularly the surface of a liquid.

tensor ('tensə, -sor) a muscle

which stretches a part.

teratogen ('terətoh,jen) an agent or influence that causes physical defects in the developing embryo.

teratogenesis (,terətoh'jenəsis) the production of deformity in the developing embryo.

teratoma (,terə'tohmə) a solid tumour containing tissues similar to those of a dermoid cyst. Found most often in the ovaries and testes, many of these tumours are malignant.

tertian ('tərshən) recurring every 48 h. *See* MALARIA.

tertiary ('tərshə·ree) third. *T. prevention* prevention of ill health, mitigating the effects of illness and disease that have already occurred. *T. syphilis* the non-infectious stage of neurosyphilis.

test (test) 1. an examination or trial. 2. analysis of the composition of a substance by the use of chemical reagents.

testicle ('testik'l) a testis; one of the two glands in the scrotum which produce spermatozoa. *Undescended t.* condition in which the organ remains in the pelvis or inguinal canal.

testis ('testis) a testicle.

testosterone (tes'tostə,rohn) the hormone produced by the testes which stimulates the development of sex characteristics. Now made synthetically. It is used medicinally in cases of failure of sex function and as a palliative treatment in some cases of advanced metastatic breast cancer in females.

tetanus ('tetənəs) an acute disease of the nervous system caused by

the contamination of wounds by the spores of a soil bacterium, *Clostridium tetani*. Muscle stiffness around the site of the wound occurs followed by rigidity of face and neck muscles; hence 'lockjaw'. All muscles are then affected and opisthotonos may occur. *T. vaccine* or *toxoid* will give an active immunity. *T. antitoxin* a serum that gives a short-term passive immunity and may be used with penicillin for immediate treatment of a case of tetanus.

tetany ('tetənee) an increased excitability of the nerves due to a lack of available calcium, accompanied by painful muscle spasm of the hands and feet (carpopedal spasm). The cause may be hypoparathyroidism or alkalosis owing to excessive vomiting or hyperventilation.

tetrachloroethylene (,tetrə,klor-·roh'ethi,leen) an anthelmintic drug widely used to treat hookworm disease.

tetracycline (,tetrə'siekleen) an antibiotic drug belonging to the group known as the tetracyclines which are effective against many different microorganisms, including rickettsiae, Gram-negative and Gram-positive organisms and certain viruses.

tetradactylous (,tetrə'daktiləs) having four digits on each hand or foot.

tetralogy (te'traləjee) a series of four. *T. of Fallot see* FALLOT'S TETRALOGY.

tetraplegia (,tetrə'pleeji·ə) quadriplegia. Paralysis of all four limbs.

thalamotomy (,thalə'motəmee)

surgical destruction of the nucleus in the thalamus to relieve intractable pain or relief of tremor and rigidity in Parkinson's disease.

thalamus ('thaləməs) a mass of nerve cells at the base of the cerebrum. Most sensory impulses from the body pass to this area and are transmitted to the cortex.

thalassaemia (,thalə'seemi·ə) a group of haemolytic anaemias mostly found in the Mediterranean region and the Far East, caused by the inheritance of abnormal haemoglobin. *T. major* Cooley's anaemia; the severest form of thalassaemia with death usually occurring before adolescence. *T. minor* a mild form of the disease with few symptoms. Those suffering from it can pass the disease on to their children.

thalassotherapy (thə,lasoh'therəpee) treatment involving sea bathing or a sea voyage.

theca ('theekə) a sheath, such as the covering of a tendon. *T. folliculi* the covering of a graafian follicle. *T. vertebralis* the membranes enclosing the spinal cord; the dura mater.

theism ('thee·izəm) chronic poisoning resulting from excessive tea drinking. Theinism.

thenar ('theenah) 1. the palm of the hand. 2. the fleshy part at the base of the thumb.

theobromine (,theeoh'brohmeen) an alkaloid derived from the cocoa bean. Used as a heart stimulant and as a mild diuretic.

theophylline (thi'ofi,leen) an alkaloid derived from tea-leaves, and with action similar to that of theobromine. Used mainly in the treatment of bronchospasm.

therapeutic (,therə'pyootik) pertaining to therapeutics or treatment of disease; curative. *T. abortion see* ABORTION. *T. community* any treatment setting (usually psychiatric) which provides a living–learning situation through group processes emphasizing social, environmental and personal interactions and which encourages the individual to learn socially from these processes. *T. use of self* the ability of the psychiatric nurse to use therapy and experimental knowledge along with self-awareness and the ability to explore, and use, one's personal impact on others.

therapeutics (,therə'pyootiks) the science and art of healing and the treatment of disease.

therapy ('therəpee) the treatment of disease. *Occupational t.* treatment by providing interesting and congenital work within the limitations of the patient in mental diseases and in order to re-educate and coordinate muscles in physical defect.

thermal ('thərməl) relating to heat.

thermocautery (,thərmoh'kawtə·ree) the deliberate destruction of tissue by means of heat. *See* CAUTERY.

thermogenesis (,thərmoh'jenəsis) the production of heat.

thermography (,thər'mogrəfee) a method of measuring the amount of heat produced by different areas of the body, using infrared photography. Used as a diagnostic aid in the detection of breast tumours and the assessment of rheumatic joints; also used in the study of pain.

thermolysis (thər'molisis) the loss of body heat by radiation, by excretion and by the evaporation of sweat.

thermometer (thə'momitə) an instrument for measuring temperature. *Clinical t.* one used to measure the body temperature. *Electronic t.* a clinical thermometer which works electrically. It contains electronic devices whose characteristics change with temperature. The reading is recorded within seconds and displayed visually.

thermoreceptor (,thəmohri'septə) a nerve ending that responds to heat and cold.

thermostat ('thərmə,stat) an apparatus which automatically regulates the temperature and maintains it at a specified level.

thermotaxis (,thərmoh'taksis) the normal regulation of body temperature by maintaining the balance between heat production and heat loss.

thermotherapy (,thərmoh'therəpee) the treatment of disease by application of heat.

thiamine ('thieə,meen) vitamin B_1, or aneurine. An essential vitamin involved in carbohydrate metabolism. A deficiency causes beriberi. The source is liver and unrefined cereals.

thiazides ('thieə,ziedz) any of a group of diuretics that act by inhibiting the reabsorption of sodium in the proximal renal tubule and stimulating chloride excretion, with resultant increase

in excretion of water.

Thiersch skin graft ('teeəsh) *I. Thiersch, German surgeon, 1822–1895.* The transplantation of areas of partial thickness skin. *See* GRAFT.

thioguanine (,thieoh'gwahneen) an antimetabolite used in the treatment of acute leukaemia.

thiopentone (,thieoh'pentohn) a basal narcotic of the barbiturate group given intravenously as a short-acting anaesthetic and in preoperative preparation.

thiopropazate (,thieoh'prohpə,zayt) a tranquillizer used in the treatment of schizophrenia and psychoneuroses.

thiotepa (,thieoh'teepə) an intravenous cytotoxic drug used in the treatment of cancer, particularly of the bladder or ovary.

thiouracil (,thieoh'yooə-rəsil) a drug used in the treatment of thyrotoxicosis. A derivative, propylthiouracil, which is more active and less toxic, is now more often used.

thirst (thərst) an uncomfortable sensation of dryness of the mouth and throat with a desire for oral fluids. *Abnormal t.* polydipsia.

Thomas splint ('tomas) *H.O. Thomas, British orthopaedic surgeon, 1834–1891.* A splint consisting of an oval iron ring which fits over the lower limb. Attached to the ring are two round iron rods which are bent into a W-shape at the lower end. It is used to support the limb and move the weight from the knee joint to the pelvis.

thoracic (thor'rasik) relating to the thorax. *T. duct* the large lym-

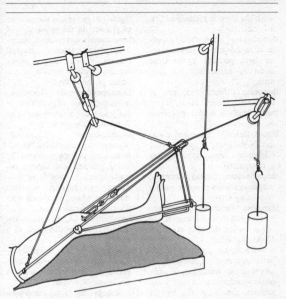

Thomas splint in use with skeletal traction.
A Pearson knee flexion piece is attached

THOMAS SPLINT

phatic vessel situated in the thorax
along the spine. It opens into the
left subclavian vein.

thoracocentesis (,thor·rəkohsen-
'teesis) puncture of the wall of the
thorax to allow aspiration of the
pleural fluid.

thoracoscopy (,thor·rə'koskəpee)
examination of the pleural cavity
by means of an endoscopic

instrument.

thoracotomy (,thor·rə'kotəmee) a
surgical incision into the thorax.

thorax ('thor·raks) the chest; a
cavity containing the heart,
lungs, bronchi and oesophagus.
It is bounded by the diaphragm,
the sternum, the dorsal vertebrae, and the ribs. *Barrel-shaped
t.* a development in emphysema,

when the chest is malformed like a barrel.

threadworm ('thred,wərm) a species of roundworm, *Enterobius vermicularis*, parasitic in the large intestine, particularly of children.

threonine ('threeə,neen) one of the essential amino acids.

thrill ('thril) a tremor discerned by palpation.

throat (throht) 1. the anterior surface of the neck. 2. the pharynx. *Clergyman's sore t*. laryngitis. *Sore t*. pharyngitis.

thrombectomy (throm'bektəmee) surgical excision of a clot from a vein or an artery.

thrombin ('thrombin) an enzyme which converts fibrinogen to fibrin during the later stages of blood clotting.

thromboangiitis (,thromboh,anji-'ietis) inflammation of blood vessels with clot formation. *T. obliterans* inflammation of the arteries, usually of the legs of young males, causing intermittent claudication and gangrene. Buerger's disease.

thrombocyte ('thromboh,siet) a blood platelet. Disc-shaped, essential for the clotting of shed blood.

thrombocytopenia (,thromboh-,sietoh'peeni·ə) a reduction in the number of platelets in the blood; bleeding may occur. Destruction of platelets can be caused by infections, certain drugs, transfusion related purpuras, idiopathic thrombocytopenic purpura and disseminated intravascular coagulation.

thrombocytosis (,thrombohsie-

'tohsis) an increase in the number of platelets in the blood.

thromboendarterectomy (,thromboh,endahtə'rektəmee) surgical removal of a clot from an artery together with a portion of the lining of the artery.

thromboendarteritis (,thromboh-,endahtə'rietis) inflammation of the lining of an artery with clot formation as a result.

thrombokinase (,thromboh-'kienayz) thromboplastin. A lipid-containing protein activated by blood platelets and injured tissues, which is capable of activating prothrombin to form thrombin which, combined with fibrinogen, forms a clot.

thrombolysis (throm'bolisis) the disintegration or dissolving of a clot.

thrombophlebitis (,thrombohfli-'bietis) the formation of a clot, associated with inflammation of the lining of the vein.

thromboplastin (,thromboh'plastin) *see* THROMBOKINASE.

thrombosis (throm'bohsis) the formation of a thrombus. *Cavernous sinus t*. thrombosis of the cavernous sinus, usually the result of infection of the face, when the veins in the sinus are affected via ophthalmic vessels. *Cerebral t*. the occlusion of a cerebral artery, the most common cause of cerebral infarction (a 'stroke'). *Coronary t*. the occlusion of a coronary vessel, by which the heart muscle is deprived of blood, causing myocardial ischaemia, and leading often to myocardial infarction (a 'heart attack'). *Lateral sinus t*. a complication of mastoiditis when infection of the lateral sinus of the dura mater occurs and there is clot formation.

thrombus ('thrombəs) a stationary blood clot caused by coagulation of the blood in the heart or in an artery or a vein.

thrush (thrush) an infection of the mucous membranes, most commonly of the mouth and vagina, by a fungus, *Candida albicans*. *See* CANDIDIASIS.

thymectomy (thie'mektəmee) surgical removal of the thymus.

thymine ('thiemeen) one of the pyrimidine bases found in DNA.

thymokesis (,thiemoh'keesis) persistence of the thymus gland in an adult.

thymol ('thiemol) an aromatic antiseptic used in solution as a mouth wash.

thymoma (thie'mohmə) a tumour that originates in thymus tissue.

thymus ('thieməs) a gland-like structure situated in the upper thorax and neck. Present in early life, it reaches its maximum development during puberty and continues to play an immunological role throughout life, even though its function declines with age.

thyrocricotomy (,thierohkrie-'kotəmee) incision of the cricothyroid membrane to achieve TRACHEOSTOMY.

thyroglobulin (,thieroh'globyuhlin) the protein in thyroxine, the endocrine secretion of the thyroid.

thyroglossal (,thieroh'glos'l) relating to the thyroid and the tongue. *T. cyst see* CYST.

thyroid ('thieroyd) 1. shaped like a shield. 2. pertaining to the thyroid gland. *T. cartilage* the largest cartilage of the larynx. It forms the 'Adam's apple' in the front of the throat. *T. gland* a ductless gland consisting of two lobes, situated in front and on either side of the trachea. It secretes the hormones thryoxine and triiodothyronine which are concerned in regulating the metabolic rate. *Intrathoracic* or *retrosternal t.* position of the gland low in the neck and wholly or in part behind the sternum. *T.-stimulating hormone* abbreviated TSH. Thyrotrophin; a hormone produced by the anterior pituitary gland which controls the activity of the thyroid gland.

thyroidectomy (,thieroy'dektəmee) partial or complete removal of the thyroid gland.

thyroiditis (,thieroy'dietis) inflammation of the thyroid. Acute thyroiditis, usually due to a virus infection, is characterized by sore throat, fever and painful enlargement of the gland. *Hashimoto's t.* a progressive autoimmune disease of the thyroid gland with degeneration of its epithelial elements and replacement by lymphoid and fibrous tissue.

thyroparathyroidectomy (,thieroh,parə,thieroy'dektəmee) surgical removal of the thyroid and parathyroid glands.

thyrotoxicosis (,thieroh,toksi-'kohsis) hyperthyroidism. The symptoms arising when there is overactivity of the thyroid gland. The metabolism is speeded up and there is enlargement of the gland and exophthalmos.

thyrotrophin (,thieroh'trohfin) *see* THYROID-STIMULATING HORMONE.

thyroxine (thie'rokseen) one of the two hormones secreted by the thyroid gland. It is used in the treatment of hypothyroidism.

TIA transient ischaemic attack.

tibia ('tibi·ə) the shin bone; the larger of the two bones of the leg, extending from knee to ankle.

tic (tik) a spasmodic twitching of certain muscles, usually of the face, neck or shoulder. *T. douloureux* paroxysmal trigeminal neuralgia.

tick (tik) a blood-sucking parasite which may transmit the organisms of disease.

tidal volume ('tied'l) the amount of gas passing into and out of the lungs in each respiratory cycle.

tincture ('tingkcha) an alcoholic solution of an animal or vegetable drug.

tine test (tien) a tuberculin skin test employing a multiple-puncture, disposable device. It is especially useful in mass screening of children, but is less accurate than the Mantoux test.

tinea ('tini·ə) a group of skin infections caused by a variety of fungi and named after the area of the body affected, thus: *T. barbae*, the beard; *T. capitis*, the head; *T. circinata* or *T. corporis*, the body; *T. cruris*, the groin; and *T. pedis*, the feet. *See* RINGWORM.

tinnitus (ti'nietəs) a ringing, buzzing or roaring sound in the ears.

tintometer (tin'tomitə) an instrument by which changes in colour of a fluid can be measured.

tissue ('tisyoo, 'tishoo) a group or layer of similarly specialized cells that together perform certain special functions.

titration (tie,trayshən) determination of a given component in solution by addition of a liquid reagent of known strength until a given end point, e.g. change in colour, is reached, indicating that the component has been consumed by reaction with the reagent.

tobramycin (,tohbrə'miesin) an antibiotic drug used chiefly in the treatment of *Pseudomonas* infection.

tocography (to'kografee) the measurement of alterations in the intrauterine pressure during labour.

tocopherol (to'kofə·rol) vitamin E, present in wheat germ, green leaves and milk.

token economy programme ('tohkən i'konəmee) a behavioural approach to modifying troublesome behaviours and restoring lost self-help behaviours by the systematic rewarding of desired behaviour by giving tokens which may be exchanged for goods or privileges.

tolazamide (to'lazə,mied) an oral hypoglycaemic drug used in the treatment of diabetes mellitus.

tolazoline (to'lazoh,leen) a vasodilator drug of the peripheral blood vessels, used in the treatment of peripheral vascular disease.

tolbutamide (tol'byootə,mied) an oral drug that stimulates the release of insulin from the pancreas. Used in the treatment of diabetes mellitus.

tolerance ('tolə·rəns) the ability to endure without effect or injury. *Drug t.* decrease of susceptibility to the effects of a drug due to its continued administration. *Immunological t.* specific non-reactivity of lymphoid tissues to a particular antigen capable, under other conditions, of inducing immunity.

tomography (toh'nogrəfee) body section radiography in which X-rays or ultrasound waves are used to produce an image of a layer of tissue at any depth.

tone (tohn) 1. the normal degree of tension, e.g. in a muscle. 2. a particular quality of sound.

tongue (tung) a muscular organ attached to the floor of the mouth and concerned in taste, mastication, swallowing and speech. It is covered by a mucous membrane from which project numerous papillae.

tonic ('tonik) 1. a term popularly applied to any drug supposed to brace or tone up the body or any particular part or organ. 2. possessing tone in a state of contraction, e.g. muscles. *T. spasm* a prolonged contraction of one or several muscles, as seen in epilepsy, for example. *See* CLONIC.

tonography (toh'nogrəfee) the measurement made by an electric tonometer recording the intraocular pressure and so, indirectly, the drainage of aqueous humour from the eye.

tonometer (toh'nomitə) an instrument for measuring intraocular pressure.

tonsil ('tonsil) a mass of lymphoid

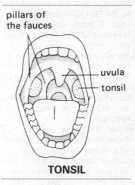

pillars of the fauces

uvula

tonsil

TONSIL

tissue, particularly one of two small almond-shaped bodies, situated one on each side between the pillars of the fauces. It is covered by mucous membrane, and its surface is pitted with follicles. *Pharyngeal t.* the lymph-adenoid tissue of the pharynx between the pharyngotympanic tubes. Adenoids.

tonsillectomy (,tonsi'lektəmee) excision of one or both tonsils.

tonus ('tohnəs) the normal state of partial contraction of the muscles.

tooth (tooth) a structure in the mouth designed for the mastication of food. Each is composed of a crown, neck and root with one or more fangs. The main bulk is of dentine enclosing a central pulp; the crown is covered with a hard white substance called enamel. *See* DENTITION.

tophus ('tohfəs) a small, hard, chalky deposit of sodium urate in the skin and cartilage occurring in gout, and sometimes appearing on the auricle of the ear.

topical ('topik'l) relating to a particular spot; local. *T. lotion* one for local or external application.

topography (tə'pogrəfee, toh-) the study of the surface of the body in relation to the underlying structures.

torpor ('tawpə) a sluggish condition, in which response to stimuli is absent or very slow.

torsion ('tawshən) twisting: (1) of an artery to arrest haemorrhage; (2) of the pedicle of a cyst which produces venous congestion in the cyst and consequent gangrene (a possible complication of ovarian cyst).

torso ('tawsoh) the body, excluding the head and the limbs; the trunk.

torticollis (,tawti'kolis) wryneck, a contracted state of the cervical muscles, producing torsion of the neck. The deformity may be congenital or hysterical, or secondary to pressure on the accessory nerve, to inflammation of glands in the neck, or to muscle spasm.

tourniquet ('tooəni,kay, 'tawni-) a constrictive band applied to a limb to arrest arterial haemorrhage. No longer used in First Aid since its use may cause permanent damage to muscles or nerve supply.

toxaemia (tok'seemi·ə) poisoning of the blood by the absorption of bacterial toxins. *T. of pregnancy* a condition affecting pregnant women and characterized by albuminuria, hypertension and oedema, with the possibility of pre-eclampsia and eclampsia developing.

toxic ('toksik) 1. poisonous, relating to a poison. 2. caused by a toxin. *T. shock syndrome* a severe illness characterized by high fever of sudden onset, vomiting, diarrhoea and, in severe cases, death. A sunburn-like rash with peeling of the skin occurs. The syndrome affects almost exclusively menstruating women using tampons, although a few women who do not use tampons and a few males have been affected. It is thought to be caused by infection with *Staphylococcus aureus*.

toxicity (tok'sisitee) the degree of virulence of a poison.

toxicology (,toksi'koləjee) the science dealing with poisons.

toxin ('toksin) any poisonous compound, usually referring to that produced by bacteria.

Toxocara (,toksoh'kair·rə) a genus of nematode worms, parasitic in the intestines of dogs and cats, which may also infest man, especially children. The spleen, liver and lungs are most often affected, but the parasite may also infest the retina, causing inflammation and granulation.

toxoid ('toksoyd) a toxin which has been deprived of some of its harmful properties but is still capable of producing immunity and may be used in a vaccine. *Diphtheria t.* toxin which has been treated with formaldehyde. Used for immunization against diphtheria. *See* TAF and APT.

Toxoplasma (,toksoh'plazmə) a

genus of protozoa which infests birds and animals and may be transmitted from them to man.

toxoplasmosis (,toksohplaz'mohsis) a disease due to *Toxoplasma gondii*. The congenital form is marked by central nervous system lesions, which may lead to blindness, brain defects and death. The acquired infection is often asymptomatic but may result in pneumonia, skin rashes and nephritis.

trabecula (trə'bekyuhlə) a dividing band or septum, extending from the capsule of an organ into its interior and holding the functioning cells in position.

trabeculectomy (trə,bekyuh'lektəmee) an operation to lower the intraocular pressure in glaucoma.

trabeculotomy (trə,bekyuh'lotəmee) an operation for glaucoma, usually performed using a laser.

tracer ('traysə) a means by which something may be followed, as (1) a mechanical device by which the outline or movements of an object can be graphically recorded, or (2) a material by which the progress of a compound through the body may be observed, e.g. a radioactive isotope tracer.

trachea (trə'keeə, 'traki·ə) the windpipe: a cartilaginous tube lined with ciliated mucous membrane, extending from the lower part of the larynx to the commencement of the bronchi.

tracheitis (,traki'ietis) inflammation of the trachea causing pain in the chest, with coughing.

trachelorrhaphy (,trakə'lo·rəfee) an operation for suturing lacerations of the cervix of the uterus.

tracheobronchitis (,trakiohbrong'kietis) acute infection of the trachea and bronchi due to viruses or bacteria.

tracheostomy (,traki'ostəmee) a surgical opening into the third and fourth cartilage rings of the trachea. *T. tubes* those used to maintain an airway following tracheotomy, either permanently or until the normal use of the air passages is regained.

tracheotomy (,traki'otəmee) surgical incision of the trachea. *Inferior* or *low t.* that in which the opening is made below the thyroid isthmus. *Superior* or *high t.* that in which the opening is made above the thyroid isthmus.

trachoma (trə'kohmə) a chronic infectious disease of the conjunctiva and cornea, producing photophobia, pain and lacrimation, caused by an organism once thought to be a virus but now classified as a strain of the bacteria *Chlamydia trachomatis*. Trachoma is more prevalent in Africa and Asia than in other parts of the world.

traction ('trakshən) the exertion of a pulling force, as that applied to a fractured bone, dislocated joint or to relieve muscle spasm to maintain proper position and facilitate healing. In obstetrics, that along the axis of the pelvis to assist in delivery of a fetal part, or the placenta and membranes. *Hamilton–Russell t.* a form of traction of the leg in which there is an upward pull over a beam and the cord is continuous with a series of pulleys attached to the

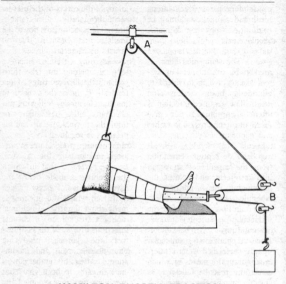

HAMILTON–RUSSELL TRACTION

limb by skin traction horizontally. *Head t.* traction exerted on the head in the treatment of cervical injury. *Skeletal t.* a method of keeping the fractured ends of bone in position by traction on the bone. A metal pin or wire is passed through the distal fragment or adjacent bone to overcome muscle contraction.

tragus ('traygəs) 1. the small prominence of cartilage at the external meatus of the ear. 2. one of the hairs at the external auditory meatus.

trait (trayt) an inherited or developed physical or mental characteristic.

trance (tranz) a condition of semi-consciousness of hysterical, cataleptic or hypnotic origin. It is not due to organic disease.

tranquillizer (,trangkwi,liezə) a drug which allays anxiety, relieves tension and has a calming effect on the patient.

transabdominal (,tranzab'domin'l, ,trahnz-) across the abdominal wall or through the abdominal cavity.

transactional analysis (tran-'zakshən'l, trahn-) a theory of personality structure and a psychotherapeutic method. The human personality is viewed as consisting of three ego states: the parent, the adult, and the child. The aim is to allow the adult ego to take control over the child and parent egos.

transaminase (tran'zami,nayz) one of a group of enzymes which catalyse the transfer of an amine group from one amino acid into another, together with a new keto acid. Transaminases include *glutamic-oxalacetic t.* (GOT) and *glutamic-pyruvic t.* (GPT).

transcendental meditation (,transen,dent'l ,medi'taytshən, 'trahn-) a technique for attaining a state of physical relaxation and psychological calm by the regular practice of a relaxation procedure which entails the repetition of a mantra. Has been successfully used by some patients to reduce hypertension.

transference (,transfə·rəns, trans-'fər·rəns, 'trahns-) in psychiatry, the unconscious transfer by the patient on to the psychiatrist of feelings which are appropriate to other people significant to the patient.

transfusion (trans'fyoozhən, trahns-) the introduction of whole blood or a blood component into a vein, performed in cases of severe loss of blood, shock, septicaemia, etc. It is used to supply

actual volume of blood, or to introduce constituents as clotting factors, or antibodies, which are deficient in the patient. *Direct t.* the transfer of blood directly from a donor to a recipient. *Exchange* or *replacement t.* the removal of most or all of the recipient's blood and its replacement with fresh blood. Often used with infants suffering from erythroblastosis. *See* RHESUS FACTOR. *Intra-arterial t.* the passing of blood into an artery under positive pressure in cases where large quantities are required rapidly, as in cardiovascular surgery.

transient ischaemic attack ('transiənt) abbreviated TIA. A sudden episode of temporary or passing symptoms due to diminished blood flow through the carotid or vertebrobasilar blood vessels.

transillumination (,tranzi,loomi-'nayshən, ,trahnz-) the illumination of a translucent body structure by a strong light as an aid to diagnosis, particularly of tumours of the retina and of abnormalities in the ethmoidal and frontal sinuses.

translocation (,tranzloh'kayshən, ,trahnz-) in morphology, the transfer of a segment of a chromosome to a different site on the same chromosome or to a different chromosome. It can be a cause of congenital abnormality.

translucent (tranz'loosn't, trahnz-) allowing light rays to pass through indistinctly.

transmigration (,tranzmie'grayshən, ,trahnz-) a movement from one place to another, as in the passage of blood cells through the walls of the capillaries. Diapedesis. *External t.* the passage of an ovum from its ovary to the uterine tube on the opposite side. *Internal t.* the movement of an ovum from one uterine tube to the other through the uterus.

transplacental (,transplə'sent'l, ,trahns-) across the placenta. Movement may be from mother to fetus or vice versa. *T. infection* may affect the unborn child.

transplant ('transplahnt, 'trahns-) 1. an organ or tissue taken from the body and grafted into another area of the same individual or another individual. 2. to transfer tissue from one part to another or from one individual to another.

transplantation (,transplahn-'tayshǝn, ,trahns-) the transfer of living organs from one part of the body to another (autotransplant) or from one individual to another (allograft). Transplantation is often called grafting, though the term grafting is more commonly used to refer to the transfer of skin.

transposition (,tranzpǝ'zishǝn, ,trahnz-) 1. displacement of any of the viscera to the opposite side of the body. 2. the operation which partially removes a piece of tissue from one part of the body to another, the complete severance being delayed until it has become established in its new position. *T. of the great vessels* a congenital abnormality of the heart in which the positions of the pulmonary artery and aorta are reversed.

transsexualism (tranz'seksyoooǝ-,lizǝm, trahnz-) a disturbance of gender identity in which the person is convinced that his or her sex is the opposite to his or her physical state.

transudate ('transyuh,dayt, 'trahn-) any fluid which passes through a membrane.

transurethral (,tranzyuh'reethrǝl, ,trahn-) passing via the urethra.

transverse (trans'vǝrz, trahnz-) cross-wise. *T. presentation* position of the fetus whereby it lies across the pelvis, which position must be corrected before normal birth can take place.

transvestite (tranz'vestiet, trahnz-) a person who experiences a habitual and strongly persistent desire to dress as a member of the opposite sex ('cross dressing'). The majority are male and have no desire to physically change sex (by surgery). Usually regarded as a relatively harmless disorder of gender identity.

tranylcypromine (,tranil'sieprohmeen) a monoamine oxidase inhibitor used in psychiatry for the treatment of depression.

trauma ('trawmǝ) injury. *Birth t.* an injury to the infant during the process of being born. In some psychiatric theories, the psychological shock produced in an infant by the experience of being born. *Psychological t.* an emotional shock that makes a lasting impression.

treatment ('treetmǝnt) the mode of dealing with a patient or disease. *Active t.* that in which specific medical or surgical treatment is undertaken. *Conservative t.* that which aims at preserving and restoring injured parts by natural means, e.g. rest, fluid replacement, etc., as opposed to radical or surgical methods. *Empirical t.* treatment based on observation of symptoms and not on science. *Palliative t.* that which relieves distressing symptoms but does not cure the disease. *Prophylactic t.* that which aims at the prevention of disease.

Trematoda (,tremə'tohdə, ,tree-) a class of fluke worms, some of which are parasitic in man. Many of them have fresh-water snails as secondary hosts.

tremor ('tremə) an involuntary, muscular quivering which may be due to fatigue, emotion or disease. Tremor, first of one hand, and later affecting the other limbs, is the first symptom of parkinsonism. *Intention t.* one which occurs on attempting a movement, as in disseminated sclerosis.

Trendelenburg's position (tren-'delən,bərgz) *F. Trendelenburg, German surgeon, 1844–1924. See* POSITION.

Trendelenburg's sign a test of the stability of the hip. The patient stands on the affected leg and flexes the other knee and hip. If there is dislocation the pelvis is lower on the side of the flexed leg, which is the reverse of normal.

trephine (tri'fien, -feen) an instrument for cutting out a circular piece of bone, usually from the skull. *Corneal t.* one used to cut out a piece of cornea in keratoplasty.

Treponema (,trepə'neemə) a genus of spirochaetes. Anaerobic bacteria, they are motile, spiral

and parasitic in man and animals. *T. careatum* the causative agent of pinta. *T. pallidum* the causative agent of syphilis. *T.p. immobilization test* a serological test for syphilis. *T. pertenue* the causative agent of yaws (framboesia).

triage (tree'ahzh) [Fr.] the assessment and classification of casualties according to the type and severity of their injuries in order to assign them for treatment.

triamcinolone (,trieam'sinə,lohn) a glucocorticoid steroid which does not cause salt and water retention.

triamterine (trie'amtə,reen) a diuretic that acts by antagonizing aldosterone and does not cause potassium loss. Used in the treatment of oedema.

triceps ('trieseps) having three heads. *T. muscle* that situated on the back of the upper arm, which extends the forearm.

trichiasis (tri'kieəsis) 1. a condition of ingrowing hairs about an orifice, or ingrowing eyelashes. 2. the appearance of hair-like filaments in the urine.

trichinosis (,triki'nohsis) a disease caused by eating underdone pork containing a parasite, *Trichinella spiralis*. This becomes deposited in muscle, and causes stiffness and painful swelling. There may also be nausea, diarrhoea and fever. Trichiniasis.

trichloroethylene (trie,klor-roh-'ethi,leen) a weak inhalation anaesthetic. Used in midwifery, for painful dressings and in general anaesthesia in combination with other anaesthetics.

trichology (tri,kolǝjee) the study

of hair.

Trichomonas (,trikoh'mohnas) a genus of flagellate protozoa that are parasitic to man. *T. hominis* infests the bowel and may cause dysentery. *T. tenax* infests the mouth and may be present in cases of pyorrhoea. *T. vaginalis* is commonly present in the vagina and may cause leukorrhoea and vaginitis.

trichomoniasis (,trikohmə'nieəsis) infestation with a parasite of the genus *Trichomonas*.

Trichophyton (,trikoh'fieton) a genus of fungi which affects the skin, nails and hair.

trichophytosis (,trikohfie'tohsis) infection of the skin, nails or hair with one of the genus *Trichophyton*. See TINEA.

trichorrhexis (,trikə'reksis) brittleness of the hair, which splits and breaks off easily.

trichosis (tri'kohsis) any abnormal growth of hair.

trichuriasis (,trikyuh'rieəsis) infestation by the whipworm.

Trichuris (tri'kyoo-ris) a genus of nematode worms which may infest the colon and cause diarrhoea. A whipworm.

tricuspid (trie'kuspid) having three flaps or cusps. *T. valve* that at the opening between the right atrium and the right ventricle of the heart.

trifluoperazine (,triefloo-oh'perə,zeen) a potent tranquillizing drug that is used in the treatment of schizophrenia and of psychoneuroses.

trifocal (trie'fohk'l) pertaining to a spectacle lens which has three foci, one for distant, one for

intermediate and one for near vision.

trigeminal (trie'jemin'l) divided into three. *T. nerves* the fifth pair of cranial nerves, each of which is divided into three main branches and supplies one side of the face. *T. neuralgia* pain in the face which is confined to branches of the trigeminal nerve. Tic douloureux.

trigeminy (trie'jeminee) the type of pulse in which there are three beats and then a missed beat. A regular irregularity. Pulsus trigeminus.

trigger finger ('trigə ,fing·gə) a stenosing of the tendon sheath at the metacarpophalangeal joint, allowing flexion of the finger but not extension without assistance, when it 'clicks' into position.

triglyceride (trie'glisə,ried) an ester of glycerol and three fatty acids.

trigone ('triegohn) a triangular area. *T. of the bladder* the triangular space on the floor of the bladder, between the ureteric openings and the urethral orifice.

tri-iodothyronine (trie,ieədoh-'thierə,neen) a hormone produced by the thyroid gland together with thyroxine.

trimeprazine (trie'meprə,zeen) a sedative drug used for preoperative medication, in the treatment of pruritus and to sedate children.

trimester (trie'mestə) a period of 3 months. *First t. of pregnancy* the first 3 months, during which rapid development is taking place.

trimipramine (trie'miprə,meen) an antidepressant drug used particularly when anxiety and insomnia accompany depression.

triplopia (tri'plohpi·ə) a condition in which three images of an object are seen at the same time.

trismus ('trizməs) lock-jaw; a tonic spasm of the muscles of the jaw.

trisomy ('triesəmee) the presence of an extra chromosome in each cell in addition to the normal paired set of 46. The cause of several chromosome disorders including Down's syndrome (mongolism) and Klinefelter's syndrome.

trocar ('trohkah) a pointed instrument used with a cannula for performing paracentesis.

trochanter (troh'kantə) either of two bony prominences below the neck of the femur. *Greater t.* that on the outer side forming the bony prominence of the hip. *Lesser t.* that on the inner side at the neck of the femur.

trochlea ('trokli·ə) any pulley-shaped structure, but particularly the fibrocartilage near the inner angular process of the frontal bone through which passes the tendon of the superior oblique muscle of the eye.

trochlear ('trokli·ə) relating to a trochlea. Pulley-shaped. *T. nerve* the fourth cranial nerve.

trophic ('trofik) relating to nutrition. *T. nerves* those which control the nutrition of a part. *T. ulcer* one arising from a failure in the nutrition of a part.

trophoblast ('trofoh,blast) the layer of cells surrounding the blastocyst at the time of and responsible for implantation.

trophoblastoma (,trofohbla-'stohmə) choriocarcinoma.

trophoneurosis (,trofohnyuh-'rohsis) malnutrition of a part, due to disturbance of the trophic nerves.

tropia ('trohpi·ə) a manifest squint, one that is present when both eyes are open.

tropical ('tropik'l) relating to the areas north and south of the equator termed the tropics. *T. medicine* that concerned with diseases that are more prevalent in hot climates.

Trousseau's sign ('troosohz) *A. Trousseau, French physician, 1801–1867.* 1. spontaneous peripheral venous thrombosis. 2. a sign for tetany in which carpal spasm can be elicited by compressing the upper arm and causing ischaemia to the nerves distally.

truancy ('trooənsee) absence of a child from school without leave. A disorder of conduct which may result from emotional insecurity or a feeling of unfairness.

truncus ('trungkəs) a trunk; the main part of the body, or a part of it, from which other parts spring. *T. arteriosus* the arterial trunk connected to the fetal heart which develops into the aortic and pulmonary arteries. *Persistent t.a.* a rare congenital deformity in which this persists, causing a mixing of the systemic and pulmonary circulations.

truss (trus) an apparatus in the form of a belt with a pressure pad for retaining a hernia in place after reduction.

Trypanosoma (,tripənoh'sohmə)

**TROUSSEAU'S SIGN (CARPOPEDAL SPASM)
WITH HYPOCALCAEMIA**

a genus of protozoan parasites which pass some of their life cycle in the blood of vertebrates, including man. *T. gambiense* and *T. rhodensiense* are transmitted by the bite of the tsetse fly, and are the cause of sleeping sickness.

trypanosomiasis (,triipənohsə-'mieəsis) a disease caused by infestation with *Trypanosoma*. Sleeping sickness.

trypsin ('tripsin) a digestive enzyme converting protein into amino acids.

trypsinogen (trip'sinəjən) the precursor of trypsin. It is secreted in the pancreatic juice, and activated by the enterokinase of the intestinal juices into trypsin.

tryptophan ('triptə,fan) one of the essential amino acids.

tsetse fly ('tetsee, 'tse-) a fly of the genus *Glossina* which transmits the parasite *Trypanosoma* to man, causing trypanosomiasis.

tsutsugamushi disease (,tsoo-tsoogə'mooshee) scrub typhus that occurs in Japan and is transmitted by the bite of a mite.

tubal ('tyoob'l) relating to a tube. *T. pregnancy* extrauterine pregnancy where the embryo develops in the uterine tube. Ectopic pregnancy.

tube feeding (tyoob) administration of liquid and semisolid foods through a nasogastric, gastrostomy, or enterostomy tube. Tube feedings are administered to patients who are unable to take foods by mouth.

Tubegauz ('tyoobi,gawz) a proprietary brand of woven circular bandage applied with a special applicator.

tubercle ('tyoobək'l) 1. a small nodule or a rounded prominence on a bone. 2. the specific lesion (a small nodule) produced by the tubercle bacillus.

tubercular (tyuh'bərkyuhlə) pertaining to tubercles.

tuberculid (tyuh'bərkyuhlid) a papular eruption usually attributed to allergy to tuberculosis.

tuberculin (tyuh'bərkyuhlin) the filtrate from a fluid medium in which *Mycobacterium tuberculosis* has been grown and which contains its toxins. *Old t.* is prepared from the human bacillus. It is used in skin tests in diagnosing tuberculosis. *See* MANTOUX TEST.

tuberculosis (tyuh'bərkyuh'lohsis) an infectious, inflammatory, notifiable disease produced by the tubercle bacillus, *Mycobacterium tuberculosis*, that is chronic in nature. *Bovine t.* a form found in cattle and spread by infected milk. *Miliary t.* a severe form with small tuberculous lesions spread throughout the body with severe toxaemia. *Open t.* any type of tuberculosis in which the organisms are being excreted from the body. *Pulmonary t.* that affecting the lungs; also termed phthisis. *T. of the spine* Pott's disease.

tuberosity (,tyoobə'rositee) an elevation or protuberance on a bone.

tuberous ('tyoobə-rəs) covered with tubers. *T. sclerosis* a familial disease with tumours on the surfaces of the lateral ventricles of the brain and sclerotic patches on its surface, and marked by mental deterioration and epileptic attacks.

tubocurarine (,tyoobohkyoo'rahreen) a preparation of curare used to secure skeletal muscle relaxation.

tubule ('tyoobyool) a small tube. *Renal* or *uriniferous t.* the essential secreting tube of the kidney.

tularaemia (,toolə'reemi·ə) a plaguelike disease of rodents, caused by *Francisella* (*Pasteurella*) *tularensis*, which is transmissible to man. The illness can be contracted by handling diseased animals or their hides, eating infected wild game or being bitten by insects that have fed on infected animals. It causes fever and headache; the lymph glands enlarge and may suppurate.

tulle gras (,tyool 'grah) a preparation of gauze impregnated with petroleum jelly. Other drugs may be added. Most useful on a granulating surface to stop a dressing adhering.

tumefaction (,tyoomi'fakshən) a swelling or the process of becoming swollen. Tumescence.

tumour ('tyoomə) an abnormal swelling. The term is usually applied to a morbid growth of tissue which may be benign or malignant. A neoplasm. *Benign* or *innocent t.* one that does not infiltrate or cause metastases, and is unlikely to recur if removed. *Malignant t.* one which invades and destroys tissue and can spread to neighbouring tissues, and to more distant sites via the blood and the lymphatic systems.

tunica ('tyoonikə) a coat, a covering, or the lining of a vessel. *T. adventitia, t. media, t. intima* the outer, middle and inner coats of an artery, respectively. *T. vaginalis* the membrane covering the front and sides of the testis.

tuning fork ('tyooning) a metal

instrument used for testing hearing by means of the sounds produced by its vibration. *See* RINNE'S and WEBER'S TESTS.

tunnel ('tun'l) in anatomy, a canal through a structure. *Carpal t.* the osteofibrous channel in the wrist between the carpal bones and tissue covering the flexor tendons. *C.t. syndrome* pain and tingling in the hand and fingers caused by compression of the median nerve in the carpal tunnel. *T. vision* vision that is restricted to the central field. Occurs in chronic glaucoma and in retinitis pigmentosa.

turbinate ('tɜrbinət, -,nayt) scroll-shaped. *T. bone* one of the three thin long plates that form the walls of the nasal cavity.

turbinectomy (,tɜrbi'nektəmee) excision of a turbinate bone.

turgid ('tɜrjid) swollen and congested.

turgor ('tɜrgə) the state of being swollen or distended.

Turner's syndrome ('tɜrnəz) *H.H. Turner, American physician, 1892–1970.* A chromosomal defect in females, causing short stature. Classically, an absence of one X chromosome. Affects 1 in 3000 live female births. The majority have streak ovaries leading to an absence of puberty and infertility. Other features may include webbing of the neck, cubitus valgus, nail abnormalities and coarctation of the aorta. Intelligence is usually normal.

tussis (,tusis) a cough.

twin (twin) one of a pair of individuals who have developed in the uterus together. *Binovular*

(dizygotic) t. each twin has developed from a separate ovum; fraternal twins. *Uniovular (monozygotic) t.* both twins have developed from the same cell; identical twins.

tylosis (tie'lohsis) the formation of a hard patch of skin. A callosity.

tympanectomy (,timpə'nektəmee) excision of the tympanic membrane.

tympanites (,timpə'nieteez) distension of the abdomen by accumulation of gas in the intestine or the peritoneal cavity.

tympanitis (,timpə'nietis) inflammation of the middle ear; otitis media.

tympanoplasty ('timpənoh,plastee) an operation to reconstruct the ear-drum and restore conductivity to the middle ear. Myringoplasty.

tympanosclerosis (,timpənoh-sklə,rohsis) fibrosis and the formation of calcified deposits in the middle ear that lead to deafness.

tympanum ('timpənəm) 1. the middle ear. 2. the ear-drum or tympanic membrane.

type (tiep) the general or prevailing character of any particular case of disease, person, substance, etc. *Asthenic t.* a type of physical constitution, with long limbs, small trunk, flat chest and weak muscles. *Athletic t.* a type of physical constitution with broad shoulders, deep chest, flat abdomen, thick neck and good muscular development. *Blood t's see* BLOOD GROUP. *Phage t.* a subgroup of a bacterial species susceptible to a particular bacteriophage and demonstrated by phage

TYPING. Called also *lysotype* and *phagotype*. *Pyknic t.* a type of physical constitution marked by rounded body, large chest, thick shoulders, broad head and short neck.

type A behaviour (tiep 'ay) a behaviour pattern associated with the development of coronary heart disease, characterized by excessive competitiveness and aggression and a fast-paced life style. Research has shown that this type of behaviour is associated with coronary artery disease and myocardial infarction. The opposite type of behaviour, exhibited by individuals who are relaxed, unhurried, and less aggressive, is called type B and is associated with a lower risk of heart disease.

typhoid fever ('tiefoyd) enteric fever. A notifiable infectious disease caused by *Salmonella typhi*, which is transmitted by water, milk or other foods, especially shellfish, that have been contaminated. There is high fever, a red rash, delirium and sometimes intestinal haemorrhage. Recovery usually begins during the 4th week of the disease. A person who has had typhoid fever gains immunity from it but may become a carrier. Although perfectly well, he harbours the bacteria and passes them out in his faeces or urine. The typhoid bacillus often lodges in the gallbladder of carriers.

typhus ('tiefəs) an acute, notifiable, infectious disease caused by species of the parasitic microorganism *Rickettsia*. There is high fever, a widespread red rash and severe headache. Typhus is likely to occur where there is overcrowding, lack of personal cleanliness and bad hygienic conditions, as the infection is spread by bites of infected lice or by rat fleas. *Scrub t.* a form spread by mites and widespread in the Far East. Tsutsugamushi disease.

tyramine ('tierə,meen, 'ti-) an enzyme present in cheese, game, broad bean pods, yeast extracts, wine and strong beer, which has a similar effect in the body to that of adrenaline. Foodstuffs containing tyramine should be avoided by patients taking monoamine oxidase inhibitors.

tyrosine ('tieroh,seen, 'ti-) an essential amino acid which is the product of phenylalanine metabolism. In some diseases, especially of the liver, it is present as a deposit in the urine. It is a precursor of catecholamines, melanin and thyroid hormones.

tyrosinosis (,tierohsi'nohsis, ,ti-) a congenital condition in which there is an error of metabolism and phenylalanine cannot be reduced to tyrosine. Hepatic failure may occur.

U

ulcer ('ulsə) an erosion or loss of continuity of the skin or of a mucous membrane, often accompanied by suppuration. *Decubitus u.* a pressure sore caused by lying immobile for long periods of time. *Duodenal u.* a peptic ulcer in the duodenum. *Gastric u.* one in the lining of the stomach. *Gravitational u.* a varicose ulcer of the leg which is difficult to heal because of its dependent position and the poor venous return. *Gummatous u.* one arising in late non-infective syphilis; it is slow to heal. *Indolent u.* one which is painless and heals slowly. *Peptic u.* one that occurs on the mucous membrane of either the stomach or duodenum. *Perforating u.* one that erodes through the thickness of the wall of an organ. *Rodent u.* a slow-growing epithelioma of the face which may cause much local destruction and ulceration, but does not give rise to metastases. Basal cell carcinoma. *Trophic u.* one due to a failure of nutrition of a part. *Varicose u.* gravitational ulcer.

ulcerative ('ulsə,raytiv) characterized by ulceration (the formation of ulcers). *U. colitis* inflammation and ulceration of the colon and rectum of unknown cause.

ultrasonic (,ultrə'sonik) relating to sound waves having a frequency range beyond the upper limit perceived by the human ear. These waves are widely used instead of X-rays, particularly in the examination of structures not opaque to X-rays.

ultrasonogram an echo picture obtained from using ultrasound.

ultrasonography (,ultrəsə'nogrəfee) a radiological technique in which deep structures of the body are visualized by recording the reflections (echoes) of ultrasonic waves directed into the tissues.

ultrasound ('ultra,sownd) ultrasonic waves used to examine the interior organs of the body. These waves can also be used in the treatment of soft-tissue pain, and to break up renal calculi or the crystalline lens when cataract is present.

ultraviolet rays (,ultrə'vieələt) short wavelength electromagnetic rays. They are present in sunlight and cause tanning and sunburn. *U. light* is used to promote vitamin D formation and for treatment of certain skin conditions.

umbilicus (um'bilikəs, ,umbi-'liekəs) the navel; the circular depressed scar in the centre of the abdomen where the umbilical cord of the fetus was attached.

unconscious (un'konshəs) 1.

insensible; incapable of responding to sensory stimuli and of having subjective experiences. 2. that part of mental activity which includes primitive or repressed wishes, concealed from consciousness by the psychological censor. *Collective u.* in jungian psychology, the portion of the unconscious which is theoretically common to mankind.

unconsciousness (un'konshəsnəs) the state of being unconscious. This may vary in depth from *deep u.*, when no response can be obtained, through to lesser degrees of unconsciousness, when the patient can be roused by painful stimuli, to a level when the patient can be roused by speech or non-painful stimuli. Deep prolonged unconsciousness is known as coma. *See* COMA.

undecenoic acid ('undekə,noh·ik) an antifungal agent used in the treatment of such infections as athlete's foot. May be used in powder, ointment, lotion or spray form.

undine ('undeen) a glass flask with a spout used for irrigation of the eye.

undulant ('undyuhlənt) rising and falling like a wave. *U. fever see* BRUCELLOSIS.

unguentum (ung'gwentəm) an ointment.

unilateral (,yooni'latə·rəl) on one side only.

union ('yooni·ən) 1. a joining together. 2. the repair of tissue after separation by incision or fracture. *See* CALLUS and HEALING.

uniovular (,yooni'ohvyuhlə, -'ov-)

from one ovum. *U. twins* identical twins, developed from one ovum.

unipara (,yooni'parə) a woman who has had only one child.

unit ('yoonit) 1. a single thing. *Intensive care u.* a hospital department reserved for those with severe medical or surgical disorders. 2. a standard of measurement. *International insulin u.* a measurement of the pure crystalline insulin arrived at by biological assay. *SI unit* one of the various units of measurement making up the Système International d'Unités (International System of Units).

urachal ('yoo'rayk'l) referring to the urachus. *U. cyst* a congenital abnormality when a small cyst persists along the course of the urachus. *U. fistula* one that forms when the urachus fails to close. Urine may leak from the umbilicus.

urachus ('yooə·rəkəs) a tubular canal existing in the fetus, connecting the bladder with the umbilicus. In the adult it persists in the form of a solid fibrous cord.

uraemia (yuh'reemi·ə) 1. an excess in the blood of urea, creatinine and other nitrogenous end products of protein and amino acid metabolism; sometimes referred to as azotaemia. 2. in current usage, the entire complex of signs and symptoms of chronic RENAL FAILURE. Depending upon the cause it may or may not be reversible. Uraemia leads to vomiting and nausea, headache, weakness, metabolic disturbances, convulsions and coma.

uraniscorrhaphy (,yooə·rənis-'ko·rəfee) suture of a cleft palate.

urataemia (,yoo·rə'teemi·ə) an accumulation of urates in the blood.

urate ('yooə·rayt) a salt of uric acid. *Sodium u.* a compound generally found in concentration around joints in cases of gout.

uraturia (,yooə·rə'tyooə·ri·ə) an excess of urates in the urine. Lithuria.

urea '(yuh'reeə, 'yooə·ri·ə) carbamide. A white crystalline substance which is an end product of protein metabolism and the chief nitrogenous constituent of urine. It is a diuretic. The normal daily output is about 33 g. *Blood u.* that which is present in the blood. Normal is 20–40 mg/ 100 ml.

urecchysis (yuh'rekisis) the extravasation of urine into cellular tissue, e.g. in rupture of the bladder as a complication of fractured pelvis.

uresis (yuh'reesis) urination.

ureter (yuh'reetə, 'yooə·ritə) one of the two long narrow tubes which convey the urine from the kidney to the bladder.

ureterectomy (yuh'reetə'rektəmee) the surgical removal of a ureter.

ureteric relating to the ureter. *U. catheter* a fine catheter for insertion via the ureter into the pelvis of the kidney, either for drainage or for retrograde urography. *U. transplantation* operation in which the ureters are divided from the bladder and implanted in the colon or loop of ileum. Congeni-

tal defects or malignant growth may make this necessary.

ureteritis (yuh,reetə'rietis) inflammation of the ureter.

ureterocele (yuh'reetə·roh,seel) a cystic enlargement of the wall of the ureter at its entry into the bladder.

ureterocolostomy (yuh,reetə·rohkə'lostəmee) anastomosis of a ureter to the colon.

ureteroenterostomy (yuh,reetə·roh,entə'rostəmee) surgical implantation of a ureter into the intestine.

ureterolith (yuh'reetə·roh,lith) a calculus in a ureter.

ureterolithotomy (yuh,reetə·rohli'thotəmee) removal of a calculus from the ureter.

ureteronephrectomy (yuh,reetə·rohnə'frektəmee) surgical removal of a kidney and its ureter.

ureterosigmoidostomy (yuh,reetə·roh,sigmoy'dostəmee) surgical implantation of the ureters into the sigmoid colon.

ureterostomy (yuh,reetə'rostəmee) the surgical creation of a permanent opening through which the ureter discharges urine.

ureterovaginal (yuh,reetə·rohvə·'jien'l, -'vajin'l) relating to the ureter and vagina. *U. fistula* an opening into the ureter by which urine escapes via the vagina.

urethra (yuh'reethrə) the canal through which the urine is discharged from the bladder. The male urethra is about 18 cm long and the female about 3.5 cm.

urethritis (,yooə·ri'thrietis) inflammation of the urethra. The condition is frequently a symptom of gonorrhoea but may be caused by other infectious organisms. *Non-specific u.* abbreviated NSU. A sexually transmitted inflammation of the urethra caused by a variety of organisms other than gonococci. *See* NON-SPECIFIC URETHRITIS.

urethrocele (yuh'reethroh,seel) a prolapse of the female urethral wall which may result from damage to the pelvic floor during childbirth.

urethrography (,yooə·ri'throg-rəfee) radiographic examination of the urethra. A radio-opaque contrast medium is inserted by catheter.

urethroplasty (yuh'reethroh,plastee) a surgical repair of the urethra.

urethroscope (yuh'reethrə,skohp) an instrument for examining the interior of the urethra.

urethrostenosis (yuh,reethroh-stə'nohsis) stricture of the urethra.

urethrostomy (,yooə·ri'throstəmee) the creation of a permanent opening of the male urethra in the perineum.

urethrotomy (,yooə·ri'throtəmee) incision of the urethra, to remedy stricture.

uric acid ('yooə·rik) lithic acid, the end product of nucleic acid metabolism, a normal constituent of urine. Its accumulation in the blood produces uricacidaemia. Renal calculi are frequently formed of it.

uricacidaemia (,yooə·rik,asi'dee-mi·ə) the presence of an excess of uric acid in the blood.

uricosuric (,yooə·rikoh'syooə·rik) a drug that promotes the excretion of uric acid in the urine.

uridrosis (,yooə·ri'drohsis) the presence of urinary constituents, such as urea and uric acid, in the perspiration. They may become deposited as crystals upon the skin. A symptom of uraemia. Uraemic snow.

urinalysis (yooə·ri'nalisis) the bacteriological or chemical examination of the urine.

urinary ('yooə·rinə·ree) relating to urine. *U. tract* the system which leads urine from the kidneys to the exterior, including the ureters, the bladder and the urethra.

urination (,yooə·ri'nayshən) micturition. The act of passing urine.

urine ('yooə·rin) the fluid secreted by the kidneys and excreted through the bladder and urethra. It is 96, water and 4, solid constituents, the most important being urea and uric acid. *Residual u.* that which remains in the bladder after micturition.

uriniferous (,yooə·ri'nifə·rəs) capable of conveying urine. *U. tubule* a renal tubule. *See* TUBULE.

urinometer (,yooə·ri'nomitə) an instrument used for measuring the specific gravity of urine.

urobilin (,yooə·roh'bielin) the main pigment of urine, derived from urobilinogen.

urobilinogen (,yooə·rohbie'linəjən) a pigment derived from bilirubin which, on oxidation, forms urobilin.

urochrome ('yooə·roh,krohm) the yellow pigment which colours urine.

urodynamics (,yooə·rohdie'namiks) the dynamics of the propulsion and flow of urine in the urinary tract.

urogenital (ˌyooə·roh'jenit'l) relating to the urinary and genital organs. Urinogenital.

urography (yuh'rogrəfee) radiographic examination of the urinary tract after the injection of a radioopaque, water-soluble, iodine-containing medium.

urogram (ˌyooə·roh,gram) a film obtained by urography.

urokinase (ˌyooə·roh'kienayz) an enzyme in urine which is secreted by the kidneys and causes fibrinolysis. In certain diseases it may cause bleeding from the kidneys.

urolith (ˌyooə·roh,lith) a calculus in the urinary tract.

urology (yuh'roləjee) the study of diseases of the urinary tract.

uropathy (yuh'ropəthee) any disease condition affecting the urinary tract.

urostomy (yuh'rostəmee) an artificial urinary conduit to deflect urine from the ureters to the abdominal wall.

urticaria (ˌərti'kair·ri·ə) nettle rash or hives. An acute or chronic skin condition characterized by the recurrent appearance of an eruption of weals, causing great irritation. The cause may be certain foods, infection, drugs or emotional stress. *See* ALLERGY.

uterine ('yootə'rien) relating to the uterus.

uterocele ('yootə·roh,seel) a hernia of the uterus; a hysterocele.

uterogestation (ˌyootə·rohje'stay-shən) development of a fetus within the uterus. A normal pregnancy.

uterography (ˌyootə'rogrəfee) radiographic examination of the uterus.

uterosalpingography (ˌyootə·roh-

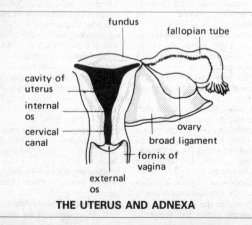

THE UTERUS AND ADNEXA

,salping'gogrəfee) radiographic examination of the uterus and the uterine tubes.

uterovesical (,yootə·roh'vesik'l) referring to the uterus and bladder. *U. pouch* the fold of peritoneum between the two organs.

uterus ('yootə·rəs) the womb: a triangular, hollow, muscle organ situated in the pelvic cavity between the bladder and the rectum. Its function is the nourishment and protection of the fetus during pregnancy and its expulsion at term. *Bicornuate u.* one having two horns. A congenital malformation. *Gravid u.* the pregnant uterus. *U. didelphys* a double uterus owing to the failure of union of the two müllerian ducts from which it is formed.

utricle ('yootrik'l) the delicate membranous sac in the bony vestibule of the ear.

uvea ('yoovi·ə) uveal tract. The pigmented layer of the eye, consisting of the iris, ciliary body and choroid.

uveitis (,yoovi'ietis) inflammation of the uveal tract.

uvula ('yoovyuhlə) the small fleshy appendage which is the free edge of the soft palate, hanging from the roof of the mouth.

uvulectomy (,yoovyuh'lektəmee) the surgical excision of the uvula.

uvulitis (,yoovyuh'lietis) inflammation of the uvula.

V

vaccination (,vaksi'nayshən) the introduction of vaccine into the body to produce immunity to a specific disease.

vaccine ('vakseen) a suspension of killed or attenuated organisms (viruses, bacteria or rickettsiae), administered for prevention, amelioration or treatment of infectious diseases. *Attenuated v.* one prepared from living organisms which, through long cultivation, have lost their virulence. *Bacille Calmette–Guérin v.* an attenuated bovine bacillus vaccine giving immunity from tuberculosis. *Triple v.* one that protects against diphtheria, tetanus and whooping cough. *Sabin v.* an attenuated poliovirus vaccine that can be administered by mouth, in a syrup or on sugar. *Salk v.* one prepared from an inactivated strain of poliomyelitis virus. *TAB v.* a sterile solution of the organisms that cause typhoid and paratyphoid A and B. Paratyphoid C may now be included.

vaccinia (vak'sini·ə) cowpox; a virus infection of cows, which may be transmitted to man by contact with the lesions. A local pustular eruption is produced.

vacuum ('vakyoom) a space from which air or gas has been extracted. *V. extractor* an instrument to assist delivery of the fetus. A suction cup is attached to the head and a vacuum created slowly. Gentle traction is applied which is synchronized with the uterine contractions.

vagal ('vayg'l) relating to the vagus nerve.

vagina (və'jienə) the canal, lined with mucous membrane, which leads from the cervix to the uterus to the vulva.

vaginismus (,vaji'nizməs) a painful spasm of the muscles of the vagina, occurring usually when the vulva or vagina is touched, resulting in painful sexual intercourse or dyspareunia.

vaginitis (,vaji'nietis) inflammation of the vagina. *Atrophic* or *postmenopausal v.* inflammation caused by degenerative changes in the mucous lining of the vagina and insufficient oestrogen secretion. Adhesions may occur, partially closing the vagina. *Trichomonas v.* infection caused by *T. vaginalis*, a protozoon which causes a thin, yellowish discharge, giving rise to local tenderness and pruritus.

vagotomy (vay'gotəmee) surgical incision of the vagus nerve or any of its branches. A treatment for gastric or duodenal ulcer. *Highly selective v.* division of only those vagal fibres supplying the acid-secreting glands of the stomach.

Medical v. interruption of impulses carried by the vagus nerve by administration of suitable drugs.

vagus ('vaygəs) the tenth cranial nerve, arising in the medulla and providing the parasympathetic nerve supply to the organs in the thorax and abdomen. *V. resection* vagotomy.

valgus (,valgəs) a displacement outwards, particularly of the feet. *Genu valgum* knock-knee, with the ankles set apart. *Hallux v.* twisting of the big toe outwards towards the other toes. *Talipes v.* club-foot with the inner edge only in contact with the ground, and the foot turned outwards.

valine ('valəen) an essential amino acid formed by the digestion of dietary protein.

Valium ('vali·əm) trade name for a preparation of diazepam, an anxiolytic and skeletal muscle relaxant.

Valsalva's manoeuvre (val'salvəz) *A.M. Valsalva, Italian anatomist, 1666–1723.* Technique for increasing the intrathoracic pressure by closing the mouth and nostrils and blowing out the cheeks, thereby forcing air back into the nasopharynx. When the breath is released, the intrathoracic pressure drops and the blood is quickly propelled through the heart, producing an increase in the heart rate (tachycardia) and the blood pressure. Immediately after this event a reflex bradycardia ensues. Valsalva's manoeuvre occurs when a person strains to defecate or urinate, uses his arm and

upper trunk muscles to move up in bed, or strains during coughing, gagging or vomiting. The increased pressure, immediate tachycardia and reflex bradycardia can bring about cardiac arrest in vulnerable heart patients.

valve (valv) 1. a means of regulating the flow of liquid or gas through a pipe. 2. a fold of membrane in a passage or tube, so placed as to permit passage of fluid in one direction only. They are important structures in the heart, in veins and in lymph vessels. *Semilunar v.* either of two valves at the junction of the pulmonary artery and aorta respectively, with the heart.

valvotomy (val'votəmee) valvulotomy. A surgical operation to open up a fibrosed valve, e.g. mitral valvotomy to relieve mitral stenosis.

valvulitis (,valvyuh'lietis) inflammation of a valve, particularly of the heart.

van den Bergh's test ('van dən ,bərgz) *A.A.H. van den Bergh, Dutch physician, 1869–1943.* A chemical test of bilirubin in serum to aid the diagnosis of jaundice.

vancomycin (,vankoh'miesin) an antibiotic highly effective against Gram-positive bacteria, especially staphylococci. The toxic effects are quite severe and may include damage to the eighth cranial (vestibulocochlear) nerve, and renal disorders.

vanillylmandelic acid (və-,niliman'delik) abbreviated VMA. A metabolite of catecholamines which is excreted in small amounts in the urine. Excessive amounts of VMA in the urine may indicate that the patient has an adrenal medullary tumour.

vaporizer ('vaypə,riezə) an apparatus for producing a very fine spray of a liquid.

varicectomy (,vari'sektəmee) phlebectomy; surgical excision of a varicose vein.

varicella (,vari'selə) chickenpox. An infectious disease of childhood having an incubation period of 12–20 days. There is slight fever and an eruption of transparent vesicles on the chest on the first day of disease, which comes out in successive crops all over the body. The vesicles soon dry up, sometimes leaving shallow pits in the skin. The disease is usually mild, but may be severe in neonates, adults and those who are immunocompromised. Chickenpox is a notifiable disease in Scotland.

varicocele ('varikoh,seel) a dilatation of the veins of the spermatic cord.

varicocelectomy (,varikohsi'lektəmee) operation for removal of dilated veins from the scrotum.

varicose (,vari,kohs) swollen or dilated. *V. veins* a dilated and twisted condition of the veins (usually those of the leg), due to structural changes in the walls or valves of the vessels. *V. ulcer* gravitational ulcer. *See* ULCER.

variola (və'rieələ) smallpox.

varix (,vair·riks) an enlarged or varicose vein.

varus (,vair·rəs) a displacement inwards. *Genu varum* bowleg, with the ankles close together.

Hallux v. twisting of the big toe inwards, away from the other toes. *Talipes v.* club-foot with the outer edge only in contact with the ground and the foot turned inwards.

vas (vas) *pl.* vasa. A vessel or duct. *V. deferens* one of a pair of excretory ducts conveying the semen from the epididymis to the urethra. *V. efferens* one of the many small tubes that convey semen from the testis to the epididymis. *Vasa vasorum* the minute nutrient vessels that supply the walls of the arteries and veins.

vascular ('vaskyuhlə) relating to, or consisting largely of blood vessels. *V. system* the cardiovascular system.

vascularization (,vaskyuhlə·rie-'zayshən) the development of new blood vessels within a tissue.

vasculitis (,vaskyuh'lietis) angiitis; inflammation of a blood vessel. *Allergic v.* a severe allergic response to drugs or to cold. Arising in small arteries or veins, with fibrosis and thrombi formation.

vasectomy (və'sektəmee) excision of a part of the vas deferens. If performed bilaterally sterility results. Now employed as a method of contraception.

vasoconstrictor (,vayzohkən-'striktə) any agent that causes contraction of a blood vessel wall, and therefore a decrease in the blood flow and a rise in the blood pressure.

vasodilator (,vayzohdie'laytə) any agent that causes an increase in the lumen of blood vessels, and therefore an increase in the blood flow and a fall in the blood pressure.

vasomotor (,vayzoh'mohtə) controlling the muscles of blood vessels, both dilator and constrictor. *V. centre* nerve cells in the medulla oblongata controlling the vasomotor nerves. *V. nerves* sympathetic nerves regulating the tension of the blood vessels.

vasopressin (,vayzoh'presin) antidiuretic hormone (**ADH**). A hormone from the posterior lobe of the pituitary gland which causes constriction of plain muscle fibres and reabsorption of water in the renal tubules. Used in the treatment of diabetes insipidus and bleeding from oesophageal varices.

vasovagal (,vayzoh'vayg'l) vascular and vagal. *V. attack* fainting or syncope stress, often evoked by emotional stress associated with fear and pain. There is postural hypotension.

vasovesiculitis (,vasohve,sikyuh-'lietis) inflammation of the vas deferens and seminal vesicles.

vector ('vektə) 1. an animal that carries organisms or parasites from one host to another, either of the same species or to one of another species. 2. a quantity with magnitude and direction. *Electrocardiographic v.* the area of the heart which is monitored during electrocardiographic investigation.

vectorcardiography (,vektə,kahdi-'ogrəfee) electrocardiographic investigation of the heart in which individual vectors are monitored.

vegan ('veegən) a vegetarian who excludes all animal protein from the diet.

vegetation (,veji'tayshən) in pathology, a plant-like outgrowth. *Adenoid v.* overgrowth of lymphoid tissue in the nasopharynx.

vehicle ('veeək'l) in pharmacy, a substance or medium in which a drug is administered.

vein (vayn) a vessel carrying blood from the capillaries back to the heart. It has thin walls and a lining endothelium from which the venous valves are formed.

venepuncture ('veni,pungkchə) the insertion of a needle into a vein for the introduction of a drug, fluid or for the withdrawal of blood.

venereal (və'nie·ri·əl) pertaining to or caused by sexual intercourse. *V. disease* a disease transmitted by sexual intercourse or other genital contact. In the UK, GONORRHOEA, SYPHILIS and CHANCROID are defined in law as venereal diseases. The term venereal disease (VD) is being replaced by the term SEXUALLY TRANSMITTED DISEASE.

venereology (və,niə·ri'oləjee) the study and treatment of venereal diseases.

venesection ('veni,sekshən) phlebotomy. Surgical blood-letting by opening a vein or introducing a wide-bore needle. Commonly performed on blood donors and occasionally to relieve venous congestion.

venoclysis (vee'noklisis) the introduction of fluids directly into veins.

venogram ('veenə,gram) 1. a graphic recording of the pulse in a vein. 2. a radiograph taken during venography.

venography (vee'nogrəfee) radiographic examination of a vein after the insertion of a contrast medium to trace its pathway.

venom ('venəm) a poison secreted by an insect, snake or other animal. *Russell's viper v.* the venom of the Russell viper (*Vipera russelli*), which acts in vitro as an intrinsic thromboplastin and is useful in defining deficiencies of clotting factor X.

venous ('veenəs) pertaining to the veins. *V. sinus* one of 14 channels, similar to veins, by which blood leaves the cerebral circulation.

ventilation (,venti'layshən) 1. the process or act of supplying a house or room continuously with fresh air. 2. in respiratory physiology, the process of exchange of air between the lungs and the ambient air. *Pulmonary v.* (usually measured in litres per minute) refers to the total exchange, whereas *alveolar v.* refers to the effective ventilation of the alveoli, where gas exchange with the blood takes place. 3. in psychiatry, the free discussion of one's problems or grievances.

ventilator ('venti,laytə) an apparatus designed to qualify the air that is breathed through it or to either intermittently or continuously control pulmonary ventilation; called also respirator.

Ventolin ('ventohlin) trade name for a salbutamol metered-dose inhaler; a bronchodilator.

Ventouse (,ven,tooz) *see* VACUUM EXTRACTION.

ventral ('ventral) pertaining to a hollow structure or belly.

ventricle ('ventrik'l) a small pouch or cavity; applied especially to the lower chambers of the heart, and to the four cavities of the brain.

ventricular (ven'trikyuhlə) pertaining to a ventricle. *V. folds* the outer folds of mucous membrane forming the false vocal cords. *V. septal defect* abbreviated VSD. Congenital abnormality in which there is communication between the two ventricles of the heart due to maldevelopment of the intraventricular septum.

ventriculocisternostomy (ven,trikyuhloh,sistər'nostəmee) surgical creation of a communication between the third ventricle and the interpeduncular cistern, for drainage of cerebrospinal fluid.

ventriculography (ven,trikyuh'logrəfee) 1. radiographic examination of the ventricles of the heart using a radio-opaque contrast medium. 2. radiographic examination of the ventricles of the brain following the injection of air or a contrast medium through a burr hole.

ventriculopuncture (ven'trikyuhloh,pungkchə) surgical puncture of a lateral ventricle of the brain.

ventriculoscope (ven'trikyuhloh,skohp) an instrument for viewing the inside of the ventricles of the brain.

ventrofixation (,ventrohfik'sayshən) stitching a retroverted uterus or other abdominal organ to the abdominal wall.

ventrosuspension (,ventrohsə-

'spenshən) an abdominal operation performed to remedy a displacement of the uterus.

Venturi mask (ven'tyooə·ree) *G.B. Venturi, Italian physicist, 1746–1822.* A type of disposable mask used to deliver a controlled oxygen concentration to a patient. The flow of 100 per cent oxygen through the mask draws in a controlled amount of room air (21 per cent oxygen). Commonly available masks deliver 24, 28, 35 or 40 per cent oxygen. At concentrations above 24 per cent, humidification may be required.

Venturi nebulizer a type of nebulizer used in AEROSOL therapy. The pressure drop of gas flowing through the nebulizer draws liquid from a capillary tube. As the liquid enters the gas stream it breaks up into a spray of small droplets.

venule ('venyool) a minute vein that collects blood from the capillaries.

verapamil (ve'rapə,mil) a coronary dilator used in the treatment of supraventricular tachycardia and of angina pectoris.

verbigeration (,vərbijə'rayshən) the monotonous repetition of phrases or meaningless words.

vermicide ('vərmi,sied) an agent which destroys intestinal worms; an anthelmintic.

vermiform ('vərmi,fawm) worm-shaped. *V. appendix* the worm-shaped structure attached to the caecum.

vermifuge ('vərmi,fyooj) an agent which expels intestinal worms; an anthelmintic.

verminous (,vərminəs) infested

with worms or other animal parasites, such as lice.

vernix ('vərniks) [L.] *varnish. V. caseosa* the fatty covering on the skin of the fetus during the last months of pregnancy. It consists of cells and sebaceous material.

verruca (və'rookə) a wart. Hypertrophy of the prickle cell layer of the epidermis and thickening of the horny layer. A virus is the causative organism. *V. acuminata* a venereal wart that appears on the external genitalia. *V. plana* a small, smooth, usually skin-coloured or light brown, slightly raised wart sometimes occurring in great numbers; seen most often in children. *V. plantaris* a viral epidermal tumour on the sole of the foot.

version ('vərshən, -zhən) the turning of a part; applied particularly to the turning of a fetus in order to facilitate delivery. *External v.* manipulation of the uterus through the abdominal wall in order to change the position of the child. *Internal v.* rotation of the fetus by means of manipulation with one hand in the vagina. *Podalic v.* turning of the fetus so that the head is uppermost and the feet presenting. *Spontaneous v.* one that occurs naturally without the application of force.

vertebra ('vərtibrə) one of the 33 irregular bones forming the spinal column. They are divided into: 7 cervical, 12 dorsal, 5 lumbar, 5 sacral (sacrum), and 4 coccygeal (coccyx) vertebrae.

vertebral ('vərtibrəl) pertaining to a vertebra. *V. column* the spine or backbone.

vertebrobasilar (,vərtibroh'basilə) pertaining to the vertebral and the basilar arteries. *V. disease* a condition affecting the flow of blood through the vertebral and basilar arteries which causes recurrent attacks of blindness, diplopia, vertigo, dysarthria and hemiparesis.

vertex ('vərteks) the crown of the head. *V. presentation* position of the fetus such that the crown of the head appears in the vagina first.

vertigo ('vərti,goh) a feeling of rotation or of going round, in either oneself or one's surroundings, particularly associated with disease of the cerebellum and the vestibular nerve of the ear. It may occur in diplopia or Menière's syndrome.

vesica ('vesikə) a bladder; usually referring to the urinary bladder.

vesicant ('vesikənt) a blistering agent.

vesicle ('vesik'l) 1. in anatomy, a small bladder usually containing fluid. *Seminal v.* one of a pair of sacs which arise from the vas deferens near the bladder and contain semen. 2. a very small blister usually containing serum.

vesicoureteric (,vesikoh·yoori-'terik) relating to the urinary bladder and the ureters. *V. reflux* the passing of urine backwards up the ureter during micturition. A cause of pyelonephritis in children.

vesicovaginal (,vesikohvə·'jien'l) relating to the bladder and vagina. *See* FISTULA.

vesicular (ve'sikyuhlə) relating to

or containing vesicles. *V. breathing* the soft murmur of normal respiration, as heard on auscultation. *V. mole* hydatidiform mole.

vesiculitis (ve,sikyuh'lietis) inflammation of a vesicle, particularly the seminal vesicles.

vesiculopapular (ve,sikyuhloh-'papyuhlə) describing an eruption of both vesicles and papules.

vesiculopustular (ve,sikyuhloh-'pustyuhlə) describing an eruption of both vesicles and pustules.

vessel ('ves'l) a tube, duct or canal for conveying fluid, usually blood or lymph.

vestibular (ve'stibyuhlə) relating to a vestibule. *V. glands* those in the vestibule of the vagina, including Bartholin's glands. *V. nerve* a branch of the auditory nerve supplying the semicircular canals and concerned with balance and equilibrium.

vestibule ('vesti,byool) a space or cavity at the entrance to another structure. *V. of the ear* the cavity at the entrance to the cochlea. *V. of the vagina* the space between the labia minora at the entrance to the vagina.

vestibulocochlear (ve,stibyuhloh'kokli·ə) pertaining to the vestibule of the ear and the cochlea. *V. nerve* the eighth cranial nerve. Also known as the auditory nerve.

vestigial (ve'stiji·al) rudimentary. Referring to the remains of an anatomical structure which, being of no further use, has atrophied.

viable ('vieəb'l) capable of independent life.

Vibrio ('vibrioh) a genus of Gram-negative bacteria, curved and motile by means of flagellae. *V. cholerae*, or *V. comma*, is that which causes cholera.

vicarious (vi'kairi·əs, vie-) substituted for another; used when one organ functions instead of another.

villus ('viləs) a small finger-like process projecting from a surface. *Chorionic v. see* CHORIONIC. *Intestinal v.* those of the mucous membrane of the small intestine, each of which contains a blood capillary and a lacteal.

vinblastine (vin'blasteen) a vinca alkaloid used as an antineoplastic in the treatment of Hodgkin's disease and testicular germinal cell cancer, usually in combination with other antineoplastic agents.

Vincent's angina ('vinsənts) *J.H. Vincent, French physician, 1862–1950. See* ANGINA.

vincristine (vin'kristeen) a vinca alkaloid used as an antineoplastic in the treatment of acute leukaemias, Hodgkin's disease, non-Hodgkin's lymphomas and some solid tumours, usually in combination with other antineoplastic agents.

vinyl ('vien'l) a plastic material now used extensively for medical equipment. *V. ether* a short-acting inhalation anaesthetic drug used mainly for inducing anaesthesia and for minor surgery.

viraemia (vie'reemi·ə) the presence of viruses in the blood.

virilism ('viri,lizəm) masculine traits exhibited by a female owing to the production of excessive

amounts of androgenic hormone either in the adrenal cortex or from an ovarian tumour. *See* ARRHENOBLASTOMA.

virology (vie'roləjee) the scientific study of viruses, their growth and the diseases caused by them.

virulence ('virələns) the power of a microorganism to produce toxins or poisons. This depends on (1) the number and power of the invading organisms, and (2) the power of the microorganism to overcome host resistance.

virulent ('virələnt) dangerously poisonous.

virus ('vierəs) any member of a unique class of infectious agents, which were originally distinguished by their smallness and their inability to replicate outside of a living host cell; because these properties are shared by other microorganisms (rickettsiae, chlamydiae), viruses are now characterized by their simple organization and their unique mode of replication. A virus consists of genetic material, which may be either DNA or RNA, and is surrounded by a protein coat and, in some viruses, by a membranous envelope. They cause many diseases, including smallpox (variola), chickenpox (varicella), herpes zoster (shingles), herpes infections, measles (rubeola), German measles (rubella), mumps, infectious mononucleosis, hepatitis A and B, yellow fever, the common cold, acquired immune deficiency disease (AIDS), influenza, certain types of pneumonia and croup and other respiratory infections, poliomyelitis, and several types of encephalitis. There is evidence that certain viruses may be capable of causing cancer.

viscera ('visə-rə) *see* VISCUS.

visceroptosis (,visə-rop'tohsis) a general tendency to prolapse of the abdominal organs.

viscid ('visid) sticky and glutinous.

viscosity (vi'skositee) resistance to flowing. A sticky and glutinous quality.

viscus ('viskəs) any of the organs contained in the body cavities, especially in the abdomen.

vision ('vishən) the faculty of seeing. Sight.

visual ('vishyooəl) relating to sight. *V. acuity* sharpness of vision. It is assessed by reading test types. *V. cells* the rods and cones of the retina. *V. field* the area within which objects can be seen when looking straight ahead. *V. purple* the pigment in the outer layers of the retina. Rhodopsin.

vital ('viet'l) relating to life. *V. capacity* the amount of air which can be expelled from the lungs after a full inspiration. *V. signs* the signs of life, namely pulse, respiration and temperature. *V. statistics* the records kept of births and deaths among the population, including the causes of death, and the factors which seem to influence their rise and fall.

vitallium (vie'tali·əm) a metal alloy used in dentistry and for prostheses in bone surgery.

vitamin ('vitəmin) any of a group of accessory food factors which

are contained in foodstuffs and are essential to life, growth and reproduction. *See* Appendix 4.

vitiligo (,viti'liegoh) a skin disease marked by an absence of pigment, producing white patches on the face and body. Leukoderma.

vitrectomy (vi'trektəmee) surgical extraction of the vitreous humour and its replacement by a physiological solution in the treatment of vitreous haemorrhage following diabetic retinopathy.

vitreous ('vitri·əs) glassy. *V. humour* the transparent jelly-like substance filling the posterior of the eye, from lens to retina.

vocal ('vohk'l) pertaining to the voice or the organs which produce the voice. *V. cords* the two folds of tissue in the larynx, formed of fibrous tissue covered with squamous epithelium. *V. resonance* the normal sounds of speech heard through the chest wall by means of a stethoscope.

volatile ('volə,tiel) having a tendency to evaporate readily.

volition (ve'lishən) the conscious adoption by the individual of a line of action.

Volkmann's contracture ('vohlkmənz) *R. von Volkmann, German surgeon, 1830–1889.* Contraction of the fingers and sometimes of the wrist or of analogous parts of the foot, with loss of power, after severe injury or improper use of a tourniquet or cast.

volume ('volyoom) the space occupied by a substance. *Minute v.* the total volume of air breathed in or out in 1 min. *Packed cell v.* that occupied by the blood cells after centrifuging (about 45% of the blood sample). *Residual v.* the amount of air left in the lungs after breathing out fully.

voluntary ('volǝntǝ·ree) under the control of the will. *See* INVOLUNTARY.

volvulus ('volvyuhlǝs) twisting of a loop of bowel causing obstruction. Most common in the sigmoid colon.

vomer ('vohmǝ) a thin plate of bone forming the posterior septum of the nose.

vomit ('vomit) 1. matter ejected from the stomach through the mouth (vomitus). 2. to eject material in this way. *Bilious v.* vomit mixed with bile. The vomit is stained yellow or green. *Coffeeground v.* ejected matter that contains small quantities of altered blood, which has this appearance. *Faecal* or *stercoraceous v.* vomit mixed with faeces. Occurs in intestinal obstruction when the contents of the upper intestine regurgitate back into the stomach. It is dark brown with an unpleasant odour.

vomiting ('vomiting) a reflex act of expulsion of the stomach contents via the oesophagus and mouth. It may be preceded by nausea and excess salivation if the cause is local irritation in the stomach. *Cyclical v.* recurrent attacks of vomiting often occurring in children and associated with acidosis. *Projectile v.* the forcible ejection of the gastric contents, usually without warning. Present in hypertrophic pyloric stenosis, and in cerebral diseases. *V. of pregnancy* vomiting occurring in the months of pregnancy. Morning sickness.

von Recklinghausen's disease (von 'rekling,howzǝnz) *see* RECKLINGHAUSEN'S DISEASE.

von Willebrand's disease (von 'vili,brants) *E.A. von Willebrand, Finnish physician, 1870–1949.* A bleeding disorder inherited as an autosomal dominant trait (rarely recessive), characterized by a prolonged bleeding time, deficiency of coagulation factor VIII, and associated with epistaxis and increased bleeding after trauma or surgery, menorrhagia, and postpartum bleeding.

vulnerability (,vulnǝ·rǝ'bilitee) weakness. Susceptibility to injury or infection.

vulva ('vulvǝ) the external female genital organs.

vulvectomy (vul'vektǝmee) excision of the vulva.

vulvitis (vul'vietis) inflammation of the vulva.

vulvovaginitis (,vulvoh,vaji'nietis) inflammation of the vulva and vagina.

W

Waldeyer's ring ('valdieəz) *H.W.G. von Waldeyer-Hartz, German anatomist, 1836–1921.* The circle of lymphoid tissue in the pharynx formed by the lingual, faucial and pharyngeal tonsils.

Wangensteen tube ('wangen‚steen) *O.H. Wangensteen, American surgeon, b. 1898.* A gastro-intestinal aspiration tube with a tip that is opaque to X-rays.

warfarin ('wawfə‧rin) an oral anticoagulant drug that depresses the prothrombin level. Used mainly in the treatment of coronary and venous thrombosis.

wart (wawt) an elevation of the skin, which is often of a brownish colour, caused by hypertrophy of papillae in the dermis due to a virus infection. *See* VERRUCA and CONDYLOMA.

Wassermann test (reaction) ('vasəmən) *A.P. von Wassermann, German bacteriologist, 1866–1925.* A complement-fixation test used in the diagnosis of syphilis.

water ('wawtə) a clear, colourless, tasteless liquid composed of hydrogen and oxygen (H_2O). *W. balance* fluid balance. That between the fluid taken in by all routes and the fluid lost by all routes. *W.-borne* descriptive of certain diseases that are spread by contaminated water. *W.-brash* the eructation of dilute acid from the stomach to the pharynx, giving a burning sensation. Pyrosis. Heartburn. *W.-seal drainage* a closed method of drainage from the pleural space allowing the escape of fluid and air but preventing air entering as the drainage tube discharges under water.

Waterhouse–Friderichsen syndrome (‚wawtəhows'freedriksən) *R. Waterhouse, British physician, 1873–1958; C. Friderichsen, Danish physician, b. 1886.* The malignant or fulminating form of meningococcal MENINGITIS, which is marked by sudden onset and short course, fever, coma, collapse, cyanosis, haemorrhages from the skin and mucous membranes, and bilateral adrenal haemorrhage.

Waterston's operation ('wawtəstənz) *D. Waterston, British paediatric surgeon, b. 1910.* A palliative operation of anastomosis of the right pulmonary artery to the ascending aorta. Used in the treatment of tricuspid atresia in the young child.

Watson–Crick helix (‚wotsən 'krik) *J.D. Watson, American geneticist, b. 1928; F. Crick, British biochemist, b. 1916.* Double helix; a representation of the structure of DEOXYRIBONUCLEIC ACID

(DNA), consisting of two coiled chains, each of which contains information completely specifying the other chain.

waxy flexibility (ˌwaksi ˌfleksiˈbilitee) a cataleptic state in which a patient's limbs are held indefinitely in any position in which they have been placed. *See* CATATONIA.

weal (weel) a raised stripe on the skin, as is caused by the lash of a whip. Typical of urticaria.

wean (ween) 1. to discontinue breast or bottle feeding and substitute other feeding habits. This should be effected gradually at about the fourth month. 2. in respiratory therapy, to gradually decrease dependence on assisted ventilation until the patient is able to breathe spontaneously.

webbing ('webing) the state of being connected by a membrane or a fold of skin. *W. of hands* or *feet* congenital abnormality in which the digits are not separated from each other. Syndactyly. *W. of neck* folds of skin in the neck, giving it a webbed appearance. Occurs in certain congenital conditions, e.g. Turner's syndrome.

Weber test ('vaybə) *F.E. Weber-Liel, German otologist, 1832–1891.* A test for hearing. A vibrating tuning fork is held in the centre of the forehead. Sound is normally heard equally in both ears. If the sound is heard louder in one ear it may be indicative of conductive deafness in that ear.

Weil's disease ('vielz) *A. Weil, German physician, 1848–1916.* Spirochaetal jaundice. The organism, *Leptospira ictero-hae-*

morrhagiae, is harboured and excreted by rats and enters through a bite or skin abrasion, or infected food or water.

Weil–Felix reaction (ˌviel'feeliks) *E. Weil, Austrian physician, 1880–1922; A. Felix, Czech bacteriologist, 1887–1956.* An agglutination test of blood serum used in the diagnosis of typhus.

well baby clinic mothers are encouraged to bring their infants to these clinics for assessment and monitoring of the child's health. Immunization is available and opportunities for 'family' health promotion.

well man clinic a 'prophylactic' clinic available for men to screen for health problems and to promote health, e.g. self-examination of the testicles.

well woman clinic a 'prophylactic' clinic available to screen women for breast and cervical cancer, anaemia, diabetes and hypertension.

wellness ('welnəs) the development of a personal lifestyle which promotes feelings of well-being, achieves the highest level of health within one's capability, and minimizes chances of becoming ill. It is guided by a developing sense of self-awareness and self-responsibility encompassing emotional, mental, physical, social, spiritual and environmental health.

wen (wen) a small sebaceous cyst; a steatoma.

Wenckebach phenomenon ('venkəˌbahk) *K.F. Wenckebach, Dutch physician, 1864–1940.* Abnormal heart rhythm in which the P-R interval gradually increases until a beat is missed.

Werdnig–Hoffmann disease (ˌvərdnig'hofmən) *G. Werdnig, Austrian neurologist, 1844–1919; J.E. Hoffmann, German neurologist, 1857–1919.* Disease characterized by progressive spinal muscular atrophy affecting the shoulder, neck, pelvis and eventually the respiratory muscles of infants.

Werner's syndrome ('vərnəz) *C.W.O. Werner, German physician, b. 1879.* A hereditary condition characterized by cataracts, osteoporosis, stuned growth and premature greying of the hair.

Wernicke's encephalopathy ('vərnikəz) *K. Wernicke, German neurologist, 1848–1905.* A neurological condition due to vitamin B_1 deficiency. Untreated it progresses from mental confusion and double vision to lethargy and coma. It is most commonly seen in chronic alcoholism.

Wernicke–Korsakoff syndrome (ˌvərnikə'kawsəkof) *K. Wernicke; S.S. Korsakoff, Russian neurologist, 1854–1900.* A disorder of the central nervous system, usually associated with chronic alcoholism, nutritional deficiency and severe deficiency of vitamin B_1. It is characterized by a combination of motor and sensory disturbances and disordered memory function.

Wertheim's operation ('vərt·hiemz) *E. Wertheim, Austrian gynaecologist, 1864–1920.* See HYSTERECTOMY.

Wharton's jelly ('wawtənz) *T. Wharton, British physician, 1614–*

1673. The connective tissue of the umbilical cord.

wheezing ('weezing) breathing with a rasp or whistling sound. It results from constriction or obstruction of the throat, pharynx, trachea or bronchi.

whiplash injury ('wip,lash) injury to the spinal cord, nerve roots, ligaments or vertebrae in the cervical region due to a sudden jerking back of the head and neck. Common in road traffic accidents where there is sudden acceleration or deceleration of the vehicle.

whiplash shake syndrome ('wip,lash shayk) a constellation of injuries to the brain and eye that may occur when a young child less than 3 years old is shaken vigorously with the head unsupported. This causes stretching and tearing of the cerebral vessels and brain substance, commonly leading to subdural haematomas and retinal haemorrhages. It may result in paralysis, blindness and other visual disturbances, convulsions and death.

Whipple's operation ('wip'lz) *A.O. Whipple, American surgeon, 1881–1963.* Radical pancreoduodenectomy performed for carcinoma of the head of the pancreas. Most of the pancreas, the pylorus, duodenum and the common bile duct are excised. Gastrojejunostomy is performed with anastomosis of the tail of the pancreas and gallbladder to the jejunum.

whipworm ('wip,wərm) *see* TRICHURIS.

white leg (wiet) milk leg. *See*

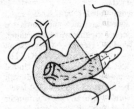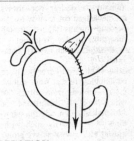

WHIPPLE'S OPERATION

PHLEGMASIA.

Whitfield's ointment ('witfeeldz) *A. Whitfield, British dermatologist, 1868–1947.* Compound ointment of benzoic acid used in the treatment of fungal diseases.

whitlow ('witloh) a felon; a suppurating inflammation of a finger near the nail. *Melanotic w.* a malignant tumour of the nail bed characterized by formation of melanotic tissue. *Subperiosteal w.* one in which the infection involves the bone covering. *Superficial w.* a pustule between the true skin and cuticle. *See* PARONYCHIA.

WHO World Health Organization.

whooping cough ('hooping ˌkof) a notifiable infectious disease characterized by catarrh of the respiratory tract and paroxysms of coughing, ending in a prolonged whooping respiration; called also pertussis. The causative organism is *Bordetella pertussis.* Whooping cough is a serious disease; most cases occur in children.

Widal reaction (vee'dahl) *G.F.I. Widal, French physician, 1862–1929.* A blood agglutination test for typhoid fever.

Wilms' tumour (vilmz) *M. Wilms, German surgeon, 1867–1918.* A highly malignant tumour of the kidney occurring in young children. A nephroblastoma.

Wilson's disease (wilsənz) *S.A.K. Wilson, British neurologist, 1878–1937.* Hepatolenticular degeneration. A congenital abnormality in the metabolism of copper leading to neurological degeneration.

wiring ('wieəring) the fixing together of a broken or split bone by the use of a wire. Commonly used for the jaw, the patella and the sternum.

wisdom teeth ('wizdəm) the back molar teeth, the appearance of which is often delayed until maturity.

wish fulfilment ('wish fuhl-

,filmənt) a desire, not always acknowledged consciously by the person, which is fulfilled through dreams or by day-dreaming.

witch-hazel ('wich,hayz'l) hamamelis.

withdrawal (widh'dror'l) 1. a pathological retreat from reality. 2. abstention from drugs to which one is habituated or addicted; also denoting the symptoms occasioned by such withdrawal. *W. symptoms* symptoms brought about by abrupt withdrawal of a narcotic or other drug to which a person has become addicted; called also abstinence syndrome. The usual reactions to withdrawal may include anxiety, weakness, gastrointestinal symptoms, nausea and vomiting, tremor, fever, rapid heartbeat, convulsions and delirium.

Wolff–Parkinson–White syndrome (,wuhlf,pahkinsən'wiet) *L. Wolff, American cardiologist, 1898–1972; Sir J. Parkinson, British physician, 1885–1976; P.D. White, American cardiologist, 1886–1973.* Abnormal heart rhythm caused by an accessory bundle between the atria and ventricles. A congenital disorder.

womb (woom) the uterus.

Wood's light (wuhdz) *R.W. Wood, American physicist, 1868–1953.* Ultraviolet light transmitted through a filter glass containing nickel oxide. It produces fluorescence of infected hairs when placed over a scalp affected with ringworm.

woolsorter's disease ('wuhlsawtəz) pulmonary anthrax.

word blindness ('wərd) *see* DYS-LEXIA.

word salad ('wərd,salad) rapid speech in which the words are strung together without meaning.

World Health Organization (wərld) abbreviated WHO. The specialized agency of the United Nations that is concerned with health on an international level.

worm (wərm) any one of a number of groups of long soft-bodied invertebrates, some of which are parasitic to man.

wound (woond) a cut or break in continuity of any tissue, caused by injury or operation. It is classified according to its nature. *Abrased w.* the skin is scraped off, but there is no deeper injury. *Contused w.* with bruising of the surrounding tissue. *W. healing* the restoration of integrity to injured tissues by replacement of dead tissue with viable tissue. The process starts immediately after an injury and may continue for months or years. *See* HEAL-ING. *Incised w.* usually the result of operation, and produced by a knife or similar instrument. The edges of the wound can remain in apposition, and it should heal by first intention. *Lacerated w.* one with torn edges and tissues, usually the result of accident or injury. It is often septic and heals by second intention. *Open w.* a gaping wound on the body surface. *Penetrating w.* often made by gunshot, shrapnel, etc. There may be an inlet and outlet hole and vital organs are often penetrated by the missile. *Punctured w.* made by a pointed or spiked instrument. *Septic w.* any type into which infection has been introduced, causing suppurative inflammation. It heals by second intention.

wrist (rist) the joint of the carpus and bones of the forearm. *W. drop* loss of power in the muscles of the hand. It may be due to nerve or tendon injury, but can result from lack of sufficient support by splint or sling.

writer's cramp (ˌrietəz 'kramp) a colloquial term for painful spasm of the hand and forearm, caused by excessive writing and poor posture.

wryneck ('rie,nek) *see* TORTI-COLLIS.

Wuchereria (ˌvookə'riə·ri·ə) a genus of nematode worms which are the principal vectors of filariasis. *W. bancrofti* is the most common species in tropical and subtropical areas.

X

X chromosome ('eks,krohmə-,sohm) the female sex chromosome, being present in all female gametes and only half the male gametes. When union takes place two *Xc's* result in a female child (XX) but one of each results in a male child (XY). *See* Y CHROMOSOME.

X-rays ('eks,rayz) electromagnetic waves of short length which are capable of penetrating many substances and of producing chemical changes and reactions in living matter. They are used both to aid diagnosis and to treat disease. Called also Röntgen rays.

xanthelasma (,zanthə'lazmə) a disease marked by the formation of flat or slightly raised yellow patches on the eyelids.

xanthine ('zantheen) a compound found in plant and animal tissues, the forerunner of uric acid in nucleoprotein metabolism.

xanthochromia (,zanthoh'krohmi-ə) 1. the presence of yellow patches on the skin. 2. the yellow colouring of cerebrospinal fluid seen in patients who have had a subarachnoid haemorrhage.

xanthoma (zan'thohmə) the presence in the skin of flat areas of yellowish pigmentation due to deposits of lipoids. There are several varieties. *X. palpebrarum* xanthelasma.

xanthopsia (zan'thopsi-ə) a disturbance of vision in which all objects appear yellow.

xanthosis (zan'thohsis) a yellow skin pigmentation, seen in some cases of diabetes and poliomyelitis.

Xenopsylla (,zenop'silə) a genus of fleas, some of which are vectors of plague. *X. cheopis* the rat flea, which transmits bubonic plague.

xeroderma (,zie·roh'dərmə) an hereditary condition in which there is excessive dryness of the skin. A mild form of ichthyosis. *X. pigmentosum* a rare hereditary and often fatal disease in which there is extreme sensitivity of the skin and eyes to light. It begins in childhood and rapidly progresses. The formation of malignant neoplasms is common.

xerophthalmia (,zie·rof'thalmi·ə) a condition in which the cornea and conjunctiva become horny and necrosed owing to a deficiency of vitamin A. Xeroma.

xerosis (zi'rohsis) a condition in which the conjunctiva appears dry and lustreless. Small white patches of horny epithelium appear on the cornea (Bitôt's spots).

xerostomia (,zie·roh'stohmi·ə) dryness of the mouth due to a failure of the salivary glands.

xylene ('zieleen) xylol; dimethyl-benzene. A clear inflammable liquid resembling benzene. Used as a solvent for rubber and in microscopy.

Xylocaine ('zieloh,kayn) a proprietary preparation of lignocaine used for local anaesthesia.

xylose ('zielohz) a pentose sugar found in connective tissue and sometimes in urine, which is not metabolized in the body.

XYY syndrome (,eks,wie'wie) an extremely rare condition in males in which there is an extra Y chromosome, making a total of 47 in each body cell. *See* KLINE-FELTER'S SYNDROME.

Y

Y chromosome ('wie,krohmə-,sohm) the male sex chromosome, being present in half the male gametes and none of the female. It carries few major genes. *See* X-CHROMOSOME.

yawning ('yawning) an involuntary act in which the mouth is opened wide and air is drawn in and exhaled. It may accompany tiredness or boredom.

yaws (yorz) framboesia. A skin infection common in tropical countries. Caused by *Treponema pertenue*, it is common among people, especially children, who live under primitive conditions in equatorial Africa, South America, and the East and West Indies.

yeast (yeest) any of the fungi of the genus *Saccharomyces*. They produce fermentation in malt, and in sweetened fruit juices, resulting in the formation of alcoholic solutions such as beer and wines.

yellow fever ('yeloh) an acute, notifiable, infectious disease of the tropics caused by a virus and transmitted by a mosquito (*Aëdes aegypti*). The virus attacks the liver and kidney and the symptoms include rigor, headache, pain in the back and limbs, high fever and black vomit. Haemorrhage from the intestinal mucous membrane may occur. There is a high mortality rate.

yttrium ('itri·əm) *symbol* Y. An element used as radioactive yttrium (^{90}Y) in the treatment of malignant effusions.

Z

Z-plasty ('zed,plastee) a plastic operation for removing and repairing deformity resulting from a contraction scar.

Ziehl–Neelsen method (,ziel-'neelsən) *F. Ziehl, German bacteriologist, 1857–1926; F.K.A. Neelsen, 1854–1894.* A method of staining tubercle bacilli for microscopic study.

Zimmer ('zimə) the trade name of a metal, light-weight walking aid, and commonly applied to other products of similar design and weight. Predominantly used by the elderly to assist in rehabilitation.

zinc (zingk) *symbol* Zn. A trace element which is essential in the body for cell growth and multiplication. The recommended daily intake of zinc is 15 mg for an adult. A severe deficiency of zinc can retard growth in children, cause a low sperm count in adult males, and retard wound healing.

Zollinger–Ellison syndrome (,zolinjə'elisən) *R.M. Zollinger, American physician, b. 1903; E.H. Ellison, American physician, 1918–1970.* A rare condition in which a pancreatic tumour causes excessive outpouring of gastric juice. Peptic ulcers may occur.

zona ('zohnə) 1. a zone. *Z. pellucida* the membrane surrounding the ovum. 2. herpes zoster; shingles. *Z. facialis* herpes of the face.

zonula ('zonyuhlə) a zonule. In anatomy, a small usually circular area. *Ciliary z.* the area surrounded by the suspensory ligaments of the eye.

zonulolysis (,zonyuh'lolisis) dissolving of the zonular fibres by zonulysin to aid cataract extraction.

zonulysin (,zonyuh'liesin) a proteolytic enzyme that may be used

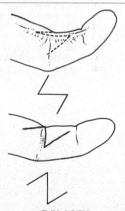

Z-PLASTY

in eye surgery to dissolve the suspensory ligament.

zoonosis (ˌzoh·əˈnohsis, ˌzooə-ˈnohsis) a disease of animals that is transmissible to man, e.g. anthrax, cat-scratch fever, etc.

zoster ('zostə) *see* HERPES

zygoma (zieˈgohmə, zi-) the arch formed by the union of the tem-poral with the malar bone in front of the ear.

zygote ('ziegoht, 'zi-) a single fertilized cell formed from the union of a male and a female gamete.

zymosis (zieˈmohsis) 1. fermen-tation. 2. the development of an infectious disease.

APPENDICES

APPENDIX 1

Primary Nursing

As nursing has developed greater competence and assurance through nursing research and nursing education, so the methods of delivering nursing care have changed over the years. There was a time when all care was provided on the basis of task allocation and nurses were allotted responsibility for performing certain common services to all patients in a ward; thus, one nurse would carry out all recordings of temperature, pulse and blood pressure, another would be responsible for the bathing of all patients, and probably the measurement of fluid balance, whilst yet another nurse would carry out all wound dressings. These tasks were performed under the direction of the ward sister who would also be responsible for the delegation of special care requirements and referrals prescribed by the doctor. As nursing developed its own body of knowledge and confidence, many nurses expressed increasing dissatisfaction at having to deliver care in such a fragmented manner, and sought better methods of meeting the total care needs of patients. The introduction of the nursing process enabled the replacement of task-oriented care with more comprehensive forms of nursing.

Team nursing was one such development. Teams of nurses, led by a qualified nurse, would deliver total care to groups of patients. The leader of the team would take responsibility for ensuring that the care planned for each patient was carried out and would also be responsible for the writing and updating of care plans. Teams and/or team leaders might change frequently, as might the groups of patients allocated to them. Sometimes in a ward there would be only one team, the ward nurses, and one leader, the ward sister, who was responsible for writing individual care plans and allocating duties to members of the team. This was task-oriented care under another name.

The most common implementation of the nursing process was the assignment of one nurse to plan and deliver care for one or more patients during a span of duty. Although this was a great improvement on previous methods, accountability for implementing and updating the care plan changed at each shift change, with resulting lack of continuity. Even with this system, especially when the designated nurse was in training, or the ward was short staffed, some functional tasks, such as the delivery of medications, remained the responsibility of one nurse.

Primary nursing has developed from these earlier experiments into different methods of delivering care; it has been described as professional nursing practice at its best, providing all the benefits to nurse, patient and family inherent in such a statement. A primary nurse is a qualified nurse who, in consultation with the patient (and family, where appropriate), plans and organizes all necessary nursing care for that patient over a 24-h period and is responsible for evaluating the effectiveness of that care. In reality, this means that the primary nurse has total responsibility for planning and organizing the care of a group of patients, perhaps four or five, from admission to discharge. The care plan is drawn up in collaboration with the patient who is encouraged to identify those deficits which impair his normal functioning. As total care co-ordinator, the primary nurse is responsible for liaising with medical staff and for all necessary referrals to other members of the caring team, i.e. dietitians, physiotherapists, occupational therapists, nurse specialists. Obviously no nurse can be on duty all the time, and therefore the primary nurse is assisted by associate nurses who carry out the plan of care in the absence of the primary nurse. Although these close professional collaborations are important, it is the primary nurse who maintains overall responsibility for planning care and, except in very exceptional circumstances, no one but the primary nurse will modify the plan of care. Often primary nurses will be associate nurses to other primary nurses in the team.

This style of nursing has many benefits: it enables the patient to be involved in decisions which affect him; the assurance of continuity of planned care enables creative and imaginative nursing in order to meet specific needs; patients, families and co-professionals all benefit from knowing who is responsible for the delivery of care to which patients, and with whom they should communicate. The primary nurse is also reminded of the need to promote high quality nursing practice, as it is she who will be called to account for her decisions and actions. The interaction between primary nurse and patient also has many potential benefits. It helps the nurse to get to know the patient and those meaningful to him and enables her to develop a picture of his home life. Learning about the patient enables the primary nurse to identify nursing problems, both actual and potential, to set goals for their resolution and to record the interventions she will prescribe to meet the goals. The planning of holistic care in this way enables the associate nurse to ensure continuity of care in the absence of the primary nurse.

In addition to raising the level of care, primary nursing enables the nurse to achieve other aspects of her role. The development of a good nurse–patient relationship facilitates education: the nurse gives information on the present illness and can teach necessary health education topics which will benefit the patient in the future. Similarly, it may be necessary to teach aspects of care to family members, and support them in helping and caring for the patient. The primary nurse must have a perspective of the patient beyond hospital and use this in discharge planning and rehabilitation strategies, thus helping the patient from dependence to independence. She also has a unique function in acting as the role model, mentor and teacher to other nurses, especially those not yet qualified. Within the caring situation she can help develop the skills and perspectives of others who will later become primary nurses.

Associate nurses are important members of the caring team; they may themselves be primary nurses to others, or they may be students. They may deliver much of the care under the direction of the primary nurse, or in her absence. In using and developing the skills of the associate nurse, the primary nurse must value the contribution of the associate and consult with her when developing or modifying a plan of care. Consultation between the two will ensure clarity of common purpose and maximize delivery of care. Working as an associate enables the nurse to develop experience and expertise in care planning under the guidance of the primary nurse which is invaluable preparation before assuming the role of primary nurse herself.

In delivering prescribed care to patients, one of the most important responsibilities of the associate nurse is the careful notation of the patient's progress and responses to interventions. The primary nurse relies upon the observations and accurate recording of the associate nurse; in this, the associate nurse plays a vital contribution in the assessment, planning and evaluation of the patient's care.

The implementation of primary nursing impinges on another role in the ward team, namely that of the charge nurse. If primary nurses are autonomous practitioners, what then is the role of the charge nurse? If primary nursing is to work well, the non-nursing responsibilities which nurses frequently undertake must be allocated to others. Manthey describes primary care systems practised in some American hospitals where those responsibilities which do not require nursing knowledge, e.g. clerical work, supplies and maintenance problems, are undertaken by administrative staff. Such a system should free the charge nurse to undertake the role of co-ordinator of care. This role is filled by a nurse of proven clinical expertise, with sound teaching skills and who has herself worked as a primary nurse. The co-ordinator can act as consultant and adviser to primary and associate nurses, and would be the referral point if there were a need to change planned care in the absence of the primary nurse. The co-ordinator would also allocate associate nurses to patients for a span of duty, allocate primary nurses to new patients, be responsible for maintaining an overall perspective of the patients and their care, and ensure the appropriate hand-over of information to nurses coming on duty. As mentor, the co-ordinator would undertake a regular review of the nursing management of patients with the appropriate primary nurse.

Many people believe that primary nursing will ultimately allow nursing to develop the 'knowledge base' needed by all professions for the treatment of patients. The expansion of the responsibilities of nurses working with this method of care exposes them to much closer working relationships with all other disciplines, helping them to work in and with interdisciplinary teams, and to value this response to patient needs. The autonomy of the primary nurse enables the development of exciting practice and encourages nurses to initiate clinically based research studies, to evaluate more closely the products they use in delivering care, and document the outcomes of nursing practice.

Further Reading

The reader is encouraged to explore the wealth of literature available on the subject of primary nursing, of which the following recommendations are but a few.

Ersser R and Tutton E (eds.) (1990) *Primary Nursing in Practice.* Scutari Press.

Felton G (1975) Increasing the quality of nursing care by introducing the concept of primary nursing: a model project. *Nursing Research* **24**: 27–32.

Manthey M (1983) *The Practice of Primary Nursing.* Blackwell Scientific.

Manthey M, Ciske K et al (1970) Primary nursing: a return to the concept 'my nurse, my patient'. *Nursing Forum* **IX** (1).

Peason A (1983) *The Clinical Nursing Unit.* Heinemann.

Pearson A (ed.) (1988) *Primary Nursing: Nursing in the Burford and Oxford Nursing Development Units.* Croom Helm.

Wright S (ed.) (1990) *My Patient, My Nurse.* Scutari Press.

APPENDIX 2

Models of Nursing

In 1966, Virginia Henderson described what she believed to be the unique functions of the nurse: 'to assist the individual, sick or well, in the performance of those activities contributing to health or its recovery – or to peaceful death – that he would perform unaided if he had the necessary strength, will or knowledge.' Viewed retrospectively, this is probably one of the first models of nursing, and one from which many later models, by other theorists, were to emerge. Many thousands of words in hundreds of articles and scores of books have been written about models; there are probably as many books on models as there are models!

A nursing model is a conceptual framework of nursing based on knowledge, ideas and beliefs. It clarifies the meaning of nursing, provides criteria for policy and gives direction to team nursing, thus providing unity of approach and the framework for continuity of care. It identifies the nurse's role, highlights areas of practice requiring research and can be the basis for a nursing curriculum. The most important aspect of any nursing model has to be its acceptability to patient and nurse; the implementation of a model of care for an individual must, whenever possible, be a partnership. Hoped-for outcomes must be planned jointly, and the patient should be encouraged to highlight those needs/deficits which he thinks are important in his life. The use of nursing models can thus be seen as restoring control to the patient and making him an active participant in his care, rather than a passive recipient.

As with the introduction of the nursing process, the emergence of nursing models was bedevilled by obscure or newly coined language and they were perceived by many nurses to have been developed by people remote from the root of nursing practice. Many of the earlier models were American and this may go some way to explaining this, especially as the terminology was foreign to many British nurses and the systems of care between the two countries differed. British nurses have now either devised their own models or adapted American models for their own use. It is not possible here to write in depth on models of nursing or to describe in detail the number of different models which have been developed. Most nursing specialities have adopted and adapted a specific model of nursing which they feel meets the needs of consumer and practitioner. Brief descriptions of four nursing models currently in use in the United Kingdom follow, together with a reading list which covers some of the excellent texts currently available on all aspects of models of nursing.

Ray adaptation model

Described as a 'biopsychosocial' model of nursing, this model is based on the assumption that each individual is a biopsychosocial being who constantly interacts with a changing environment, using innate and acquired mechanisms which are biological, psychological and social in origin. Health and illness are viewed as inevitable dimensions of the individual's life, and in order to respond positively to environmental change, the individual must adapt. Adaptation is a function of the stimulus to which the individual is exposed and of the individual's adaptation level. According to Ray, the individual has four modes of adaptation: physiological needs, role functions, 'self' concept, and interdependence relations.

Orem's self-care model

This model, based on Orem's extensive work over many years, reflects her belief that individuals, who are rational, thinking biological organisms, interact with and are affected by their environment and are capable of actions which affect themselves, other individuals and the environment in which they live. Thus they have control! She theorizes that most individuals can meet their own self-care needs, i.e. breathing, eating, excreting, exercising, resting, the need for interaction with others, and for solitude, and the avoidance of stress, by feeling and being normal. Therefore, the role of nursing is to assess whether the individual can meet 'unusual self-care demands' and to give direct assistance when he is unable to do so.

Roper, Logan and Tierney: Activities of living

This model describes 12 activities of living concerned with an individual's life span from birth to death, and which from time to time the individual will be able to perform unaided and at other times will require help; thus, the individual, during his life span, will fluctuate from total independence in performing any one or all of the activities to total dependence. The nurse uses this model to assist patients in times of need, handing back control when the patient is able to manage. The essential activities of living described by Roper, Logan and Tierney are: maintaining a safe environment, communicating, breathing, eating and drinking, eliminating, personal hygiene and dressing, controlling body temperature, mobilizing, working and playing, expressing sexuality, sleeping, and dying.

King: An interaction model

King based her model of care on many years of research and observation of interactions between nurses and patients. King says that nursing is a process of action, reaction, interaction and transaction, and by using this process, together with the four concepts which form the basis of her model (social systems, health, perception and interpersonal relationships), the nurse can meet the care needs of individuals, whatever their background or circumstances.

Further Reading

Chapman CM (1985) *Theory of Nursing – Practical Application*. Harper and Row.

Henderson V (1966) *The Nature of Nursing*. Collier MacMillan.

Kershaw B (1988) Nursing in cancer care: introducing the Henderson model. In Tschudin V (ed.) *Nursing the Patient with Cancer*. Prentice Hall.

Kershaw B & Salvage J (eds) (1986) *Models for Nursing*. John Wiley & Sons.

Orem D (1980) *Nursing – Concepts of Practice*, 2nd edn. McGraw-Hill.

Pearson A & Vaughan B (1986) *Nursing Models for Practice*. Heinemann.

Peplau HE (1952) *Interpersonal Relations in Nursing*. GP Putman.

Roy C (1976) *Introduction to Nursing: An Adaptation Model*. Prentice Hall.

Rogers M (1970) *An Introduction to the Theoretical Basis of Nursing*. FA Davis.

Roper N, Logan W & Tierney A (1980) *The Elements of Nursing*. Churchill Livingstone.

Walsh M (ed.) *Nursing Models in Clinical Practice*. Baillière Tindall (forthcoming, early 1991).

Wright SG (1986) *Building and Using a Model of Nursing*. Edward Arnold.

APPENDIX 3

Transcultural Nursing

(Co-authored by Jennifer Barclay, Senior Nurse, HIV Support Team, St Mary's Hospital, London W2 1NY)

The United Kingdom today has a multiracial society. Many people settled in this country a number of years ago, and there are now members of second, third and maybe more generations of immigrant families who are British subjects but continue to maintain links with their cultural heritage. Not only are there people who have settled in and adopted the UK as their home, but there are also visiting businessmen and women, students seeking further education, and short-term residents. The length of time an individual resides in a cultural environment different from his root culture will, to some extent, create in that individual a mixture of attitudes. That mix of attitudes will include some created by both his root culture and his new environmental culture. The UK is still essentially a Christian country and the laws of the land are thus in keeping with the Christian philosophy. Hospitals, and health care services, follow this same ethic, and nursing therefore is taught in accordance with this. Unless there is an ethnic community in the vicinity of a hospital, or there are members of staff from non-Western cultures, there is very little opportunity for staff to gain insight into the differing needs of people from religious and cultural backgrounds other than their own.

Contact with the health care services can be an anxious time for all, but for those individuals who have a different perspective of health care, and are unused to Western health perspectives, it may cause greater anxieties. For the nurse to be able to assess a patient's individual needs accurately and implement appropriate care, there is thus a need to acknowledge cultural and religious differences. Initial contact with the patient, either in the hospital or in the community, is the time at which the health care professional will identify some of the various cultural differences.

Name

Mr, Miss, Ms and Mrs are Western titles and may not be used by individuals from other cultures. Many documents in the UK continue to require an individual to place their Christian name before their surname. It would be inappropriate to ask a non-Christian for the same information; to ask the individual for their family name and first name would be more appropriate and eliminates any potential embarrassment. In addition, it is not unknown for a patient to have more than one set of clinical notes because the family name was not accurately ascertained on registration.

Language/communication

Any difficulty with communication will normally be obvious at the initial meeting with the individual. First-generation immigrants are likely to be the people who may present with difficulty in communication if their first language is not English. This is particularly so with Asian and Middle Eastern women.

It is as well to remember that when an individual has a second language, no matter how well they speak it, anxiety and stress can cause them to lose that language, albeit temporarily. It is not uncommon for an individual to be assessed initially as not being able to communicate in English, only for it to become apparent, when they have settled into their new environment and the stresses and anxieties have lessened, that they can speak English perfectly. It is common practice amongst health workers to use the second and third generation members of the family, often children or young adults, to act as interpreters, as they are often bilingual. This is a good idea when asking everyday questions, but should there be a need to ask intimate questions or communicate bad news, it would be more considerate to involve the skills of a third party, as family members or close friends are likely to avoid interpreting the truth and may tell the patient something else, rather than be the bearer of bad tidings. Therefore, using the skills of a suitable interpreter who understands medical terminology, and who is prepared to impart this information, will avoid the creation of unnecessary additional stress. It is also important to note that, in some cultures, only women may ask personal questions of women, and men of men. If this practice is not respected, the wrong information may be given to avoid embarrassment to both the interpreter and the patient.

Religion

For many people such as Sikhs, Muslims, Hindus, Buddhists, Christians and Jews, religion is a way of life and has a direct impact upon their activities of daily living. It is not necessary to understand fully the detailed facts of differing religions, but the health care worker needs to be aware that there are differences in order to prevent assumptions being made incorrectly. It is also vital that generalizations are avoided. There is a need to identify early on whether the patient will want his own religious representative present or to visit. Involving the family from the beginning will facilitate this requirement, as they will know how and when to contact the appropriate person.

Many Eastern religions require people to pray at certain times, fast on certain days and wear certain religious objects. Many of the religious objects or symbols worn can be mistaken for jewellery. If medical intervention or a nursing procedure is likely to compromise these religious requirements, inform the patient and his family as to the reason prior to any action. Many religious observances may be waived during illness; however, if there is any doubt in the individual's mind, he will become anxious. Whenever possible, the religious advisor/teacher should be consulted on these occasions so that permission for and explanation of such exemptions may be obtained.

Dietary considerations

Both Jews and Muslims are forbidden to eat pork or any pork products. Furthermore, Muslims may eat the meat of other animals only if they have been ritually slaughtered by the halal method. This does not, however, mean that *all* Jews will want kosher food (food prepared according to the Jewish ordinances to make it 'pure') and all Muslims halal meat (meat that has been ritually slaughtered according to Muslim law), but consultation with the patient will make his or her preferences clear.

If an individual is reluctant to eat, it is often assumed that the hospital food is unsuitable, although this may not always be so. However, many individuals, especially those from Eastern cultures are accustomed to eating their meals with their family. As this is a time when family matters are discussed, to be alone and away from the family environment may be the cause of loss of appetite. Where possible, therefore, invite the family to bring food, or to be present at meal times.

Personal hygiene

Washing in still water is considered unclean by many people, particularly Muslims, Sikhs and Hindus. As most hospitals have baths, and the advent of legionellosis has required the use of showers to be considered carefully, some patients would prefer to remain unwashed. If this is the case, then all that is needed is to supply the individual with a jug of water and a bowl for hand and face washing, or an empty jug with the bath or basin tap running for body washing. If the patient is more dependent, exceptions will be made.

The Muslim religion requires that the right hand be used for the eating and preparing of food and the left hand for other procedures, such as cleaning the perineum; thus, one often refers to either the 'clean' or 'dirty' hand. This has certain implications for the individual who has one hand incapacitated. In such circumstances, the individual will not be able to eat with his left hand, nor may he use the right hand for cleaning the perineum. This, therefore, has particularly serious implications for the individual with a colostomy, as a colostomy cannot be tended with one hand, although wearing disposable gloves for stoma care may be an acceptable alternative for some. There is thus a need for special preoperative counselling and discussion.

Modesty

Dignity and modesty are often compromised in the hospital setting and great sensitivity is called for. Many women, regardless of their cultural origins, will have never exposed their bodies to a stranger. A male doctor or other health care professional examining a woman, or vice versa, can thus cause great distress, particularly to women of certain cultures where modesty is highly valued, and for those in purdah. In mixed ward settings, therefore, women should be offered separate bays or rooms when available, and priority should always be given to those women in purdah. Hospital gowns, which are notoriously skimpy, are unacceptable to many individuals. Exposing an arm to accommodate an intravenous infusion, or fractured arm with a splint, may cause some individuals to remain in bed rather than to mobilize, as this may cause them to lose their dignity. Additional covering may solve this problem.

Skin and hair care

Caring for the hair and skin, as with other areas of care, needs to be assessed individually. People with naturally tight, curly hair, need to have their hair cared for in a different way to those with straight or wavy hair. 'Afro' hair, for example, can be dry and brittle and, if long, may tangle very easily. It may need to be moisturized or oiled at the scalp and combed frequently, sometimes with a wide-toothed comb, preferably in small sections at a time.

All people have skin that differs in colour and type and in order to provide satisfactory skin care the patient's skin type must be assessed individually. For example, if dry skin is neglected, lesions and cracks can soon develop, and it is therefore advisable to ask patients what they usually use to keep their skin moist. Some brown or black skin is prone to keloid scarring (hyperkeratinization), whereby the most simple of invasive treatments can cause excessive and pigmented scarring to appear. Thoughtful positioning of vaccinations, immunizations and, where possible, other surgical procedures, will reduce visible disfigurement should keloid scarring develop. Newborn babies and preschool children, particularly of Asian, southern European and African descent, often have areas of hyperpigmentation that resemble bruises. These are correctly referred to as 'Mongolian blue spots', and can range from 1 to 15 cm in diameter. The areas where these lesions are often seen are around the sacrum, on the buttocks and on the back of the hands and wrists. Although they tend to fade as the child grows, there have been instances when a family has been investigated for non-accidental injury to a child because of ignorance of such hyperpigmentation. Mongolian blue spots should be borne in mind, therefore, whenever a black or dark-skinned child is being investigated for child abuse as a false allegation may be made.

Hospital procedures

Careful thought should be given to all hospital routines and procedures for all patients as some may particularly create difficulties for people with other cultural backgrounds. Discussing elimination or other intimate health issues may be culturally offensive to some. As with all areas of nursing care, and with all patients, a sensitive approach is necessary to ensure privacy and the maintenance of self-respect.

Medications and treatments may be offensive or taboo for some religious groups. Blood transfusions for Jehovah's Witnesses, for example, are forbidden. Iron injections are usually derived from pigs and would therefore be unacceptable to many Muslims, Jews and vegetarians. Insulin, although now less of a problem because of the availability of Humulin, can offend Hindus, and possibly Sikhs, if it is bovine in origin, and Jews and Muslims if porcine. There are also many emollients derived from animals that may offend some people. Medications with an alcohol base may similarly be refused by those to whom alcohol is forbidden. Thus, nurses need to be aware of all preparations likely to contain potentially taboo or offensive elements.

Visiting hours

In some hospitals, visits continue to be limited to two persons per patient and have time restrictions. This may cause some distress to many patients. The extended family is evident within many cultural groups. Generally speaking, West Indian, Asian and Middle Eastern families like to visit as a family where possible. Such visits will include children and grandchildren, uncles and aunts, parents and grandparents. To allow a large family to visit one patient may distress other patients, and yet to restrict numbers of visitors will distress the patient himself. Coming to a compromise is all that can be done in circumstances in which visiting restrictions have to be imposed. Open visiting is more accommodating in these situations, and to allow the family to have a hand in the care of their relative is also beneficial to both family and patient.

Myths

There is still a belief that people of different races or parts of the world have different pain thresholds, but this is not so. It is the *expression* of pain that differs within cultures. For example, Japanese individuals may smile or laugh when experiencing pain, in order to not 'lose face'. Those of Anglo-Saxon origin sometimes tend to be stoical, withdraw socially, and express a 'stiff upper lip'. Some southern Europeans, for example Italians and Greeks, vocally express their pain far more freely. However, it is important to remember that every individual will have a different pain tolerance, regardless of culture or country of origin.

Death and bereavement

This will always be a difficult matter to deal with correctly if the patient and his family are not consulted and involved in care. Most people from Eastern cultures will wish to be involved in the care of the dying, and particularly the last offices. Death is perceived as a continuum of life for many and there are certain customs and practices which need to be followed; naturally it is very important that nurses fully acquaint themselves with the specific cultural requirements associated with death, bereavement, and the last offices. Nurses in the UK consider that last offices are the final act that they can perform for a patient, and rarely is this duty offered to relatives. This may be appropriate in the absence of a family, but families of different cultures will often want to be involved, and to deny them that right may cause them greater grief when trying to come to terms with their loss. The wishes of some families, however, may conflict with standard hospital procedures and need to be anticipated; negotiation may need to take place in order to minimize the stress and anxiety for the family, hospital staff and other patients in the ward. It might be that, if nurses were to offer all relatives and partners the option of assisting at the time of death, people would find it easier to come to terms with their loss sooner and it would assist them with their grieving process. However, if this approach is adopted there will also be a need for nurses to learn to 'let go'. The need for staff support here is essential, particularly when the patient has been in hospital for some time and a bond has developed between nurse and patient.

Caring for people from cultural and religious backgrounds other than one's own is rewarding. By adding newly found cultural knowledge to existing theory and practice, the nurse will be able to design the delivery of care appropriately, without assumptions or value judgements, at an individual and more holistic level.

Further Reading

Baxter C (1987) *Hair Care of African, Afro-Caribbean and Asia Hair Types*. National Extension College.

Baxter C (1988) *The Black Nurse: An Endangered Species*. National Extension College.

Fuller J & Toon P (1988) *Medical Practice in a Multiracial Society*. Heinemann.

Karseras P & Hopkins E (1987) *British Asians' Health in the Community*. Scutari Press.

Mares P, Henley A & Baxter C (1985) *Health Care in Multiracial Britain*. National Extension College.

Neuberger J (1987) *Caring for the Dying People of Different Faiths*. Austin Cornish (Lisa Sainsbury Foundation).

Sampson C (1982) *The Neglected Ethic: Religious and Cultural Factors in the Care of Patients*. McGraw-Hill.

APPENDIX 4

Nutrition

(Co-authored by Elizabeth Janes, Health Visitor Student, South Bank Polytechnic, London SE1 0AA)

The following section has been designed to provide useful information related to nutrition. Detailed dietary advice has been purposely omitted and readers are recommended to consult a dietitian if this is required.

Definitions
Nutrition is the combination of processes by which the body receives and uses food for growth, development and maintenance. Nutrients are substances that nourish the body. The six classes of nutrients are: fats, carbohydrates, proteins, minerals, vitamins and water.
Nutritional status is the condition of the body as a result of its receiving and using nutrients.
Dietetics is the science of applying the principles of nutrition to the feeding of individuals or groups.

A healthier diet: Recent publications

The NACINE Report (1983)
A discussion paper drawn up by the National Advisory Committee on Nutrition Education (NACINE), under the chairmanship of Professor WPT James, entitled *Proposals for Nutritional Guidelines for Health Education in Britain*. Based on a number of major official, academic and international reports on nutrition, this report sets out short and long-term goals for dietary change. It is hoped that the short-term changes will be adopted by the end of the 1980s and the long-term goals by the year 2000.

The COMA Report (1984)
'*Diet and Cardiovascular Disease*', a report proposed by the Committee on Medical Aspects of Food Policy (COMA) which concentrates on aspects of the diet related to cardiovascular disease. Its main recommendations concern dietary fat.

The JACNE Report (1985)
'*Eating for a Healthier Heart*' based on the COMA report (above) was produced under the auspices of the British Nutrition Foundation and Health Education Council. It is a brief practical guide to altering our

fat consumption, particularly saturated fat, which is thought to be strongly related to the high incidence of heart disease.

British Diabetic Association recommendations for diabetics (1982)

1. *Energy intake.* This should be based on individual need with suitable adjustments for the overweight.
2. *Increased intake of fibre-rich (slowly absorbed) carbohydrate.* At least 50% of the dietary energy should be obtained from fibre-rich foods, e.g. wholemeal bread, wholegrain cereal, pulses and potatoes. Rapidly absorbed carbohydrates, e.g. sugar, sweets, sweetened drinks and fibre-free starch, should only be taken in small quantities or exchanges as part of a fibre-rich meal or in special circumstances, i.e. illness, hypoglycaemic emergency, in conjunction with strenuous exercise.
3. *Decreased fat intake.* Ideally fat intake should be reduced to 35% of total energy intake, primarily by reducing fat-rich meat and dairy products.
4. *Balance between carbohydrate intake and medication.* Regularly spaced meals are important for all diabetics, especially those requiring insulin or oral hypoglycaemic agents. Carbohydrate portions or exchanges remain the simplest way of distributing the daily carbohydrate intake.
5. *Weight reduction.* Effective weight loss is the most important dietary goal for the overweight, non-insulin-dependent diabetic. A low fat, fibre-rich diet is recommended.
6. *Salt.* Diabetics should not consume more sodium than the non-diabetic.
7. *Alcohol.* Unless medically contraindicated, diabetics may consume alcohol so long as its energy contribution to the diet is noted.
8. *Sorbitol, fructose and products containing them.* These foods should be regarded with caution. Guidance should be sought if a diabetic wishes to include them in the diet.
9. *Diet prescription.* This must be based on individualized eating habits. Insulin should ideally be prescribed to fit in with existing eating habits rather than vice versa. Professional dietetic advice is essential.

Dietary fibre

This is a class of carbohydrate defined as non-starch polysaccharides (NSP) which are composed of a number of constituents, the physiological significance of which is not always clear. Dietary fibre is difficult to measure, especially in starch-rich foods such as potatoes and cereals. Several different methods of analysis are available and give different results. A number of collaborative trials are currently in progress to establish the most accurate method for reference purposes. It is probable that the Englyst technique will be chosen for the standard (see Further Reading).

Table 1. Practical suggestions for healthy eating.

Ways to increase fibre intake

Eat more: Wholemeal bread
and cakes and
biscuits

Wholemeal flour (in
cooking)

Brown rice

Wholemeal pasta

High fibre cereal,
e.g. muesli,
porridge, bran

Pulses, fruit,
vegetables

Dried fruit and nuts

Ways to reduce fat intake

Eat more:	Eat less:
Low fat spread	Butter, oil, lard, margarine
Cottage and curd cheese	Hard cheese
Skimmed or semi-skimmed milk	Full cream milk, cream
Low fat yoghurt	Red meat
Low fat meat, e.g. chicken	Fatty meat, e.g. pork, sausages, bacon
Fish	Fried foods
Pulses	Pastries
Fruit, vegetables	Rich puddings
Cereal products	

Ways to cut down on sugar

Eat more:	Eat less:
Unsweetened breakfast cereals	Sugar, honey, jam
Sugar-free squash and fruit juice	Cakes, biscuits
Unsweetened fruit, e.g. canned in natural juice or fresh	Sweet puddings
	Sweetened breakfast cereals
	Tinned fruit (in syrup)
	Sweetened squash/carbonated drinks
	Sweet alcohol, e.g. sweet sherry, etc.

Table 2. A guide to the contribution of common foods to the diet.

High fat

Fat and oils	(lard, butter, margarine, oil, dripping)
Dairy foods	(cream, evaporated milk, whole milk, hard cheese, full cream yoghurt, egg yolk)
Meat	(especially mince, sausages and offal)
Nuts	(including peanut butter)
Fish	(oily fish, e.g. sardines, mackerel)

Pastry, cakes and biscuits made with fat, chocolate, cocoa, fudge, toffee, avocado pears

High sugar

Sugar, jam, honey, marmalade, treacle, syrup, molasses
Fruit cordials, squash, chocolate, sweets
Cakes, biscuits, sweet pastry
Dried fruit, tinned fruit in syrup
Sweet wine, sherry
Sweetened breakfast cereals, e.g. sugar-coated

High fibre

Wholegrain cereal and wholemeal flour products
Dried fruit, nuts
Fresh fruit and vegetables
Pulses, e.g. baked beans, butter beans, chick peas, lentils

High protein

Meat, fish, cheese, eggs
Pulses, nuts
Milk, milk powder

High potassium

Fruit and vegetables
Digestive biscuits
Fruit juice, tomato juice, salad cream
Brown sugar
Dried fruit
Wholemeal bread
Bovril, Marmite, Oxo
Nuts, crisps, Twiglets
All alcohol (except spirits)
Salt substitutes, e.g. Selora, Ruthmol

Strong coffee, Horlicks, Ovaltine, malted milk drinks
Chocolate, cocoa, cocoa products
Wholemeal flour
Liquorice, fruit gums

High sodium
Table salt and sea salt
Bacon, ham, tongue, sausages
Cheese
Tinned vegetables
Tinned or packet soups
Meat and yeast extracts, e.g. Bovril, Marmite, stock cubes
Tinned meat and tinned fish
Smoked fish
Potato crisps, etc.
Tinned vegetable juice
Pickles, chutney, bottled sauce

Enteral nutrition

Enteral nutrition is the provision of nutrition via the gastrointestinal tract. It includes nutrition taken orally or administered via a tube. The term is usually only applied to the feeding of patients who are unable or unwilling to feed themselves and/or who require additional or total nutritional support.

Tube feeding involves the administration of a fluid diet via a fine plastic tube. Several routes may be used to reach the gut, e.g. nasogastric, nasoduodenal, oesophagostomy, gastrostomy or jejunostomy. Specialized plastic tubes have now been developed for each of these sites and the relative merits of each should be carefully considered in relation to the patient's needs.

Home-made feeds are rarely used nowadays as they are easily contaminated during preparation, can block tubes with particulate matter and may not be nutritionally complete. Manufactured feeds are available in a great variety and can be selected to meet individual patient requirements.

Complications of tube feeding

1. *Gastrointestinal complications*: nausea, diarrhoea, abdominal distension and discomfort. Diarrhoea can be avoided by: (1) gradual introduction of feeds, especially in malnourished patients or those whose gut has been rested; (2) use of low lactose feeds, especially

Table 3. Non-starch polysaccharide (fibre) content of some foods analysed using the Englyst method.

Foods	g/100 g fresh weight
Cereals (good sources)	
Wheat bran	41.9
Allbran	22.9
Weetabix	9.8
Shredded Wheat	9.8
Oats	6.6
Wholemeal bread	5.8
Brown bread	4.3
Wholewheat spaghetti (cooked value)	3.0
Vegetables	
Dried peas (cooked value)	5.6
Dried haricot beans (cooked value)	5.0
Cabbage	3.3
Lunnen beans	3.1
Brussels sprouts	1.8
Tomatoes	1.1
Hazel-nuts	2.8
Potatoes	1.0*
Poor sources	
Brown rice (cooked value)	1.7
White bread	1.6*
Cornflakes	0.6
Rice Krispies	0.6
White rice (cooked value)	0.5
Sago	0.5
Cornflour	0.1
Tapioca	0.4
Arrowroot	0.1

* On cooking or storing, resistant starch is formed. This remains undigested and a significant quantity therefore enters the large bowel and will increase faecal weight by acting as an energy source for bacterial growth.
Source: Manual of Dietetic Practice (ed. Briony Thomas). Blackwell Scientific Publications (1988).

Table 4. Patient monitoring during enteral feeding.

Parameter	Frequency
Body weight	Daily, twice weekly or weekly (according to nursing time)
Urinalysis	4–6 hourly
Blood glucose	4–6 hourly if glycosuria is present
24-h urine for urinary urea	Twice weekly (daily if required for nitrogen balance studies)
Full serum profile and electrolytes	Twice weekly
Accurate fluid balance	Daily

in Asian, African and Mediterranean patients; (3) care in avoiding contamination of the feed; (4) continuous drip feeding rather than bolus feeding; and (5) use of sterile proprietary feed. Antibiotic therapy is a common cause of diarrhoea in tube fed patients. It should be treated with an antidiarrhoeal agent in preference to stopping the feed.

2. *Nasal necrosis and oesophageal erosions/strictures.* These are more often associated with the long-term use of wide bore tubes, e.g. Ryles tubes. Soft, fine bore tubes should always be used in preference for feeding purposes.

3. *Metabolic complications*: hyperglycaemia, electrolyte abnormalities, dehydration (especially if diarrhoea is present).

Parenteral feeding
Total parenteral nutrition (TPN) is the aseptic delivery of nutritional substitutes directly into the circulatory system.

This route may be necessary when:

1. The gastrointestinal tract is inaccessible e.g. oesophageal stricture.
2. Complete rest of the gastrointestinal tract is indicated, e.g. gastrointestinal fistula and exacerbation of inflammatory bowel disease.
3. The gastrointestinal tract is not working, e.g. postoperative ileus, malabsorption, short bowel syndrome.
4. The patient's requirements are greatly increased and cannot be met by enteral feeding, e.g. premature infants, severely burned patients.

There are several aspects of management:

1. Establishing and maintaining access.
2. Method of administration.
3. Selection of the type and quality of feeding solutions.
4. Observation, monitoring and assessment.

Table 5 summarizes the main points under these areas. The reader is referred to specialized texts for details of this method of feeding (see Further Reading).

Parenteral feeding lines are at great risk of contamination and therefore any procedures involving them should be kept to a minimum and be carried out by a small number of specially trained nurses. This practice has been found to significantly reduce the infection rate in parenteral feeding lines.

Miscellaneous diets

Bristol diet
An unorthodox diet restricting fat, sugar, salt and animal protein. Based on fresh raw foods. Sometimes used in the treatment of cancer. It remains controversial.

Cambridge diet
A proprietary, very low calorie diet designed for weight loss. Should only be used under medical supervision.

Oxford diet
A high-fibre diet for diabetic patients that has been used to achieve good diabetic control.

Gunsen diet
An anticancer diet involving an intensive detoxification programme followed by an intensive nutrition programme that floods the body with easily assimilated nutrients needed for improving metabolism and healing. The therapy includes high potassium, low sodium foods, no fats or oils, minimal animal protein, large amounts of raw fruit and vegetable juices, and raw liver.

Macrobiotic diet
A philosophy for a healthy way of life and dietary reform rediscovered by Georges Obswana, it is based on the Chinese principles of yin (centrifugal) and yan (centripetal) force. Foods are classified as yin and yan and consumption of these should be balanced for good health.

Table 5. Management of parenteral feeding.

Aspect	Main points
1. Access	Feeding solutions are hyperosmolar and damaging to veins. Solutions should be administered into a central vein, e.g. via the subclavian. Strict asepsis is essential. Peripheral access may be used in certain circumstances
2. Administration	Strict flow control essential using electromechanical devices, e.g. peristaltic purges, flow controllers, volumetric pumps (preferable because drop size of parenteral nutrition solutions varies with composition)
	Feed may be given using:
	(a) A sequential, single bottle regimen
	(b) A multiple bottle regimen using a Y or W connector
	(c) A 2–3 litre bag
3. Feeding solutions	Combinations of the following are used in order to meet patient requirements. They must be given strictly according to a doctor's prescription.
	10%, 20%, 50% glucose
	10%, 20% lipid solutions
	Amino acid solutions
	Electrolytes and water
	Water soluble vitamins
	Fat soluble vitamins
	Trace elements, e.g. zinc
	A range of commercial products is available. Strict asepsis is required for preparation of 2–3 litre bags or when making additions to proprietary feeds. This should be carried out under laminar flow conditions

4. Monitoring	Suggested initial frequency
Urinalysis for glycosuria	6-hourly
Serum glucose	As required
Serum urea and electrolytes	Daily
Serum magnesium	Weekly
Liver function tests	Weekly
Temperature, pulse, respiration	4-hourly
Weight	Daily
Strict fluid balance	Daily

Cultural differences in diet

Food habits vary according to race, religion and culture. It is important to try and accommodate these individual preferences when a patient is in hospital. The following points may be useful guidelines, although an effort should be made to discover personal preferences where possible.

Jews

Orthodox Jews eat a kosher diet (kosher = clear or pure). This refers to the method of food preparation, including animal slaughter. The following are normally avoided:

1. Flesh from animals with cloven feet (e.g. pigs, deer).
2. Shellfish (e.g. crabs, oysters) and fish without fins and scales (e.g. eels).
3. The consumption of milk and meat products at the same meal.
4. Strict orthodox Jews may avoid ordinary cheese, which is prepared from rennet obtained from the stomach of animals.

Roman Catholics

Meat may be avoided on Fridays, although this is no longer subject to papal decree.

Seventh-Day Adventists

Members of this group are usually ovolactovegetarians. Intake of iron and calcium is potentially unsatisfactory unless the diet is well balanced.

Muslims
Pork is usually avoided by most Muslims as it is considered unclean and thus taboo. Traditionally eaten foods include rice and mutton (which is the preferred meat). Many Muslims prefer only to eat meat that has been ritually slaughtered by the halal method. The evening meal is often light and consists of white cheese, olives and bread. Some Muslims use their 'clean hand' to eat in preference to cutlery, as their religion requires that the right hand be used for the eating and preparation of food, whereas the left hand is used for other, unclean procedures, such as cleaning the perineum. Scrupulous washing is normally performed before meals.

Hindus
The cow is usually regarded as a sacred animal. Some Hindus may eat fish, eggs and milk, while others restrict themselves to milk as their only source of animal protein.

Vegans
A vegan eats no animal foods or any product of an animal. Therefore, whereas vegetarians will eat dairy produce, vegans will not. A very carefully balanced and varied diet is required in order to avoid nutrient deficiency, especially in children.

Manufacturers of dietetic products
Abbott Laboratories Ltd, Queensborough, Kent ME11 5EL

Bayer UK Ltd, Bayer House, Strawberry Hill, Newbury, Berkshire RG13 1JA

Beecham Products, Beecham House, Great West Road, Brentford, Middlesex TW8 9BD

Boots Co. Plc, 1 Thane Road West, Nottingham NG2 3AA

Bristol-Myers Pharmaceuticals, Swakeley House, Milton Road, Ickenham, Uxbridge, Middlesex UB10 8NS

Britannia Pharmaceuticals Ltd, Forum House, 41–75 Brighton Road, Redhill, Surrey RH1 6YS

E. Brown (Medical) Ltd, Evett Close, Stocklake, Aylesbury, Buckinghamshire HP20 1DN

Carnation Foods Co. Ltd, Danesford House, Medmenham, Marlow, Buckinghamshire SL7 2ES

Cow & Gate Ltd, Cow & Gate House, Trowbridge, Wiltshire BA14 8YX

Farley Health Products Ltd, Torr Lane, Plymouth PL3 5UA

Fresenius Ltd, 6/7 Christleton Court, Stuart Road, Manor Park, Runcorn, Cheshire

Kabi-Vitrium Ltd, Kabi-Vitrium House, Riverside Way, Uxbridge, Middlesex UB8 2YF

E. Merck Ltd, Winchester Road, Four Marks, Alton, Hampshire GU34 5HG

Nestlé Co. Ltd, Health Care Division, St George's House, Croydon, Surrey CR9 1NR

Norwich Eaton Ltd, Hedley House, St Nicholas Avenue, Gosforth, Newcastle-upon-Tyne NE99 1EE

Rourch Labs Ltd, Rourch House, North End Road, Wembley Park, Middlesex HA9 0NF

Scientific Hospital Supplies Ltd, 38 Queensland Street, Liverpool L7 3JG

Further Reading

Cannon G & Einzig H (1984) *Dieting Makes You Fat*. Sphere.

Davidson S, Passmore R, Brock JF & Trusswell AS (1979) *Human Nutrition and Dietetics*. Churchill Livingstone.

Dickerson JWT & Lee HA (1978) *Nutrition in the Clinical Management of Disease*. Edward Arnold.

Englyst HN & Cummings JH (1984) Simplified method for the measurement of total NSP by GLC. *Analyst* **109**: 937–942.

Englyst H, Wiggins HS & Cummings JH (1982) Determination of NSP in plant foods by GLC of constituent sugars as alditol acetates. *Analyst* **107**: 307–318.

Englyst HN, Anderson V & Cummings JH (1983) Starch and NSP in some cereal foods. *Journal of the Science of Food and Agriculture* **34**: 1434–1440.

Francis D (1986) *Nutrition for Children*. Blackwell Scientific.

Green ML & Harr J (1981) *Nutrition in Contemporary Nursing Practice*. John Wiley & Sons.

Huskisson J (1985) *Applied Nutrition and Dietetics*, 2nd edn (Current Nursing Practice Series). Baillière Tindall.

McLaren DS & Burnson D (1982) *Textbook of Paediatric Nutrition*. Churchill Livingstone.

Moghissi K & Boone J (1983) *Parenteral and Enteral Nutrition for Nurses*. Heinemann.

Paul AA & Southgate DAT (1978) *McCane and Widdowson, The Composition of Food*. HMSO.

Thomas B (1988) *Manual of Dietetic Practice*. Blackwell Scientific.

Walker C & Cannon C (1984) *The Food Scandal*. Century.

APPENDIX 5

Innovative Therapies

During the twentieth century there have been enormous technical and pharmaceutical developments which have changed the face of health care. Transplantation of vital organs has become a reality; prebirth detection of many congenital and inherited abnormalities is possible and means that defects can be treated before birth. The work of scientists in the development of new drugs ensures the cure of many conditions and improved longevity for others. There are, however, many people for whom cure is not possible, or who are left with long-term residual defects as a result of treatment. For these, there is often a poor quality of life or shortened life expectancy. Increasingly this latter group seeks interventions which will enable them to cope with the manifestations of illness or treatment, and allow them to function at an optimum level. These interventions are variously described as alternative, complementary or supportive, and in this section are referred to as innovative therapies.

Alongside the developments in health care technology we have seen a greater awareness and knowledge of health care by the consumer. The burgeoning of all forms of communication media has ensured greater access to information for the general public, and in recent years much of this has been about many aspects of health care. These improved communications have exposed the public to methods of health care and health promotion which were, and often still are, viewed with great suspicion, and dismissed as quackery, dangerous, fad medicine, or mumbo-jumbo, and yet there are an increasing number of people who embrace these various therapies and incorporate them into their daily lives, and an equally large number of nurses and other health care providers who are undertaking further education in order to learn the various skills required to help patients. This development may be due to demands made by patients who wish to continue therapies they were undergoing before coming into hospital.

One of the main objections of health care providers to innovative therapies is the lack of scientific research to support the claims made about them. With the increase of the number of innovative practitioners, and the incorporation of many therapies into the patient's plan of care, this research is now beginning to be undertaken.

It is important to distinguish between invasive and non-invasive innovative therapies, and it is not within the scope of this text to discuss the burgeoning pharmacopeia of complementary drug therapies, or the innovative interventions viewed as invasive procedures. This section will deal with those therapies used to improve quality of life and which can be incorporated into treatments and practices by appropriately qualified nurses. It is, of course, not possible to describe all therapies in current use; the intention is to stimulate further investigation into the subject.

Aromatherapy

Aromatherapy is an ancient therapeutic art used throughout history in the medical practices of the great civilizations of the world. It aims to enhance feelings of well-being, reduce stress, and assist in the rejuvenation and regeneration of the human body by using different massage techniques to relieve specific symptoms.

Vital to the art of aromatherapy are the essential oils. These oils are obtained from a wide range of plants, trees, herbs, flowers and fruit, each with its own unique properties and aroma; they are used for a variety of purposes, including the relief of stress or nervous-related disorders, some stimulate and rejuvenate whilst others aid circulation. The essential oils are combined with a base oil and are then massaged into the skin, where they are absorbed into the bloodstream and distributed throughout the body. In order for this to be beneficial, the therapist needs extensive knowledge of blood and lymph pressure flow, stress and release points and relaxation points.

Therapeutic massage

Therapeutic massage can have many physical and psychological benefits for patients, including alleviation of anxiety and mind/body tension, and a re-harmonizing of the 'whole' person. Following therapeutic massage, patients often notice a reduction of pain or the absence of previous pain for a short time. It has also been seen to be valuable in improving sleep patterns, increasing appetite and renewing feelings of general well-being. It can also help reduce feelings of nausea, relieve muscle stiffness and tension following surgery, and assist the circulation and sensation in paralysed or semi-mobile limbs. Therapeutic massage can be of particular benefit to those experiencing depressive feelings who have difficulty talking about their feelings.

The technique of therapeutic massage involves gentle stroking and kneading movements combined with acupressure using essential oils (pure extracts of plants and herbs), and the use of a relaxation tape to enhance the effects of the massage.

Relaxation and visualization

Most people at some point in their lives are exposed to stress and anxiety which may arise for a variety of reasons: problems at work, unemployment, financial problems, personal crises or emotional upsets. Stress may present in a variety of symptomatic manifestations which disappear on resolution of the problem causing the stress, or they may be masked by the administration of anxiolytic agents. There has been much evidence in recent years of the dangers of resorting to drugs, many of which can be addictive, in the long-term management of stress and anxiety. Illness is a particularly stressful time for many people. Concerns about diagnosis, treatment and outcomes can cause intense anxiety for the individual and family; it may be alleviated by an optimistic prognosis or may go unnoticed or misdiagnosed as an illness-related symptom.

Relaxation exercises, often combined with visualization, have become used increasingly in the management of stress and anxiety in recent years, particularly for people with chronic stress problems, and chronic or life-threatening conditions. There are different schools of relaxation techniques, using different approaches to achieve the same end. Common to all is that the exercises take place in a quiet, comfortable ambience. One example of a relaxation exercise is that during which the individual sits or lies in a comfortable position with eyes closed and is asked to imagine a beautiful scene which gives him pleasure; soothing music may or may not be used. He is gradually asked to notice his breathing and to control its rate and depth. Once this has been achieved, various sets of muscles are alternately relaxed and tensed until all muscles have been exercised. Following the exercises, the individual rests for a short time, or may even take a nap, before continuing with his normal activities.

Relaxation is sometimes combined with imagery in helping people with stress, or symptoms associated with long-term illness or the sequelae of its treatment. Imagery is based on the assumption that mind and emotions can stimulate the body's systems to combat symptoms or the disease itself. During the imagery phase the patient imagines his illness or symptoms and the treatments being used to combat them, and visualizes the interaction of the two, i.e. he imagines the chemotherapy attacking the cancer cells, or the anti-inflammatory drugs attacking the rheumatic joints. There is increasing evidence that under the guidance of a qualified practitioner, imagery can be beneficial to some patients.

Relaxation and visualization can also be valuable in counteracting the effects of certain treatments, particularly those which cause nausea, headache, muscle tension and pain. Often the relaxation exercises are combined with an audio-tape of sounds which are pleasing to the individual; this may be one or several pieces of music, the sounds of the voices of friends or loved ones, or the sounds of nature (for example, jungle noises or waves lapping the sea shore). The aim is for the relaxation exercises and sounds to increase feelings of well-being by evoking pleasant former memories and diverting the attention from the symptoms of the treatment.

Reflexology

Reflexology is the technique of deep massage of the soles of the feet, and occasionally the palms of the hands, to relieve somatic symptoms. It has been practised for thousands of years and works on a similar basis to acupuncture, without using needles. Most areas of the body have reflex zones on the foot, and by feeling the foot the qualified reflexologist can diagnose disorders of various organs of the body. After diagnosis the somatic disturbance is treated by deep massage of the appropriate area of the feet. It is said that functional disorders such as migraine, sinusitis, stress, headaches, constipation and bladder disorders respond well to reflexology.

Hypnotherapy

Hypnosis is a state of profound relaxation during which the individual is susceptible to suggestion. Hypnotherapy carried out by a qualified and experienced therapist can produce anaesthesia, elevate the pain threshold and improve mental attitude.

Hypnotherapy can be carried out individually or in groups. The therapist first ensures a state of relaxation and then, with direct or indirect suggestion, deals with the problem troubling the patient. It is possible for an experienced therapist to provide pain relief equal to that given by pharmacological preparations, or even displace pain to a less troublesome area. Mood elevation can be achieved by suggestions which return the individual to happier times in their lives, helping them to relive pleasant experiences.

Individuals can be taught self-hypnosis to manage future pain and stress.

Further Reading

Kaptchuk T & Croucher M (1986) *The Healing Arts*. BBC.
Shone R (1984) *Creative Visualisation*. Thorsons.
Stanway A (1986) *Alternative Medicines*. Penguin.
Tisserand R (1988) *The Art of Aromatherapy*. CW Daniel.

APPENDIX 6

Human Immunodeficiency Virus (HIV) and the Acquired Immune Deficiency Syndrome (AIDS)

Historical perspective

In 1981, in the United States of America, large numbers of young men in New York and California began to succumb to illnesses which had previously responded to treatment, or had only been seen in people suffering gross impairment of the immune system. At first, these deaths were regarded as isolated incidents but, as the numbers increased, there came the realization that health care faced a tremendous challenge.

Those affected early in the epidemic presented a number of correlating factors: the patients were either young homosexual men, male or female intravenous drug abusers, recipients of blood or blood products (such as coagulating agents), or refugees from Haiti living in the United States. At about the same time there was also evidence of a similar epidemic emerging in sub-Saharan Africa.

As now, the majority of those affected in the earliest days of the epidemic in the West were young homosexual/bisexual men, and the early investigations into the cause concentrated on the sexual and social behaviour of this group. It was believed that perhaps the presence of certain infectious agents in semen, such as cytomegalovirus or Epstein–Barr virus, were transmitted during sexual intercourse through lesions in the anal mucosa. It was also thought that the use during sexual intercourse of stimulants, such as butyl or amyl nitrate, might have affected the immune system. Early investigators named the condition Gay Related Immune Deficiency Syndrome or GRIDS.

The virus

In 1982 and 1983, Dr Luc Montagnier and Dr Robert Gallo, working independently of each other in Paris and Washington, discovered the causative organisms of what by now had become known as acquired immune deficiency syndrome (AIDS): human immunodeficiency virus I and human immunodeficiency virus II (HIV I and HIV II). These discoveries enabled us to understand better the progression of the condition and the likely routes of transmission. From this original work scientists have been able to develop tests which can detect antibodies to the virus in an infected person's blood, and thus increase the ability to monitor the spread of the virus.

AIDS describes the spectrum of diseases caused by HIV infection. The virus causes an impairment of the body's cellular immune system which may result in infection by organisms of no or low pathogenicity for those in good health (opportunistic infections), pulmonary *Pneumocystis carinii* pneumonia (PCP), or the development of unusual tumours, principally Kaposi's sarcoma (KS). In addition, there are many other organisms found in people with AIDS which can result in localized or disseminated manifestations affecting all areas of the body.

Manifestation of HIV infection

Infection with HIV occurs after virus in the blood, semen, vaginal secretions or breast milk of a carrier gains entry to a particular form of host lymphocyte, the helper T lymphocyte. After a variable period, antibodies to the virus appear in the blood. This seroconversion may coincide with a transient glandular fever-like illness. These antibodies do not seem to be protective as the virus continues to be found in the helper T lymphocytes, where its continued replication destroys these cells and causes disordered immune function. At present it appears that many HIV-infected individuals remain asymptomatic, although they have the potential to infect others by the previously described routes. Some of the remainder may be asymptomatic but develop persistent generalized lymphadenopathy (PGL). Others, in addition to having enlarged lymph nodes, develop symptoms such as night sweats, diarrhoea, weight loss and malaise, a condition known as AIDS-related complex (ARC). Examination of the blood may show abnormally low platelet and neutrophil counts in addition to low lymphocyte counts.

Only individuals with an opportunistic infection or unusual tumour can be diagnosed as having AIDS. At present the majority of those known to be infected with HIV are asymptomatic for these conditions; this demonstrates the error of calling the HIV antibody test the 'AIDS test'.

A more recently recognized phenomenon is the effect of HIV on the nervous system. The early manifestations include personality changes and memory disturbances, whilst in the late stages there may be fits, AIDS encephalopathy (dementia) and painful peripheral neuropathy. It must be realized that, as control of HIV depends to a great extent on behavioural modifications, the onset of dementia carries with it serious implications.

There are several important things to remember about infection with HIV. Not everyone who is infected will produce detectable antibodies and, although infected and infectious, will be negative on testing. Similarly, there may be a decrease in detectable antibodies in people with advanced manifestations of AIDS. For those who do progress to AIDS-related illness, there may be a time lag from infection with HIV to discernible illness, varying from a few weeks to 5 years or more. Because of this extraordinarily long incubation period, all those who wish to be tested for antibodies to the virus should first be exposed to in-depth counselling, by experienced counsellors, about the implications which may result from a positive test. The reactions of society to this condition has, on very many occasions, been alarming and those known to be infected with HIV have sometimes been rejected by society, with consequent loss of employment, housing and insurance.

Caring for a person with AIDS

There are at present few biomedical therapies to help combat the manifestations of AIDS, and therefore the challenges to nursing are those of excellence: excellent education, excellent managerial leadership and excellent nursing skills. If nursing is to respond well to the challenges presented by AIDS, it must address the issues of continuing education of all nurses on the subject, meaningful and sensitive managerial support, and the delivery of appropriate and meaningful care, whilst the recognition of the role of the nurse as an educator in further preventing the spread of HIV must be provided for, as required by the UKCC *Code of Professional Conduct for the Nurse, Midwife and Health Visitor*. It is essential that education for all health care providers, especially nurses, is mandatory and not optional. Nurses with a sound knowledge base can do much to ameliorate the sometimes devastating manifestations of this condition by working alongside the person with AIDS and those closest to him.

The onset of AIDS, and the potential for transmission from body fluid to body fluid, serves to remind us of the need to ensure a high level of clinical practice which will significantly reduce the risk of infection of health care providers by any pathogenic organism. This can be achieved without implementing outrageous infection control procedures in the delivery of care. Nurses must be aware of the fact that all body fluids are potentially hazardous and must therefore be treated accordingly. Sound and safe practice in the handling of sharp devices will minimize risks of needle-stick injuries, etc.

Careful assessment of the needs of each individual should determine the care setting. Some, especially those who are bleeding, producing copious sputum, suffering chronic diarrhoea, or who have low blood counts exposing them to possible infections, will benefit from the use of a single room. Those who do not fit this category may, unless they request otherwise, be cared for in the normal ward setting. Nurses who, for whatever reason, are themselves immune compromised should not care for other immune compromised people; this applies equally to nurses who have exposed eczema lesions which might become contaminated with body fluids. Similarly, nurses with lesions on the hand or any other part of the body which could be contaminated should ensure that such abrasions are properly covered as part of general good practice before nursing any patient.

At present, the majority of people with AIDS presenting for care (homosexual/bisexual men and intravenous drug abusers) follow life-styles of which nurses have little or no knowledge. In order to meet the challenges of this situation, nurses must not be judgemental of their patients' life-styles or their health deficits. To be so would be very likely to lead to rejection of the nurse by the patient, resulting in failure to deliver effective care. It is important to remember that, even now, the majority of people with AIDS became infected with the virus before we were aware of its existence.

Growing numbers of children are also being infected, either as a result of the mother being HIV antibody positive, or as a result of treatment with infected blood products (i.e. haemophiliacs) or blood transfusions. The paediatric presentation is different to that of adults, just as children themselves are different, but the challenge is to provide a high level of care to the individual child and his family situation.

The real challenge of care in the clinical setting is to leave control with the patient, to participate in those clinical regimens which it is hoped will make him well again, and give him knowledge so that he can care for himself. This can be interpreted as knowing when to lead, when to follow, and when to be at the side. In order to do this effectively the development of an appropriate care model is essential. Often, for people with AIDS, 'getting better' is not feasible; therefore, nurses must concentrate on the patient feeling better and feeling in control, as far as he is able, and using those interventions and skills which will enhance this.

Often when people with AIDS come into hospital for the first time they have already amassed a great deal of knowledge about their condition and its likely outcome. They may have the experience of having many friends who have been similarly affected, some of whom have died, and they may have preconceptions of health care providers based on the experiences of their friends. Knowledgeable patients make many more demands on the nurse than those with little knowledge. They are often seeking partnership rather than paternalism, and may expect, or even demand, a measure of control over decisions affecting their care. An acceptance of this partnership can be a good learning experience for both carer and cared for. This condition has resulted in many people with AIDS resorting to other potential remedies, either to keep them well or treat symptoms; many of these substances are homeopathic in origin, some are recently developed but not available on drug tariffs. Nurses will need knowledge of these preparations, their modes of action, side-effects, and hoped-for outcomes. Obviously patients place great hope in these therapies and will expect to be supported in their choices. They may also have become involved in and be benefiting from other supportive, but non-traditional, interventions, the 'complementary therapies' such as relaxation/visualization, reflexology, aromatherapy, therapeutic massage, hypnotherapy and shiatsu.

These interventions, used to improve quality of life, are often extremely important to the patient who will want them recognized as such and continued in hospital or at home. Nurses will be expected to ensure continued access to these services and could learn new skills from such practitioners.

Caring for someone with AIDS frequently involves caring for many people: the partner, family and friends. All of them will have unique experiences of what this condition has meant to them and how it has affected them; the partner may also be infected with HIV; knowledge of the illness may have exposed previously unknown life-styles or habits to family members, causing stress, conflict and division. The nurse is in a unique position to help keep people together or to reunite them to face the stressful times which might lie ahead.

Advocacy

In addition to delivering high standards of physical and psychological support, the nurse may need to act as advocate for the person with AIDS. No condition in recent times has received as much publicity as that apportioned to people with AIDS. Much of it, particularly in the general media, has been demeaning and derogatory to people unable to defend themselves. The sometimes sensational coverage of the condition has had a deleterious effect on efforts to educate the general public on what it means to have AIDS. The ethic of caring involves advocacy, which means ensuring that the needs, rights and humanity of patients are not usurped. Therefore nurses have a responsibility to ensure that those they care for are dealt with fairly by other professionals by protecting patients' rights, and by non-professionals by ensuring confidentiality of patient information.

Prevention

Nursing forms the basis of health care and as such not only has a significant impact on the quality of care received by people with AIDS, it also impacts, through preventative education, on the extent of the HIV epidemic itself. Nurses are in a unique position to reduce transmission of HIV through health promotion. In some parts of the world, especially amongst homosexual communities, there has been a dramatic response to the health education message, often initiated by the community itself and resulting in fast and effective changes in behaviour in populations at risk of infection. In these same places, but amongst other groups, there has not been this response and the numbers of people infected with HIV increases inexorably.

In order to perform as health promoters, nurses must first understand the illness, and next understand that AIDS has a potential to be a problem for everyone in society. Therefore, educational strategies on safer sexual practices and harm-reduction behaviour must be devised for all sections of society, including drug users. In educating the public about AIDS, there is a need to develop the trust of those who must be reached. Education must be targeted carefully; thus, it is essential to be aware of who needs to be reached and why. Influencing the behaviour of young people is a high priority. Coming to sexual awareness is often a very difficult time, contradictory messages cause confusion and can be dangerous; if these effects are to be prevented, empathy and sensitivity will be vital in addressing the values of trust, love, respect and concern for others in human relationships.

The future
The exact number of people in the world currently infected with HIV is not known; it affects many millions, of whom a large proportion will progress to symptomatic disease and die. The lack of resources in some countries, and the conflict of opinion between health care and the media in others, may mean that even more millions will be touched by this virus before it is contained. All these people will be dependent on the realism and humanity of nursing to help them in their personal battle with HIV and AIDS.

Further Reading
In order to cope effectively with the wide physical and psychological manifestations of AIDS, nurses will need to refer to a wide variety of texts on this subject; those listed below are particularly recommended.

Chaitow L & Martin S (1988) *A World Without AIDS*. Thorsons.

Department of Health and Social Security *AIDS and Drug Misuse, Part 1*. Report of the Advisory Committee on the Misuse of Drugs. DHSS.

Flaskerud JH (1989) *AIDS/HIV Infection – A Reference Guide for Nursing Professionals*. WB Saunders.

Freedman-Kien AE (1989) *Colour Atlas of AIDS*. WB Saunders.

Miller D (1987) *Living with AIDS and HIV*. MacMillan.

Miller R & Bor R (1988) *AIDS – A Guide to Clinical Counselling*. Science Press.

Pratt RJ (1988) *AIDS – A Strategy for Nursing Care*, 2nd edn. Edward Arnold.

Royal College of Nursing (1990) *AIDS Nursing Guidelines*, 3rd edn. RCN.

Sande MA & Volberding PA (eds) (1988) *The Medical Management of AIDS*. WB Saunders.

Shiltz R (1988) *And The Band Played On – Politics, People and the AIDS Epidemic*. Penguin.

Stalcht J & Dale R (1988) *Understanding AIDS*. Which Books.

Youle M, Clarbow J et al (1988) *AIDS – Therapeutics in HIV Disease*. Churchill Livingstone.

APPENDIX 7

Resuscitation

Prompt action in dealing with the unconscious patient may save a life. However, in order to intervene effectively, it is important to try to establish why unconsciousness occurred. In most instances the cause will be known, but what about the occasions when a seemingly unconscious patient is discovered? What to do? Take the pulse, and note the rate and calibre. Lift the eye-lids (are the pupils dilated or pin-point?), and smell the breath (is there evidence of alcohol or ketones or some other odour?). Look for evidence of drug overdose. Gently shake and try to rouse the person. If no response occurs begin the resuscitation procedure.

The unconscious patient should be cared for in the lateral or semi-prone position. This enables the tongue to lie forwards and facilitates the exit of secretions through the mouth. Any dentures or vomit, etc. should be removed from the mouth to prevent their inhalation. Observations should ensure that air intake is neither excessive nor shallow and that there is no evidence of cyanosis. The breathing patterns of the unconscious patient can change almost instantly and, to counteract untoward changes, essential equipment must be readily avilable to facilitate intervention. This should include: oxygen, and the equipment necessary to administer it, suction apparatus to remove excessive secretions, a mouth gag, angled spatula, tongue clip, sponge holding forceps and gauze swabs. In addition, equipment necessary for intubation and cardioversion should be easily accessible.

The unconscious patient must be observed at all times, and if changes in the breathing pattern occur, help should be summoned and action initiated. Obstructed airway is not uncommon in such patients and may manifest with difficulty in air intake, dilated nostrils, or the sucking inwards of the soft tissues of the neck and upper thorax. When this occurs, access to the mouth should be gained using the mouth gag; ensure the tongue is forward and remove excess secretions using suction apparatus, then ensure that no foreign body is impeding the airway. An obstructed airway most frequently occurs if the patient is cared for in the wrong position, or if he moves from the lateral or semi-prone position.

The cessation of breathing or apnoea is a medical crisis requiring immediate and vigorous action. If the brain is without oxygen for more than 2 or 3 min then irreparable damage will occur to the brain tissue. Resuscitation must therefore begin immediately. Three methods of artificial respiration are described here.

Mouth-to-nose respiration (Figure 1)

1. Ensure that no foreign matter occludes the airway.
2. Grasp the patient's head with one hand and extend his neck by pressing his head backwards and at the same time lifting his jaw upwards and forwards with the other hand. Close his mouth with the thumb.
3. Inhale deeply, place the mouth over the patient's nose and blow until the chest rises. Open the mouth for exhalation, as the patient may have expiratory nasopharyngeal obstruction.
4. Withdraw the mouth and take another deep breath while the patient exhales. Repeat the cycle 12 times a minute. The first six breaths should be given as rapidly as possible.
5. In a child, both his mouth and nose may be covered by the lips and the breaths should be gentler; in infants, only puffs should be used to avoid lung rupture.

Mouth-to-mouth respiration

This method may be preferred, in which case the patient's nostrils should be closed by pressing with the finger and thumb and the breath exhaled into his mouth. Apart from this, the procedure is the same as for mouth-to-nose respiration.

An artificial mouthpiece and airway should be used if there is damage to the oral cavity resulting in excessive bleeding. Draw the patient's jaw forward, open his mouth and insert the airway, directing it first towards the roof of the mouth (so that it curves upwards towards the palate) and then rotating it downwards behind the tongue.

The stomach may become blown up with air, especially if the head is not properly extended. If this occurs, briefly apply pressure over the upper part of the abdomen (epigastrium, between the sternum and umbilicus).

Holger–Nielsen method of artificial respiration

This method (Figure 2) should be used only when it is impossible to use the expired air method of artificial respiration because of damage to the head and neck region or in cases of severe facial trauma.

1. With the patient prone, flex his arms and rest his forehead on his hands, so as to keep the nose and mouth free.
2. Kneel at the head, placing one knee near the head and the other foot by the elbow.
3. Place the hands over the shoulder blades, with the thumbs touching on the midline and the fingers spread out, the arms being kept straight (Figure 2a).
4. Bend forward with arms straight, applying light pressure, while counting 'one, two, three' (Figure 2b). This is expiration.

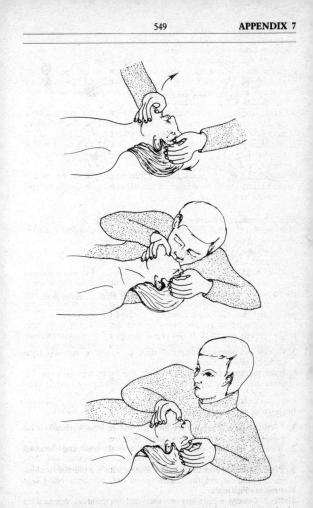

Figure 1. Expired air artificial respiration by the mouth-to-nose method.

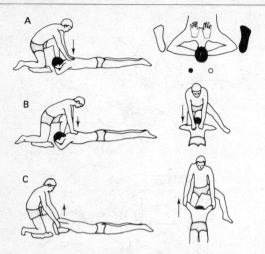

Figure 2. The Holger–Nielsen method of artificial respiration.

5. Release pressure gradually and slide the hands to just above the patient's elbows. Count 'four'.
6. Raise the arms and shoulders by bending backwards until you feel resistance and tension, without lifting the chest off the ground, while counting 'five, six, seven' (Figure 2c). This is inspiration.
7. Lay the arms down and replace your hands on the patient's back while counting 'eight'.
8. Repeat (3) to (7) with a rhythmic movement at the rate of nine times a minute.
9. When breathing is re-established, carry out arm raising and lowering (6 and 7 above) alone, 12 times a minute. Arm raising: one, two, three (inspiration). Arm lowering: four, five, six (expiration).

Manual resuscitators

There are many simple devices that can be manually operated to maintain respiration by blowing air into the lungs. The most commonly

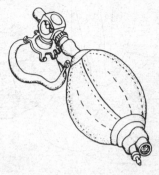

Figure 3. Ambu resuscitator bag.

available is the Ambu resuscitator bag (Figure 3). Where artificial respiration has to be maintained for a prolonged period, such methods are inadequate and a power-driven mechanical respirator is required.

Cardiopulmonary resuscitation (Figure 4)
After the lungs have been inflated several times ensure, by feeling the carotid or femoral artery, that a pulse is present. If no pulse can be felt at these points then the heart has ceased beating and cardiopulmonary resuscitation procedures must be commenced without delay.

1. Summon help.
2. Ensure that the patient's airway is open and continue pulmonary resuscitation using mouth-to-mouth/nose methods or an Ambu bag.
3. Ensure that the patient is on a firm surface, if necessary place a board under the upper half of the patient.
4. Place the heel of the hand on the lower two-thirds of the sternum, place your other hand on top, make sure your arms are perfectly straight, thus bringing your shoulders in line with your hands. If there is only one operator, commence alternating two lung inflations with 15 sternal compressions. If there are two operators, and one operator is focusing on lung inflations and the other is delivering

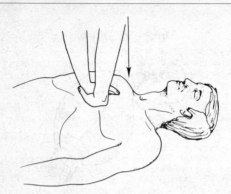

Figure 4. External cardiac massage.

external cardiac massage, alternate one lung inflation with five sternal compressions (the latter at 80–100 compressions per minute).
5. Pause after 15 depressions of the sternum and deliver one deep breath to the patient.
6. Continually monitor to ensure that external cardiac massage is generating an artificial pulse.
7. Assess patient after each 15 depressions of the sternum, to monitor restoration of spontaneous cardiac function.

Vigorous cardiopulmonary resuscitation is frequently not without hazards, and may result in the patient sustaining fractured ribs or sternum; these, however, will heal and such injuries are often unavoidable.

Early and effective cardiopulmonary resuscitation can save lives by maintaining breathing and heartbeat until more technical methods can be brought to the patient. It is therefore essential to ensure that resuscitation practice is carried out in all hospital departments on a regular basis.

Further Reading

Safar P & Bircher NG (1988) *Cardiopulmonary Cerebral Resuscitation*, 3rd edn. WB Saunders.
Woolf N & Laverack G (1987) *Ambulance Aid*. Baillière Tindall.

APPENDIX 8

Drugs and Their Control

(Co-authored by Tim Root, Chief Pharmacist, Royal Marsden Hospital, London SW3 6JJ)

The two acts which control the manufacture, supply and use of drugs are the Medicines Act 1968 and the Misuse of Drugs Act 1971.

The Medicines Act
The Act defines 'medicinal products' as substances sold or supplied for administration to humans or animals for medicinal purposes. Part 3 of the Act, and orders made under it, control the manufacture and sale or supply of medicines, and for this purpose broadly classify them into 3 classes:

1. Prescription-only medicines (POM)
2. Pharmacy medicines (P)
3. General sales list medicines (GSL)

Different legal requirements apply to the sale, supply and labelling of each class.

In hospitals and other institutions, all medicines should be appropriately and securely stored in order to ensure that they remain safe and effective in use and to deter unauthorized access to them and hence possible misuse. (See *Guidelines for the Safe and Secure Handling of Medicines: 'The Duthie Report'* published by the Department of Health 1988.)

The Misuse of Drugs Act
This Act designates and defines as Controlled Drugs a number of 'dangerous or otherwise harmful' substances. These substances are all also by definition Prescription-only medicines under the Medicines Act. The controls imposed by the Misuse of Drugs Act are therefore additional to those under the Medicines Act. The main purpose of the Misuse of Drugs Act is to prevent abuse of Controlled Drugs by prohibiting their manufacture or supply except in accordance with various regulations made under the act. Other regulations govern requirements for safe custody, destruction and supply to addicts.

For these purposes, under the current (1985) Regulations, Controlled Drugs are classified into five Schedules, each representing a different level of control. For practical purposes *Schedule 2* is the most relevant to hospital and community nursing practice. It includes: cocaine; the major opioids such as diamorphine, methadone, morphine, papaveretum and pethidine; and the major stimulant amphetamine (and related drugs). (Amendments to this list and the list of drugs in the other Schedules, may be made from time to time.)

Prescriptions for Schedule 2 drugs (and for those in Schedules 1 and 3) must:

1. Be handwritten, signed and dated by the prescriber.
2. Be in ink or be otherwise indelible.
3. Include the name and address of the patient.
4. State (in words and figures) the total quantity of the drug to be supplied.
5. State the dose to be taken.

(Some of these requirements may be relaxed for the prescription of some Controlled Drugs to addicts, for the treatment of their addiction, by doctors who hold a special Home Office Licence.)

In hospitals, ordering, supply and storage of Controlled Drugs is subject to tight control.

1. They are stored separately in a locked cupboard (which may be within a second outer cupboard) to which access is restricted. The key to the cupboard is held by a first level nurse.
2. Supply from the pharmacy is made to a ward or department only on receipt of a written order signed by a responsible nurse.
3. A record is kept of stock held and details of doses given. A special register is used for this and no other purpose, and it is usually the case that each entry is countersigned by two nurses. The records should be regularly checked by the nurse in charge and by a pharmacist, according to Health Authority policy.

Abbreviations used in prescriptions

Abbreviations of Latin are being replaced by English versions, which is considered safer. However, the nurse may still meet these Latin abbreviations.

Abbreviation	Latin	English
a.c.	ante cibum	before food
ad lib.	ad libitum	to the desired amount
b.d. or b.i.d.	bis in die	twice a day
c.	cum	with
o.m.	omni mane	every morning
o.n.	omni nocte	every night
p.c.	post cibum	after food
p.r.n.	pro re nata	whenever necessary
q.d.	quaque die	every day

q.d.s.	quaque die sumendum	four times daily
q.i.d.	quater in die	four times a day
q.q.h.	quater quaque hora	every four hours
R	recipe	take
s.o.s.	si opus sit	if necessary
stat.	statim	at once
t.d.s.	ter die sumendum	three times a day
t.i.d.	ter in die	three times a day

Administering (the role of the nurse, midwife and health visitor)

The United Kingdom Central Council (UKCC), in an advisory paper on the administration of medicines, clearly states the role and responsibility of the nurse, midwife and health visitor in the administration of prescribed drugs. This is reproduced in full below.

(a) The exercise of professional judgement (which involves the application of his/her knowledge and experience to the situation faced) will lead the practitioner to satisfy himself/herself that he/she is competent to administer the medicine and prepared to be accountable for that action. Once that decision has been made, the practitioner follows a sequence of steps to ensure the safety and well-being of the patient, and which must as a prerequisite be based on a sound knowledge of the patient's assessment and the environment in which care is given.

(b) *Correctness*. This involves interpretation of the prescription and container information in terms of what has been prescribed. Illegibility and lack of clarity of the instruction must be questioned. It also involves ensuring that the medicine is to be administered to the patient for whom it has been prescribed, and in the form and by the method prescribed.

Certain of these points do not usually apply in the context of a patient's home where the patient is receiving medicines from a personalized container. The visiting practitioner does, however, have a responsibility to assist the patient's understanding and help ensure safe administration.

Where a patient is in possession of a range of medicines in containers which are not labelled with precise instructions, and the danger of over- or under-administration exists, it may be necessary for the practitioner to advise the prescribing doctor so that he/she may consider whether any action is required.

(c) *Appropriateness and the possible need to withhold*. This involves checking the expiry date of the medicine, careful consideration of the dosage and the method, route and timing of administration in the context of the condition of each specific patient. It may be necessary or deemed advisable at the time when a medicine is due to be administered to withhold it in order to seek further verification from the prescribing doctor, or confirmation from the responsible senior nurse that it should be given. Where, in the opinion of the administering nurse or responsible senior nurse (i.e. the nurse on duty to whom the administering nurse is in line responsibility at the time), contraindications to the administration of the medicine are observed the prescribing doctor should be contacted without delay. (In respect of this point and that at (b) above the advice of the relevant pharmacist will often be helpful in those situations where the prescribing doctor or an appropriate alternative doctor cannot be contacted.)

(d) *Reinforcement.* The positive effect of treatment may need to be reinforced by the nurse. Every occasion on which a medicine is administered is an opportunity for such reinforcement and for reassurance. In the community particularly it is also an opportunity to help ensure avoidance of misuse of self-medication, and the misuse of the prescribed drugs by others who reside in or are visiting the household.

(e) *Recording/reporting.* As part of the ongoing process (not solely at the times of administration of medicines) the effects and side-effects of the treatment should be noted. Taking appropriate action in relation to side-effects is essential. Positive and negative effects should be reported to the appropriate doctor and recorded.

(f) *Record of administration.* Where a practitioner is involved in the administration of medicines thorough and accurate records of the administration must be maintained. In hospital settings this will normally be achieved by initialling the appropriate box on a treatment record at the time of administration, which together with the administering practitioner's signature are essential minimum requirements, and all must be legibly written. If (as a result of consideration as in (c) above) a medicine is not administered a record to that effect should be made.

(g) The UKCC is of the view that practitioners whose names are on the first level parts of the register, and midwives, should be seen as competent to administer medicines on their own, and responsible for their actions in so doing. The involvement of a second person in the administration of medicines with a first level practitioner need only occur where that practitioner is instructing a learner or the patient's condition makes it necessary or in such other circumstances as are locally determined. Where two persons are involved responsibility still attaches to the senior person.

(h) The UKCC is totally opposed to the involvement of personnel who are not professionally registered such as nursing auxiliaries or assistants in the administration of medicines since it gives a false sense of security, undermines true responsibility, and fails to satisfy points (c) and (d) of this section.

(i) Given the wording of Rule 18 (2) of Statutory Instrument 1983 No. 873, the UKCC is opposed to the use of a second level practitioner for the administration of medicines other than under the direction of a first level nurse. It is recommended that employers adopt the same stance unless:

1. they have provided additional instruction relevant to the medicines likely to be encountered in a particular setting;
2. they have undertaken an assessment of the individual's knowledge and competence to perform the task; and
3. they are prepared to accept the responsibility for any errors that are consequential upon using a second level practitioner beyond the role for which training prepared him/her.

(j) The principles enunciated in this section are equally applicable to a medicine round or to the administration of medicines within individual care.

(k) The responsibility of the nurse varies in the setting of a patient's home, where he/she needs to be cognizant of the 'freedom' of the patient in his own setting, and the implications of self-medication and the possession of 'over the counter' medicines. Where a nurse working in the community becomes involved in obtaining prescribed medicines for patients he/she must recognize his/her responsibility for their safe transit and correct delivery.

(l) In accordance with the requirements of the Medicines Act 1968 and the Misuse of Drugs Act 1971 and subsequent regulations there are specific arrangements for midwives working in the community, and occupational health nurses, to obtain and administer medicines. Those relating to midwives are contained in the UKCC Midwife's Code of Practice and those to occupational health nurses in the Royal College of Nursing Society of Occupational Health Nursing Information Leaflet No. 11 dated November 1983. Also in pursuance of Regulation 10 (3) of the Misuse of Drugs Regulations 1973 specific 'Group Authority' is given to certain registered nurses employed at places of work.

The foregoing guidance applies to the administration of drugs in all health care settings.

Further Reading

ABPI Data Sheet Compendium (current edition). Datapharm Publications Limited.

British National Formulary (current edition). British Medical Association and The Pharmaceutical Society of Great Britain.

Connechen J, Shanley E & Robson H (1983) *Pharmacology for Nurses*, 5th edn. Nurses' Aids Series. Baillière Tindall.
Jefferies P (1983) *Mathematics in Nursing*, 6th edn. Nurses' Aids Series. Baillière Tindall.
Pirie S (1985) *Maths for Nursing*. Baillière Tindall.
Wellington FM et al (1987) *Baillière's Pharmacology for Nurses*, 2nd edn. Baillière Tindall.

APPENDIX 9

Legal and Ethical Issues

Florence Nightingale said 'The hospital should be seen to do the patient no harm' and this is as true today as it was when she said it. With the advancement in high technology treatments for many conditions, with the resulting rapid throughput of patients and concomitant pressure of work upon the nurse, the tendency for mistakes to happen is likely to increase, and the nurse shares responsibility for ensuring that these are kept to a minimum by following well tried procedures.

As the role of nursing has developed over the years, so the involvement of nurses in ethical issues concerning health care and its delivery have increased. The *Code of Professional Conduct for the Nurse, Midwife and Health Visitor* issued by the UKCC, leaves nurses in no doubt of their responsibility: 'Each registered nurse, midwife and health visitor shall act at all times in such a manner as to justify public trust and confidence . . . to serve the interests of society, and above all to safeguard the interests of individual patients and clients.' Patients calling upon the services of health care professionals, in whatever setting, have a right to expect to be treated with equity and honesty regarding their condition and its treatment. No one member of the team has the authority to deny patients these rights.

One of the greatest responsibilities of nurses working in hospital settings is to ensure the safety of patients; thus, the work environment must be as free as possible from hazards which might harm patients, and patients likely to come to harm should be protected at all times.

Consent to treatment
Entry into hospital signifies that an individual, realizing he has a health problem, is seeking advice and help. It does not in any way indicate that he has implicitly consented to treatment, or that he has relinquished his rights as a citizen. Therefore throughout his stay in hospital the patient should be informed of what is to happen and his agreement obtained. Often this can be achieved informally, e.g. 'Mr Jones we wish to take a sample of blood to measure the haemoglobin level.' By rolling up his sleeve, Mr Jones has given consent, but only for that particular test to be done. To do more, or to carry out tests to which consent has not been given may be construed as an assault, and as such answerable in court and before the UKCC. Other procedures, which carry with them a reasonable hazard, may not be performed without the written consent of the individual.

Surgery

Any individual having attained the age of 16 years and considered to be of sound mind can consent to an anaesthetic prior to a surgical procedure. He must not, of course, be allowed to sign such a consent in ignorance, and therefore has the right to be informed of his diagnosis, the procedure to be performed, the consequences this might have on his future functional ability, and the hoped-for outcome of the procedure. The patient has a right to limit the extent of the surgery should he so wish.

Consent should be obtained, whenever possible well in advance of the procedure, by a doctor and in the presence of a nurse. This enables the nurse to be aware of what has been said and to offer the patient supplementary information as requested. Where the patient is under the age of consent, unconscious or mentally incapacitated, the consent may be obtained from the next of kin, who should also have access to the nurse to obtain additional information if necessary.

Clinical trials

All patients invited to participate in clinical drug trials must give written consent before entering into the trial. Again, this is obtained in the presence of a nurse by a doctor, who should explain the nature of the drug, the potential side-effects, the previous results of the use of the drug, the hoped-for outcomes and benefits for the patient. A copy of the protocol of the trial should be lodged on the ward where the treatment is to occur so that it is accessible to all nurses caring for the patient. The patient should always be informed of his right not to participate, the right to know of other treatments for his condition, and the right to withdraw from the trial at any time without jeopardizing his access to other treatments.

Other treatments

Those treatments which do not require written consent should none the less be carefully explained to the patient and his verbal agreement to participate should be recorded in his notes. In order to make a rational decision the patient will require information on the mode and action of the treatment, and all the side-effects which will or might occur, how these will be managed, and how they will affect the quality of his life.

Correct identity

It is sadly not uncommon for mistakes involving identity of patients to be made, resulting in wrong drugs being administered or treatments carried out. This can easily be overcome by ensuring that all patients in general and maternity hospitals wear identity bands on which their name is easily decipherable. Newly born babies must be correctly labelled at birth to ensure that children are not handed to the wrong mother or placed in the wrong cot.

In all instances the label should bear the individual's name and hospital number, and should be checked routinely before the administration of any drug or any treatment. Obviously this check system is most important prior to surgery. The patient's name should be checked against the prescription chart before administration of the premedication; when the porter arrives to transport the patient to theatre the patient should be asked 'What is your name?' and the reply checked with the identity band, the notes and the operating list. The responsibility for marking a site prior to surgery does not rest with the nurse, who should under no circumstances participate in this.

Theatre count

During operative procedures it is the responsibility of the 'scrubbed nurse' to ascertain the numbers of instruments, blades, needles, swabs and packs laid out prior to commencement of surgery and to check these numbers with a colleague. During surgery the nurse ensures that all equipment and swabs handed to the surgeon are returned to her, and that additional equipment and swabs brought into use during the operation are recorded. Before the operation site is closed the nurse must undertake a final check to ensure that all equipment is accounted for. If numbers do not tally, the surgeon must be informed and closure delayed until a satisfactory recount has taken place.

Administration of drugs

The responsibilities of the nurse in the administration and storage of drugs is discussed in Appendix 8.

Accidents to patients and visitors

Everyone working in hospital, of whatever discipline, has a responsibility to ensure a safe environment for patients and visitors. They can do this by bringing to the attention of those responsible any defects in furniture or equipment, the negligence of others resulting in equipment obstructing public areas, or unsafe floor surfaces. It is best when reporting such matters to note the time and date they were reported and to whom.

Although the hospital does have some responsibility for those it employs, the individual can be held responsible for culpable negligence or incompetence resulting in loss or injury to the patient and may have damages awarded against him personally. This highlights the importance of all health care workers belonging to an appropriate professional organization or trade union. If the accident involves a student nurse or support worker, it may have to be demonstrated that she has received proper instruction in the procedure undertaken, e.g. where a patient has suffered due to bad lifting techniques.

As an action against a hospital may be brought several years after the incident, or a hearing may take a long time to come to court, it is essential that all untoward incidents involving patients and visitors are fully recorded on an appropriate accident form which is then lodged with the hospital administrator.

In order to reduce the likelihood of accidents in hospitals, the Health and Safety at Work Act 1974 recommends the appointment of health and safety officers to monitor and ensure safe working conditions within the area in which they work.

Self-discharge of patients

When the patient demands to discharge himself, the nurse on duty should try to dissuade him and should inform the medical officer concerned with his care. If the patient is adamant, each hospital will follow its own procedure. It is probable that a senior administrative officer will see the patient and ask him to sign a written statement to the effect that he is discharging himself against medical advice. Should he refuse to sign, a note to this effect will have to be made and signed by two witnesses, one of whom is usually the administrative officer concerned and the other the nurse in charge at the time. The patient must be allowed to leave, except in the case of a mentally disordered patient who is subject to a restriction order or where it is felt he may be a danger to himself or others, when he may be detained for 3 days to enable an order to be obtained.

Mentally disordered patients

The proper care and treatment of these patients, which includes those with mental illness, mental impairment, severe mental impairment and psychopathic disorder, and the safeguarding of their property and affairs is laid down in the Mental Health Act 1983, and the rules made thereunder. Most of these patients are now admitted without legal formality (informal admission) provided that they are not unwilling to enter hospital. They may leave when they wish, unless detained for 3 days. A person may be liable to detention in hospital or guardianship under the Act only if he is suffering from one of the named forms of disorder and if, for his own health or safety or for the protection of others, he needs restraint or control.

Unless subject to a court order, mentally impaired or psychopathic patients can first be made subject to detention or guardianship only before the age of 21 years. This ceases at 25 years unless a report has been furnished by the responsible medical officer that they would be likely to act in a manner dangerous to themselves or others. Except in criminal cases, and subject to the aforesaid, detention in hospital or guardianship is for two consecutive periods of 1 year and then for 2-yearly periods. Renewal of authority in each instance is on report by the responsible medical officer that continuance of the detention or guardianship is necessary for the patient's own health or safety or for the protection of others.

Confidentiality

The protection of confidential information pertaining to the illness or condition of a patient, or the protection of information divulged by a patient, is an ethical duty of the medical and nursing professions and the nurse must ensure never to discuss information received by nature of her position, except with other colleagues involved with the patient when the knowledge may assist in the patient's treatment. Even in such instances the nurse must ask the permission of the patient before divulging such information.

Confidential information should not be divulged to relatives or friends, nor should information on the patient's condition be passed to his employers as this may cause loss to the patient for which the nurse may be held legally liable. Telephone requests for information on the progress of the patient must be handled with discretion. It could save many problems if, on admission, the patient is asked to whom information may be divulged, and to ascertain the extent of information to be given.

Most breaches of confidentiality occur without thinking. The nurse must ensure that she never discusses a patient or his problems anywhere outside the ward.

Patients' property

The Department of Health requires all hospitals under its care to inform patients that the hospital cannot accept responsibility for valuables or money unless these have been handed over for safe keeping. Where it is known that a patient has an excess of money, he should be invited to hand it over against a signed receipt so that it may be placed in the hospital safe. The valuables and money of an unconscious patient admitted as an emergency should be listed, checked by two nurses and put in safe-keeping.

While a patient is in hospital, the nurse has no right to go through his locker or personal property without his consent. Searching his possessions may be justified if it is suspected that the patient intends to injure himself or others and has the means to do so. Even in such a case, the nurse will be wise to have a witness.

When a patient dies in hospital, his possessions must be recorded in the property book; money and valuables should be listed and packed separately. The property will then be checked and the book signed by two persons, usually a nurse and the sister or her deputy. Strictly speaking, the property should be handed over to the executors of the deceased, but unless property of considerable value is involved it is usual to hand it over, against a receipt, to the next of kin. This may be the responsibility of an administrative officer and in this case the nurse should on no account give property or valuables to relatives or friends of the deceased. Care must be taken in the descriptive terms used; for example, 'yellow metal' is a safer term to use than gold, and 'white metal' than silver or platinum, since the relatives may refuse to accept an article made of base metal that has been incorrectly described.

Making of wills and signing of legal documents

Most hospitals have a rule against or discourage nurses from signing legal documents or witnessing signatures during their professional duties. This is to protect the nurse should the document be challenged later on the ground of the unfitness of the patient. However, the nurse has the duty to pass on immediately any request of this nature on the part of the patient so that the services of a solicitor may be obtained, or those of a hospital administrative officer, who will assist the patient in every way, even in drawing up a simple will if so required.

Further Reading

Protection of the rights of patients whilst receiving treatment and care is an integral part of the role of the nurse. To assist the nurse in the exercise of this responsibility, the following publications are recommended.

Finch JD (1981) *Health Services Law.* Sweet & Maxwell.
Health and Safety at Work Act (1974) HMSO.
Rumbold G (1986) *Ethics in Nursing Practice.* Baillière Tindall.
Safeguards Against Failure to Remove Swabs and Instruments from Patients (1978) Medical Defence Council and Royal College of Nursing.
Safeguards Against Wrong Operations (1978) Medical Defence Council and Royal College of Nursing.
Seedhouse D (1988) *Ethics: The Heart of Health Care.* John Wiley & Sons.
Watchdog: For the Record (1978) Royal College of Nursing.

APPENDIX 10

The National Health Service

The National Health Service of the United Kingdom is the largest employer of labour in Europe, with the exception of the armed forces of the USSR, and is allocated approximately 6% of the gross domestic product.

The face of health care has changed dramatically since the National Health Service was founded in 1948. There is now a thriving private health sector, due mainly to the number of people either purchasing private health insurance or receiving such incentive benefits from employers. This development has accessed a wider choice for consumers and has widened the employment opportunities for health care personnel.

No other group of employees has experienced more radical change brought about by constant reorganization. Since 1948, a succession of reports commissioned by different governments, some of which aided development of the services and some of which were viewed as change for the sake of change, have dramatically altered the original concept of the National Health Service: free for all at the point of delivery.

The recent changes began in 1966 with the publication and hasty implementation of the Salmon report which addressed issues of nursing management. A further reorganization followed in 1974. This encompassed some of the recommendations of the Salmon report and recommended management of services on a three-tier system at District, Area and Regional levels. A Royal Commission of the National Health Service, which published its findings in 1979, was highly critical of the structure of the health services, saying that there were too many tiers, too many administrators of all disciplines, too much wastage of money and an inability to make speedy decisions. Consequently the report, *Patients First* (1979), recommended further changes in an attempt to make the system less unwieldy.

The most dramatic change in the 1980s was the implementation of the Griffiths Report (1983) on the general management of the health services, which largely came about due to the failure of the 1974 reorganization. The report opened management of health services, which previously had operated on something akin to a closed-shop policy, to a much wider range of people, and attracted into health care managers from industry and commerce as well as from the health care professions. The ethos of the report was twofold: cost effectiveness and accountability.

The simultaneous publication, in 1986, of the Green Paper on Primary Health Care and the Cumberlege Report addressed health care issues in the community. The Green Paper concentrated attention on the services provided by general practitioners, dentists and pharmacists, and addressed in depth how these practitioners might provide better services to patients. A good practice allowance was envisaged for general practitioners to encourage the development of a wider range of services, thus encouraging patients to join their lists. Incentives for dentists to participate more fully in health service treatments, with more emphasis on preventative services and advice, were envisaged. Pharmacists were perceived as providing an increased advisory service to both patients and doctors. The Green Paper also proposed improvements to help deal with primary health care problems in inner city areas.

The Cumberledge Report recommended the setting up of neighbourhood nursing services, based on a health centre or geographically defined area; the report emphasized amongst other things the need to encourage the nurse manager back into clinical practice, the creation of the nurse practitioner who would work alongside her general practitioner colleagues with her own case-load, and the provision for community based nurses to have limited prescribing powers.

In 1988, Sir Roy Griffiths produced a report, *Community Care – Agenda for Action*, in which he envisaged that much of the care currently provided by the health services to people in the community could be provided on a much more cost-effective basis by local authority social services. The basic premise behind the suggestion was that in the future there will be fewer qualified nurses available, and that such scarce resources should be channelled to those consumers who really need them.

In 1989, the Chief Nursing Officer issued a report, *A Strategy for Nursing*. The report had its genesis in 1986 when leaders of nursing were brought together to examine how the profession should progress in a health service which would undergo many changes in the future, and the impact such changes would have on nursing. Demographic changes mean that there will be fewer nurses available in the future and the aim of the strategy is to ensure that nurses, midwives and health visitors are used to maximum effect. A 'strategy for nursing' identifies 44 targets affecting clinical practice, manpower, education, management and leadership. The report expresses the opinion that at least 14 of these targets are achievable by 1991. The targets of the strategy encompass extended clinical roles, setting of standards and measurement of outcomes, research-based practice, and the development of the nurse as a manager. Skill mix, recruitment, support workers are also amongst the achievable targets listed, whilst education and leadership are viewed as paramount in achieving the strategies laid down in the document.

Also in 1989, the Secretary of State for Health published a White Paper, *Working for Patients*, which contained proposals for the most radical reorganization of health care ever. The report stated that, although the health service in the United Kingdom was amongst the best in the world, the cost of providing such a service for 1988/89 would be 26 billion pounds, an increase of 40% on 1978/79 figures. The report added that the increasing demands on the service could not be met solely by the provision of more money, and therefore a radical overhaul of the service with wide-ranging changes was necessary. The implementation of the report is intended to improve the performances of all hospitals and general practice, thus obliterating wide variations in the quality and quantity of services which currently exist throughout the United Kingdom. The stated aim of the report is to give more control at local level so that services can respond to local needs and be locally accountable for the provision of services. The main aim is to give people health care and choices of health care in the locality where they live, and to reward those health care staff who respond appropriately and effectively to such demands and needs.

The White Paper contains seven key measures: hospitals are to have greater control of their own affairs; hospitals are encouraged to become self-governing trusts within the NHS with greater power for local pay bargaining and obtaining finance; health authorities/self-governing hospitals will be enabled and encouraged to offer their services to other health authorities and to private hospitals, thus improving availability of services in areas where there may be long waiting lists, and improving income to the hospital/authority; general practitioners will be encouraged to become budget holders in order to purchase a defined range of services from hospitals of their choice; patients will be able to change their general practitioner much more easily; management structures at regional, district and family practitioner level will be reformed along business lines and reduced in size; medical audit and measurement of standards of care and services will be introduced throughout the health service.

Self-governing hospitals are seen as providing greater patient choice and enhanced efficiency, and acting as a spur to other hospitals to do better. It is envisaged that such hospitals will form a National Health Service Trust with a board of executive and non-executive directors (as in public companies), the executive members to include: the general manager, the senior nurse manager, a medical director, and the director of finance. Self-governing hospitals will be dependent for revenue on the quality and quantity of the services they market, principally to health authorities, general practitioners and the private sector. Self-governing hospitals will be empowered to determine pay and conditions of service for their staff. It is intended that the first self-governing hospitals will be operational in 1991.

The implications of *Working for Patients* extend into all areas of health care and nurses working in every discipline will be affected by the proposals.

Further Reading

Clay TC (1987) *Nurses, Power and Politics*. Heinemann.

Department of Health and Social Services (1983) *NHS Management Inquiry Report (Griffiths Report)*. HMSO.

Department of Health and Social Services (1988) *Community Call – Agenda for Action*. HMSO.

Department of Health (1989) *Working for Patients*. HMSO.

Department of Health (Nursing Division) (1989) *A Strategy for Nursing*. HMSO.

Moores B (ed.) (1986) *Are They Being Served?* Philip Alan.

Neighbourhood Nursing: a Focus for Care (Cumberledge Report) (1986) HMSO.

Primary Health Care: An Agenda for Discussion (Green Paper) (1986) HMSO.

Report of the Committee of Senior Nursing Staff Structure (Salmon Report) (1966) HMSO.

Royal Commission on the National Health Service (1979) HMSO.

White R (ed.) (1986) *Political Issues in Nursing – Past, Present and Future*, vol. 2. John Wiley & Sons.

APPENDIX 11

United Kingdom Central Council for Nursing, Midwifery and Health Visiting

The United Kingdom Central Council for Nursing, Midwifery and Health Visiting (UKCC) was established in November 1980 and assumed its full functions in July 1983, taking over the responsibilities of the General Nursing Council for England and Wales, the Central Midwives Board, the Council for the Training of Health Visitors, the Panel of Assessors for District Nurse Training and the Joint Board of Clinical Nursing Studies.

The UKCC is the statutory body responsible for the regulation of the nursing, midwifery and health visiting professions. Its main duties are to define educational policies and standards and to monitor and advise on professional conduct. In each of the four countries of the United Kingdom there is a National Board of Nursing, Midwifery and Health Visiting, which works in close liaison with the UKCC to ensure that policies are implemented.

The 1979 Nurses and Midwives Act states that 'the principal function of the Central Council shall be to establish and improve standards of professional conduct' and 'the powers of the Council shall include that of providing, in such manner as it thinks fit, advice for nurses, midwives and health visitors on standards of professional conduct'. As a result of this, the Council produced a *Code of Professional Conduct for the Nurse, Midwife and Health Visitor*. This document, issued to all newly qualified nurses, lays down the rules which nurses must observe in their professional practice. A midwives' Code of Practice was subsequently published. To assist nurses to achieve and maintain standards of professional conduct, the UKCC has also published a number of advisory documents in recent years; details are given in the Further Reading list at the end of this section.

When allegations of professional misconduct are made, they are investigated by the National Board of the country concerned and, where appropriate, referred to the Professional Conduct Committee for hearing. This committee, which is open to observers, meets in different locations across the United Kingdom.

Education
In 1984, the UKCC established a project which was the responsibility of its Educational Policy Advisory Committee (EPAC); the terms of

reference were 'to determine the education and training required for the professional practice of nursing, midwifery and health visiting in relation to the projected health care needs in the 1990s and beyond and to make recommendations'. This was to become known as Project 2000.

After wide consultations between EPAC and interested professionals and groups, the final recommendations of the committee were submitted to Ministers early in 1987. The submission recommended dramatic changes to the educational system in order to meet the projected reduction in numbers of those entering nursing during the next two decades, to ensure cost effectiveness and value for money, and to support the shift towards provision of health care in the community and the increased emphasis on the prevention of ill-health. In order to meet these factors, the committee believed a more appropriately prepared practitioner was needed.

The major proposal of the document was to have only a single level of registered nurses, with the recommendation that the training of enrolled nurses (second level nurses) cease as soon as possible. The report envisaged that the new nurse would embrace much of the work previously shared by first and second level nurses. They perceived the nurse of the future as a 'knowledgeable doer' who will have a support worker to help her, and a specialist practitioner to help and advise her. Project 2000 recommends that in future all nurses will have a 3-year preparation programme and will share a common foundation programme, which will last for up to 18 months, before nurses 'branch out' into their chosen area of care. These branches will initially be the nursing care of the adult, the child, mentally handicapped persons, and mental health; other areas might be added later. The preparation for all branches will place strong emphasis on health promotion and health care. The report re-emphasized nursing as a practice-based profession, but recommended that students of nursing be supernumerary during their training and that they should deliver care under supervision, according to the level of their theoretical grounding and practical experience. It agreed that student nurses should receive non-means-tested bursaries and that closer links with further and higher education should be established. The report also discusses in great detail the types and numbers of teachers it envisages for the future, and the facilities in which they will teach.

Vehement opposition from midwives resulted in the following recommendations from the committee: that separate and distinct competencies for midwives be maintained; that the existing 18-month post-registration education and training be maintained; and that a direct entry programme to midwifery be developed and encouraged. New and experimental programmes in midwifery training are also to be encouraged.

Registration

From 1987 onwards, all nurses, midwives and health visitors have been required to re-register periodically with the UKCC in order to continue practising. Those who have lapsed or been absent from the profession for more than 5 years will be required to undergo a period of re-training and re-orientation before being allowed to register or practise.

Those nurses who trained for the enrolled part of the register, and who wish and are able to undertake studies to enable them to become first level nurses, should be encouraged and assisted in their efforts.

Further Reading

UKCC (1984) *Annual Report 1953–84.*

UKCC (1984) *The Code of Professional Conduct for the Nurse, Midwife and Health Visitor*, 2nd edn.

UKCC (1985) *Advertising by Registered Nurses, Midwives and Health Visitors.*

UKCC (1986) *Administration of Medicines.*

UKCC (1986) *Handbook of Midwives Rules.*

UKCC (1987) *Confidentiality – An elaboration of Clause 9 of the Code of Professional Conduct.*

UKCC (1988) *The First Five Years 1983–88.*

UKCC (1989) *Exercising Accountability.*

UKCC (1989) *A Midwives Code of Practice for Midwives Practising in the UK.*

APPENDIX 12

Professional Organizations and Trade Unions

There are a variety of organizations available to meet the specific professional/labour relations needs of the nurse. Some of them concentrate only on professional issues pertinent to a specific area of practice, others combine professional and industrial relations functions, and some concentrate almost exclusively on issues surrounding pay and conditions of service. It is important that all nurses join an organization which will offer them protection and support to enable them to function effectively in their practice. Some nurses belong to more than one organization, joining a large organization to represent their interest in areas of pay and conditions of service, legal protection, and for the other services available (mortgages, insurance, etc.), and smaller, more focused professional groups which address issues related to their area of practice.

Association of Professional and Executive Staffs (APEX)
APEX recently combined forces with MATSA the white collar section of the General and Municipal Boiler Makers Union (GMB; membership 800 000). It is committed to issues of equal pay and rights, and works for better pay and conditions of service and a healthier working environment. APEX, through GMB, sponsors Members of Parliament (MPs) and is affiliated to the Trades Union Congress (TUC).

Association of Professions for Mentally Handicapped People (APMH)
APMH is a multidisciplinary organization committed to improving the services available to people with mental handicap, to promoting their general welfare by encouraging high standards of care and a unified professional view on strategies for mental handicap, and to educating the public to understand, accept and respect people with a mental handicap. APMH is not affiliated to the TUC, nor does it sponsor MPs.

Confederation of Health Service Employees (COHSE)
COHSE is among the larger health service unions and membership is open to anyone working in health services; it therefore represents, amongst others, nurses, nursing auxiliaries, ambulance personnel, engineers and porters. The organization is committed to improved pay and conditions of service in the health service, especially for lower paid workers. COHSE sponsors MPs and is affiliated to the TUC.

District Nursing Association UK (DNA)

The DNA is a professional organization and trade union which addresses the specific needs of nurses working in the district. Since it was formed in 1971, the association has enjoyed continued growth and is consulted by government on all matters relating to district nursing. It organizes regular conferences and communicates with its members through a quarterly newsletter. The DNA is not affiliated to the TUC and does not sponsor MPs.

Health Visitors' Association (HVA)

The HVA is the main professional organization representing the interests of health visitors and school nurses; it has some 15 000 members. It was the first health organization to affiliate to the TUC (in 1924) and combine the roles of trade union and professional association.

The HVA's professional service to members includes update and refresher education courses and the provision of a specialist library and information service. It is also closely concerned with professional development and standards of practice. It provides industrial advice to members through its labour relations department and network of local representatives. It publishes a monthly professional journal, *Health Visitor*, which is distributed free to all members.

Infection Control Nurses' Association (ICNA)

The ICNA was formed in 1970 to meet the professional needs of infection control nurses. The association comprises a network of regional groups which acts as a support network and information source for members. The national executive committee manages the business affairs of the association and supports regional groups in organizing study days and conferences. The association publishes the *Journal of Infection Control Nursing* as a supplement to *Nursing Times* four times a year. It is not affiliated to the TUC and does not sponsor MPs.

National Association of Local Government Officers (NALGO)

NALGO was formed in 1905; it is a specialist trade union dealing with administrative and clerical, nursing, midwifery, and professional and technical staff in the public services. It has in excess of 750 000 members, making it the fourth largest trade union in the United Kingdom. It negotiates for its members on all relevant committees and offers legal and wide-ranging welfare services; and publishes *NALGO News* which is distributed free to members. NALGO is affiliated to the TUC but does not sponsor MPs.

National Association of Theatre Nurses (NATN)

NATN was formed in 1964 to promote the improvement of care and service to the patient in the operating theatre and to promote the exchange of professional information between members. The association has 47 branches in the United Kingdom and associate members throughout the world. The NATN journal, the *British Journal of Theatre Nursing*, is published monthly and distributed to all members. An education and research fellowship was founded in 1983 to enable theatre nurses to undertake research and further education. NATN is not affiliated to the TUC and does not sponsor MPs.

National Union of Public Employees (NUPE)

NUPE is one of the largest public sector trade unions and accepts into membership anyone working in the public sector. Within health care, its largest membership is amongst ancillary staffs, although it does have a nursing section. The organization is particularly committed to improving pay and conditions of service amongst low paid hospital and local authority workers. NUPE sponsors MPs and is affiliated to the TUC.

Royal College of Midwives (RCM)

The RCM functions as a trade union and professional organization for 80% of the country's practising midwives (34 000 members). It is the only organization which represents all categories of midwife, and offers services to meet educational, professional and labour relations needs. In recent years its membership has increased by 25%.

The RCM has board offices in each of the four countries of the United Kingdom. Each country elects its own board, three members of which serve on the council of the college; a further 12 council members are elected by the whole UK membership. The interests of members at local level are served by a wide network of stewards and branch officers.

The organization is committed to encouraging high standards of care in midwifery, and to the reduction of social deprivation and deficits in health.

The Royal College of Midwives is an independent trade union, is not affiliated to the TUC, and does not sponsor MPs.

Royal College of Nursing of the United Kingdom (Rcn)

The Rcn is the largest organization in the United Kingdom representing the interests of qualified nurses and students of nursing. It has in excess of 250 000 members. The organization is committed to meeting the professional, educational and labour relations needs of its members through its board offices at country level and regional offices in each of the counties. The structure of the membership is based on local branches, members of which elect officers to represent their interests, and also elect to the council of the college on a regional basis. The college comprises departments which meet the specific needs of its membership: labour relations/legal, professional, international, welfare, students and education.

The Education Department is controlled by the Rcn Institute of Advanced Nursing Education in London, Birmingham and Belfast, who offer a wide variety of educational programmes and courses for nurses.

The professional needs of its members are addressed by the Department of Nursing Policy and Practice. The diverse interests of nurses are reflected by the wide variety of professional associations, societies, forums and special interest groups run by the professional officers in this department.

The International Department liaises closely with nursing organizations in other countries, and with international organizations. Through this department, the Rcn represents the interests of British nurses on the Standing Nursing/Midwifery Committee of the EEC. The International Department is available to offer practical advice and help with contracts and conditions of service for those nurses wishing to work overseas. It can also help in arranging overseas study visits.

The Labour Relations/Legal Department offers a service to those experiencing difficulties in their place of work. It is concerned with salaries/conditions of service, health and safety at work and legal problems of nurses. The department co-ordinates a nationwide stewards' scheme and a network of health and safety representatives.

CHAT (Counselling Help and Advice Together) is a confidential counselling service available to all nurses.

The headquarters building of the Rcn houses the largest nursing library in the United Kingdom with 40 000 volumes and 220 regular journals. The specialist collections of literature and nursing research (the Historical Collection and the Sternberg Collection) can be found here.

The Rcn operates a wide range of membership services, has its own housing association for retired nurses, and confers fellowships upon nurses who are deemed to have made a significant contribution to the art and science of nursing.

The organization is an independent trade union, is not affiliated to the TUC and does not sponsor MPs. The Rcn represents UK nursing on the board of the International Council of Nurses.

International Council of Nurses (ICN)

Founded in 1899, the ICN is the oldest international professional organization in the health care field. ICN accepts into membership one association of nurses per country. There are 95 national nurses' organizations in membership. In addition, ICN works with approximately 50 other national associations or groups of nurses with a view to their future membership.

The governing body of the ICN is the Council of National Representatives (CNR) elected on the principle of one country, one vote. The CNR meets every 2 years to determine policy matters affecting the nursing profession. Every fourth year this meeting is held in conjunction with an ICN quadrennial congress, open to nurses throughout the world.

ICN is in official relationship with the World Health Organization (WHO), is included on the special list of non-governmental organizations maintained by the International Labour Organization (ILO), for consultative purposes is in relationship with the United Nations Educational, Scientific and Cultural Organization (UNESCO) and with the United Nations International Children's Emergency Fund (UNICEF), is on the Consultative Register of the Economics and Social Council (ECOSOC), and is in relationship with the International Committee of the Red Cross, the League of Red Cross Societies, the World Medical Association, the International Hospital Federation and the Union of International Associations.

APPENDIX 13

Useful Addresses

Age Concern England (National Old Peoples' Welfare Council), 60 Pitcairn Road, Mitcham, Surrey CR4 3LL

Alcohol Concern (The National Agency of Alcohol Misuse), 305 Grays Inn Road, London WC1X 8QF

Alzheimer's Disease Society, 3rd Floor, Bank Building, Fulham Broadway, London SW6 1EP

Arthritis and Rheumatism Council (ARC), 41 Eagle Street, London WC1R 4AR

Association of British Paediatric Nurses (ABPN), c/o Central Nursing Office, The Hospital for Sick Children, Great Ormond Street, London WC1

Association of Carers, First Floor, 21–23 New Road, Chatham, Kent ME4 4JQ

Association for Improvements in the Maternity Services (AIMS), 163 Liverpool Road, London N1 0RF

Asthma Society, 300 Upper Street, London N1 2XX

Back Pain Association, 31–33 Park Road, Teddington, Middlesex TW11 0AB

Breast Care and Mastectomy Association, 26a Harrison Street, London WC1H 8JG

British Association for Cancer United Patients (BACUP), 121 Charterhouse Street, London EC1

British Association for Counselling, 37a Sheep Street, Rugby, Warwickshire CV21 3BX

British Colostomy Association, 38–39 Eccleston Square, London SW1V 1PB

British Council for the Rehabilitation of the Disabled, 25 Mortimer Street, London W1

British Deaf Association, 38 Victoria Place, Carlisle, Cumbria CA1 1HU

British Diabetic Association, 10 Queen Anne Street, London W1M 0BD

British Dietetic Association, Daimler House, Paradise Circus, Queensway, Birmingham B1 2BJ

British Epilepsy Association, Anstey House, 40 Hanover Square, Leeds LS3 1BE

British Geriatrics Society (BGS), 1 St Andrew's Place, London NW1 4LB

British Heart Foundation, 102 Gloucester Place, London W1H 4DH

British Kidney Patients' Association, Bonden, Hampshire

British Nutrition Foundation, 15 Belgrave Square, London SW1X 8PS

British Pregnancy Advisory Service, Austry Manor, Wooten Wawen, Solihull, West Midlands B95 6DA

British Red Cross Society (BRCS), 9 Grosvenor Crescent, London SW1X 7EJ

Cancer Link, 17 Britannia Street, London WC1X 9JN

Carer's National Association, 29 Chilwalk Mews, London W2 3RG

Coeliac Society, PO Box 220, High Wycombe, Buckinghamshire HP11 2HY

Committee on Safety of Drugs, Finsbury Square House, 33–37a Finsbury Square, London EC2

Compassionate Friends, 6 Denmark Street, Bristol BS1 5DG

Coronary Prevention Group, Central Middlesex Hospital, Acton Lane, London NW10

Cruse (National Association for the Widowed and their Children), Cruse House, 126 Sheen Road, Richmond, Surrey TW9 1UR

Department of Health, Richmond House, 79 Whitehall, London SW1A 2NS

English National Board for Nursing, Midwifery and Health Visiting (ENB), Victory House, 170 Tottenham Court Road, London W1P 0HA

Family Planning Association (FPA), Margaret Pyke House, 27–35 Mortimer Street, London W1N 7RJ

Food and Drink Federation, 6 Catherine Street, London WC2B 5JJ

Foresight – the Association for the Promotion of Preconceptual Care, The Old Vicarage, Church Lane, Witley, Godalming, Surrey GU8 5PN

Gamblers Anonymous and Gam-Anon, 17–23 Blantyre Street, Cheyne Walk, London SW10 0DT

General Medical Council (GMC), 44 Hallam Street, London W1

Gerontology Nutrition Unit, Royal Free Hospital, School of Medicine, 21 Pond Street, London NW3 2PN

Haemophilia Society, 123 Westminster Bridge Road, London SE1 7HR

Health Education Authority, 78 New Oxford Street, London WC1A 1AH

Health Visitors' Association, 36 Eccleston Square, London SW1V 1PF

Help the Aged, 16–18 St James's Walk, London EC1R 0BE

Hospice Information Service, St Christopher's Hospice, 51–59 Lawrie Park Road, Sydenham, London SE26 6DZ

Hospital Caterers' Association, 43 Royston Road, Penge, London SE20 7QW

Ileostomy Association of Great Britain and Ireland, Amblehurst House, Chobham, Woking, Surrey GU24 8PZ

Institute of Complementary Medicine, 21 Portland Place, London W1N 3AF

International Council of Nurses, 37 rue Vermont, 1202 Geneva, Switzerland

Invalids at Home, 23 Farm Avenue, London NW2 2BJ

King's Fund Centre (KFC), 126 Albert Street, London NW1 7NF

Lady Hoare Trust for Physically Disabled Children (Associated with Arthritis Care), 7 North Street, Midhurst, West Sussex

GU29 9DJ

Leukaemia Society, 28 Eastern Road, London N2

London Food Commission, PO Box 291, London N5 1DU

MacMillan Cancer Relief, Anchor House, 15–19 Britten Street, London SW3 3TY

Malcolm Sargent Cancer Fund for Children, 14 Abingdon Road, London W8 6AF

Marie Curie Memorial Foundation, 28 Belgrave Square, London SW1X 8QG

Medic-Alert Foundation, 11–13 Alfton Terrace, London N4 3JP

MIND (National Association for Mental Health), 22 Harley Street, London W1N 2ED

Multiple Sclerosis Society of Great Britain and Northern Ireland, 25 Effie Road, Fulham, London SW4 0QP

Narcotics Anonymous, PO Box 246, London SW1

National Advisory Centre on the Battered Child, Denver House, The Drive, Bounds Green Road, London N11

National Association for the Welfare of Children in Hospital (NAWCH), Argyle House, 29–31 Euston Road, London NW1 2SD

National Board for Nursing, Midwifery and Health Visiting for Northern Ireland, RAC House, 79 Chichester Street, Belfast BT1 4JE

National Board for Nursing, Midwifery and Health Visiting for Scotland, 22 Queens Street, Edinburgh EH2 1GX

National Childbirth Trust (NCT), 9 Queensborough Terrace, London W2 3TB

National Council for One Parent Families, 255 Kentish Town Road, London NW5 2LX

National Federation of Kidney Patients' Associations, Acorn Lodge, Woodsets, Nr Worksop, Notts S81 8AT

National Schizophrenia Fellowship, 79 Victoria Road, Surbiton, Surrey KT6 4NS

National Society for Epilepsy, Chalfont Centre for Epilepsy, Chalfont St Peter, Gerrards Cross, Bucks SL9 0RJ

National Society for PKU and Allied Disorders, 26 Towngate Grove, Mirfield, West Yorkshire

National Society for the Prevention of Cruelty to Children (NSPCC), 67 Saffron Hill, London EC1N 8RS

Nursing and Hospital Careers Information Centre, 121 Edgware Road, London W2 2HX

Nutrition Society, Grosvenor Gardens House, 35–37 Grosvenor Gardens, London SW1W 0BS

Oxford Nutrition, PO Box 31, Oxford OX2 6HB

Parkinson's Disease Society, 36 Portland Place, London W1N 3DG

Pregnancy Advisory Service, 13 Charlotte Street, London W1P 1HD

Primary Nursing Network, c/o Jane Salvage, Nursing Developments, King's Fund Centre, 126 Albert Street, London NW1 7NF

Renal Society, 64 South Hill Park, London NW3 2SJ

Royal Association in Aid of the Deaf and Dumb, 27 Old Oak Road, London W3 7SL

Royal College of Midwives (RCM), 15 Mansfield Street, London W1M 0BE

Royal College of Nursing and Council of Nurses of the United Kingdom (Rcn), 20 Cavendish Square, London W1M 0BE

Royal Institute of Public Health and Hygiene, 28 Portland Place, London W1N 4DE

Royal National Institute for the Blind (RNIB), 224 Great Portland Place, London W1N 6AA

Royal National Institute for the Deaf (RNID), 105 Gower Street, London WC1E 6AH

Royal Society of Health, 13 Grosvenor Place, London SW1X 7EN

Royal Society for the Prevention of Accidents (RoSPA), Cannon House, The Priory, Queensway, Birmingham B4 6BS

St John Ambulance Association (StJAA), 1 Grosvenor Crescent, London SW1X 7EF

Samaritans Incorporated, 17 Uxbridge Road, Slough, Berkshire SL1 1SN

Sickle Cell Society, Green Lodge, Barretts Green Road, London NW10 7AP

Spastics Society, 12 Park Crescent, London W1N 4EQ

Standing Conference on Drug Abuse, 1–4 Hatton Place, Hatton Garden, London EC1N 8ND

Stillbirth and Neonatal Death Society (SANDS), Argyle House, 29–31 Euston Road, London NW1 2SD

Stress Syndrome Foundation, Cedar House, Yalding, Kent ME18 6JD

Sue Ryder Foundation, Cavendish, Sudbury, Suffolk CO10 8AY

Terrence Higgins Trust, BM AIDS, London WC1N 3XX

Tranquilizer Withdrawal Support, 160 Tosson Terrace, Heaton, Newcastle-upon-Tyne NE6 5EA

Twins and Multiple Births Association, 54 Broad Lane, Hampton, Middlesex TW12 3BG

United Kingdom Central Council for Nursing, Midwifery and Health Visiting (UKCC), 23 Portland Place, London W1N 3AF

Vegan Society, 47 Highlands Road, Leatherhead, Surrey

Vegetarian Society, Parkdale, Denham Road, Altrincham, Cheshire

Welsh National Board for Nursing, Midwifery and Health Visiting, 13th Floor, Pearl Assurance House, Greyfriars Road, Cardiff CF1 3AG

Women's Health Concern (WHC), Ground Floor, 17 Earls Terrace, London W8 6LP

Women's Royal Voluntary Service (WRVS), 17 Old Park Lane, London W1Y 4AJ

World Health Organization, Geneva, Switzerland

APPENDIX 14

Degrees, Diplomas and Organizations

ABPN	Association of British Paediatric Nurses
AIMSW	Association of the Institute of Medical Social Workers
APEX	Association of Professional and Executive Staffs
APMH	Association of Professions for Mentally Handicapped People
ARRC	Associate, Royal Red Cross
BA	Bachelor of Arts
BAON	British Association of Orthopaedic Nurses
BDA	British Dental Association
BDSc	Bachelor of Dental Science
BITA	British Intravenous Therapy Association
BN	Bachelor of Nursing
BPOG	British Psychosocial Oncology Group
BSc (Soc SC-Nurs)	Bachelor of Science (Nursing)
CCHE	Central Council for Health Education
CMT	Clinical Midwife Teacher
CNAA	Council for National Academic Awards
COHSE	Confederation of Health Service Employees
CPH	Certificate of Public Health
CSP	Chartered Society of Physiotherapists
DCH	Diploma in Child Health
DDA	Dangerous Drugs Act
DipEd	Diploma in Education
DipNEd	Diploma in Nursing Education
DN	Diploma in Nursing
DNA	District Nursing Association
DNE	Diploma in Nursing Education
DPH	Diploma in Public Health
DPhil	Doctor of Philosophy
DPM	Diploma in Psychological Medicine
DSc	Doctor of Science
DTM&H	Diploma in Tropical Medicine and Hygiene
EN(G)	Enrolled Nurse (General)
EN(M)	Enrolled Nurse (Mental)
EN(MH)	Enrolled Nurse (Mental Handicap)
ENB	English National Board for Nursing, Midwifery and Health Visiting

FCSP	Fellow of the Chartered Society of Physiotherapists
FETC	Further Education Teaching Certificate
FNIF	Florence Nightingale International Foundation
FPA	Family Planning Association
FRcn	Fellow of the Royal College of Nursing
FRS	Fellow of the Royal Society
FRSH	Fellow of the Royal Society of Health
GMC	General Medical Council
HSA	Hospital Savings Association
HV	Health Visitor
HVA	Health Visitors' Association
ICN	International Council of Nurses
ICNA	Infection Control Nurses' Association
ICW	International Council of Women
IHF	International Hospital Federation
INR	Index of Nursing Research
MA	Master of Arts
MAO	Master of the Art of Obstetrics
MAOT	Member of the Association of Occupational Therapists
MBA	Master of Business Administration
MBIM	Member of the British Institute of Management
MCSP	Member of the Chartered Society of Physiotherapists
MIND	National Association for Mental Health
MPhil	Master of Philosophy
MRC	Medical Research Council
MRSH	Member of the Royal Society for the Promotion of Health
MSF	Manufacturing Science and Finance
MSRG	Member of the Society of Remedial Gymnasts
MSR(R)	Member of the Society of Radiographers (Radiography)
MSR(T)	Member of the Society of Radiographers (Radiotherapy)
MSc	Master of Science
MTD	Midwife Teachers' Diploma
NALGO	National Association of Local Government Officers
NAMCW	National Association for Maternal and Child Welfare
NAMH	National Association for Mental Health
NATN	National Association of Theatre Nurses

NAWCH	National Association for the Welfare of Children in Hospital
NHS	National Health Service
NIB	Northern Ireland Board for Nursing, Midwifery and Health Visiting
NNEB	National Nursery Education Board
NUMINE	Network of Users of Microcomputers in Nurse Education
NUPE	National Union of Public Employees
OHNC	Occupational Health Nursing Certificate
ONC	Orthopaedic Nurses' Certificate
OND	Ophthalmic Nursing Diploma
OT	Occupational Therapist
PhD	Doctor of Philosophy
PMRAFNS	Princess Mary's Royal Air Force Nursing Service
PNA	Psychiatric Nurses' Association
QARANC	Queen Alexandra's Royal Army Nursing Service
QARNNS	Queen Alexandra's Royal Naval Nursing Service
QIDN	Queen's Institute of District Nursing
QNI	Queen's Nursing Institute
RCM	Royal College of Midwives
Rcn	Royal College of Nursing
RCNT	Registered Clinical Nurse Tutor
RGN	Registered General Nurse
RHV	Regional Health Visitor
RM	Registered Midwife
RMN	Registered Mental Nurse
RN	Registered Nurse (USA and other overseas countries)
RNMD	Registered Nurse for Mental Defectives
RNMH	Registered Nurse for the Mentally Handicapped
RNMS	Registered Nurse for the Mentally Subnormal
RNPFN	Royal National Pension Fund for Nurses
RNT	Registered Nurse Tutor
RRC	Royal Red Cross
RSCN	Registered Sick Children's Nurse
StAAA	St Andrew's Ambulance Association
StJAA	St John Ambulance Association
StJAB	St John Ambulance Brigade
SCM	State Certified Midwife
SEN	State Enrolled Nurse

SNB	Scottish National Board for Nursing, Midwifery and Health Visiting
SNNEB	Scottish National Nursing Examination Board
SRN	State Registered Nurse
SSStJ	Serving Sister of the Order of St John of Jerusalem
UKCC	United Kingdom Central Council for Nursing, Midwifery and Health Visiting
VSO	Voluntary Service Overseas
WHO	World Health Organization
WNB	Welsh National Board for Nursing, Midwifery and Health Visiting
WPHOA	Women's Public Health Officers' Association
WRVS	Women's Royal Voluntary Service

APPENDIX 15

Units of Measurement and Tables of Normal Values

SI Units (Système Internationale d'Unités)

Base units

Physical quantity	Name of unit	Symbol
Mass	kilogram	kg
Length	metre	m
Time	second	s
Electric current	ampere	A
Temperature	kelvin	K
Luminous intensity	candela	cd
Amount of substance	mole	mol

Derived units
Derived units to measure other quantities are obtained by multiplying or dividing any two or more of the seven base units. Some of these have their own names and symbols. For example:

Physical quantity	Name of unit	Symbol	Base or derived units
Force	newton	N	$kg \cdot m \cdot s^{-2}$
Pressure	pascal	Pa	$N \cdot m^{-2}$
Energy, work, heat	joule	J	$N \cdot m$
Power	watt	W	$J \cdot s^{-1}$

Prefixes used for multiples

Factor	Prefix	Symbol
10^{-12}	pico	p
10^{-9}	nano	n
10^{-6}	micro	μ
10^{-3}	milli	m
10^{-2}	centi	c
10^{-1}	deci	d
10	deca	da
10^2	hecto	h
10^3	kilo	k
10^6	mega	M
10^9	giga	G
10^{12}	tera	T

Capacity

The SI unit of *volume* is the cubic metre (m^3), but the litre (l) is more commonly used and accepted (it is equivalent to 1 dm^3).

1000 microlitres (μl)	= 1 millilitre (ml)		
10 millilitres	= 1 centilitre (cl)		
100 millilitres	= 10 centilitres		
1000 millilitres	= 100 centilitres	= 1 decilitre (dl)	
		= 10 decilitres	= 1 litre (l)

1 cubic centimetre (cm^3 *or* cc) = 1 millilitre
1 cubic decimetre (dm^3)   = 1 litre

Domestic equivalents (approximate)

1 teaspoon	=	5 ml
1 dessertspoon	=	10 ml
1 tablespoon	=	20 ml
1 sherryglass	=	60 ml
1 teacup	=	142 ml
1 breakfastcup	=	230 ml
1 tumbler	=	285 ml

Weights

1000 micrograms (μg)	= 1 milligram (mg)
1000 milligrams	= 1 gram (g)
1000 grams	= 1 kilogram (kg)
1000 kilograms	= 1 metric tonne

Energy

A dietetic calorie is the amount of heat required to raise the temperature of 1 litre of water by 1 °C and is equal to 4.184 kilojoules.

1 g fat will produce 38 kilojoules or 9 calories.
1 g protein will produce 17 kilojoules or 4 calories.
1 g carbohydrate will produce 17 kilojoules or 4 calories.

Comparative temperatures

Celsius (°C)	Fahrenheit (°F)	Celsius (°C)	Fahrenheit (°F)
100 Boiling point	212	38.5	101.3
95	203	38	100.4
90	194	37.5	99.5
85	185	37	98.6
80	176	36.5	97.7
75	167	36	96.8
70	158	35.5	95.9
65	149	35	95
60	140	34	93.2
55	131	33	91.4
50	122	32	89.6
45	113	31	87.8
44	112.2	30	86
43	109.4	25	77
42	107.6	20	68
41	105.8	15	59
40	104	10	50
39.5	103.1	5	41
39	102.2	0 Freezing point	32

To convert readings of the Fahrenheit scale into Celsius degrees subtract 32, multiply by 5, and divide by 9, for example:

$$98 - 32 = 66 \times 5 = 330 \div 9 = 36.6.$$
Therefore 98 °F = 36.6 °C.

To convert readings of the Celsius scale into Fahrenheit degrees multiply by 9, divide by 5, and add 32, for example:

$$36.6 \times 9 = 330 \div 5 = 66 + 32 = 98.$$
Therefore 36.6 °C = 98 °F.

The term 'Celsius' (from the name of the Swede who invented the scale in 1742) is now being internationally used instead of 'centigrade', which term is employed in some countries to denote fractions of an angle.

Normal values

These normal values were compiled by Ruth Halliday SRN, St Bartholomew's Hospital, London.

Haematology

Basophil granulocytes	$0.01–0.1 \times 10^9/l$
Eosinophil granulocytes	$0.04–0.4 \times 10^9/l$
Erythrocyte sedimentation rate (ESR)	< 20 mm in 1 h
Haemoglobin	
male	$14.0–17.7 \ g \cdot dl^{-1}$
female	$12.2–15.2 \ g \cdot dl^{-1}$
Leukocytes	$4.3–10.8 \times 10^9/l$
Mean corpuscular haemoglobin (MCH)	27–33 pg
Mean corpuscular haemoglobin concentration (MCHC)	$32–35 \ g \cdot dl^{-1}$
Mean corpuscular volume (MCV)	80–96 fl
Monocytes	$0.2–0.8 \times 10^9/l$
Neutrophil granulocytes	$3.5–7.5 \times 10^9/l$
Packed cell volume (PCV)	
male	$0.42–0.53 \ 1 \cdot 1^{-1}$
female	$0.36–0.45 \ 1 \cdot 1^{-1}$
Plasma volume	$45 \pm 5 \ ml \cdot kg^{-1}$
Platelet count	$150–400 \times 10^9/l$
Red cell folate	$> 160 \ \mu g \cdot l^{-1}$
Red cell mass	
male	$30 \pm 5 \ ml \cdot kg^{-1}$
female	$25 \pm 5 \ ml \cdot kg^{-1}$
Reticulocyte count	0.5–2.5% of red cells
Serum B_{12}	$150–675 \ pmol \cdot l^{-1}$ (160–925 $ng \cdot l^{-1}$)
Serum folate	$5–63 \ nmol \cdot l^{-1}$ (3–20 $\mu g \cdot l^{-1}$)

Total blood volume
    male 75 ± 10 ml·kg^{-1}
    female 70 ± 10 ml·kg^{-1}

Coagulation

Bleeding time (Ivy method)	3–8 min
Partial thromboplastin time (PTTK)	30–40 s
Prothrombin time	10–14 s

Biochemistry

Acid phosphatase	1–5 U·l^{-1}
Alanine aminotransferase (ALT)	5–30 U·l^{-1}
Albumin	34–48 g·l^{-1}
Alkaline phosphatase	25–115 U·l^{-1}
Alpha-l-antitrypsin	2–4 g·l^{-1}
Alpha-fetoprotein	< 10 kU·l^{-1}
Amylase	70–300 U·l^{-1}
Angiotensin-converting enzyme	204–360 U·l^{-1}
Aspartate aminotransferase (AST)	10–40 U·l^{-1}
Bicarbonate	22–30 mmol·l^{-1} (22–30 mEq·l^{-1})
Bilirubin	< 17 µmol·l^{-1} (0.3–1.5 mg·dl^{-1})
Calcium	2.2–2.67 mmol·l^{-1} (8.5–10.5 ng·dl^{-1})
Chloride	100–106 mmol·l^{-1} (100–106 mEq·l^{-1})
Cholinesterase	2.25–7.0 U·l^{-1}
Copper	12–25 µmol·l^{-1} (100–200 mg·dl^{-1})
Complement – total haemolytic	150–250 U·mol^{-1}
Creatinine	0.06–0.12 mmol·l^{-1} (0.6–1.5 mg·dl^{-1})
Creatinine kinase (CPK)	24–195 U·l^{-1}
Ferritin	5.8–120 nmol·l^{-1} (15–250 µg·l^{-1})
Gamma glutamyl transferase (γ-GT)	10–40 iu·l^{-1}
Glucose	4.5–5.6 mmol·l^{-1} (70–110 mg·dl^{-1})
Glycosylated haemoglobin (Hb$_1$Ac)	3.8–6.4%
Hydroxybutyric dehydrogenase (HBD)	40–125 U·l^{-1}
Iron	13–32 µmol·l^{-1} (509–150 µg·dl^{-1})

Iron binding capacity (total)	42–80 μmol·l^{-1} (250–410 μg·dl^{-1})
Lactate dehydrogenase	240–525 U·l^{-1}
Lead	1.8 μmol·l^{-1}
Magnesium	0.7–1.1 mmol·l^{-1}
Osmolality	280–296 mmol·kg^{-1} (280–296 mosmol·kg^{-1})
Phosphate	0.8–1.4 mmol·l^{-1}
Potassium	3.5–5.0 mmol·l^{-1} (3.5–5.0 mEq·l^{-1})
Protein (total)	62–80 g·l^{-1} (6.2–8.0 g·dl^{-1})
Sodium	135–146 mmol·l^{-1} (135–146 mEq·l^{-1})
Urate	0.18–0.42 mmol·l^{-1} (3.0–7.0 mg·dl^{-1})
Urea	2.5–6.7 mmol·l^{-1} (8–25 mg·dl^{-1})
Vitamin A	0.5–2.1 μmol·l^{-1} (0.15–0.6 μg·ml^{-1})
Vitamin D	
25-hydroxy	19.4–137 nmol·l^{-1} (8–55 ng·l^{-1})
1,25-dihydroxy	62–155 pmol·l^{-1} (26–65 pg·l^{-1})
Zinc	7–18 μmol·l^{-1}
Blood gases	
Arterial PCO$_2$	4.8–6.1 kPa (36–46 mmHg)
Arterial PO$_2$	10–13.3 kPa (75–100 mmHg); for every year over 60, *add* 0.13 kPa
Arterial [H$^+$]	35–45 nmol·l^{-1}
Arterial pH	7.35–7.45
Cerebrospinal fluid	
Pressure (adult)	50–200 mm water
Cells	0–5 lymphocytes/mm^3
Glucose	3.3–4.4 mmol·l^{-1}
Protein	100–400 mg·l^{-1}

Faeces
Normal fat content
    Daily output on normal diet   < 7 g
    Fat (as stearic acid)   11–18 mmol/24 h

Lipids and lipoproteins
Cholesterol   3.9–7.8 nmol·l^{-1}
Triglyceride   0.5–2.1 nmol·l^{-1}
Phospholipid   2.9–5.2 nmol·l^{-1}
Non-esterified fatty acids
    male   0.19–0.78 nmol·l^{-1}
    female   0.06–0.9 nmol·l^{-1}
Lipoproteins
    VLDL   0.128–0.645 nmol·l^{-1}
    LDL   1.55–4.4 nmol·l^{-1}
    HDL – male   0.7–2.0 nmol·l^{-1}
        – female   0.95–2.15 nmol·l^{-1}
Lipids (total)   4.0–10 g·l^{-1}
                         (400–1000 mg·dl^{-1})

Urine
Total quantity in 24 h   1000–1500 ml
Specific gravity   1.012–1.030
pH   4–8
Average solids excreted in 24 h
    Calcium   2.5–7.5 mmol
    Copper   0–1.6 μmol
    Creatinine   9–17 mmol
    5-Hydroxyindole acetic acid   15–75 μmol
    4-Hydroxy-3-methoxymandelic acid 10–35 μmol
    Hydroxyproline   0.08–0.25 mmol
    Lead   0.39 μmol·l^{-1} or less
    Magnesium   3.3–5.0 mmol
    Oestriol   varies widely during
                         pregnancy (μmol)
    Phosphate   15–50 mmol
    Protein (quantitative)   < 0.15 g
    Urea   250–500 mmol
    17-Ketosteroids
        Men   8–15 mg
        Women   5–12 mg

Thyroid function tests

Total serum thyroxine (T_4)	60–160 nmol·l^{-1}
Total serum triiodothyronine (T_3)	1.2–3.1 nmol·l^{-1}
Free serum thyroxine (T_4)	13–30 pmol·l^{-1}
Thyroid-stimulating hormone (TSH)	0.5–5.0 mu·l^{-1} (lower limit not definable on older assays)

Acceptable weights

Acceptable weights as recommended by the Fogarty Conference (USA, 1979) and the Royal College of Physicians (1983).

Height without shoes (m)	MEN Weight without clothes (kg)			WOMEN Weight without clothes (kg)		
	Acceptable average	Acceptable weight range	Obese	Acceptable average	Acceptable weight range	Obese
1.45				46.0	42–53	64
1.48				46.5	42–54	65
1.50				47.0	43–55	66
1.52				48.5	44–57	68
1.54				49.5	44–58	70
1.56				50.4	45–58	70
1.58	55.8	51–64	77	51.3	46–59	71
1.60	57.6	52–65	78	52.6	48–61	73
1.62	58.6	53–66	79	54.0	49–62	74
1.64	59.6	54–67	80	55.4	50–64	77
1.66	60.6	55–69	83	56.8	51–65	78
1.68	61.7	56–71	85	58.1	52–66	79
1.70	63.5	58–73	88	60.0	53–67	80

1.72	65.0	59–74	89	61.3	55–69	83
1.74	66.5	60–75	90	62.6	56–70	84
1.76	68.0	62–77	92	64.0	58–72	86
1.78	69.4	64–79	95	65.3	59–74	89
1.80	71.0	65–80	96			
1.82	72.6	66–82	98			
1.84	74.2	67–84	101			
1.86	75.8	69–86	103			
1.88	77.6	71–88	106			
1.90	79.3	73–90	108			
1.92	81.0	75–93	112			
BMI*	22.0	20.1–25.0	30.0	20.8	18.7–23.8	28.6

* Body mass index = weight/height^2 (kg/m^2).

From Bray GA (ed.) (1979) *Obesity in America*, Proceedings of the Second Fogarty International Center Conference on Obesity, No. 79, Washington DC: DHEW.